a LANGE medical book

SURGERY ON CALL

Fourth Edition

Edited by

Alan T. Lefor, MD, MPH, FACS
Director, Division of Surgical Oncology
Director, Surgical Education and Academic Affairs
Cedars-Sinai Medical Center
Los Angeles, California
Professor of Clinical Surgery
Department of Surgery
David Geffen School of Medicine at UCLA
Los Angeles, California
Visiting Professor, Center for Graduate Medical Education
Jichi Medical School
Tochigi, Japan

Leonard G. Gomella, MD, FACS
The Bernard W. Goodw
Chairman
Department of Urology
Jefferson Medical Colle
Thomas Jefferson Unive
Philadelphia, Pennsylvai

Lange Medical Books/McGraw-Hill
Medical Publishing Division

New York   Chicago   San Francisco   Lisbon   London
Madrid   Mexico City   Milan   New Delhi   San Juan
Seoul   Singapore   Sydney   Toronto

The McGraw·Hill Companies

Surgery On Call, Fourth Edition

Copyright © 2006, 2001 by the **McGraw-Hill Companies, Inc.** All rights reserved. Printed in the United States of America. Except as permitted under the United States Copyright Act of 1976, no part of this publication may be reproduced or distributed in any form or by any means, or stored in a database or retrieval system, without the prior written permission of the publisher.

Previous edition copyright © 1996,1990 by Appleton & Lange

1 2 3 4 5 6 7 8 9 0 DOCDOC 0 9 8 7 6 5

ISSN 1-44-4033
ISBN 0-07-140254-3

This book was set in Helvetica by Pine Tree Composition, Inc.
The editors were Janet Foltin, James Shanahan, Harriet Lebowitz, and Peter J. Boyle; the production supervisor was Catherine Saggese; Patricia Perrier prepared the index.
RR Donnelley was printer and binder.

This book is printed on acid-free paper.

INTERNATIONAL EDITION ISBN 0-07-110494-1

Copyright © 2006. Exclusive rights by the McGraw-Hill Companies, Inc. for manufacture and export. This book cannot be re-exported from the country to which it is consigned by McGraw-Hill. The International Edition is not available in North America.

To Sheila and Maarten, and to Tricia, Leonard, Patrick, Andrew, and Michael for their gift of time.

Contents

Associate Editors

Contributors

Aimee Gelhot Adams, PharmD
Director, Primary Care Pharmacy Practice Residency
University of Kentucky Medical Center
Assistant Professor
College of Pharmacy and Department of Medicine
University of Kentucky
Lexington, Kentucky

Rodrigo F. Alban, MD
Resident in Surgery
Department of Surgery
Cedars-Sinai Medical Center
Los Angeles, California

Takeshi Aoki, MD
Assistant Professor of Surgery
Showa University School of Medicine
Tokyo, Japan

Eraj Basseri, MD
Resident in Surgery
Department of Surgery
Cedars-Sinai Medical Center
Los Angeles, California

Marjorie R. Chelly, MD
Resident in Surgery
Department of Surgery
Cedars-Sinai Medical Center
Los Angeles, California

Ritu Chopra, MD
Resident in Surgery
Department of Surgery
Cedars-Sinai Medical Center
Los Angeles, California

Alice Chung, MD
Resident in Surgery
Department of Surgery
Cedars-Sinai Medical Center
Los Angeles, California

David Feldmar, MD
Resident in Surgery
Department of Surgery
Cedars-Sinai Medical Center
Los Angeles, California

Douglas L. Fraker, MD, FACS
Jonathan E. Rhoads Professor of Surgery
Vice Chairman, Clinical Affairs
Director, General Surgery
Department of Surgery
University of Pennsylvania
Philadelphia, Pennsylvania

Fumihiko Fujita, MD
Assistant Professor of Surgery
Nagasaki University School of Medicine
Nagasaki, Japan

Joubin S. Gabbay, MD
Resident in Surgery
Department of Surgery
Cedars-Sinai Medical Center
Los Angeles, California

Mark D. Gaon, MD
Resident in Surgery
Department of Surgery
Cedars-Sinai Medical Center
Los Angeles, California

Tewodros Gedebou, MD
Los Angeles, California

Leonard G. Gomella, MD, FACS
The Bernard W. Goodwin Jr. Professor
Chairman, Department of Urology
Jefferson Medical College
Thomas Jefferson University
Philadelphia, Pennsylvania

Masanobu Hagiike, MD PhD
Fellow in Minimally Invasive Surgery
Department of Surgery
Cedars-Sinai Medical Center
Los Angeles, California
Assistant Professor of Surgery
Faculty of Medicine
Kagawa University
Kagawa, Japan

Steven Haist, MD, MS, FACP
Professor of Medicine
Division of General Medicine
Department of Internal Medicine
University of Kentucky Medical Center
Lexington, Kentucky

Yukiharu Hayase, MD
Associate Professor
Center for Graduate Medical Education
Jichi Medical School
Tochigi, Japan

John C. Kairys, MD
Assistant Professor
Program Director, Department of Surgery
Thomas Jefferson University
Philadelphia, Pennsylvania

Samuel M. Keim, MD
Program Director
Associate Professor
Department of Surgery, Division of Emergency Medicine
University of Arizona Health Sciences Center
Tucson, Arizona

Kelly Killeen, MD
Resident in Surgery
Department of Surgery
Cedars-Sinai Medical Center
Los Angeles, California

Yoshiaki Kita, MD
Associate Professor
Department of Surgery
Jikei Medical School
Tokyo, Japan

Wega Koss, MD
Assistant Professor of Surgery
John A. Burns School of Medicine
University of Hawaii
Honolulu, Hawaii

Alan T. Lefor, MD, MPH, FACS
Director, Division of Surgical Oncology
Director, Surgical Education and Academic Affairs
Cedars-Sinai Medical Center
Los Angeles, California
Professor of Clinical Surgery
Department of Surgery
David Geffen School of Medicine at UCLA
Los Angeles, California
Visiting Professor, Center for Graduate Medical Education
Jichi Medical School
Tochigi, Japan

Sergey Lyass, MD
Chief Resident in Surgery
Department of Surgery
Cedars-Sinai Medical Center
Los Angeles, California

Carie McVay, MD
Resident in Surgery
Department of Surgery
Cedars-Sinai Medical Center
Los Angeles, California

Gregg Nishi, MD
Chief Resident in General Surgery
Department of Surgery
Cedars-Sinai Medical Center
Los Angeles, California

Abraham A. Nisim, MD
Resident in Surgery
Department of Surgery
Cedars-Sinai Medical Center
Los Angeles, California

Koji Otsuka, MD
Assistant Professor of Surgery
Showa University School of Medicine
Tokyo, Japan

Nicholas A. Pavona, MD
Professor, Department of Surgery
Division of Urology
Benjamin Franklin University Medical Center
Chadds Ford, Pennsylvania

Nakaya Saito MD, MS
Office of Medical Education
John A. Burns School of Medicine
University of Hawaii at Manoa
Honolulu, Hawaii

Atsushi Shimizu, MD
Assistant Professor
Department of Surgery
Jichi Medical School
Tochigi, Japan

Kelly M. Smith, PharmD
Associate Professor
Division of Pharmacy Practice and Science
University of Kentucky College of Pharmacy
Director, Drug Information Center
University of Kentucky Medical Center
Lexington, Kentucky

Harmik J. Soukiasian, MD
Chief Resident in General Surgery
Cedars-Sinai Medical Center
Los Angeles, California

Jacob Spivak, MD
Chief Resident in Surgery
Department of Surgery
Cedars-Sinai Medical Center
Los Angeles, California

Stephanie Tretiak, PharmD
SICU Clinical Pharmacist
Department of Pharmacy
Cedars-Sinai Medical Center
Los Angeles, California

Eric A. Wiebke, MD, MBA, FACS
Professor
Department of Surgery
Indiana University
Indianapolis, Indiana

Makiko Yoshida, Pharmacist
Aoyama Second Hospital
Department of Pharmacy
Osaka, Japan

Preface

We are grateful to be able to bring to you the fourth edition of *Surgery On Call*. The "On Call" series is based on Dr. Tricia Gomella's concept that first appeared in 1988 in *Neonatology: Basic Management, On-call Problems, Diseases, and Drugs*. *Surgery On Call* was the first developed for the series and debuted in 1990. There are now several "On Call" books in this McGraw-Hill series including Internal Medicine, OB/GYN, Emergency Medicine, Critical Care, and Pediatrics. Many have been translated into foreign languages. The PDA version is available for *Internal Medicine On Call* and is in development for others in the series.

The idea is a simple one: house officers are not usually presented with a diagnosis when on call, but with a specific complaint or problem that requires action and ultimately leads to a diagnosis. Most medical books approach diseases from the diagnosis and disease perspective. Medical education requires a careful synthesis of the practicality of dealing with patient issues on a day-to-day basis with the essentials of medicine. We hope that this manual will provide the house officer and student with the tools to provide well thought out initial care to the patient. This initial care should be followed by a more detailed study of the patient's problem available in standard textbooks of surgery.

In general, the problems reflect those of adult patients, with consideration to pediatric surgical issues supplied where appropriate. Contributions of house staff are invaluable in identifying the issues addressed while on call on a given surgical service. We take great pride in the fact that most of the contributors to this book are residents working daily "in the trenches." This book reflects generally accepted practices from major medical centers around the country. All sections of the book have been updated from the previous edition to reflect the ever-changing practice of medicine. All of the clinical problems have been revised and refined to reflect current practices that are fairly standard across the United States. New medications have been added to the existing comprehensive list to make it a more useful reference.

Surgery On Call has found itself at home in the international medical community as well. It has been translated into Portuguese and the third edition has been specifically revised for use in Australia. Several other foreign versions are in development.

We would like to acknowledge our contributors for their efforts, McGraw-Hill for their encouragement and patience, and Janet

Foltin and James Shanahan for their outstanding editorial assistance. Please contact us with any suggestions you may have so that the book will be able to provide our readership with the essential skills needed to make the all important on-call experience one of efficient patient care and a sound educational opportunity.

Alan T. Lefor, MD, MPH, FACS
Leonard G. Gomella, MD, FACS

Los Angeles and Philadelphia
July 2005

I. On-Call Problems

1. ABDOMINAL DISTENTION

I. Problem. A 42-year-old female patient is complaining of abdominal bloating.

II. Immediate Questions

A. Was the patient recently operated upon? Immediate postoperative abdominal distention is common and may be related to ileus or gastric distention.

B. Is a nasogastric (NG) tube in place? NG tubes can relieve gastric distention but will be of little use in decompressing colonic gas.

C. What medications is the patient taking? Certain medications such as narcotics and anticholinergics will slow intestinal motility. Diuretic induced hypokalemia may also cause decreased motility.

D. What previous operations has the patient had? The cause of the distention may be obstruction from adhesions or tumor. Bowel obstruction in the adult is remembered by the mnemonic HAM (hernia, adhesions, malignancy).

E. What are the vital signs? Abdominal distention may restrict pulmonary function and cause tachypnea. Fever may suggest an infectious process such as peritonitis or pneumonia, which may cause a reflex ileus. Fever or tachycardia associated with bowel obstruction may indicate ischemia, thus requiring immediate surgical intervention.

F. When was the most recent bowel movement or flatus? Bowel movements and the passage of flatus are useful indicators of bowel activity. Their absence suggests ileus, which can be mechanical (obstruction) or functional (adynamic ileus) in origin. The patient may have a partial small bowel obstruction and still be able to pass flatus.

G. Has the patient been vomiting? Vomiting is often a sign of obstruction. The characteristics of the material may aid in diagnosing the site of obstruction. In gastric outlet obstruction, there is little, if any, bile in the vomitus, whereas distal small bowel obstruction tends to be bilious or feculent.

III. Differential Diagnosis

A. Gastrointestinal (GI) Tract Obstruction

1. **Stomach**. Gastric outlet obstruction by tumor, ulcer, or gastric atony can lead to gastric dilatation and a sensa-

tion of bloating. This is common in pediatric patients who tend to swallow large amounts of air while crying.

2. **Small intestine**. Mechanical causes such as adhesions after previous abdominal surgery, intraluminal obstruction (tumor, foreign body, gallstone, etc), or extraluminal obstruction commonly cause small bowel obstruction. Internal hernias or strangulated/incarcerated external hernias can also cause small bowel obstruction. A gallstone ileus is due to a large gallstone impacted at the ileocecal valve, usually seen in the elderly. This is usually preceded by an attack of acute cholecystitis with a cholecystoduodenal fistula. Intussusception is telescoping of 1 piece of bowel into another, usually associated with a lead point. Usually occurring in the pediatric population, the most common area of intussusception is the ileocecal valve.

3. **Large intestine**. Causes include tumors, volvulus, foreign bodies, and fecal impaction (particularly in elderly, bedridden patients). Pseudoobstruction of the colon (Ogilvie's syndrome) should also be included in the differential.

4. **Problems not in the GI tract.** Although rare, gynecologic tumors, retroperitoneal sarcomas, lymphomas, or genitourinary tumors (in addition to others) may cause obstruction. Pneumonia can cause a reflex ileus across the diaphragm.

B. **Intestinal Ischemia**. This is usually diagnosed by acidosis, high white blood cell (WBC) count, and "pain out of proportion to physical findings" on physical examination. High amylase and lactic acid levels may also aid in the diagnosis.

C. **Paralytic Ileus** (adynamic ileus). This can be secondary to intra-abdominal infection (peritonitis), systemic disease (sepsis), or inflammatory processes (pancreatitis, cholecystitis). This is frequently seen in the postoperative period, after blunt abdominal trauma, and secondary to certain medications (see page 1). "Reflex" ileus is often associated with pneumonia or urinary tract infection (pyelonephritis). Electrolyte abnormalities (K^+, Ca^{++}, Mg^{++}) can also cause ileus.

D. **Organomegaly**. Massive hepatomegaly and splenomegaly may be confused with distention.

E. **Intra-abdominal Mass**. Different lesions such as cysts (mesenteric, ovarian, renal), tumors, aneurysms, or even an unrecognized pregnancy can lead to complaints of distention.

F. Bladder Distention. Bladder outlet obstruction, most often because of prostatic enlargement or neurogenic bladder (spinal cord injury, diabetic) may cause massive bladder distention. Placement of a Foley catheter can immediately diagnose and control this problem.

G. Abdominal Wall or Groin Hernia. These may cause an obstructed loop of bowel that may also be strangulated and thus ischemic.

H. Ascites. Usually a chronic condition related to liver diseases (alcoholic cirrhosis) or carcinoma (malignant ascites). Inquire about any history of alcohol abuse.

IV. Database
A. Physical Examination Key Points

1. **Vital signs.** Fever suggests an inflammatory process, and tachypnea may represent respiratory compromise. Tachycardia and hypotension are usually present with more serious causes of obstruction.

2. **Heart.** Irregular rhythms, including atrial fibrillation, can lead to arterial embolization and bowel ischemia.

3. **Lungs.** Auscultation may reveal evidence of pneumonia.

4. **Abdomen.** Perform auscultation, percussion, inspection, and palpation. Evaluate for the presence of bowel sounds (usually absent with peritonitis, increased and high pitched with small bowel obstruction). Direct special attention to the left upper quadrant for evidence of gastric distention such as tympany. Note any old surgical scars and palpate for any tenderness to suggest peritoneal irritation (generalized with peritonitis or localized with other causes of an acute abdomen such as cholecystitis; see Problem 2, page 6). Abdominal wall herniation may be present. Costovertebral angle tenderness suggests an inflammatory process involving the diaphragm, liver, spleen, or kidney. A fluid wave is seen in ascites. Check for organomegaly.

5. **Rectal examination.** Digital examination may reveal fecal impaction, foreign body, or rectal tenderness. Determine the presence of occult blood on a fecal sample.

6. **Inguinal.** Check for hernias in groin and femoral areas.

7. **Skin.** Changes consistent with alcohol abuse, such as spider angiomata; palmar erythema may occur with ascites.

8. **Peripheral vascular.** Sign of embolization that may have accompanying emboli leading to intestinal is-

chemia (eg, absent pulses in the lower extremities or multiple sites of ischemia distally).

   9. **Pelvic examination.** Adnexal masses or tenderness may suggest ovarian tumors as a cause of ascites or pelvic inflammatory disease.
   10. **Intake/output.** Check for fluid sequestration, a sign of possible ischemia.

B. Laboratory Data
   1. **Hemogram.** Left shift and leukocytosis may suggest an infectious process or ischemic bowel.
   2. **Serum electrolytes.** Severe hypokalemia may cause an ileus. Third spacing of fluid with an obstruction may cause serious electrolyte imbalances.
   3. **Liver function tests.** These tests help in the evaluation of patients with liver and biliary disease and include bilirubin, alkaline phosphatase, alanine aminotransferase, and aspartate aminotransferase.
   4. **Urinalysis.** White cells and positive leukocyte esterase suggest a urinary tract infection.
   5. **Serum amylase and lipase.** These are typically high in patients with pancreatitis. Amylase may also be increased with a perforated viscus, intestinal obstruction, or mesenteric ischemia.
   6. **Arterial blood gas.** Acidosis can be present with bowel ischemia.
   7. **Lactic acid level.** Can be increased with bowel ischemia.

C. Radiologic and Other Studies
   1. **Abdominal radiography**. Supine and upright abdominal radiographs should be ordered (in addition, an upright chest radiograph should always be included in the evaluation; see below). A "ground glass" appearance is seen with ascites, air-fluid levels on the upright film can be seen with ileus or obstruction, and a large gastric bubble may suggest postoperative gastric atony or gastric outlet obstruction. If the cecum is markedly dilated (10–12 cm across), cecal perforation may result, and emergent intervention is needed. Other things to look for are distended loops of bowel, presence of air in the colon, signs of volvulus, coiled springs (intussusception), and sentinel loop (pancreatitis).
   2. **Chest radiography**. An upright chest radiograph is often the best film to detect free air under the diaphragm. Free air may be normal in the immediate postoperative period after a laparotomy; otherwise, this suggests a perforation. Pneumonia may also be diag-

nosed. Pleural effusion directs attention to a subdiaphragmatic inflammatory process.

3. **Barium studies**. These should not be obtained without very careful consideration if obstruction is suspected. Conversely, in the case of an intussusception, a barium enema may also be curative (in infants only). These studies are particularly hazardous in the presence of a perforation because extravasated barium is a terrible complication ("barium peritonitis"). Water-soluble contrast medium (Gastrografin) is a good alternative if there is any chance of perforation.

4. **Ultrasound and computed tomography (CT)**. This can help establish the diagnosis especially if a tumor, ascites, or organomegaly is suspected. Cholelithiasis with resulting cholecystitis may be detected on ultrasound.

5. **Endoscopy**. Esophagogastroduodenoscopy (EGD) is invaluable in evaluating gastroduodenal obstruction. Colonoscopy is helpful in evaluating colon masses and colon distention.

V. Plan. Relieve the distention first and then identify and treat the underlying cause.

A. **Initial Management**. In most cases, keeping the patient off oral nutrition (NPO) with adequate intravenous hydration is acceptable initial therapy while the workup is in progress (see Section IV, page 385).

B. **GI Decompression**. When GI obstruction is the cause or vomiting is present, a functioning NG tube is essential. In the absence of gastric distention, a NG tube may be less useful at relieving distention but should be used empirically (see Section III, page 354).

C. **Fluid Balance**. Carefully monitor fluid intake and output, especially if an NG tube is in place. Replacement of NG tube aspirate may be indicated if large volumes are being evacuated.

D. **Specific Treatment Plans**. The underlying cause must be clearly identified and appropriately managed. Common treatment plans include:
   1. Correct any electrolyte abnormalities, especially hypokalemia. Use intravenous (IV) potassium chloride (see page 170).
   2. Review medications and dosing intervals for any agents that may slow intestinal motility and adjust accordingly.
   3. Fecal impaction should be cleared with gentle digital extraction.

4. Ascites is usually managed medically (sodium restriction, spironolactone) with paracentesis used therapeutically if respiratory compromise is present.
5. Postoperative ileus usually clears spontaneously unless complications such as infection intervene.
6. Operative intervention is indicated in many cases of abdominal distention including bowel ischemia, obstructing hernia, perforation, or mechanical obstruction.
7. Colonoscopy can be used to manage volvulus and pseudo-obstruction. Neostigmine can be used to manage pseudo-obstruction.

REFERENCES

Doherty GM, et al. The acute abdomen. In: Way LW, Doherty GM, eds. *Current Surgical Diagnosis and Treatment*, 11th ed. New York: McGraw-Hill; 2003, p 503–16.
Richards WO, Williams LF. Obstruction of the large and small intestine. *Surg Clin North Am* 68:355–76, 1988.
Silen W. *Cope's Early Diagnosis of the Acute Abdomen.* Oxford: Oxford University Press; 1990, p 150–74.

2. ABDOMINAL PAIN

I. **Problem**. Seven days after a 40% burn, a 60-year-old male patient complains of pain in the right upper quadrant.

II. **Immediate Questions**

A. **What are the vital signs?** Fever indicates an inflammatory process. Hypotension and tachycardia may indicate shock owing to sepsis or hemorrhage. Fever may be absent in the elderly or in those patients receiving immunosuppressive or antipyretic medications.

B. **Where is the pain located?** Early in the course of the illness, pain may be "shifted" away from the actual site of pathology, and late in the course pain may become generalized. The classic example is appendicitis, in which discomfort is initially periumbilical or epigastric and later localized in the right lower quadrant. If the process goes unchecked, generalized abdominal pain (peritonitis) may result. Referred pain to the groin can be seen with ureteral colic and with pancreatitis or a ruptured abdominal aneurysm (Figures I–1 and I–2).

C. **When did the pain start?** The onset, frequency, and duration of the pain are helpful features. Acute, explosive pain is typical of a perforated viscus, ruptured aneurysm or abscess, or ectopic pregnancy. Pain intensifying over 1–2 hours is typical of acute cholecystitis, acute pancreatitis,

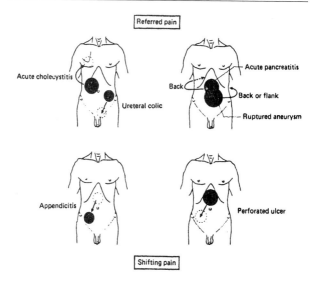

Referred pain

Acute cholecystitis

Ureteral colic

Acute pancreatitis

Back

Back or flank

Ruptured aneurysm

Appendicitis

Perforated ulcer

Shifting pain

Figure I–1. Referred and shifting pain in the acute abdomen. Solid circles indicate the site of maximum pain, and dashed circles show the sites of lesser pain. *(Reproduced, with permission, from Doherty GM, Boey JH. Acute abdomen. In: Way LW, Doherty GM, eds.* Current Surgical Diagnosis & Treatment, *11th ed. Copyright (c) 2003 by The McGraw-Hill Companies, Inc.)*

strangulated bowel, mesenteric thrombosis, proximal small bowel obstruction, or renal or ureteral colic. Vague pain that increases over several hours is most often seen with acute appendicitis, distal small bowel and large bowel obstructions, uncomplicated peptic ulcer disease, and various gynecologic and genitourinary conditions (see Figure I–2).

D. **What is the quality of the pain (dull, sharp, intermittent, constant, worst in life, burning)?** Classically described patterns include "burning" (eg, peptic ulcer disease), "searing" (eg, ruptured aortic aneurysm), and "intermittent" (eg, renal or ureteral colic; see Figure I–2). Have the patient scale the severity of the pain from 1 (least painful) to 10 (most painful). This provides a guide to follow the course more objectively.

E. **What makes the pain better or worse?** Pain that increases with deep inspiration is associated with diaphragmatic irritation (eg, pleurisy or inflammatory lesions of the

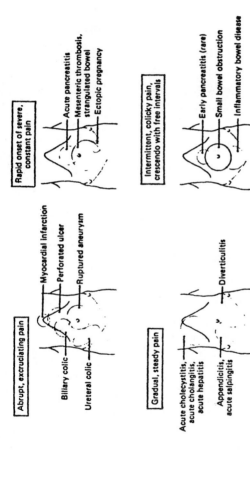

Figure I–2. The location and character of the pain are useful in the differential diagnosis of the acute abdomen. *(Reproduced, with permission, from Doherty GM, Boey JH. Acute abdomen. In: Way LW, Doherty GM, eds. Current Surgical Diagnosis & Treatment, 11th ed. Copyright (c) 2003 by The McGraw-Hill Companies, Inc.)*

upper abdomen). Food often relieves the pain of peptic ulcer disease. Narcotics relieve colic but provide little relief for pain caused by strangulated bowel or mesenteric thrombosis. Bending forward often relieves the pain of pancreatitis. Peritonitis often causes the patient to lie motionless on the back because any movement causes pain.

F. What are the associated symptoms, if any? Vomiting with onset of pain is seen in peritoneal irritation or perforation of a hollow viscus and is a prominent feature of upper abdominal diseases such as Boerhaave's syndrome (esophageal perforation after forceful vomiting), acute gastritis, or pancreatitis. In distal small bowel or large bowel obstruction, nausea is usually present long before vomiting begins. Hematemesis suggests upper GI (UGI) bleeding (ulcer disease, Mallory-Weiss syndrome). Diarrhea, if severe and associated with abdominal pain, suggests infectious gastroenteritis, and if bloody, may represent ischemic colitis, ulcerative colitis, Crohn's disease, or amebic dysentery. Constipation alternating with diarrhea may be seen with diverticular disease. Although constipation is often nonspecific, obstipation (absence of passage of stool and flatus) is strongly suggestive of mechanical bowel obstruction. Hematuria suggests a genitourinary cause.

G. What are the characteristics of the vomitus? (see Problem 54, page 197.)

H. When did the patient eat last? Allows an assessment of the time course of the illness and is particularly important if anesthesia is planned.

I. What is a female patient's menstrual history? Missed or late period may suggest an ectopic pregnancy. Mittelschmerz is pain due to a ruptured ovarian follicle.

J. What is the patient's medical and surgical history? Knowledge of a history of ulcers, gallstones, alcohol abuse, or operations and a list of current medications aids in establishing the cause. A history of blunt abdominal trauma 1–3 days before onset of pain may signify subcapsular hemorrhage of the liver, spleen, or kidney.

III. Differential Diagnosis. Abdominal pain has intra-abdominal and extra-abdominal sources and can be associated with medical and surgical diseases. The list is too long to reproduce in its entirety here, but listed are some of the more frequently encountered causes.

A. Intra-abdominal
  1. Hollow viscera. Hollow viscera can perforate in the face of obstruction, and perforation represents an acute surgical emergency.
    a. Upper abdominal: esophagitis, gastritis, peptic ulcer disease, cholecystitis.
    b. Midgut: small bowel obstruction or infarction; obstruction may be a result of adhesions (benign and malignant), hernias (internal and external), or volvulus.
    c. Lower abdominal: inflammatory bowel disease, appendicitis, mesenteric lymphadenitis, obstruction.
    d. Gastroenteritis, colitis.
  2. Solid organs.
    a. Liver: hepatitis.
    b. Pancreas: pancreatitis.
    c. Spleen: splenic infarction.
    d. Kidney: stones, pyelonephritis, abscess.
  3. Pelvic.
    a. Pelvic inflammatory disease.
    b. Ectopic pregnancy (rupture is a surgical emergency).
    c. Other: fibroid torsion, cysts, endometriosis.
  4. Vascular. Vascular catastrophes are often surgical emergencies.
    a. Ruptured aneurysm.
    b. Dissecting aneurysm.
    c. Mesenteric thrombosis or embolism.
    d. Splenic or hepatic rupture; usually post-traumatic.

B. Extra-abdominal. Pathology in extra-abdominal diseases may rarely present as referred abdominal pain. The most important pathologies to remember are sickle cell crisis, pneumonia (especially lower lobe), myocardial infarction (MI), and, rarely, diabetic ketoacidosis.

C. Other
  1. Trauma patient. Blunt trauma may cause injuries to solid viscera (spleen, liver, kidney, pancreas) or to fixed structures such as the duodenum. Penetrating trauma may injure any intra-abdominal structure.
  2. Postoperative. Postoperative abdominal pain usually decreases significantly in uncomplicated cases during the first 2–3 postoperative days. Persistent pain may indicate a problem such as obstruction or abscess formation. Uncomplicated postoperative pain is derived from both visceral fibers because of surgical injury to peritoneal linings and to somatic fibers innervating the abdominal wall.

   3. **Critically ill patient.** Patients who have severe stress from such serious insults as multiple trauma or burns, often complicated by sepsis, may develop potentially life-threatening intra-abdominal events.
      a. Acute stress gastritis (usually manifested as massive UGI bleeding).
      b. Curling's ulcer with or without perforation (after burn).
      c. Acalculous cholecystitis and cholestasis from long-term use of total parenteral nutrition.
   4. **Special populations.** Special populations of patients, including the elderly, those with acquired immuno-deficiency syndrome (AIDS), and those with hemophilia may present with unusual causes of abdominal pain or may have unusual presentations of common disorders.

IV. Database

A. Physical Examination Key Points

   1. **Overall appearance.** Writhing in agony is typical of colic, whereas a motionless patient is suggestive of problems that cause peritoneal irritation.
   2. **Lungs.** Listen for basilar rales or rhonchi indicating possible pneumonia. Dullness to percussion may represent pleural effusion or consolidation.
   3. **Heart.** Look for evidence of cardiac decompensation (distended neck veins, S_3 gallop, peripheral edema), especially in the patient with pre-existing coronary disease, which may direct attention toward an MI or atrial fibrillation to suggest emboli.
   4. **Abdomen.**
      a. **Inspection:** Note presence of distention (obstruction, ileus, ascites), scaphoid (perforated ulcer), flank ecchymoses (hemorrhagic pancreatitis), caput medusae (portal hypertension), and surgical scars (adhesions, tumor).
      b. **Auscultation:** Listen for bowel sounds (absent or occasional tinkle with obstruction or ileus; hyperperistaltic with gastroenteritis; rushes with small bowel obstruction).
      c. **Percussion:** Tympany is associated with distended loops of bowel; dullness and a fluid wave with ascites; loss of liver dullness is associated with free air.
      d. **Palpation:** Guarding, rigidity, and rebound tenderness are hallmarks of peritonitis. Localized tenderness is often seen with cholecystitis, appendicitis,

salpingitis, and diverticulitis. Costovertebral angle tenderness is common with pyelonephritis. Murphy's sign is inspiratory arrest while palpating the gallbladder in acute cholecystitis. Pain with active hip flexion (psoas sign) can represent a retrocecal appendix or psoas abscess. The obturator sign (pain on internal and external rotation of the flexed thigh) can be found with a retrocecal appendix or obturator herniation. Masses may also be detected.

5. **Rectal examination.** A mass suggests a rectal carcinoma, a fissure indicates Crohn's disease, and unilateral tenderness suggests appendicitis (usually retrocecal) or an abscess. If stool is present, evaluate for occult blood (see page 320).

6. **Pelvic examination.** Examine for cervical motion tenderness and purulent cervical discharge that suggests pelvic inflammatory disease (salpingitis, tuboovarian abscess). Other masses may be felt (ectopic pregnancy, ovarian cyst, neoplasm).

7. **Extremities.** Evaluate for asymmetric pedal pulses, pain, pallor, and paresthesias as evidence of ischemia that may be associated with an embolic phenomenon.

8. **Skin.** Look for jaundice and spider angiomata seen with liver disease. Cool and clammy skin from peripheral vasoconstriction is an ominous sign of severe hypotension.

B. **Laboratory Data**

1. **Hemogram.** Anemia may indicate hemorrhage from an ulcer, colon cancer, or leaking aneurysm. Leukocytosis indicates presence of inflammation. A low WBC count is more typical of viral infections such as gastroenteritis or mesenteric adenitis.

2. **Serum electrolytes, urea nitrogen (BUN), and creatinine.** Bowel obstruction with vomiting can cause hypokalemia, dehydration, or both (BUN/creatinine ratio 20:1).

3. **Bilirubin, aspartate and alanine aminotransferases, and alkaline phosphatase.** Hepatitis, cholecystitis, and other liver diseases may be diagnosed through these tests.

4. **Amylase.** Markedly high levels are associated with pancreatitis. Amylase can also be increased with perforated ulcer and small bowel obstruction; occasionally, a pseudocyst or hemorrhagic pancreatitis may result in a normal amylase level.

5. **Arterial blood gases.** Hypoxia is often an early sign of sepsis. Acidosis may be present in ischemic bowel.

6. **Pregnancy test.** Premenopausal women should be tested to rule out ectopic pregnancy, whether or not they use contraceptives.
7. **Urinalysis.** Hematuria may indicate urolithiasis; pyuria and hematuria can be present in urinary tract infections or, rarely, in appendicitis.
8. **Cervical culture.** Send specimen specifically for gonorrhea (anaerobic) testing if pelvic inflammatory disease is suspected.

C. Radiologic and Other Studies
   1. **Flat and upright abdominal films.** Observe for the following key elements: gas pattern, bowel dilatation, air-fluid levels, presence of air in rectum, pancreatic calcifications, loss of psoas margin, displacement of hollow viscera, gallstones and renal stones, portal vein air, or aortic calcifications.
   2. **Chest film.** May demonstrate pneumonia, widened mediastinum, pleural effusion, or a raised hemidiaphragm (subdiaphragmatic inflammatory process). Free air under the diaphragm suggests a perforation and is most often seen on the upright chest film.
   3. **Ultrasound.** May show gallstones, ectopic pregnancy, or other pathology.
   4. **Abdominal CT scan.** Most sensitive when evaluating patients with acute abdominal pain and a wide variety of diagnosis are being considered.
   5. **Other studies as clinically indicated.**
      a. **Intravenous pyelogram (IVP).** Excretory urogram is helpful in the workup of urolithiasis.
      b. **Electrocardiogram (ECG).** Rules out MI as a cause of upper abdominal distress and nausea.
      c. **Biliary scintigram.**
      d. **Contrast bowel studies.** UGI swallow and enemas (barium, dilute barium, Gastrografin).
      e. **Endoscopic studies.** EGD, colonoscopy, or endoscopic retrograde cholangiopancreatography.
      f. **Arteriography.**
      g. **Peritoneal lavage (page 373) or paracentesis (page 367).**

V. **Plan.** Abdominal pain can present a diagnostic dilemma, especially in patients at the extremes of age or in those unable to communicate. It is essential to recognize that certain conditions are life threatening and require urgent operation (Table I–1). The surgeon's goal is to determine whether abdominal pain requires acute surgical intervention. Pain that is present for at least 6 hours without relief is likely to require surgery to

TABLE I–1. INDICATIONS FOR URGENT OPERATION IN PATIENTS WITH ACUTE ABDOMEN.

Physical findings

Involuntary guarding or rigidity, especially if spreading
Increasing or severe localized tenderness
Tense or progressive distention
Tender abdominal or rectal mass with high fever or hypotension
Rectal bleeding with shock or acidosis
Equivocal abdominal findings with—
    Septicemia (high fever, marked or increasing leukocytosis, mental changes, or
       increasing glucose intolerance in a diabetic patient)
    Bleeding (unexplained shock or acidosis, decreasing hematocrit)
    Suspected ischemia (acidosis, fever, tachycardia)
    Deterioration on conservative therapy

Radiologic findings

Pneumoperitoneum
Gross or progressive bowel distention
Free extravasation of contrast material
Space-occupying lesion on scan, with fever
Mesenteric occlusion on angiography

Endoscopic findings

Perforated or uncontrollably bleeding lesion

Paracentesis findings

Blood, bile, pus, bowel contents, or urine.

Source: Reproduced, with permission, from Doherty GM, Boey JH: Acute Abdomen. In: Current Surgical Diagnosis and Treatment, 11/e. LW Way, GM Doherty (editors). McGraw-Hill 2003.

prevent further morbidity. Diagnostic laparotomy or laparoscopy is routinely performed in cases where a definite diagnosis is not present. Analgesic use remains controversial, but moderate doses will not mask symptoms and will make the patient more comfortable. Specific types of therapy and operations for each possible diagnosis cannot be described here but can be found in surgical and medical textbooks.

A. Observation. With the exception of catastrophes that require urgent surgical exploration (see Table I–1), most cases of abdominal pain require close observation, medical management, and judicious use of analgesics. Patients should be kept NPO and given IV hydration, with careful attention to intake and output. GI decompression should be considered, especially if distention or vomiting is present. In addition, serial physical examinations by the same examiner are useful in determining progression of symptoms and aid in securing the diagnosis.

    B. Surgery. Perforated viscus, vascular catastrophes, high-grade bowel obstruction, certain splenic and hepatic injuries, ruptured ectopic pregnancies, and appendicitis require emergency surgery. Indications for urgent operation without a precise preoperative diagnosis are outlined in Table I–1.

REFERENCES

Fischer JE, et al. Manifestation of gastrointestinal disease. In: Schwartz SI, et al, eds. *Principles of Surgery,* 7th ed. New York: McGraw-Hill, 1999; p 1033–80.

Purcell T. Nonsurgical and extraperitoneal causes of abdominal pain. *Emerg Med Clin North Am* 7:721–40, 1989.

Silen W. *Cope's Early Diagnosis of the Acute Abdomen.* Oxford: Oxford University Press; 1990, p 231–9.

3. ACIDOSIS

(See also Section II, page 268)

  I. Problem. A patient with fulminant acute pancreatitis and accompanying acute respiratory distress syndrome (ARDS) requires intubation and mechanical ventilation. The initial arterial blood gas after intubation demonstrates a pH of 7.14.

  II. Immediate Questions

    A. Is the acidosis respiratory, metabolic, or a combination of both? Evaluation of any acid-base disorder begins with an arterial blood gas report. If the base excess is negative (or a positive deficit), the acidosis is at least partly metabolic. If the partial pressure of carbon dioxide (PCO_2) is <40 mm Hg, then acidosis is metabolic, possibly with respiratory compensation. If the PCO_2 >40, then acidosis is at least partly respiratory. For every 10 torr that the PCO_2 is >40, the pH will be lowered by 0.08 under normal circumstances. For example, if the PCO_2 is 60, one would expect an acidotic pH of 7.24; therefore, any additional acidosis can be attributed to metabolic causes. Expected compensatory adjustments for acute acidosis disturbances can be calculated as follows:

$$PCO_2 = 1.5 \ (\text{serum } HCO_3) + 8 \ (\pm 2)$$

    B. What is the volume status of the patient? A common cause of metabolic acidosis in the acute setting is lactic acidosis due to poor perfusion of tissues. Examine the patient, look at recent urine output, and assess cardiac filling

an acidotic pH of pressures (if available) to gauge the intravascular volume of the patient.

C. **Is there any problem with the ventilator circuit?** In a nonintubated patient with a respiratory acidosis, there is usually apparent difficulty in breathing. In a patient on a ventilator, a respiratory acidosis may not be clinically apparent in a sedated or obtunded patient. Check the ventilator circuit, the exhaled volume, and check the settings on the ventilator to make certain there is no technical explanation for the acidosis. Verify the position of the endotracheal tube on chest radiograph because it can slip distally into the right mainstem bronchus.

D. **Are there any arrhythmias or ectopy?** With a profound acidosis of any cause, there may be disturbances of the cardiac rhythm or ventricular ectopy. Obtain an ECG and monitor the patient.

III. **Differential Diagnosis**. The most important initial distinction in diagnosing the cause of acidosis is between respiratory and metabolic causes. In the acutely ill patient, both causes may be present as in the patient example cited above.

A. **Respiratory Acidosis**. By definition, this is alveolar hypoventilation. There are 2 main categories, acute and chronic, and these have relative compensatory adjustments depending on their chronicity. Acute occurs within 24 hours and the expected pH is $0.008 \times$ change in P_{CO_2}. If chronic, ie, after 24 hours, the expected pH is $0.003 \times$ change in P_{CO_2}.

1. **Pulmonary conditions.** Common etiologies include (a) asthma, (b) mechanical upper airway obstruction, (c) space-occupying lesions, (d) severe pulmonary edema, and (e) pneumonia.

2. **Drugs/toxins.** Hypoventilation secondary to (a) alcohol ingestion, (b) narcotics/sedative overdose, and (c) neuromuscular blocking agents.

3. **Neuromuscular conditions.** Differential includes (a) myasthenia gravis, (b) pickwickian syndrome, (c) cerebrovascular accident, and (d) Guillain-Barré syndrome.

B. **Metabolic Acidosis.** This can be subdivided into conditions with a normal anion gap and those with an increased anion gap, implying a high unmeasured anion level. The anion gap is calculated as $([Na] + [Cl]) - [HCO_3]$. The normal range is 8–12 mEq/L.

1. **Normal anion gap.**
   a. **Loss of bicarbonate.** Usually from the GI tract as diarrhea, small bowel fistula, pancreatic-cutaneous fistula, or a large amount of external biliary drainage.

      b. Renal tubular acidosis. If the patient has a normal anion gap and loss of bicarbonate is evident, calculation of a urinary cation gap may be helpful. It is calculated as (urine Na + urine K) − urine Cl. A positive value indicates renal tubular acidosis, and a negative value indicates GI losses.

  2. Increased anion gap.

    a. Lactic acidosis: poor perfusion with interference with the normal oxidative metabolism.

    b. Diabetic ketoacidosis

    c. Alcoholic ketoacidosis

    d. Chronic renal insufficiency: increased unmeasured anions include sulfates and phosphates.

    e. Drugs and poisoning. Overdose of aspirin or ingestion of methyl alcohol, ethylene glycol, or paraldehyde.

IV. Database

A. Physical Examination Key Points

1. **Vital signs.** Look for evidence of hypoventilation, hypotension, tachycardia, or fever. Sepsis can cause shock, a common cause of acidosis.

2. **Skin.** Cool, clammy extremities and mottled skin occur in shock when peripheral perfusion is poor.

3. **HEENT.** Head, eyes, ears, nose, throat (HEENT) ketosis or fruity odor on breath suggests diabetic ketoacidosis. Look for tracheal shift from a space-occupying lesion or jugular venous distention (eg, congestive heart failure [CHF] or tension pneumothorax).

4. **Pulmonary.** Evaluate for absent or decreased breath sounds, stridor in upper airway obstruction, wheezes, or rales, and evidence of accessory muscle use (sternocleidomastoid, rectus)

5. **Abdomen.** Peritoneal signs indicate an acute abdomen, and marked distention may inhibit respiration. Look for evidence of paradoxical motion (abdominal breathing)

6. **Neuromuscular.** Generalized weakness or focal neurologic signs, depressed level of consciousness, obtundation, or coma should be noted.

B. Laboratory Data

1. **Hemogram.** Leukocytosis is seen with sepsis and anemia is common with chronic renal insufficiency.

2. **Electrolytes, BUN, and creatinine.** Calculate the anion gap from the electrolytes. A high serum level of chloride is present in non-anion gap metabolic acidosis. Renal insufficiency may be present.

3. **Blood glucose, ketone levels.** Increases are associated with diabetic ketoacidosis.
4. **Lactate levels.** Levels are increased with sepsis and poor perfusion.
5. **Arterial blood gas (ABG).** Repeat the ABG to follow therapeutic interventions.

C. **Radiologic and Other Studies**
   1. **Chest radiograph.** To evaluate for infiltrates, pulmonary edema, effusions, and endotracheal tube position (ideal position is approximately 2 cm above the carina).
   2. **ECG with rhythm strip.** To evaluate for arrhythmias; consider heart failure or MI; check cardiac enzymes (creatine kinase and troponin I).
   3. **Electromyelogram.** This and other specialized neurologic tests may be needed to diagnose primary neurologic conditions.

V. **Plan.** In general, for respiratory and metabolic acidoses, cure of the underlying cause of the acidosis is the primary goal. In emergent situations, the 2 methods to reverse the acidosis are to administer sodium bicarbonate intravenously (reserved for severe acidemia, ie, pH <7.2) and to hyperventilate the patient. Be sure to check serial pH values to monitor the progress of therapy.

A. **Metabolic Acidosis**
   1. **Bicarbonate therapy.** In general, administer IV bicarbonate if the pH <7.20.
      a. Calculate the bicarbonate need for the entire body:

Patient's body weight (in kg) $\times 0.40 \times (24 - [HCO_3]) =$ Total number of mEq of HCO_3 needed

      b. Administer 50% of this amount over the first 12 hours as a mixture of bicarbonate with 5% dextrose with water (D5W).
      c. Complications of bicarbonate therapy include:
         i. Hypernatremia
         ii. Volume overload
         iii. Hypokalemia, which is caused by intracellular shifts of potassium as the pH increases.
   2. Control underlying causes
      a. Volume resuscitate in sepsis, hemorrhagic shock, and other causes of lactic acidosis.
      b. Insulin and saline for diabetic ketoacidosis (see page 493).
      c. Dialysis as needed for renal failure.

B. **Respiratory Acidosis.** The main goal is to cure the underlying cause.

   1. If necessary, intubate the patient and treat with mechanical ventilation. If a patient is already intubated and has a significant respiratory acidosis, then increase alveolar ventilation by increasing tidal volume (up to 10–15 mL/kg) while following peak inspiratory pressures or increase the respiratory rate.

   2. In an emergent situation, disconnect the patient from the ventilator and hyperventilate by hand with the bag device. The importance of good pulmonary toilet, ie, suctioning of secretions, cannot be overemphasized.

REFERENCES

Adrogué HJ, Madias N. Management of life-threatening acid-base disorders. *N Engl J Med* 338:26–34, 1998.

Hood VL, Tannen RL. Lactic acidosis. In: Adrogué HJ, ed. *Contemporary Management in Critical Care, vol 1, no 2. Acid-base and electrolyte disorder.* New York: Churchill Livingstone; 1991, p 1–19.

Rose BD, Post TW. *Clinical Physiology of Acid-Base and Electrolyte Disorders,* 5th ed. New York: McGraw-Hill; 2001, p 328–47.

4. ALKALOSIS

(See also Section II, page 268)

I. **Problem.** A 47-year-old female is on a ventilator in the intensive care unit (ICU) and has a pH of 7.56 1 day after thoracotomy for a Belsey antireflux procedure.

II. **Immediate Questions**

A. **Is the patient on a ventilator and, if so, what is the respiratory rate and tidal volume?** Alkalosis may be a result of over ventilation ("blowing off CO_2"). Rate (intermittent mandatory ventilation [IMV] or assist control mode) and volume for each delivered breath (tidal volume) are important. The tidal volume should be set at 6–10 mL/kg. Minute ventilation equals rate multiplied by tidal volume, so a change in either parameter will affect the minute ventilation.

B. **What medication is the patient taking?** Thiazide diuretics can result in a "contraction" alkalosis and excess bicarbonate and bicarbonate precursors.

C. **What is the composition of the IV fluids?** Be sure there is no added bicarbonate (avoid Ringer's lactate) and make sure the patient is receiving sufficient chloride (80–100 mEq/day as NaCl, plus losses).

D. Is there a NG tube in place, or is there vomiting? The NG tube drainage of the GI tract is a common cause of alkalosis. The most common metabolic abnormality in surgical patients is hypokalemic hypochloremic metabolic alkalosis. The alkalosis is a result of renal exchange of K^+ for H^+ and **not** the loss of HCl from the stomach. These patients are alkalotic and yet have aciduria ("paradoxical aciduria"). As K^+ is removed by the NG tube, the kidney attempts to hold onto K^+, so it exchanges K^+ with H^+, thereby leaving the patient alkalotic. Thus, therapy is directed at volume repletion and K^+ repletion.

III. Differential Diagnosis. The key differential point is similar to that of acidosis: Is the origin of the disturbance metabolic or respiratory?

A. Metabolic Alkalosis. This is seen usually as increased serum bicarbonate. Compensation is usually by hypoventilation and increased renal excretion of bicarbonate. It is diagnosed by an increased pH, with a normal or increased arterial P_{CO_2}.

1. Loss of HCl (chloride responsive), urine Cl <10 mEq/L;
   a. NG suction, vomiting.
   b. Villous adenoma (potassium wasting).
   c. Diuretics (especially thiazides).
   d. Post-hypercapnia.
   e. Cystic fibrosis.
2. Chloride resistant (chloride unresponsive), urine Cl >10 mEq/L.
   a. Bicarbonate administration (oral and parenteral).
   b. Chronic hypokalemia.
   c. Primary hyperaldosteronism.
   d. Cushing's syndrome, exogenous steroids.
   e. Bartter's syndrome.
   f. Hypercalcemia and hypoparathyroidism.

B. Respiratory Alkalosis. Hyperventilation results in decreased P_{CO_2}, and the compensatory mechanism is through increased renal bicarbonate excretion.

1. Anxiety.
2. Hypermetabolic states (eg, fever, early sepsis).
3. Iatrogenic. Ventilator rate or tidal volume is too high.
4. Pregnancy.
5. Cirrhosis.
6. Cardiac disease (refer to Problem 12, page 54).
7. Pulmonary disease (refer to Problem 26, page 106).
8. Salicylate intoxication (alkalosis early, with metabolic acidosis later).

IV. Database

A. Physical Examination Key Points

1. **Vital signs.** Pay particular attention to the respiratory rate. Tachypnea may signify a respiratory cause.
2. **Lungs.** Check for signs of pulmonary edema (rales).
3. **Skin.** Look for changes associated with alcohol abuse such as palmar erythema, spider angiomata, etc. Signs of sepsis or decreased perfusion may be present.

B. Laboratory Data.
Obtain simultaneous ABG and electrolyte levels.

1. **Arterial blood gases.** As noted above.
2. **Serum electrolytes.** Pay particular attention to hypokalemia, which may accompany alkalosis (low serum H^+ balanced by exchange of K^+ in the kidney).
3. **Serum salicylate levels.** If aspirin intoxication is suspected.

C. Radiologic and Other Studies.
In general, none are indicated. Patients on a ventilator should have chest radiographs as indicated.

V. Plan.
It is essential to identify the underlying cause of alkalosis and control it.

A. Discontinue Exogenous Bicarbonate.
Bicarbonate precursors such as acetate salts (amino acids) found in hyperalimentation solutions should also be evaluated. If hyperalimentation is essential, attempt to increase the chloride salts in the solution, and the amino acid content may need to be decreased.

B. IV Fluid Replacement.
For alkalosis resulting from the loss of HCl, administer NaCl as normal saline IV. For alkalosis that is chloride resistant, administer IV KCl.

C. Sedation.
Sedate for anxiety in ventilated patients that may be causing respiratory alkalosis with agents such as diazepam, lorazepam, or midazolam.

D. Decreased Minute Ventilation.
Use a rebreathing mask in the nonintubated patient with respiratory alkalosis, or decrease the minute ventilation by decreasing the rate or the tidal volume. Be sure that the tidal volume is set for 6–10 mL/kg.

E. Control Hypokalemia.
Use KCl supplementation.

F. Replace Volume Losses.
Replace fluid volume lost through the NG tube or vomiting, usually using D5 1/2 normal saline (NS) with 20 mEq KCl/L.

REFERENCES

Galla JH. Metabolic alkalosis. *J Am Soc Nephrol* 11:369–74, 2000.
Rose BD, Post TW. *Clinical Physiology of Acid-Base and Electrolyte Disorders, 5th ed.* New York: McGraw-Hill; 2001, p 328–47.

5. ANAPHYLAXIS (DRUG REACTION)

Immediate Actions

1. Stop administration of allergen (eg, blood, medication, IV contrast).
2. Assess airway and intubate if necessary (may be difficult secondary to laryngeal edema or laryngospasm).
3. Check breathing and administer O_2.
4. Ensure adequate IV access (14 or 16 gauge) and begin fluids (LR 500 mL bolus).
5. Place on continuous cardiac monitor and pulse oximetry.
6. Treat with epinephrine, Benadryl, or steroids (see Subsection V, "Plan").

I. **Problem.** A postoperative patient has developed severe dyspnea and a generalized rash after receiving IV penicillin.

II. **Immediate Questions.** Respiratory distress and hypotension can be life threatening and should be controlled immediately.

   A. **What are the patient's vital signs?** Tachycardia is a common finding and could represent a response to hypoxia, fear, hypotension, or arrhythmia. Hypotension requires immediate management in this setting (IV crystalloid, epinephrine, and Benadryl as soon as available).

   B. **Can the patient communicate appropriately?** Appropriate answers to simple questions indicate that cerebral oxygenation is adequate. An inability to speak suggests severe respiratory deterioration leading to upper airway obstruction from laryngospasm or laryngeal edema.

   C. **What medication is the patient taking?** Many medications can cause anaphylaxis, but the most common in this setting are penicillin, other β-lactamase antibiotics (cephalosporins), and IV contrast.

III. **Differential Diagnosis.** *Anaphylaxis* technically refers to the signs and symptoms caused by an antigen-mediated release of IgE-induced mediators. It can be localized (as in allergic rhinitis) or systemic and life threatening.

A. Acute Allergic Reaction (Anaphylaxis). Most often caused by medications noted in Subsection II–C. Less frequently, anaphylaxis may be caused by food, environmental agents (dust, pollen), or insects.

B. Upper Airway Obstruction. May be caused by a foreign body or laryngeal edema and classically presents as stridor.

C. Acute Asthmatic Attack. Wheezing with a history of asthma is usually present.

D. Pulmonary Embolus. Especially in the postoperative setting, this must be considered in the patient who is acutely short of breath.

E. Pulmonary Edema. To be considered in the elderly patient who has underlying coronary artery disease. Can present with dyspnea, "cardiac" wheezes, and, sometimes, hypotension. Chest radiograph confirms the diagnosis.

F. Other Causes. Other causes for this constellation of symptoms are discussed in other sections: dyspnea (Problem xxx, page xxx), hypotension (Problem xxx, page xxx), pruritus (Problem xxx, page xxx), and wheezing (Problem xxx, page xxx).

IV. Database. Knowledge of patient allergies and current medications is essential. Relation of medication administration to onset of symptoms is also important.

A. Physical Examination Key Points

1. **Vital signs.** Tachycardia is an early sign. Hypotension must be recognized early and may present as syncope.
2. **Lungs.** Listen for wheezing (suggests bronchospasm), stridor (suggests laryngospasm), and adequacy of air movement.
3. **Skin.** Generalized rash, urticaria, and pruritus are the most common signs seen in an anaphylactic reaction.
4. **Extremities.** Look for evidence of cyanosis. A medic-alert bracelet may relate causes of allergic reaction.
5. **Mental status.** Somnolence in this setting demands immediate respiratory support and is frequently indicative of severe hypercapnia.
6. **Gastrointestinal.** Nausea, vomiting, abdominal pain, tenesmus, or diarrhea may accompany anaphylaxis.

B. Laboratory Data

1. **Arterial blood gas.** Usually has no role in the management of a patient with acute respiratory distress.

C. Radiologic and Other Studies
   1. **Chest radiograph.** When time permits, a chest radiograph will rule out other causes of respiratory distress (CHF, pneumonia, etc).
   2. **Electrocardiogram.** Acute MI can present as pulmonary edema with severe dyspnea. Right ventricular strain can be seen in pulmonary embolus (PE).

V. Plan. Therapy should be initiated quickly based on clinical findings and **before** performing other studies and laboratory examinations. Therapy is dictated by the severity of reaction. Be prepared to initiate cardiopulmonary resuscitation.

   A. Laryngeal Edema. Oxygen by face mask should be instituted for moderate to severe dyspnea. Intubation (or surgical airway) may be required if the patient is in severe respiratory distress (stridor), is severely somnolent, or is desaturating. Sedation and paralysis are contraindicated. Racemic epinephrine in a nebulizer may temporize laryngeal edema. Consider steroids (methylprednisolone 125–250 mg every 6 hours) for protracted mild to moderate laryngeal edema. Epinephrine (as outlined in Subsection V-C, below) and diphenhydramine (Benadryl) 25–50 mg orally (PO) or intramuscularly (IM) for mild reactions and 50–100 mg IV for severe reactions should be given immediately.

   B. Bronchospasm. In addition to oxygen, Benadryl, epinephrine, and albuterol by inhalation should be given. Consider the use of aminophylline, ipratropium bromide, and steroids (as outlined above).

   C. Hypotension. Epinephrine 1:1000 solution 0.3–0.5 mL (0.01 mL/kg for children) *SC* or IM (improved absorption with generalized urticaria) should be given immediately for moderate to severe anaphylaxis (laryngospasm, bronchospasm, or hypotension) with dramatic improvement often seen. Repeat the dose in 5–10 minutes as needed. *The epinephrine used for cardiopulmonary resuscitation (CPR) is a 1:10,000 solution given IV and should not be used in this situation.* Use epinephrine with caution in patients >40 years (due to a risk of arrhythmia and cardiac ischemia). In severe hypotension, acute respiratory failure from bronchospasm, or upper airway obstruction, *IV* epinephrine is administered (10 mL of 1:100,000 solution over 10 minutes followed by continuous drip at 1–4 µg/min). Volume repletion should start immediately with crystalloid. In refractory hypotension, consider vasopressors (dopamine, isoproterenol, or Levophed), glucagon (1 mg IV), or steroids (as above).

D. **Other Considerations**. Consider activated charcoal for in-
gested antigens. Cimetidine (300 mg IV every 6 hours)
should be given for persistent anaphylaxis.

E. **Monitoring.** Resolution of the respiratory distress associated with anaphylaxis is usually so dramatic that ICU monitoring after the episode is often unnecessary. Patients
who are given epinephrine need cardiac monitoring for at
least 30 minutes. Benadryl should be continued for the
next 48 hours and steroids should be tapered in cases of
persistent bronchospasm or hypotension.

F. **Prophylaxis.** Patients known to have an allergy to IV contrast medium should be premedicated with prednisone (50
mg for 13 hours, 7 hours, and 1 hour before the procedure)
and Benadryl (50 mg IM 1 hour before the procedure) and
receive low-osmolality dye.

REFERENCES

Bochner BS, Lichtenstein LM. Anaphylaxis. *N Engl J Med* 324:1785–90,
1991.
Dejarnatt AC, Grant JA. Basic mechanisms of anaphylaxis and anaphylac-
toid reactions. *Immunol Allergy Clin North Am* 12:501–11, 1992.
Yocum MW, Khan DA. Assessment of patients who have experienced anaphylaxis: a 3–year survey. *Mayo Clin Proc* 69:16–23, 1994.

6. ANEMIA

I. **Problem.** A patient admitted for a varicose vein stripping has
a hematocrit of 19% on preoperative laboratory evaluation.

II. **Immediate Questions**

A. **Is the patient hemodynamically stable?** A patient with a
chronic anemia has already compensated for volume loss.
The evaluation and therapy of those patients can proceed
in an orderly fashion. Patients with a low hematocrit secondary to an acute bleed may need urgent volume resuscitation. However, those patients almost always present with
clinically apparent bleeding as opposed to being diagnosed on a routine laboratory study. Tachycardia and determination of postural hypotension are important signs of
hypovolemia.

B. **Is the patient's stool positive for occult blood?** On a
surgical service, a patient with a newly decreased hematocrit should be assumed to have GI bleeding until proved
otherwise. Ask about melena (tarry stools) or change in
bowel habits.

C. **Does the patient have a history of anemia?** Review the chart or clinic records to find the most recent hematocrit. Ask if the patient has knowledge of an anemia or if there is a family history of anemia.

D. **Is the low hematocrit result correct?** If the laboratory result is unexpected or if it does not correlate with the clinical appearance of the patient, question the validity of the test. Sources of laboratory error regarding a low hematocrit include (1) the sample is from a different patient; (2) a technical problem with the machine; and (3) blood drawn proximal to an open IV line. Incorrect laboratory results are unusual, but it is worth repeating the test before embarking on an extensive workup.

III. **Differential diagnosis.** Anemia is present in many disease states. Chronic anemia can be categorized as microcytic or macrocytic. Microcytic anemias are easily to remember by the acronym TAILS (thalassemia, anemia of chronic disease, iron deficiency, lead poisoning, sideroblastic). Macrocytic anemias are usually due to vitamin B_{12} or folate deficiencies, usually in alcoholic patients. Acute anemia due to blood loss can be from many different sources and must be dealt with in a timely fashion.

IV. **Database**

A. **Physical Examination Key Points**

1. **Vital signs.** Orthostatic hypotension and tachycardia indicate hemodynamically significant anemia.

2. **Skin.** Pallor, pale conjunctiva, and pale nail beds correlate with the degree of anemia reported by the laboratory.

3. **Abdomen.** Splenomegaly is present in hemolytic anemias, in disorders with intracorpuscular defects leading to destruction of red blood cells (RBCs), and myeloid metaplasia. A mass may be present with malignancy.

4. **Rectal examination.** Pay close attention to any mass or the presence of occult blood.

5. **Dressings, drains, and surgical sites** should be inspected.

6. **Am NG tube** can used to rule out an UGI source of bleeding (ulcer, varices, etc).

B. **Laboratory data (see Section II, page 268 for more details)**

1. **Hemogram.** In addition to the hematocrit, assess the WBC and platelet counts for evidence of general bone marrow depression or leukemia.

2. **RBC indices.** MCV and MCHC allow a classification of anemia according to RBC size and hemoglobin content. Iron deficiency anemia is microcytic and hypochromic, whereas megaloblastic anemia is typically macrocytic.

3. **Peripheral blood smear.** This can also be used to assess the actual size of RBCs because indices may be misleading. Examining the shape of the cells (spherocytosis, elliptocytosis, RBC fragments) is sometimes helpful. An RBC distribution width is available in some centers, which can help determine a mixed population of macrocytic and microcytic cells.

4. **Reticulocyte count.** This provides a measurement of the production of RBCs at the level of the marrow. A low reticulocyte count suggests inadequate production of RBCs, whereas an increased count is associated with increased destruction of RBCs.

5. **Serum chemistries, BUN, and creatinine.** This may show evidence of renal failure or increased indirect bilirubin in hemolytic anemias.

6. **Iron, total iron binding capacity (TIBC).** In iron deficiency, serum iron is decreased and TIBC is increased. In anemia of chronic disease, serum iron is decreased or normal and TIBC is decreased.

7. **Haptoglobin.** Often decreased in hemolytic anemia.

8. **Folate, vitamin B$_{12}$ levels.** These levels measure deficiencies of specific metabolites.

9. **Coombs' test.** This measures immunoglobulin M and G antibodies in hemolytic anemias.

C. **Radiologic and Other Studies**

1. **Bone marrow biopsy.** If reticulocyte count is low, this biopsy assesses erythrocyte precursors, iron stores, and bone marrow replacement by infiltrative disease processes.

2. **GI workup.** May include UGI series, barium enema, upper endoscopy, colonoscopy, angiography, or tagged RBC nuclear scans if workup indicates a GI source of anemia.

3. **Ultrasound and CT scans.** May be useful in the evaluation for a tumor.

V. **Plan.** Notify senior staff because elective operations will often be postponed when an anemia is identified.

A. **Acute Management.** If hemodynamically significant anemia is present, start a large-bore IV (≥18 gauge and draw necessary blood samples for the laboratory and blood bank at the same time) and begin fluid resuscitation. Check stools for occult blood and, if heme-positive, consider passing an NG tube as an initial diagnostic maneuver to check for a UGI source of bleeding. Blood transfusions should be initiated if indicated.

B. Evaluation. Continue with GI workup as described above. If anemia is due to causes other than acute blood loss, gather laboratory data as discussed above, and a hematology consultation.

C. Specific Therapies

1. **Iron deficiency.** Ferrous sulfate or gluconate 325 mg 3 times a day given with a stool softener (eg, Colace) because iron pills cause constipation.
2. **Folate deficiency.** Folate 1 mg PO or mixed with IV fluids every day.
3. **Vitamin B$_{12}$ deficiency.** Vitamin B12 1000 mg IM daily for 14 days and then 1000 mg IM monthly.
4. **Hemolytic anemia.** Often controlled with glucocorticoids such as prednisone 60–100 mg/day and may require splenectomy.
5. **Intracorpuscular RBC defect.** Often splenectomy will be helpful.
6. Transfusions as needed.
7. Operation may be needed depending on GI tract evaluation.
8. H$_2$-receptor blockers (eg, Tagamet or Zantac) and antacids for ulcer disease.

REFERENCES

Fischer JE, et al. Manifestation of gastrointestinal disease. In: Schwartz SI, et al, eds. *Principles of Surgery.* New York: McGraw-Hill, 1999; p 1033–80.

Tefferi A. Anemia in adults: A contemporary approach to diagnosis. *Mayo Clin Proc* 78:1274–80, 2003.

Weintraub SL, et al. Principles of preoperative and operative surgery. In: Townsend C, ed. *Sabiston's Textbook of Surgery,* 16th ed. Philadelphia: WB Saunders; 2001, p 221–42.

7. ARTERIAL LINE PROBLEMS

(Technique for arterial line placement is discussed in Section III, page 334).

I. Problem. The arterial line is not functioning in a 65-year-old patient on the first postoperative day after pulmonary lobectomy.

II. Immediate Questions

A. What is the appearance of the tracing? An absent tracing may indicate clotting of the catheter. A normal tracing indicates at least adequate arterial flow in the catheter. A dampened tracing may indicate air in the system or a clot. If this is noted, flush the tubing after disconnecting it from the arterial line.

B. Is the extremity distal to the line compromised? Be sure that the extremity is not ischemic. Checking the pulse oximeter on the extremity with the arterial line may be helpful in discerning whether the problem lies at the extremity or in the arterial line setup. If there is any question, the line should be removed.

C. Can blood be drawn back through the catheter? Even if the catheter cannot be used to draw blood, it can often function as a blood pressure monitor.

D. Does the arterial pressure measured correlate with a cuff pressure? In general, cuff measurements should be 10–15 mm Hg of the arterial line reading.

III. Differential Diagnosis

A. Mechanical
1. **Kinked catheter.**
2. **Clotted catheter.** Often caused by insufficient heparin in the flush solution.
3. **Faulty monitor or transducer.** The ICU staff will be helpful in solving this problem.
4. **Positional catheter.** This is often a problem with the way the catheter was sutured in place or the positioning of the extremity on the armboard.

B. Vascular
1. **Thrombosed vessel.** Check the pulse proximally with a Doppler probe, if necessary. Risk factors include (1) hypotension, (2) mechanical pressure to control bleeding at the site, (3) use of a catheter too large for the vessel, and (4) a catheter left in place for too long.
2. **Torn artery around the catheter that is causing bleeding.** Most common after a problematic cutdown. Application of pressure, as for any bleeding, should control the problem and prevent a large periarterial hematoma that may result in a pseudoaneurysm later.

IV. Database

A. Physical Examination Key Points
1. Examine the insertion site for signs of infection or bleeding. Correlate waveforms and measurements with noninvasive cuff measurements.

2. The distal extremity (hand or foot) should be examined for evidence of ischemia. Place a pulse oximeter on a digit of the extremity in question.
3. The entire tubing, transducer, and monitoring system should be checked for mechanical problems.

B. Laboratory Data. The only useful laboratory data concern the setting of bleeding from the site. Prothrombin time (PT) and partial thromboplastin time (PTT), platelets, and fibrin split products are helpful if diffuse bleeding is present. Hematocrit is essential if bleeding has been excessive.

V. Plan. Check the pressure tracing against a standard blood pressure cuff measurement. Verify the acceptable withdrawal of arterial blood. Occasionally, a catheter may be used to withdraw arterial blood but not provide reliable pressure monitoring and vice versa.

A. Bleeding
1. Apply direct pressure or a pressure dressing if bleeding from the site is a problem. Bleeding from other sites may signify disseminated intravascular coagulation (DIC).
2. After a catheter is removed, pressure should be applied to the site for at least 10 minutes to prevent bleeding with resultant hematoma and subsequent pseudoaneurysm formation.

B. Mechanical Problems
1. The use of an armboard will help prevent many mechanical problems. Positional catheter problems may be solved with an armboard or resuturing the catheter.
2. Kinked or clotted catheters usually must be replaced.
   a. If a catheter clots, verify that there is sufficient heparin in the flush bag (usually heparin 2–4 U/mL).
   b. If the vessel appears undamaged, consider changing the catheter over a guidewire by using a sterile technique. Be sure to carefully suture it in place to avoid kinking the catheter.
3. A dampened waveform usually indicates air in the transducer system or a clot in the catheter. Air bubbles can usually be flushed clear.

C. Reading Errors. The difference between the cuff and arterial line pressure is usually less than 10–15 mm Hg. Using an appropriate sized blood pressure cuff, keeping tubing lengths as short as possible, and verifying that there is a properly "zeroed" transducer and no air in the system should minimize the differences.

D. Thrombosis. Usually requires removal of the catheter and observation for ischemic changes. If there are ischemic changes, a careful follow-up examination is warranted to avoid progression of ischemia.

REFERENCES

Frezza EE, Mezghebe H. Indications and complications of arterial catheter use in surgical or medical intensive care units: analysis of 4932 patients. *Am Surg* 64:127–35, 1998.

Gardner RM. Direct arterial pressure monitoring. *Curr Anaesth Crit Care* 1:239–44, 1990.

Weiss BM, Galtiker RI. Complications during and following radial artery cannulation: a prospective study. *Intensive Care Med* 14:424–31, 1986.

8. ASPIRATION

I. **Problem.** A patient with obtunded trauma in the emergency room is being evaluated for a head injury; the patient vomits and develops acute respiratory distress.

II. **Immediate Questions**

A. **What are the vital signs?** Significant respiratory distress (tachypnea and tachycardia) may indicate massive aspiration of gastric contents. A decrease in oxygen saturation should alert the physician to respiratory decompensation. Fever may indicate underlying infectious process.

B. **Is the airway protected?** If the patient cannot protect the airway, then intubation is indicated. Check the patient's Glasgow Coma Scale (GCS); a score <8 is an indication for emergent intubation.

C. **Is the patient cyanotic?** Cyanosis and tachypnea after aspiration usually require intubation.

D. **What is the patient's neurologic status?** Patients who are unconscious or obtunded are at higher risk for pulmonary aspiration.

III. **Differential Diagnosis**

A. **Aspiration Pneumonitis.** Risk factors include (1) altered mental status (due to head injury, drugs, or alcohol), (2) reflux disease, (3) NG tube placement, (4) tracheostomy, and (5) vomiting. Emergency intubation has a high incidence of aspiration. Emergent intubation for pregnant patients, patients who recently ate, or patients with bowel obstruction requires rapid sequence induction with cricoid pressure to decrease aspiration risk.

B. **Asthma.** Wheezing from aspiration, especially chronic aspiration, can mimic asthma.

 C. **Pneumonia.** May precede aspiration or be caused by aspiration.

 D. **Pulmonary Embolus and Infarction.** Acute dyspnea and respiratory failure are common presentations of PE (refer to Problem 26, page 106).

 E. **Foreign Body Aspiration.** A problem most common in children. Older patients with poor dentition may aspirate loose teeth.

 F. **Pneumothorax.** This can also mimic an aspiration situation, especially in a trauma patient.

IV. **Database.** History of asthma should be ruled out. Evaluate for risk factors of PE (birth control pills, recent operation with prolonged bedrest, previous deep venous thrombosis [DVT]).

 A. **Physical Examination Key Points**
 1. **Vital signs.** Pay close attention to respiratory rate and oxygen saturation.
 2. **HEENT.** Check dentition for loose or missing teeth. If an NG or feeding tube is present, check its position.
 3. **Neck.** Evidence of tumor involvement of the pharynx, tracheostomy, surgery of the head and neck, trauma, and radiation to the head and neck should be sought. Also, check for jugular venous distention (JVD) that may indicate a pneumothorax.
 4. **Lungs.** Wheezing occurs when airways are irritated by stomach contents. Rales can also be present when a large volume of aspiration has occurred.
 5. **Skin.** Look for cyanosis to suggest hypoxia.
 6. **Extremities.** Look for evidence of DVT.
 7. **Neurologic examination.** Careful evaluation of mental status and presence of gag reflex are important. A GCS should be determined.

 B. **Laboratory Data**
 1. **Arterial blood gas.** Intubation should be performed if adequate oxygenation cannot be maintained.
 2. **Hemogram.** Pay particular attention to the WBC count.
 3. **Sputum Gram stain and culture.** Pathogenic organisms may grow in cases of chronic aspiration or in acute aspiration pneumonia.

 C. **Radiologic and Other Studies**
 1. Chest radiograph may show the following features.
 a. Air trapping ("hyperaeration") on the side of foreign body aspiration.
 b. Infiltrate in an area of the superior segment of the lower lobes (midlung fields) with aspiration in bedridden patients or the right lower lobe in upright

patients. These segmental bronchi course directly posteriorly and are thus most dependent in the supine patient. Infiltrates may not be seen immediately after aspiration.

    c. Wedge-shaped infarct in some cases of PE; free air with a pneumothorax.

    d. Clear fields and flattened diaphragm in uncomplicated asthma or chronic obstructive pulmonary disease (COPD).

    e. Aspiration can result in infiltrates in any portion of either lung or no infiltrate depending on quantity and quality of the material aspirated.

  2. Other studies. Ventilation/perfusion (V/Q) scan if venous thrombosis or pulmonary emboli is suspected. Subsequent barium swallow will show signs of reflux. If reflux is suspected, it is important that Gastrografin not be used due to its severe pulmonary toxicity.

V. Plan. Aspiration should be suspected in patients who may be unable to protect their airway, with neurologic or oncologic disease affecting swallowing and coughing and with depressed mental status, obtundation, or absent gag reflex (eg, head trauma or alcohol intoxication), and in those patients who have required intubation on a full stomach.

  A. Prevention

    1. For emergent intubation, it may be advisable to administer IV agents such as cimetidine to attempt to increase gastric pH and rapid sequence induction with cricoid pressure.

    2. For patients being fed via NG tube, gastric emptying should be confirmed (by checking residuals every 4 hours) and the head of the bed should be elevated.

    3. Unconscious patients should be placed in a lateral, slightly head-down position, whenever possible.

    4. NG tubes should be placed to suction if in place.

  B. Oxygenation. Supplemental oxygen is usually given by mask initially. Carefully monitor oxygenation with a transcutaneous oxygen saturation monitor or repeatABG tests.

C. Intubation and Pulmonary Toilet. These will be needed if oxygenation is poor or in a patient who is obtunded or unconscious.

  D. Medications

    1. Start antibiotics based on culture results when there is evidence of established pneumonia. Acute aspiration pneumonia may be aerobic or mixed anaerobic-aerobic flora.

    2. Anaerobic organisms are more likely with poor denti-
tion. Empiric antibiotic therapy recommended.

  E. Bronchoscopy. Performed when foreign body aspiration
is suspected or in those patients who aspirated particulate
gastric material that cannot be adequately suctioned.

  F. Chest Tube or CT-Guided Aspiration. May be needed
later for drainage of an empyema. Chronic aspiration
pneumonia may be necrotizing with formation of a lung abscess or progression to empyema.

  G. Respiratory Therapy. This is the most important aspect of
management. Every 2 to 4 hours, albuterol treatments
should be administered to control bronchospasm. This
should be accompanied by frequent tracheal suctioning.

REFERENCES

Depaso WJ. Aspiration pneumonia. *Clin Chest Med* 12:269–84, 1991.
Fischer JE, et al. Surgical complications. In: Schwartz SI, et al, eds. *Principles of Surgery,* 7th ed. New York: McGraw-Hill; 1999, p 441–84.
Marik PE. Aspiration pneumonitis and aspiration pneumonia. *N Engl J Med*
344:665–71, 2001.

9. BRADYCARDIA

  I. Problem. After a hernia operation, a patient is found to have a
heart rate of 42 beats/min on a routine vital signs check.

 II. Immediate Questions

  **A. What is the patient's blood pressure and is the patient
alert and oriented?** The initial questions define the severity of the problem. Because the clinical relevance of a significant bradycardia is decreased perfusion pressure, the
rapid assessment of perfusion, ie, blood pressure and
mental status, should be performed.

  B. What is the patient's normal resting heart rate? The
range of normal heart rates is wide and a rate of 42
beats/min in a patient at rest may not be abnormal in some
people, eg, highly conditioned athletes.

  **C. Are there any associated symptoms of chest pain or
pressure, dyspnea, diaphoresis, nausea, or lightheadedness?** A new bradydysrhythmia may be a manifestation
of an acute cardiac event such as an inferior MI.

  **D. What medication is the patient taking, and does the
patient have a pacemaker?** Certain medications, such as
β blockers (eg, propranolol), verapamil, digitalis, and oth-

ers can lead to bradycardia. A patient with a pacemaker may have pacer malfunction.

   E. Does the patient have a history of cardiovascular disease? This may further clarify the nature of the slow heart rate.

III. Differential Diagnosis. Disturbances in the cardiac conduction pathway that lead to bradydysrhythmia are due to dysfunction at the level of the sinus node or at the level of the atrioventricular (AV) node/His Purkinje system. Within these 2 categories different conditions exist and are defined by characteristic ECG patterns and associated with particular clinical conditions.

   A. Sinus Node Disease
   1. **Sinus bradycardia.**
      a. **Vasovagal syncope.**
      b. **High vagal tone.** More common in conditioned athletes and in the elderly.
      c. **Increased intracranial pressure.** Cushing's reflex results in bradycardia (and hypertension).
   2. **Sinus node dysfunction.** Sick sinus syndrome and tachycardia-bradycardia syndrome are variants of sinus node disease.
      a. Ischemic cardiomyopathy.
      b. Hypertensive cardiomyopathy.
      c. Hypothyroidism.
      d. Hypothermia.
      e. Infiltrative diseases (amyloidosis, etc).

   B. AV Node Disease
   1. **First-degree AV block.** PR interval longer than 0.2 second.
   2. **Second-degree AV block Mobitz type I (Wenckebach).** Successive prolongation of the PR interval with eventual decreased ventricular beat (Figure I–3).
      a. **Inferior MI.**
      b. **Drug toxicity.** Frequently implicated drugs are digoxin, β blockers (propranolol), and calcium channel blockers (verapamil).
   3. **Second-degree AV block Mobitz type II.** Intermittent missed ventricular beat. Associated conditions are the same as those for third-degree AV block and this condition may progress to third-degree AV block.
   4. **Third-degree AV block.** Also called "AV dissociation."
      a. **Myocardial infarction:** most common sites are anteroseptal or inferior.
      b. **Primary degenerative disease** of the conducting system.

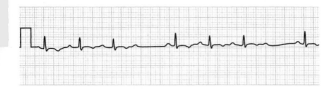

Figure I–3. Second-degree atrioventricular block Mobitz type I (Wenckebach) with 4.3 conduction. *(Reproduced, with permission, from Lefor AT. Critical Care On Call. Copyright (c) 2002 by The McGraw-Hill Companies, Inc.)*

    c. Infiltrative conditions: sarcoidosis, amyloidosis, neoplasms.
    d. Infectious diseases: viral myocarditis, acute rheumatic fever, Lyme disease.

IV. Database. The primary focus to diagnose a bradycardia is the 12-lead ECG and rhythm strip, which should be obtained concurrently with the initial history and physical examination.

  A. Physical Examination Key Points
    1. Vital signs. Note heart rate, blood pressure, respiratory rate.
    2. Lungs. Listen for evidence of failure (crackles).
    3. Cardiac. Note new murmurs or gallops. Is rhythm regular or irregular?
    4. Skin. Pallor, cool, moist skin as evidence of poor perfusion.
    5. Neurologic. Look for evidence of increased intracranial pressure (papilledema). Decreased mental status is a measurement of inadequate perfusion pressure.

  B. Laboratory Data
    1. Electrolytes. Hypokalemia can potentiate digoxin toxicity and hypocalcemia can result in a prolonged QT interval and bradycardia.
    2. Troponin I/creatine phosphokinase (CPK) with isoenzymes to evaluate myocardial injury (see Section II, page 323).
    3. Digoxin level if indicated. Toxicity is often manifested as bradycardia. Toxic levels usually 2.5 ng/mL.
    4. Thyroid hormone levels. Hypothyroidism can cause bradycardia.
    5. ABG levels if indicated by respiratory distress or dyspnea.

  C. Radiologic and Other Studies
    1. Electrocardiogram. This is analyzed systematically in the usual manner.

2. **Chest radiograph.** Change in cardiac silhouette and lung fields may be associated with myocardial dysfunction.
3. **Specialized tests** conducted by cardiologists include electrophysiologic mapping to define the precise location of blocks and complete autonomic blockade (using atropine and propranolol) to determine the intrinsic heart rate and document the contribution of vagal tone to the bradycardia.

V. Plan. The treatment plan will be dictated by the type and degree of bradycardia and any underlying clinical condition. Remember that not all bradycardia is clinically significant. Use extreme caution, especially in the elderly, when managing bradycardia. In urgent situations treat with IV fluids, IV atropine, administer oxygen, and obtain an ECG as soon as possible. The management of critical bradycardia can be found in the advanced cardiac life support (ACLS) algorithm for bradycardia (Figure I–4, page 38).

A. Critical Symptomatic Bradycardia. The treatment algorithm should be used in cases of acute, clinically significant bradycardia usually associated with hypotension in the following sequence:
  1. Atropine 0.5–1.0 mg IV (0.01 mg/kg). May be repeated every 5–10 minutes to a total dose of 2 mg.
  2. Transcutaneous pacing if available.
  3. Dopamine 5–20 mg/kg/min.
  4. Epinephrine 2–10 mg/min.
  5. Isoproterenol (isuprel) 1–3 mg/min IV continuous infusion (small dose).
  6. Consider IV fluid bolus to ensure adequate preload if patient does not appear in pulmonary edema.

B. Treat the Underlying Condition
  1. **Myocardial ischemia.** Should be managed with nitrates and oxygen and the usual protocol for myocardial ischemia.
  2. **Increased intracranial pressure.** Maneuvers to decrease pressure include mannitol diuresis, elevation of the head of the bed, and mechanical hyperventilation.

C. Pacemaker therapy. If the bradydysrhythmia does not respond to medical therapy, ventricular pacing should be used. External pacer pads are the quickest method of pacing the heart but do not "capture" consistently. Transvenous pacers (eg, Pacing Swan-Ganz catheter) should be used for more prolonged pacing. If this option is needed, contact the cardiology consultant.
  1. Indications for temporary pacemaker.
    a. Transient second-degree AV block with an inferior MI.

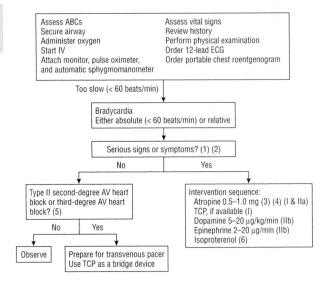

Footnotes

(1) Serious signs or symptoms must be related to the slow rate.
 Clinical manifestations include:
  Symptoms (chest pain, shortness of breath, decreased level of consciousness) and
  signs (low BP, shock, pulmonary congestions, CHF, acute MI).
(2) Do not delay TCP while awaiting IV access or for atropine to take effect if patient is
 symptomatic.
(3) Denervated transplanted hearts will not respond to atropine. Go at once to pacing,
 catecholamine infusion, or both.
(4) Atropine should be given in repeat doses in 3–5 min up to a total of 0.04 mg/kg.
 Consider shorter dosing intervals in severe clinical conditions. It has been suggested
 that atropine should be used with caution in atrioventricular (AV) block at the His-
 Purkinje level (type II AV block and new third degree block with wide QRS complexes)
 (class IIb).
(5) Never treat third-degree heart block plus ventricular escape beats with Lidocaine.
(6) Isoproterenol should be used, if at all, with extreme caution. At low doses it is class IIb
 (possibly helpful); at higher doses it is class III (harmful).
(7) Verify patient tolerance and mechanical capture. Use analgesia and sedation as needed.

Figure I–4. Bradycardia algorithm (patient not in cardiac arrest). *(Reproduced, with permission, from Adult Advanced Cardiac Life Support. JAMA 268:16, 1992. Updated according to American Heart Association Guidelines, 2000.).*

      b. AV block as a result of drug toxicity.

      c. As temporizing measure before permanent pacemaker.

    2. Indications for permanent pacemaker.

      a. Sinus node dysfunction: must be documented to be symptomatic.

      b. Second- or third-degree AV block associated with an acute MI.

      c. Symptomatic Mobitz type II and third-degree AV block.

  D. Digoxin toxicity. Check level, hold medication, and consider digoxin antibody (Digibind) 60 mg per digoxin 1 mg IV.

REFERENCES

Alpert MA, Flaker GC. Arrhythmias associated with sinus node dysfunction. *JAMA* 250:2160–8, 1983.

Josephson ME, Zimetbaum P. The bradyarrhythmias: disorders of sinus node function and AV conduction disturbances. In: Braunwald E, et al, eds. *Harrison's Principles of Internal Medicine*, 16th ed. New York: McGraw-Hill; 2005, p 1333–41.

Mangrum JM, Dimarco JP. The evaluation and management of bradycardia. *N Engl J Med* 342:703–9, 2000.

10. BRIGHT RED BLOOD PER RECTUM (HEMATOCHEZIA)

I. Problem. You are called to see a 60-year-old female patient who is passing red blood through the rectum 3 days after undergoing a modified radical mastectomy.

II. Immediate Questions

  A. What are the vital signs? Look for signs of hemodynamically significant blood loss such as tachycardia and hypotension.

  B. What volume of blood has been passed and over what period? The volume of blood may help assess the significance of the bleed because the hematocrit may not decrease until later.

  C. What was the most recent hematocrit? A baseline value is needed to assess the amount of bleeding.

  D. What is the nature of the stool? Coating of the stool often indicates an anal process such as hemorrhoids, but may also suggest a lower GI tumor. Bright red blood is more likely to be from the distal left colon. Melena usually signifies bleeding proximal to the right colon.

E. What medication is the patient taking, and is there any history of alcohol abuse? Alcoholism may suggest varices; ulcerogenic medications include aspirin and other nonsteroidal antl-inflammatory drugs (NSAIDS); overuse of warfarin (Coumadin) may cause GI tract bleeding.

F. Has the patient had recent GI tract surgery? It is common to have some bloody bowel movements immediately after GI tract surgery.

III. Differential Diagnosis

A. Diverticular Disease. A common cause (up to 70%) of massive lower GI bleeding and usually on the left side.

B. Angiodysplasia. These are usually right-sided lesions and thus most often associated with melena. More frequent in the elderly. The natural history of bleeding from angiodysplasia usually includes rebleeding.

C. Polyps. Villous adenomas can also cause potassium loss.

D. Carcinoma. Usually large intestinal adenocarcinoma.

E. Inflammatory Bowel Disease. Ulcerative colitis is more frequently associated with bloody diarrhea than is Crohn's disease.

F. Hemorrhoids. Although their presence may be common, this does not preclude the presence of simultaneous tumor or angiodysplasia.

G. Mesenteric Thrombosis. This may lead to ischemic bowel presenting initially as ischemic colitis. Remember "abdominal pain out of proportion to findings on physical examination" as an indicator of bowel ischemia.

H. Meckel's Diverticulitis. Meckel's scan may be diagnostic.

I. Anal Fissures. Usually have severe pain at anus with bowel movements.

J. Massive UGI Bleeding. This usually results in rapid intestinal transit and resulting hematochezia. Blood is an excellent cathartic. Remember that lower GI bleeding can originate anywhere in the GI tract.

K. Infectious Colitis. *Shigella*, *Yersinia*, enteroinvasive *Escherichia coli*, and *Salmonella* often cause bloody diarrhea. Consider stool culture with a history of chronic diarrhea.

IV. Database

A. Physical Examination Key Points

1. **Vital signs.** Look for evidence of hypovolemia (tachycardia and hypotension). Fever may represent inflammatory bowel disease or an infectious gastroenteritis.

   2. **Abdomen.** Palpate for masses or tenderness. Left lower quadrant mass that may be associated with diverticulitis or right lower quadrant mass is often associated with Crohn's disease.
   3. **Rectal.** Hemorrhoids, fissures, or masses may be detected.
   4. Is bleeding present at other sites to suggest a systemic cause?
   5. Check for signs of cirrhosis (palmar erythema, caput medusae) to suggest a possible UGI source.

B. **Laboratory Studies**
   1. **Hemogram.** Serial hematocrit checks are helpful because a massive bleed may not reflect itself in a change in hematocrit for some time.
   2. **Clotting studies.** PT/PTT and platelet count may reveal a coagulation disorder.
   3. **Blood bank.** Send a specimen for type and cross-match.

C. **Radiologic and Other Studies**
   1. **NG tube.** Pass an NG tube to rule out UGI bleeding.
   2. **Colonoscopy**. Should be done as soon as possible to evaluate the cause (cancer, inflammatory bowel disease [IBD], ischemic colitis) and location of bleeding and possibly control lesions such as polyps or angiodysplasia. A quick rigid sigmoidoscopy may be helpful.
   3. **Angiography.** Is indicated for the diagnosis of lower GI bleeding in any patient who requires more than 2 U of blood to maintain hematocrit or becomes hypotensive. Remember that angiography is impossible with barium in the gut. To be helpful, bleeding must usually be 0.0.5–1.0 mL/min.
   4. **Radiolabeled red cell study (usually technetium 99m).** This can sometimes localize lesions in the GI tract, especially with slower rates of bleeding than needed for angiography (0.2 mL/min).
   5. **UGI endoscopy (EGD).** Although an NG tube can usually rule out UGI sources of bleeding, an inconclusive workup for lower GI bleeding necessitates a definitive look at the UGI tract.

V. **Plan.** Approximately 80% of patients with lower GI bleeding stop bleeding spontaneously. Acute, severe hemorrhage is potentially life threatening and should be controlled first.

A. **Acute Intervention.** Large-bore IVs (16 gauge) should be placed for volume repletion. Use crystalloid or blood if hematocrit is low. In general, attempt to keep hematocrit >30%. Use hemodynamic parameters to guide fluid and

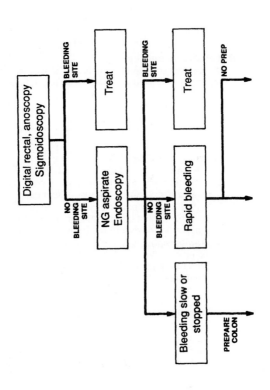

Digital rectal, anoscopy Sigmoidoscopy

BLEEDING SITE → Treat

NO BLEEDING SITE → NG aspirate Endoscopy

BLEEDING SITE → Treat → **NO PREP**

NO BLEEDING SITE → Rapid bleeding → **NO PREP**

Bleeding slow or stopped → **PREPARE COLON**

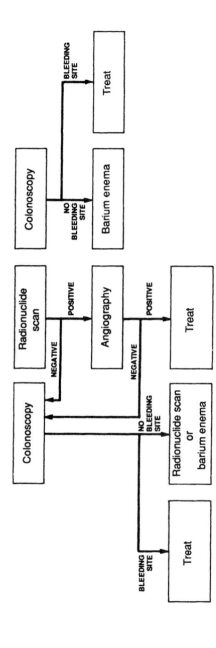

Figure I–5. Suggested scheme for the management of lower gastrointestinal hemorrhage. NG = nasogastric tube. *(Reproduced, with permission, from Chang GJ, Shelton A, Schrock TR, Welton ML. Large intestine. In: Way LW, Doherty GM, eds. Current Surgical Diagnosis & Treatment, 11th ed. Originally published by Appleton & Lange. Copyright (c) 2003 by The McGraw-Hill Companies, Inc.)*

blood replacement. A Foley catheter will allow more accurate assessment of volume status. Consider a central venous pressure (CVP) line if there is any instability and in the elderly patient. The philosophy should be to treat these people like trauma patients (ABCs: Airway, ie, intubate whenever possible, Breathing, ie, ventilate, and Circulation, ie, chest compression; etc; see below).

   B. Diagnosis and Treatment. A suggested algorithm for the diagnosis and management of acute lower GI bleeding is outlined in Figure I–5.
   1. Treatment is directed at the cause. If a bleeding diverticulum is found, initial therapy is the intra-arterial infusion of vasopressin rather than resection.
   2. The combined approach of angiography and colonoscopy can usually localize the bleeding site. In cases where the site cannot be identified, subtotal colectomy is usually indicated.
   3. Surgery eventually may be needed to control lesions such as carcinoma, polyps, hemorrhoids, and the lesions of inflammatory bowel disease.
   4. Local care for hemorrhoids includes sitz baths, stool softeners, and suppositories (Anusol, etc). Chronic anal fissures may require lateral sphincterotomy.

REFERENCES

Fischer JE, et al. Manifestation of gastrointestinal disease. In: Schwartz SI, et al, eds. *Principles of Surgery.* New York: McGraw-Hill, 1999; p 1033–80.

Mcguire HH. Bleeding colonic diverticula: a reappraisal of natural history and management. *Ann Surg* 220:653–6, 1994.

Zuccaro G. Management of the adult patient with acute lower gastrointestinal bleeding. *Am J Gastroenterol* 93:1202–8, 1998.

11. CARDIOPULMONARY ARREST

Immediate Actions

   1. Assess responsiveness.
   2. If unresponsive, follow algorithm shown in Figure I–6.

 I. Problem. One week after amputation above the knee, a patient is found unresponsive and pulseless in bed,

 II. Immediate Questions
   A. Is the patient responsive? Basic CPR begins with an attempt to arouse the patient. Always call for help.
   B. Is the airway obstructed? Finger sweep or suction out the patient's mouth. Listen for air movement.

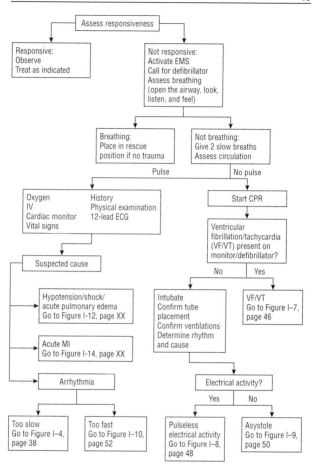

Figure I–6. Universal algorithm for adult emergency cardiac care (ECC). *(Reproduced, with permission, from Adult Advanced Cardiac Life Support. JAMA 268:16, 1992. Updated according to American Heart Associationn Guidelines, 2000.)*

C. **Are there vital signs?** Check for carotid pulse and blood pressure. After these basic questions are asked and maneuvers performed, begin ventilation with 100% oxygen by bag and mask and chest compressions. The following questions are then asked as ACLS is started.

D. **What medication is the patient taking?** Cardiac medications are particularly important, especially antiarrhythmics and digoxin. An adverse reaction to a recently administered medication may be determined. Have someone obtain the most recent medication list for the patient.

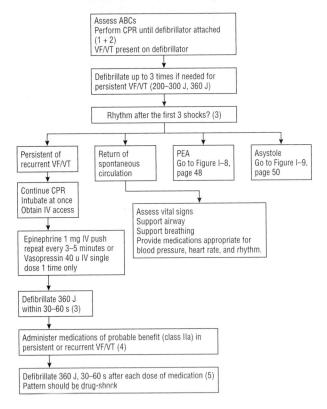

Figure I–7. Algorithm for ventricular fibrillation and pulseless ventricular tachycardia (VF/VT). *(Reproduced, with permission, from Adult Advanced Cardiac Life Support. JAMA 268:16, 1992. Updated according to American Heart Association Guidelines, 2000.)*

E. **Are there any recent laboratory values, particularly potassium or hematocrit?** Hyperkalemia (usually >7 mEq/L), hypercalcemia (>11 mEq/dL), or severe anemia may cause cardiac arrest.

F. **What are the patient's major medical problems?** Ask about coronary artery disease, previous MI, hypertension, previous PE, and recent operation.

III. **Differential Diagnosis.** Arrest rhythms include ventricular fibrillation and tachycardia, asystole, bradycardia, and electromechanical dissociation. Causes of cardiopulmonary arrest may include:

A. **Cardiac**
  1. MI
  2. CHF
  3. Ventricular arrhythmias
  4. Cardiac tamponade

B. **Pulmonary**
  1. Pulmonary embolus
  2. Acute respiratory failure

Footnotes to Figure I–7
Class I: Definitely helpful.
Class IIa: Acceptable, probably helpful.
Class IIb: Acceptable, possibly helpful.
Class III: Not indicated, may be harmful.

(1) Precordial thump is a class IIb action in witnessed arrest, no pulse, and no defibrillator available.
(2) Hypothermic cardiac arrest is treated differently after this point. See section on hypothermia.
(3) Multiple sequenced shocks (200 J, 200–300 J, 360 J) are acceptable here (class I), especially when medications are delayed.
(4) Lidocaine 1.5 mg/kg IV push. Repeat in 3–5 min to total loading dose of 3 mg/kg; then use:
  Bretylium 5 mg/kg IV push. Repeat in 5 min at 10 mg/kg.
  Magnesium sulfate 1–2 g IV in torsades de pointes or suspected hypomagnesemic state or severe refractory VF.
  Procainamide 30 mg/min in refractory VF (maximum total 17 mg/kg).
(5) Sodium bicarbonate (1 mEq/kg IV):
  Class IIa
  If known preexisting bicarbonate-responsive acidosis.
  If overdose with tricyclic antidepressants.
  To alkalinize the urine in drug overdoses.
  Class IIb
  If intubated and continued long arrest interval.
  Upon return of spontaneous circulation after long arrest interval.
  Class III
  Hypoxic lactic acids.

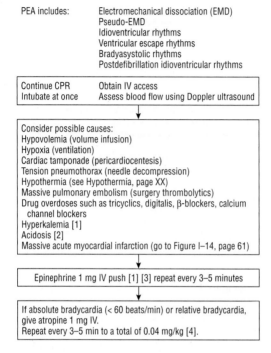

PEA includes: Electromechanical dissociation (EMD)
                    Pseudo-EMD
                    Idioventricular rhythms
                    Ventricular escape rhythms
                    Bradyasystolic rhythms
                    Postdefibrillation idioventricular rhythms

| Continue CPR | Obtain IV access |
| Intubate at once | Assess blood flow using Doppler ultrasound |

Consider possible causes:
Hypovolemia (volume infusion)
Hypoxia (ventilation)
Cardiac tamponade (pericardiocentesis)
Tension pneumothorax (needle decompression)
Hypothermia (see Hypothermia, page XX)
Massive pulmonary embolism (surgery thrombolytics)
Drug overdoses such as tricyclics, digitalis, β-blockers, calcium
   channel blockers
Hyperkalemia [1]
Acidosis [2]
Massive acute myocardial infarction (go to Figure I–14, page 61)

Epinephrine 1 mg IV push [1] [3] repeat every 3–5 minutes

If absolute bradycardia (< 60 beats/min) or relative bradycardia,
give atropine 1 mg IV.
Repeat every 3–5 min to a total of 0.04 mg/kg [4].

Figure I–8. Algorithm for pulseless electrical activity (PEA) (electromechanical dissociation [EMD]). *(Reproduced, with permission, from Adult Advanced Cardiac Life Support. JAMA 268:16, 1992. Updated according to American Heart Association Guidelines, 2000.)*

      3. Aspiration
      4. Tension pneumothorax
   C. Hemorrhagic. Undiagnosed severe bleeding, eg, rupture aortic aneurysm, can result in cardiac arrest.
   D. Metabolic
      1. Hypokalemia, hyperkalemia. These may induce arrhythmias.
      2. Acidosis. Severe acidosis may suppress myocardial function.
      3. Warming from hypothermia. Arrhythmias may be induced.

Footnotes to Figure I–8
Class I: Definitely helpful.
Class IIa: Acceptable, probably helpful.
Class IIb: Acceptable, possibly helpful.
Class III: Not indicated, may be harmful.

[1] Sodium bicarbonate 1 mEq/kg is class I if patient has known preexisting hyperkalemia.
[2] Sodium bicarbonate 1 mEq/kg:
  Class IIa
    If known preexisting bicarbonate-responsive acidosis.
    If overdose with tricyclic antidepressants.
    To alkalinize the urine in drug overdoses.
  Class IIb
    If intubated and continued long arrest interval.
    Upon return of spontaneous circulation after long arrest interval.
  Class III
    Hypoxic lactic acids.
[3] The recommended dose of epinephrine is 1 mg IV push every 3–5 min. If this approach fails, several class IIb dosing regimens can be considered:
    Intermediate: epinephrine 2–5 mg IV push, every 3–5 min.
    Escalating: epinephrine 1 mg–3 mg–5 mg IV push (3 min apart).
    High: epinephrine 0.1 mg/kg IV push, every 3–5 min.
[4] Shorter atropine dosing intervals are possibly helpful in cardiac arrest (class IIb).

IV. Database

A. Physical Examination Key Points. As described, check responsiveness and vital signs. Resuscitation should always be initiated before a detailed physical examination is performed. Always remember the ABCs.

1. Check ventilation and perform airway opening maneuvers (jaw thrust or chin lift) as needed.
2. Look for tracheal deviation as evidence of a tension pneumothorax.
3. Distended neck veins may indicate pericardial tamponade or pneumothorax.

B. Laboratory Data. These should be obtained as soon as possible, but should not delay the start of therapy.

1. ABG.
2. Serum electrolytes, with special attention to potassium.
3. Complete blood cell (CBC) count, especially the hematocrit.

C. Radiologic and Other Studies

1. Continuous cardiac monitoring and frequently checking lead placement.
2. Other studies may be performed after the patient has been resuscitated. A chest radiograph may be the single most

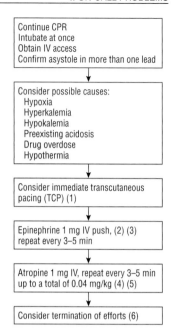

> Continue CPR
> Intubate at once
> Obtain IV access
> Confirm asystole in more than one lead

> Consider possible causes:
>   Hypoxia
>   Hyperkalemia
>   Hypokalemia
>   Preexisting acidosis
>   Drug overdose
>   Hypothermia

> Consider immediate transcutaneous pacing (TCP) (1)

> Epinephrine 1 mg IV push, (2) (3) repeat every 3–5 min

> Atropine 1 mg IV, repeat every 3–5 min up to a total of 0.04 mg/kg (4) (5)

> Consider termination of efforts (6)

Figure I–9. Asystole treatment algorithm. *(Reproduced, with permission, from Adult Advanced Cardiac Life Support. JAMA 268:16, 1992. Updated according to American Heart Association Guidelines, 2000.)*

important immediate study because it may help diagnose a pneumothorax, hemothorax, or pericardial effusion.

V. Plan. Therapy for cardiac arrest is based on specific algorithms outlined by the American Heart Association (AHA). Specific AHA algorithms for ventricular fibrillation, ventricular tachycardia, bradycardia asystole, and electromechanical dissociation are shown in Figures I–6 through I–10. Frequently used resuscitation medications are located inside the back cover. Every physician should have these memorized.

In addition, successful resuscitation is based on a team approach with 1 leader monitoring the rhythm and ordering therapy according to the appropriate algorithm. Everyone must remain calm and must be assigned to a specific job.

Resuscitation begins with the ABCs. For adults, the ratio of 5 compressions to 1 breath is used in 2-person CPR.

A. Ventricular Fibrillation and Pulseless Tachycardia (see Figure I–7). Torsade de pointes, a rare ventricular arrhythmia, is managed with a temporary pacemaker, rarely bretylium, but never lidocaine. Most often congenital or

Footnotes to Figure I–9

Class I: Definitely helpful.

Class IIa: Acceptable, probably helpful.

Class IIb: Acceptable, possibly helpful.

Class III: Not indicated, may be harmful.

(1) TCP is a class IIb intervention. Lack of success may be due to delays in pacing. To be effective TCP must be performed early, simultaneously with drugs. Evidence does not support routine use of TCP for asystole.

(2) The recommended dose of epinephrine is 1 mg IV push every 3–5 min. If this approach fails, several class IIb dosing regimens can be considered:

Intermediate: epinephrine 2–5 mg IV push, every 3–5 min.

Escalating: epinephrine 1 mg–3 mg–5 mg IV push (3 min apart).

High: epinephrine 0.1 mg/kg IV push, every 3–5 min.

(3) Sodium bicarbonate 1 mEq/kg is class I if patient has known preexisting hyperkalemia.

(4) Shorter atropine dosing intervals are class IIb in asystolic arrest.

(5) Sodium bicarbonate 1 mEq/kg IV:

Class IIa

If known preexisting bicarbonate-responsive acidosis.

If overdose with tricyclic antidepressants.

To alkalinize the urine in drug overdoses.

Class IIb

If intubated and continued long arrest interval.

Upon return of spontaneous circulation after long arrest interval.

Class III

Hypoxic lactic acids.

(6) If patient remains in asystole or other agonal rhythms after successful intubation and initial medications and no reversible causes are identified, consider termination of resuscitative efforts by a physician.

Consider interval since arrest.

drug induced, it is characterized by "twisting" or direction changes of the QRS complex around the isoelectric line.

B. Pulseless Electrical Activity (see Figure I–8). In surgical patients, always consider PE, especially in high-risk patients (obese, previous PE, certain pelvic and orthopedic cases), and hypovolemia as causes of pulseless electrical activity. In trauma patients, consider tension pneumothorax and cardiac tamponade.

C. Asystole. See algorithm in Figure I–9. The prognosis is very poor in cases of asystole. Defibrillate if there is any question about the rhythm being fine ventricular tachycardia.

D. Bradycardia. See Figure I–4 and Problem 9, page 34.

E. Tachycardia. See Figure I–10 and Problem 68, page 234. Emergency cardioversion is reviewed in Figure I–11.

F. Hypotension, Shock, and Acute Pulmonary Edema. May arise independently or may be associated with a cardiac event (see Figure I–12 and Problem 48, page 178).

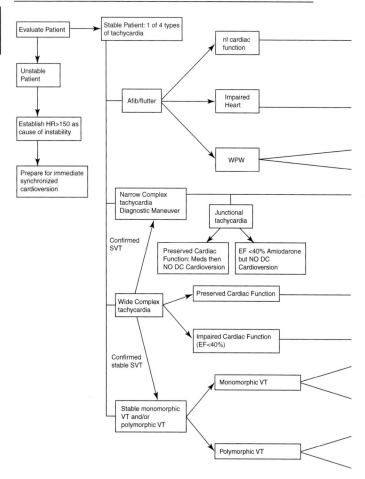

Figure I–10. Tachycardia algorithm. *(Modified with permission from American Heart Association 2000 Handbook of Emergency Cardiovascular Care.)*

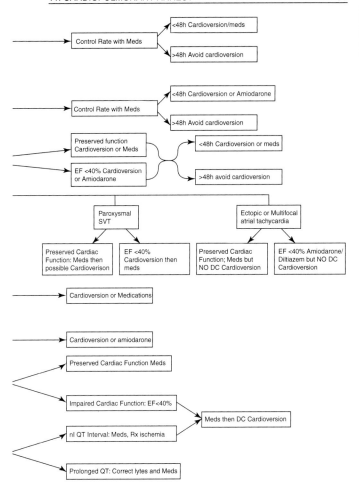

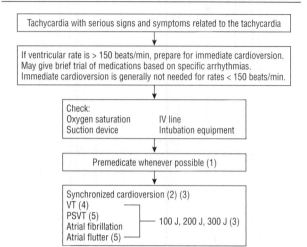

Tachycardia with serious signs and symptoms related to the tachycardia

If ventricular rate is > 150 beats/min, prepare for immediate cardioversion.
May give brief trial of medications based on specific arrhythmias.
Immediate cardioversion is generally not needed for rates < 150 beats/min.

Check:
Oxygen saturation   IV line
Suction device   Intubation equipment

Premedicate whenever possible (1)

Synchronized cardioversion (2) (3)
VT (4)
PSVT (5)
Atrial fibrillation
Atrial flutter (5)   100 J, 200 J, 300 J (3)

Footnotes
(1) Effective regimens have included a sedative (eg, diazepam, midazolam, barbituates, etomidate, ketamine, methohexital) with or without an analgesic agent (eg, fentanyl, morphine, meperidine).
     Many experts recommend anesthesia if service is readily available.
(2) Note possible need to resynchronize after each cardioversion.
(3) If delays in synchronization occur and clinical conditions are critical, go to immediate unsynchronized shocks.
(4) Treat polymorphic VT (irregular form and rate) like VF:
     200 J, 200–300 J, 260 J.
(5) PSVT and atrial flutter often respond to lower energy levels (start with 50 J).

Figure I–11. Electrical cardioversion algorithm (patient not in cardiac arrest). *(Reproduced, with permission, from Adult Advanced Cardiac Life Support. JAMA 268:16, 1992. Updated according to American Heart Association Guidelines, 2000.)*

REFERENCE

Cummins RO. *ACLS Provider Manual.* New York: American Heart Association; 2001.

12. CHEST PAIN

I. **Problem.** Four days after a radical nephrectomy, a 62-year-old patient tells the nurse of an ongoing episode of chest pain that has lasted for 10 minutes.

II. **Immediate Questions.** The conditions that lead a patient to complain of "chest pain" range from inconsequential to life threatening. The purpose of the immediate questions is to determine the urgency of response and to ascertain whether ischemic heart disease is causing the pain.

A. **Does the patient have a history of coronary artery disease?** If so, does the current pain resemble previous episodes of angina pectoris? In patients with documented cardiac disease, particularly if the current episode resembles previous known angina episodes, the pain should be treated as myocardial ischemia with sublingual nitroglycerin (0.4 mg typical initial dose) immediately. The patient should be transferred to at least a telemetry unit, and a cardiology consultation should be obtained.

B. **What is the location, nature, and severity of the pain?** The location of the pain (substernal, epigastric), presence of radiation of the pain to other areas (jaw, arms, flank, abdomen), nature of the pain (burning, crushing, tearing, stabbing), and the severity of the pain (mild, moderate, severe) can help define patterns of chest pain that fit certain diagnostic categories. However, chest pain cannot be defined by clinical criteria alone because there is considerable overlap in pain from different causes due to thoracic viscera sharing common neural pathways. Classic angina is a retrosternal crushing pain ("an elephant sitting on my chest") and may radiate to the jaw or left arm. Thoracic aortic dissection is usually described as tearing or ripping, and peptic ulcer is often burning or gnawing.

C. **What was the patient doing when the pain began?** The inciting activity at the onset of an episode of chest pain is helpful in defining the diagnosis. Classic angina is brought on by exertion. Pleuritic pain is exacerbated by coughing. Esophagitis is often exacerbated by recumbency.

D. **Are there any symptoms associated with the episode of chest pain?** Inquire specifically about nausea, dyspnea, diaphoresis, dizziness, syncope, abdominal pain, pleuritic pain, palpitations, and presence of acid taste in the mouth.

III. **Differential Diagnosis**

A. **Cardiac/Vascular**

1. **Acute MI.** Crushing retrosternal chest pain lasting >1 hour and unrelieved by nitroglycerin; usually associated with signs of CHF, ECG changes, and hypotension.

2. **Angina pectoris.** The pain of angina is typically described as crushing, substernal, often with radiation to

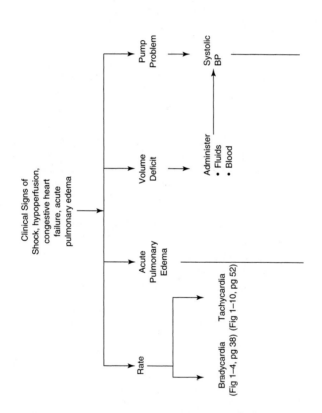

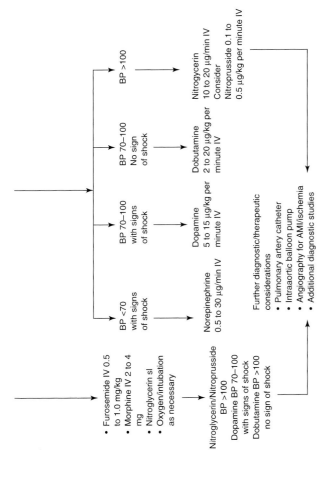

Figure I–12. Algorithm for hypotension, shock, and acute pulmonary edema. *(Modified, with permission from American Heart Association Guidelines, 2000.)*

the arms or jaw. There is often associated nausea, diaphoresis, dyspnea, or palpitations and usually relieved by nitroglycerin.

3. **Aortic dissection.** The pain is tearing in nature and radiates to the back and is usually associated with a recent history of hypertension.

4. **Acute pericarditis.** A friction rub may be present and an effusion typically seen on echocardiogram.
   a. **Infectious:** most commonly viral or tuberculosis (TB).
   b. **Myocardial infarction:** there can be early pericarditis in the first few days or pericarditis 1–4 weeks after MI (Dressler's syndrome).
   c. **Uremia.**
   d. **Malignant neoplasm:** most often breast or bronchogenic.
   e. **Connective tissue diseases.**

5. **Primary pulmonary hypertension.** The pain is mild, and dyspnea on exertion is a prominent symptom.

B. **Pulmonary**
   1. **Pulmonary embolus/infarction.**
   2. **Pneumothorax.** Acute onset, often with dyspnea; suspect in young patients or those with COPD.
   3. **Pleurodynia.** Bornholm's disease caused by Coxsackie viral illnesses.
   4. **Pneumonia/pleuritis.** This pain is typically pleuritic (made worse on deep inspiration).

C. **Gastrointestinal**
   1. **Gastroesophageal reflux.** The patient often describes an acid taste in the mouth, associated with recumbency.
   2. **Esophageal spasm.** Easily confused with angina pectoris because it may cause substernal pain that is relieved by nitrates.
   3. **Gastritis.** Alcoholism or results from overuse of medications such as NSAIDs.
   4. **Peptic ulcer disease.** Typically epigastric pain that is relieved by eating.
   5. **Biliary colic.** Usually associated with eating fatty foods and is located in the epigastrium or right upper quadrant.
   6. **Pancreatitis.** Often relieved by sitting forward.

D. **Musculoskeletal.** Pain is reproduced by palpation of the chest wall.
   1. **Costochondritis.** Point tenderness over the costochondral junction.

    2. Muscle strain/spasm. There is often a history of exercise or exertion.

    3. Rib fractures after trauma.

IV. Database

A. Physical Examination Key Points

1. **Vital signs.** Hypotension is an ominous sign and may represent cardiovascular collapse (extensive MI, dissecting aneurysm, PE, or tension pneumothorax). Hypertension in the face of an MI or aortic dissection requires emergency therapy to decrease pressure. Fever (usually low grade) may represent an embolus or other inflammatory process (eg, pneumonia, pleurisy, or pericarditis). Tachycardia may also require urgent cardioversion or may be due to hypovolemia. Tachypnea may be due to pleural effusions or CHF.

2. **HEENT.** Thrush (especially in immunosuppressed patients) may represent *Candida* esophagitis.

3. **Neck.** Venous distention with CHF or pneumothorax.

4. **Chest.** Chest wall tenderness or contusion with rib fracture; sternal instability after median sternotomy may indicate infection. Point costochondral tenderness with costochondritis.

5. **Lungs.** Rales with CHF, dullness to percussion with fluid or pneumonic consolidation, friction rub with pleural inflammation, decreased breath sounds with fluid or pneumothorax.

6. **Heart.** Murmur with valvular disease, friction rub with pericarditis (*note:* a "normal finding" immediately after open heart surgery), and displaced point of maximal impact (PMI) with CHF.

7. **Abdomen.** Determine presence or absence of bowel sounds, inflammation, or other evidence of intra-abdominal pathology. Right upper quadrant pain with deep inspiration (Murphy's sign) indicates biliary colic. Hepatomegaly may be due to CHF.

8. **Neurologic.** Aortic dissection may cause a characteristic hemiplegia.

9. **Extremities.** Edema with CHF or asymmetric swelling with venous thrombosis.

B. Laboratory Studies

1. **Hemogram.** Leukocytosis in infectious illnesses, particularly lymphocytosis in viral conditions.

2. CPK and troponin I every 6 hours to evaluate myocardial injury.

3. ABG in most cases and always if there is any dyspnea.

C. Radiologic and Other Studies

1. **Electrocardiogram.** Obtain a baseline study. Evaluate systematically and compare with previous ECGs. Document the presence and degree of pain at the time of the ECG. ECG findings of an MI may include Q waves, ST-wave changes (depression or elevation), or T-wave inversions. With a subendocardial infarction, the Q wave may not be present. Arrhythmias may also be present. Note the leads in which changes are present. Changes in ECG leads II, III, and aVF usually indicate an inferior wall MI (Figure I–13), whereas changes in leads V_1–V_6 indicate an anterior MI.

2. **Chest radiograph.** If there is any possibility of myocardial ischemia, obtain a portable chest radiograph so that the patient is not left unmonitored in the radiology department. Look for pneumothorax, effusions, infiltrates, globular heart shadow (pericardial effusion), and silhouette of the thoracic aorta and mediastinum (widened with aneurysm or dissection).

3. **Echocardiogram.** This evaluates the patient for pericardial effusion, cardiac wall motion, valvular disease, and aortic dissection.

4. **Aortogram/contrast spiral CT scan.** To diagnose aortic dissection.

5. **Bilateral lower extremity Doppler study V/Q scan/pulmonary angiogram** to diagnose pulmonary emboli. A negative V/Q scan can be used to out a PE, but spiral CT of the chest or pulmonary angiogram may be better modalities to use. An "indeterminate" scan requires further study with pulmonary arteriography or spiral CT of the chest.

V. Plan. The treatment plan is dictated by establishing the correct diagnosis. Of the conditions previously listed, myocardial ischemia, aortic dissection, tension pneumothorax, and PE are

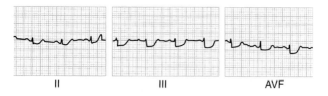

Figure I–13. ST-segment depression in leads II, III, and aVF in a patient with acute inferior subendocardial ischemia infarction. *(Reproduced, with permission, from Lefor AT. Critical Care On Call. Copyright (c) 2002 by The McGraw-Hill Companies, Inc.)*

most immediately life threatening but manageable. If a reasonable suspicion of myocardial ischemia as the source of pain exists, do not hesitate to treat the patient accordingly (Figure I–14).

A. Emergency Management

1. Treat with oxygen therapy by mask or nasal cannula.

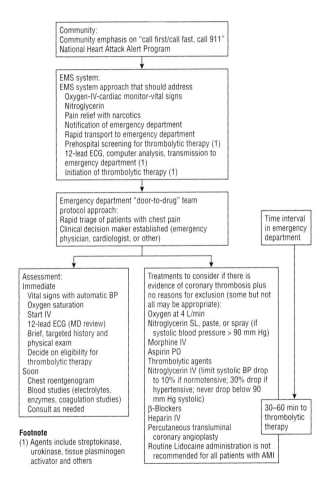

Figure I–14. Acute myocardial infarction (AMI) algorithm. Recommendations for early treatment of patients with chest pain and possible AMI. *(Reproduced, with permission, from Adult Advanced Cardiac Life Support. JAMA 268:16, 1992.)*

2. Obtain an ECG and leave the leads in place to serve as a monitor and to repeat the ECG if pain recurs or increases.
3. Request an immediate portable chest radiograph and a room air blood gas.
4. If myocardial ischemia is a possibility, treat with sublingual nitroglycerin as a diagnostic and therapeutic trial.

B. Myocardial Ischemia
   1. **Nitrates.** Sublingual nitroglycerin 0.4 mg (1/150 grain) is a typical starting dose. Monitor symptomatic relief and blood pressure. Repeat every 5–10 minutes up to 3 doses. If nitroglycerin is effective but pain recurs, establish a nitroglycerin drip at 10/20 mg/min and titrate to pain relief. Keep systolic blood pressure >90 mm Hg.
   2. **Morphine.** If pain is not relieved by nitroglycerin or if the patient cannot tolerate nitrates, treat with morphine 1–3 mg IV.
   3. **Oxygen.** Four liters by nasal prongs (approximately equal to 35% mask).
   4. **Lidocaine.** If clear-cut infarction by ECG or if prominent ectopy, treat with 75–100 mg bolus IV, then begin a continuous IV infusion at 2 mg/min.
   5. Continue monitoring and make arrangement to admit to critical care unit or ICU.
   6. Coronary thrombolysis or emergent coronary angiogram may be indicated and is coordinated by the cardiologist.

C. Aortic Dissection or Rupture. Initial treatment attempts to eliminate pain and decrease systolic blood pressure. Surgical correction is indicated for all symptomatic aneurysms.
   1. **Nitroprusside (Nipride).** A continuous infusion of 0.5–1.0 mg/kg/min titrated to control blood pressure.
   2. **Esmolol drip** Keeping the systolic blood pressure <120 mm Hg is very important to prevent further dissection.
   3. **Morphine.** Use 1–3 mg IV prn to relieve pain.

D. Pulmonary Embolus
   1. Check baseline coagulation parameters (PT/PTT).
   2. Give heparin IV bolus of 80 IU/kg and then begin a continuous IV infusion of 18 IU/kg/h. Check the PTT in 6 hours and adjust heparin to keep PTT at 1.5–2.5 times normal. Low-molecular-weight heparin (Lovenox) may also be considered.
   3. If anticoagulation is contraindicated, then Greenfield filter placement is indicated.

E. Pneumothorax. If this is strongly suspected, then establish immediate emergency needle thoracostomy or place a chest tube (page 347).

F. Pericarditis. Monitor for tamponade, indomethacin or other anti-inflammatory agents, needle aspiration may be indicated.

G. Gastritis/Esophagitis
   a. Antacids
   b. IV H_2-receptor blockers (cimetidine, ranitidine).

H. Costochondritis. Treat with NSAIDs (ibuprofen, etc).

REFERENCE

Marino PL. *The ICU Book,* 2nd ed. Philadelphia: Williams & Wilkins; 1997, p 301–16.

13. CHEST TUBE PROBLEMS

(Chest tube placement is discussed in Section III, page 347.)

Immediate Actions

Suspicion of a tension pneumothorax (based on tachycardia, hypotension, jugular venous distention, and absent or diminished breath sounds) in a patient with a chest tube already in place necessitates immediate insertion of a large-bore needle (14 gauge) at the anterior axillary line to allow egress of the air. Do not waste time obtaining a chest radiograph.

I. Problem. The chest tube in a 20-year-old male admitted for spontaneous pneumothorax is malfunctioning.

II. Immediate Questions

   A. What are the vital signs? Tachycardia, tachypnea, and hypotension may indicate a tension pneumothorax in a patient with a malfunctioning chest tube.

   B. What is the problem? Problems may include changes in drainage quality or quantity, persistent air leak, drainage around the tube dressing, increasing subcutaneous emphysema, or a patient's complaints of discomfort.

   C. When and why was the tube inserted? The problem will be approached differently if the tube was put in during an operation, or emergently to drain an effusion, or to evacuate air from a spontaneous pneumothorax.

   D. When was the last radiograph obtained? If recently, immediately check the film; if not, obtain a current one.

E. Is the chest tube plugged? Sometimes an obvious clot can be seen in the chest tube. This can be removed by "stripping" the chest tube tubing.

III. Differential Diagnosis

A. Faulty Drainage System. Collection containers may be full, tubing may be kinked, or the wall suction may not be adequate.

B. Continuous Air Leak. Indicated by persistent bubbling in the water seal chamber of the chest tube drainage system.
   1. Cracked tube, loose or leaking connections, or other mechanical problem.
   2. Last hole (hole closest to the drainage system) is outside the pleural space.
   3. Lung parenchymal injury with persistent leak (bronchopleural fistula). May be posttraumatic lung injury (penetrating injury) or iatrogenic during tube placement.

C. Bloody Drainage
   1. **Intercostal vessel injury.** Avoided by placing the tube over the top of the rib and directly abutting the bone.
   2. **Bloody effusion.** Malignant effusions are often bloody.
   3. **Pulmonary artery injury.** A rare problem.
   4. **Post-traumatic.** Most traumatic pneumothoraces are associated with some degree of bleeding.
   5. **Parenchymal lung injury.** Possibly at the time of tube placement.

D. Decreased Drainage
   1. Clotted tube.
   2. Resolution of the problem that led to tube placement.

E. Subcutaneous Emphysema
   1. Migration of the last hole outside the chest cavity.
   2. Improper placement (subcutaneous tube).
   3. Significant air leak requiring placement of a second chest tube.
   4. Tension pneumothorax.

IV. Database

A. Physical Examination Key Points
   1. **Vital signs.** Tachypnea, decreased oxygen saturation, may indicate a pneumothorax or respiratory compromise. Tension pneumothorax may decrease blood pressure.
   2. **Neck.** Tracheal deviation may indicate a tension pneumothorax (trachea deviates away from the side of the tension pneumothorax). JVD can also be caused by a tension pneumothorax.

      3. Lungs. Check for symmetric breath sounds. Hyperresonance may signify a pneumothorax, whereas dullness may suggest an effusion or hemothorax.

      4. Chest wall. Determine whether there is crepitans that signifies subcutaneous emphysema. Examine the insertion site for signs of tube migration, infection, or skin bleeding. Watch for unequal chest rise.

  B. Laboratory Data

      1. Arterial blood gases. Are usually not necessary.

      2. Coagulation studies (PT/PTT/platelets) especially in cases of severe bleeding.

      3. CBC count and serial hematocrit for hemothorax.

  C. Radiologic and Other Studies

      1. Obtain a chest radiograph. This is probably the most important diagnostic maneuver. Check tube position, see where the last hole of the tube is located, and note if there is any effusion (new or recurrent) or any residual pneumothorax.

V. Plan.

  A. Air Leak

      1. Be sure that the last hole is in the chest cavity (on radiograph). One may notice a rush of air at the site, which usually indicates that the last hole is outside the chest. If the last hole is outside the chest, replace the tube. Pushing the tube in is associated with a significant risk of empyema and is strongly contraindicated.

      2. To differentiate tube problems from system problems, try clamping the tube *briefly* at the entry site. A persistent air leak indicates a problem in the drainage system, not in the patient or tube. Remember to unclamp the chest tube once you are done.

  B. Drainage Around the Tube. An enormous effusion is controlled simply by reinforcing the dressing. Be sure the last hole is in the chest. Tight closure of skin around the tube at the entry site may cause subcutaneous dissection of fluid or air.

  C. Change in Drainage Quality

      1. The sudden appearance of bloody drainage after inserting a tube can indicate damage to intercostal vessels or, more significantly, may indicate damage to lung parenchyma. This may also represent bleeding after repeated attempts at placement of an ipsilateral subclavian line.

      2. Intercostal vessel damage may stop on its own but, if persistent, will require operative exposure and ligation.

3. Blood tingeing of a previously straw-colored effusion is usually of little significance.

4. In general, after initial chest tube placement for hemothorax, >1500 mL of blood or >200 mL/h for 2 hours is an indication for emergent thoracotomy.

D. **Change in Drainage Quantity.** A sudden increase in drainage is rare, unless the drainage becomes bloody and is related to a vascular mishap. This should be correlated with the recent radiograph. Is there a new effusion on that side? A sudden decrease in drainage with appearance of a new effusion usually warrants removal of the tube and/or placement of a new one.

E. **Subcutaneous Emphysema.** A pneumothorax is often associated with subcutaneous air, and there is often some air after placement of the tube. However, new subcutaneous emphysema, especially after a tube has been in for a while, may indicate migration of the tube, such that the last hole is now out of the chest. This usually indicates a poorly functioning tube and necessitates replacement. The appearance of a great deal of subcutaneous air right after tube placement may be alleviated by enlarging the tube entrance site, to allow egress of the air rather than forcing the air (from a pneumothorax) to track SC. Large air leaks may require a second tube. Also, check for a concomitant contralateral pneumothorax.

F. **Patient Discomfort.** There is always some pleuritic pain after placement of a tube, especially at the entrance site. Such pain must be differentiated from chest pain from other causes. Sudden onset of new pain must be investigated by examining the position of the end of the tube, looking for evidence of pneumothorax, and examining the entrance site. Occasionally narcotics may be needed. A patient-controlled analgesia machine is often a good choice for patients with chest tubes.

REFERENCE

Cerforlio R. General principles of postoperative care. In: Shields T, et al, eds. *General Thoracic Surgery,* 5th ed. Philadelphia: Lippincott Williams & Wilkins; 2000, p 509–15.

14. CHANGING NEUROLOGIC STATUS

I. **Problem.** You are called to evaluate a 34-year-old woman for somnolence 2 days after a modified radical mastectomy.

II. **Immediate Questions**

A. **What are the vital signs?** Shock of any cause can lead to poor cerebral perfusion and altered mental status. A changing respiratory pattern may indicate increased intracranial pressure. Tachycardia or fever may represent sepsis. Hypotension may cause cerebral hypoperfusion.

B. Was the patient fully awake at any time since surgery? Get an idea of the time course for the change in neurologic status.

C. What medication is the patient taking? Look at the medication records to see how much pain medicine and sedation the patient has received, not just how much has been ordered.

D. Does the patient have diabetes? Hypoglycemia or hyperglycemia may cause altered mental status.

E. Was there a traumatic event? For example, did the patient fall out of bed, or is the problem a result of a motor vehicle accident (closed head injury)? Long bone fractures may cause fat embolism syndrome.

III. Differential Diagnosis

A. Trauma

1. **Subdural hematoma.** The most common intracranial mass lesion caused by a head injury.
2. **Epidural hematoma.** Usually associated with a skull fracture and a lacerated meningeal vessel.
3. **Concussion.** A clinical diagnosis of cerebral dysfunction that resolves within 24 hours of the injury.
4. **Contusion.** Usually associated with neurologic deficits that persist >24 hours after injury and that demonstrate small hemorrhages in the cerebral parenchyma on CT scan.
5. **Fat embolus syndrome.** After long bone fracture. Look for petechial rash.

B. Metabolic Causes

1. **Exogenous.** Alcohol (including withdrawal "delirium tremens"), drugs (including drug withdrawal), narcotics, anesthetic agents (delayed clearance postop), poisoning.
2. **Endogenous**
   a. **Endocrine**
      i. **Pancreas:** insulin, hypo- and hyperglycemia
      ii. **Pituitary:** hyper- and hypopituitarism
      iii. **Thyroid:** hyper- and hypothyroid
      iv. Adrenal insufficiency
      v. **Parathyroid:** hyper- or hypocalcemia
      vi. **Postictal state:** seizure disorder
   b. **Fluids/electrolytes**
      i. **Sodium:** hypo- and hypernatremia may cause confusion.

      ii. **Potassium:** hypo- and hyperkalemia
     iii. **Calcium:** hypo- and hypercalcemia
     iv. **Magnesium:** hypo- and hypermagnesemia
      v. Acidosis (especially respiratory) or alkalosis
     vi. **Osmolarity disturbances:** hyperosmolar coma
  c. Organ failure: including renal, hepatic, or pulmonary (hypoxia, hypercarbia, fat embolism syndrome)

C. Infection
  1. Central nervous system (CNS) infections (meningitis, encephalitis).
  2. Systemic sepsis.

D. Tumors
  1. Primary or metastatic to CNS.
  2. Paraneoplastic syndromes.

E. Psychiatric Causes. In psychogenic coma, the neurologic and laboratory profile is completely normal. Depression may also cause dementia especially in the elderly. ICU psychosis and postcardiotomy delirium are occasionally seen. ICU psychosis is seen frequently in the elderly patient and can be brought on by sleep deprivation or medications.

F. Miscellaneous
  1. Seizures. Including postictal states.
  2. Cerebrovascular disease. Infarction or hemorrhage, arteriovenous malformation, hypertensive encephalopathy.
  3. Syncope (see Problem 67, page 232).
  4. Decreased cardiac output (shock).
  5. Other CNS diseases. These are usually more chronic: Alzheimer's disease, normal pressure hydrocephalus, Wernicke's encephalopathy (thiamine deficiency).

IV. Database. If the event occurs during the postoperative period, determine the nature, onset, and duration of event. Further, ascertain anesthetic used, medications given, and IV fluids administered.

A. Physical Examination Key Points
  1. Vital signs. Hyper- or hypotension, tachy- or bradycardia, temperature, and respiratory rate may give a clue to the diagnosis.
  2. HEENT. Papilledema (increased intracranial pressure from a mass or hypertensive encephalopathy), meningeal signs such as nuchal rigidity, pupillary reaction (pinpoint with narcotic), unilateral fixed and dilated, suggest herniation, dilated and fixed (anoxia). Conjunc-

tival and fundal petechiae suggest fat embolism. Fruity breath is associated with ketoacidosis. Hemiplegia or aphasia may indicate a stroke. Look for evidence of head trauma.

3. **Skin.** Jaundice, spider angiomata, palmar erythema with liver disease. Petechiae in neck and upper chest. Bruising around the head as evidence of head trauma.

4. **Neurologic examination.** (See Appendix for GCS, page 541.) Evaluate patient for spontaneous movements, response to pain, cranial nerve function.

B. **Laboratory Data**
1. **CBC and platelet counts.** To evaluate for infection or anemia.
2. **Complete blood chemistry.** Includes electrolytes, BUN, creatinine, calcium, magnesium, osmolality; glucose can be rapidly checked with a "finger-stick" glucometer available on most nursing units.
3. **Arterial blood gases.** A respiratory or metabolic cause may be found. Hypoxia or hypercarbia may also cause delirium. Check oxygen saturation with pulse oximeter.
4. Urine and serum toxicology screening, if indicated.
5. Cultures for sepsis, if indicated.

C. **Radiologic and Other Studies**
1. **Chest radiograph.** Especially if infectious or pulmonary source possible.
2. **CT of the head.** If there is any indication of a CNS cause of coma-especially focal neurologic signs or presence of papilledema.
3. **Lumbar puncture** (see page 363).
4. **Electrocardiogram.** Myocardial infarction or atrial fibrillation (mural thrombi with emboli).
5. **Electroencephalogram.**

V. **Plan.** Although the therapy of changing neurologic status must be directed at the underlying cause, certain initial steps should be taken immediately. Ensure adequate airway, breathing, and circulation. Intubation may be necessary to protect the airway.

A. **Metabolic Causes.** Manage the defect shown on laboratory studies. Refer to the specific abnormality in the index. A single ample of 50% dextrose can be given IV if there is any suspicion of hypoglycemia. The effect on a patient in diabetic ketoacidosis is minimal, so it is always safer to administer the dextrose.

B. **Exogenous Causes.** Any suspicion of narcotic-induced somnolence can be safely managed with naloxone,

0.4–0.8 mg IV push. Repeat dose may be necessary (up to 4–5 ampules are commonly administered in this situation).

C. **Tumor.** Somnolence in the presence of metastatic or primary CNS tumors is an emergency that is usually controlled by radiotherapy. Administer dexamethasone bolus 0.1–0.2 mg/kg.

D. **Infection.** Controlled with large-dose antibiotics as appropriate to the Gram's stain organisms.

E. **Cardiac syncope or low cardiac output.** Managed by approaching the underlying cardiac problem.

F. **Vascular.** Intracranial bleeding is usually managed like other causes of increased intracranial pressure. Contact the neurosurgeon. Increased intracranial pressure should be emergently controlled because herniation may occur. Intubation with hyperventilation (Pco_2 28–34 mm Hg), osmotic diuresis with mannitol (1–1.5 g/kg over 20 minutes).

G. **ICU psychosis.** This is a diagnosis of exclusion and based on clinical suspicion. Provide the patient with a companion and use restraints as a last resort. Haloperidol (Haldol) may be needed (risk of ventricular dysrhythmias). Avoid benzodiazepines because these may have a paradoxical effect.

REFERENCES

Beers R, Berkow M. *The Merck Manual of Diagnosis and Therapy,* 17th ed. West Point: Merck & Company; 1999, p 1385–1400.

Degowin R, Degowin R. Neuropsychiatric examination impaired consciousness. In: *Diagnostic Examination,* 7th ed. New York: McGraw-Hill; 2000, p 126–9.

15. COAGULOPATHY

I. **Problem.** After placement of a LeVeen shunt, a patient has bleeding from peritoneal and neck incisions and oozing from an intravenous site.

II. **Immediate Questions**

A. **What are the patient's vital signs?** Determine if the bleeding episode is extensive enough to cause hypovolemia and shock. Assess volume status by blood pressure, heart rate, urine output, and CVP. Do not place central venous access until the extent of coagulopathy has been determined.

B. **How much external bleeding is there?** One way to separate clinically significant bleeding episodes from insignificant ones is to quantitate the bleeding. Look at the wound to see if there is active bleeding. Check any old dressings saved so that you can see the quantity and quality of the wound drainage.

C. **Are there factors that increase the likelihood of generalized bleeding?** In general, when confronted with a bleeding or oozing wound, ask the patient about liver disease, relatives with bleeding disorders, and use of medications such as aspirin, NSAIDs, or anticoagulants. Look for easy bruising or petechia. Post-trauma patients may also be coagulopathic from extensive blood loss.

D. **Could the hematoma cause compression of a major anatomic structure?** This question is pertinent to neck wounds where a wound hematoma can compress the trachea, and mediastinal wounds where undrained bleeding could cause pericardial tamponade. In both cases be prepared to open the wound quickly if problems develop.

III. Differential Diagnosis

A. **Inadequate Surgical Hemostasis.** This is the most common cause of localized bleeding in the postoperative patient.

B. **Platelet Disorders**
   1. **Thrombocytopenia**
      a. **Decreased production:** often secondary to chemotherapy or bone marrow replacement by fibrosis or neoplasia.
      b. **Sequestration:** caused by splenic enlargement due to portal hypertension, neoplasia, or storage diseases.
      c. **Destruction:** idiopathic thrombocytopenic purpura, thrombotic thrombocytopenic purpura, and drug reactions (eg, heparin) can cause platelet destruction.
   2. **Qualitative platelet disorders**
      a. **von Willebrand's disease:** an autosomal dominant disease with decreased platelet adhesion.
      b. **Platelet release defects:** due to interference with cyclooxygenase metabolism by aspirin and NSAID.
      c. **Glanzmann's disease.**
      d. **Bernard-Soulier syndrome.**

C. **Coagulation Defects**
   1. **Congenital**
      a. **Hemophilia A:** a factor VII deficiency, X-linked, with an incidence of 1 in 10,000 male births.
      b. **Hemophilia B:** a factor IX deficiency, X-linked, with an incidence of 1 in 100,000 male births.
   2. **Acquired**

    a. Disseminated intravascular coagulation: A consumptive coagulopathy in which clotting factors are depleted. Associated with sepsis, trauma, burns, disseminated malignancy, obstetric catastrophes, and following peritoneovenous (LeVeen) shunt (due to proteinaceous material entering the venous system).

    b. Vitamin K deficiency: Vitamin K is needed for synthesis of coagulation factors II, VII, IX, and X. Patients who remain NPO for prolonged periods may develop a deficiency.

    c. Hepatic failure: Not only vitamin K-dependent factors but factors I, V, and XI are synthesized by the liver.

IV. Database. The keystone in diagnosing a coagulopathy is understanding and using the appropriate laboratory tests. It is important to draw blood for needed tests before instituting therapy or transfusions.

  A. Physical Examination Key Points

    1. Vital signs. Tachycardia and orthostatic hypotension signify a major loss of blood.

    2. Skin. Paleness of the skin signifies significant blood loss. Petechia, purpura, easy bruising, and oozing from IV sites suggest a systemic rather than a local cause.

    3. Incision. Examine the incision for hematoma or active bleeding.

    4. Abdomen. Splenomegaly, hepatomegaly, or ascites may suggest a diagnosis.

    5. Extremity. Hemarthrosis may be seen with hemophilia.

    6. Neurologic examination. Needed as a baseline and to assess CNS bleeding, if present.

  B. Laboratory Data

    1. Hemogram. Follow serial hematocrits in ongoing bleeding.

    2. Platelet count. Adequate numbers do not imply adequate platelet function.

    3. PT and PTT. PT is high if there is a deficiency of factors I, II, V, VII, or X. PTT assesses all coagulation proteins except factors VII and XIII. Factor VII has the shortest half-life and is the usual cause in generalized problems, such as liver disease. Heparin increases PTT, whereas Coumadin increases PT and international normalized ratio.

    4. Thrombin time. Assays functional fibrinogen level and can assay for heparin effect.

    5. Fibrinogen and fibrin split products. In DIC fibrinogen is decreased and fibrin split products are increased.

6. **Bleeding time.** Evaluates platelet function. Not reproducible and not sensitive.
7. **Ristocetin test.** Screening test for patients with suspected von Willebrand's disease.
8. **Peripheral blood smears.** May reveal fragments and helmet cells in DIC and thrombotic thrombocytopenic purpura.
9. **Type and crossmatch** to the blood bank, if needed.
10. Save 1 or 2 tubes of blood before therapy to assay for any coagulation factors that may be needed.

C. **Radiologic and Other Studies**
   1. **Chest radiograph.** If there are indications of intrathoracic or mediastinal bleeding.
   2. **Bone marrow biopsy.** May be performed at some point to assess platelet production.

V. **Plan.** Assess the rate of bleeding and differentiate between mechanical bleeding and true coagulopathy. Almost all external bleeding that is mechanical can be controlled by applying direct pressure and elevation. Management of a medical coagulopathy requires the laboratory results previously discussed to make the correct diagnosis and institute treatment. In the acute setting, assess all cases for the amount of blood loss and the volume status and manage with intravenous fluids and blood.

A. **Thrombocytopenia**
   1. Use random donor platelet transfusion usually 5–10 units at a time for a platelet count of 20,000 or less. More can be given if there is ongoing bleeding. Patients receiving multiple platelet transfusions will develop antibodies and do better with HLA-matched single donor platelets. Immunocompromised patients should receive irradiated platelets to avoid a graft-vs-host reaction.
   2. **Drug reaction.** Discontinue the drug and transfuse platelets if necessary. Penicillins (infrequently) and heparin can cause thrombocytopenia.
   3. **Idiopathic thrombocytopenic purpura.** No management is usually needed until the platelet count is <10,000. Chronic idiopathic thrombocytopenic purpura is controlled with prednisone, cyclophosphamide (Cytoxan), azathioprine, or danazol. The best long-term results are with splenectomy. Platelet transfusions before splenectomy in these patients will be very short-lived.
   4. Document functional defect with bleeding time.

B. **Von Willebrand's Disease**
   1. **Cryoprecipitate** (see Section V, page 390).
   2. **DDAVP.** A vasopressin analog that increases von Willebrand factor levels (see Section VII, page 478).

C. **Hemophilia A.** The half-life of factor VIII is about 12 hours. One unit per kilogram of factor VIII transfused increases body activity about 2%. Load a patient with 50 U/kg IV and then give 25 U/kg every 12 hours. Cryoprecipitate contains a 20-fold increase in factor VII activity compared with FFP = fresh frozen plasma. There is also factor VIII concentrate.

D. **Hemophilia B.** FFP or plasma enriched in prothrombin complex is frequently used.

E. **Disseminated intravascular coagulation.** Manage the underlying cause. Support the bleeding patient with FFP, platelet transfusions, and blood transfusions.

F. **Vitamin K deficiency/liver disease.** If immediate treatment is needed, transfuse with FFP 2–4 U and follow PT/PTT. In all cases begin treatment with vitamin K 10 mg subcutaneously (SC) every day for 3 days in a row.

REFERENCES

Fressinaud R, et al. Therapeutic monitoring of von Willebrand Disease: interest and limits of a platelet function analyzer at high shear rates. *Br J Haematol* 106:777–83, 1999.

Lusher J. Screeening and diagnosis of coagulation disorders. *Am J Obstet Gynecol* 175:778–83, 1996.

Peterson A, et al . The preoperative bleeding time test lacks clinical benefit: College of American Pathologists and American Society of Clinical Pathologists positions paper. *Arch Surg* 133:134–9, 1998.

16. COLOSTOMY PROBLEMS

I. **Problem.** A 68-year-old patient 6 days after abdominoperineal resection has problems with the function of his colostomy.

II. **Immediate Questions**

A. **How old is the colostomy, and what type of colostomy is it?** A new colostomy can retract into the wound, whereas obstruction tends to be a problem with an older colostomy. Loop or "double barrel" colostomies are temporary and usually are decompressive, whereas "end" colostomies are usually permanent.

B. **What color is the mucosa?** Mucosal ischemia can occur in the immediate postoperative period. The mucosa may appear pale and edematous or dusky.

C. **What is the volume and nature of the output?** A colostomy that has been working and suddenly stops can be approached differently than one that has never worked. In the first few postoperative days, the output is scant and usually blood-tinged. When peristalsis resumes, the appliance will become filled with gas before the discharge of liquid feces, usually around the third or fourth postoperative day. If the output is liquid and frequent, one should think about an outlet stenosis, intra-abdominal infection, recurrence of disease, or resection of an excessive length of bowel.

D. Is there a mass in the area of the colostomy? Parastomal hernia and abscess must be ruled out.

III. **Differential Diagnosis.** There are different potential problems with stomas that are discussed in 2 groups: new stomas and existing stomas. Problems with new stomas are likely to arise in the first few days after surgery.

A. New Stoma Problems
1. **Stomal retraction.** A surgical emergency because a stoma that retracts into the peritoneal cavity can lead to fecal spillage.
2. **Stomal necrosis.** The outcome of a necrotic stoma depends on how much necrosis is present. This can lead to a superficial slough of the mucosa or progress to complete full-thickness necrosis necessitating reoperation for creation of a new stoma.
3. **Stomal bleeding.** Can be from inadequate hemostasis at operation, peristomal bleeding due to intra-abdominal hemorrhage, skin bleeding, intraluminal bleeding, or mucosal irritation.
4. **Parastomal hernia or prolapse.** Usually due to a large fascial defect. May require recreation of the stoma.

B. Existing Stoma Problems
1. **Impaction/obstruction.** Obvious from history and examination of the stoma with a gloved finger.
2. **Bleeding.** See Problem 10, page 39.
3. Mucosal slough.
4. Poor fitting appliance/skin irritation.
5. Parastomal hernia.
6. **Stenosis.** Often associated with high output of liquid and detected by examination with a gloved, well-lubricated finger. Can be at skin level or at the fascia.
7. **Abscess.** Leakage of stool into the surrounding subcutaneous tissue can cause an abscess. An immediate incision and drainage is required before necrotizing fasciitis develops.

IV. **Database**

A. Physical Examination Key Points
1. Examine the abdomen for signs of peritonitis or signs of obstruction.

2. Examine the stoma for ischemia by carefully evaluating the color and presence/absence of retraction. Most often, this can be accomplished by pressing the transparent colostomy bag gently against the stoma and using a penlight. A viable stoma will transilluminate and a nonviable stoma often will not transilluminate. A pale tan color usually signifies ischemia. Black mucosa with a faint greenish tint signifies necrosis, and no mucosa visible signifies retraction. If the mucosa or surrounding site is bloody, quantitate and look for a local source. After a few postoperative days, the stoma normally will appear edematous with a dull pink-brown color. Look for an abscess or a parastomal hernia. Digital examination of the stoma should be done if stenosis is suspected.

B. Laboratory Data. These are usually helpful only if excessive bleeding is a problem (clotting studies [PT/PTT] and hemogram). WBC count is useful if an abscess is suspected.

C. Radiologic and Other Studies
   1. **Abdominal films.** Look for obstructive pattern of bowel at the level of the stoma or proximally (air-fluid levels, etc).
   2. **Gastrografin** enema through the colostomy to evaluate obstructing lesions. Gastrografin is also a cathartic.

V. Plan. Management of stomal problems depends on the nature of the problem and its etiology.

A. Stomal Ischemia. A truly ischemic stoma requires careful evaluation and then reoperation to revise the stoma.

B. Stomal Retraction. If the stoma retracts fully into the abdominal cavity, immediate operation is required.

C. Fecal Impaction. Usually caused by dehydration, narcotics, or lack of bulk in the diet. It is usually managed by warm colostomy irrigation, gentle cathartics, and it is prevented long term by stool softeners, bulk laxatives, and adequate fluid intake.

D. Bleeding. If a site of bleeding in the skin or on the mucosa is clearly visible, it can often be corrected with silver nitrate or a suture. If bleeding results from any of the causes of GI bleeding, a full evaluation is indicated (see Problem 10, page 39).

E. Appliance Problems. Consultation with an enterostomal care specialist can often be helpful to select the best appliance for the patient. Protective paste or Stomahesive may be applied to protect skin.

    F. Stenosis. Usually responds to early digital dilatation. Re-operation sometimes is needed only if the stenotic area is at the level of the fascia.

    G. Obstruction. Fecal impaction may be cleared as previously discussed. More serious causes may represent recurrent tumor.

    H. Parastomal abscess requires incision and drainage.

    I. Parastomal hernia can present with pain and can be left alone if the stoma still functions well. Repair may be indicated if the stoma is permanent and very symptomatic.

REFERENCES

Cain K, et al. Care of stomas. In: Baker R, Fischer J, eds. *Mastery of Surgery.* New York: Lippincott Williams & Wilkins; 2001, p 1490–506.

Keighly M. Ostomy management. In: Pemberton J, ed. *Shackelfords Surgery of the Alimentary Tract, vol IV,* 5th ed. Philadelphia: WB Saunders; 1996, p 305–23.

17. COMA & ACUTE MENTAL STATUS CHANGES

(See also Problem 14, page 66)

  I. Problem. The night nurse wants an order to sedate an elderly patient who is agitated, uncooperative, and confused.

  II. Immediate Questions

    A. What is the patient's baseline mental status? If this behavior deviates from the patient's normal level of function, then it indicates an underlying cause.

    B. What medication is the patient taking? Many medications have a primary effect on the CNS (eg, pain medications and sedatives) or can affect neurologic changes due to their side effects, overdosage, or an adverse drug reaction.

    C. Does the patient have a history of alcohol, narcotic, or prescription drug abuse? Surreptitious use while in the hospital or withdrawal symptoms can occur.

    D. Has the patient had any recent trauma, especially head injury? This may suggest the cause.

    E. Are there any other associated symptoms? Such as wheezing, tachypnea, chest pain, paresthesias, or bleeding.

    F. What is the patient's state of consciousness? Coma is unresponsiveness to external stimuli. Stupor and lethargy represent states of gradually less impairment. Delirium is acute confusion and decreased alertness and occurs often with agitation and hallucinations. Dementia is a chronic condition of mental deterioration with loss of memory and cognitive functions.

III. Differential Diagnosis

A. Traumatic
1. Subdural or epidural hematoma.
2. Contusion.
3. Concussion.

B. Cerebrovascular
1. Subarachnoid hemorrhage.
2. Intracerebral hemorrhage.
3. Hypertensive encephalopathy.
4. Eclampsia.

C. Metabolic
1. **Exogenous**
   a. Narcotic or alcohol abuse
   b. Medication overdose
   c. Poisoning
2. **Endogenous**
   a. **Endocrine:** Hypoglycemia, diabetic ketoacidosis (DKA), hypo- and hyperglycemia (pituitary, thyroid, parathyroid, and adrenal).
   b. **Organ failure:** Hepatic, renal, respiratory, and cardiac.
   c. **Vitamin deficiency:** Thiamine, B_{12}
   d. **Acid-base, fluid, and electrolyte disorders:** Hypo- and hyperglycemia (kalemia, natremia, calcemia, magnesemia, and osmolarity).

D. Infectious. Meningitis, encephalitis, abscess.

E. Neoplasm. Space-occupying lesion or hydrocephalus.

F. Syncope or Postictal State.

G. Psychiatric. Depression, Alzheimer's disease.

IV. Database

A. Physical Examination Key Points
1. **Vital signs.** Fever suggests infection, brady- or tachy-arrhythmia, hypotension in shock or intoxication, respiratory rate and pattern (Cheyne-Stokes in transtentorial herniation, ataxic with medullary lesion).
2. **HEENT.** Especially pupils for reactivity, shape, size (pinpoint with narcotics), and fundi for papilledema or

retinopathy; cranial nerves; odor of breath (alcohol, uremia, fruity with DKA).
3. **Skin.** Cyanosis, turgor, bruising, and bleeding.
4. **Chest.** Breath sounds, cardiac murmurs
5. **Neurologic.** Include observations on posturing, level of consciousness, cranial and peripheral nerve functions, reflexes, and motor function. Evaluate GCS.

B. **Laboratory Data**
1. **Serum glucose.** Glucose is the primary brain substrate.
2. **Serum electrolytes.** To evaluate obvious metabolic causes.
3. **Drug screen.** Barbiturates, narcotics, and alcohol.
4. **Arterial blood gas.** Check for acidosis, hypoxia, and hyperpnea.
5. **PT/PTT and platelet count.** For coagulation study.
6. **Hemogram.** Leukocytosis in infection, assess anemia.

C. **Radiologic and Other Studies**
1. **Chest radiograph.** Pneumothorax, pleural effusion.
2. **Electrocardiogram.** To diagnose MI or arrhythmia.
3. **Head CT.** To evaluate stroke, mass lesion, edema, shift.
4. **Lumbar puncture.** Hemorrhage or infection.
5. **Electroencephalogram.** Seizure activity, cerebral cortical function.

V. **Plan.** As diagnostic information is being collected, therapy should be provided simultaneously to correct obvious abnormalities. History should be obtained from family, friends, or caregiver, with particular attention to head trauma, especially a lucid interval after initial loss of consciousness, illicit drug usage, poison ingestion, seizure, respiratory distress, history of diabetes, and heart, lung or kidney disease. Patients with changes in mental status on the wards may need to be moved to a unit for closer monitoring. Resuscitation should follow general guidelines.

A. **Ventilatory Support.** Supplemental oxygen, positioning, intubation, and mechanical ventilation if necessary (airway, breathing). Threshold for intubation is *low*.

B. **Circulatory Support.** IV access and fluid administration, if appropriate. Any source of bleeding should be identified and controlled, and blood products given as needed.

C. **Dextrose.** 50 mL 50% solution IV if serum glucose is unknown or 50 mg/dL.

D. **Thiamine.** 10 mg IV initially and 100 mg IM for 3 days if alcoholism is suspected.

   E. Naloxone. 0.4–0.8 mg IV for unknown cause of coma or opiate intoxication. Repeat dosage may be necessary.

   F. Flumazenil (Romazicon). 0.2 mg IV over 60 seconds, repeat as needed up to 3–5 mg for suspected benzodiazepine overdose. **Caution:** Can precipitate seizures in patients with history of seizures.

   G. Supportive Care. Including nutrition, hydration, and joint range of motion. Prophylaxis for stress ulcers (H_2-receptor blockers, antacids), pressure sores (turn every 2 hours, air mattress, heal pads), and corneal abrasions (tape eyes shut).

REFERENCES

Lycette J, et al. Neurosurgical critical care. In: Bongard F, ed. *Current Critical Care Diagnosis and Treatment,* 2nd ed. New York: McGraw-Hill; 2003, p 407–15.

Wijdicks E. Neurologic complications in critically ill patients. *Anesth Analg* 83:411–9, 1996.

18. CONSTIPATION

  I. Problem. A 75-year-old bedridden woman from a nursing home has not had a bowel movement in 7 days.

  II. Immediate Questions

    A. What are the patient's vital signs? Fever, tachycardia, and hypotension may indicate infection or sepsis.

    B. Is the patient's abdomen tense, tender, or distended, and is the patient passing flatus? Bowel obstruction, perforation, and infarction are life-threatening emergencies. Obstipation (failure to pass flatus and stool) is often a sign of an ominous problem.

    C. What is the patient's bowel history? Nursing home patients are often laxative dependent. Surgical history may suggest obstruction from tumor or adhesions.

    D. What medication is the patient taking? Narcotics and anticholinergics use can decrease bowel motility.

  III. Differential Diagnosis

    A. Mechanical Obstruction

      1. Mild constipation. Can also be caused by painful perianal disease (eg, hemorrhoids or fissure) that causes spasm.

      2. Fecal impaction. This is common in the elderly and related to dehydration, poor diet, and inactivity.

      3. Obstruction due to a hernia, adhesions, mass (inflammatory or neoplastic) or volvulus,

B. **Pharmacologic.** Medications that commonly cause constipation include narcotics and iron supplements. Low residue diets can also cause constipation.

C. **Neurologic.** Pelvic or spinal trauma can result in anal sphincter dysfunction. Neoplastic involvement of pelvic nerve roots can result in colonic dysmotility.

D. **Other Causes.** Inactivity, poor fluid intake, and laxative abuse predispose to constipation. Electrolyte disturbances rarely may cause dysmotility (eg, hypokalemia).

IV. **Database**

A. **Physical Examination Key Points**
1. **Vital signs.** Fever and tachycardia suggest an infectious cause.
2. **Abdominal examination.** Look for distention and palpate for masses. Determine presence or absence and quality of bowel sounds. Determine if pain is present at rest or with palpation. Determine if there are any peritoneal signs.
3. **Rectal examination.** Determine if there is hard stool, blood, or a mass.
4. **Neurologic examination.** Examine for evidence of previous stroke or other neurologic disease.

B. **Laboratory Data**
1. **Fecal occult blood.** Suggests mass or ischemia.
2. **Serum electrolytes.** Hypokalemia is an infrequent cause of bowel dysmotility.
3. **Hemogram.** Leukocytosis may indicate infection. Anemia may indicate GI bleed.
4. **Arterial blood gas.** Indicated if obstruction and bowel infarction are suspected (hallmark is refractory metabolic acidosis). Lactic acid level may also be obtained if bowel infarction is suspected.

C. **Radiologic and Other Studies**
1. Mild constipation and impaction usually need no further studies.
2. Abdominal films, especially if obstruction is suspected (see Problem 1, page 1).
3. **Contrast studies and abdominal CT scan.** These are usually needed if there is evidence of chronic constipation or if there is evidence of blood in the stool (see Problem 10, page 39).

V. **Plan.** Medications that predispose patients to constipation (narcotics, anticholinergics) should be stopped whenever possible. Correct existing electrolyte abnormalities, with specific attention paid to hypokalemia.

A. Prevention. Postoperative and bedridden patients benefit from stool softeners (sodium docusate), fiber-rich diet (fruits, vegetables, or bran or supplemented with agents such as psyllium), and adequate fluid intake. The patient should also be out of bed and ambulating as soon as possible.

B. Laxatives and Enemas. Mild constipation can be treated in different ways depending on physician preference: motility stimulant (bisacodyl), laxative (milk of magnesia), or gentle enemas (fleets, tap water, soap suds). Gastrografin enemas can be used if all else fails. Doses can be found in Section VII (Commonly Used Medications). Laxatives are *contraindicated* in the presence of obstruction or in the patient whose obstruction is being considered in the differential diagnosis.

C. Disimpaction. Gentle digital disimpaction (well-lubricated, *double*-gloved finger) is required when hard stool in the rectum cannot be passed. This procedure can be followed up with careful retention enemas (soap suds or mineral oil may be used) and then with stool softeners to prevent recurrence.

D. Other. Perforation, acute obstruction, and sepsis require emergency operation. If partial obstruction (no obstipation) is present, gentle clearing with enemas followed by contrast studies or colonoscopy is indicated.

REFERENCES

Lembo A, Camilleri M. Current concepts: chronic constipation. *N Engl J Med* 349:1360–8, 2003.
Prather C, Ortiz-Camacho C. Evaluation and treatment of constipation and fecal impaction in adults. *Mayo Clin Proc* 73:881–7, 1998.

19. COUGH

I. Problem. A patient being treated with IV antibiotics for cellulitis complains of a cough.

II. Immediate Questions

A. Is the patient bringing up sputum with the cough? What are the characteristics of the sputum? A productive cough is more suggestive of significant infection than a nonproductive one, particularly if the sputum appears purulent. The presence of blood in the sputum raises a host of other issues (see Problem 36, page 136).

B. Is the patient tachypneic or dyspneic? A cough does not usually require emergent or urgent action unless the patient has chronic pulmonary or cardiac disease because these patients may develop respiratory compromise with a new acute pulmonary event.

C. Is the cough acute or chronic? In patients with a chronic cough, determine whether there is a change in the nature or characteristic of the cough.

D. Is the patient immunocompromised? Ask specifically about medications (steroids, chemotherapeutics) or secondary conditions (diabetes, AIDS, cancer) that predispose to serious pulmonary infections.

E. Is the cough associated with any specific activity? A cough that occurs with recumbency may signify pulmonary edema. A coughing spasm during sleep may be aspiration pneumonitis. A cough after eating or drinking could be a tracheoesophageal fistula or neurologic disorder.

III. **Differential Diagnosis.** The differential diagnosis for a cough can be structured by the causative agent that is stimulating the cough reflex.

A. **Inflammatory**
   1. **Acute.** Bacterial, viral, fungal, and acid-fast organisms are causative agents, as are associated systemic signs of infection such as leukocytosis, fever, viral exanthem, and purulent sputum. Certain sputa are characteristic such as rust-colored for pneumococci, currant-jelly for *Klebsiella,* and foul-smelling for anaerobic organisms.
   2. **Chronic.** Chronic bronchitis occurs almost exclusively in smokers and is defined as a chronic productive cough for ≥3 months a year for 2 years. Patients on angiotensin-converting enzyme inhibitor therapy for hypertension may have a chronic cough.

B. **Mechanical.** Mechanical stimulation of the cough reflex can occur with inhalation or intrinsic or extrinsic mechanical stimuli.
   1. **Inhalation**
      a. **Foreign body aspiration:** Localized wheezing with risk factors of depressed level of consciousness.
      b. Particulate aerosols.
      c. **Aspiration of GI secretions:** Night-time or early morning coughing spells are characteristic.
      d. Allergens in sensitive persons.
   2. **Intrinsic**
      a. **Pulmonary edema:** Typical symptoms include acute dyspnea and copious frothy sputum.

  b. Interstitial lung disease: Restrictive disease by pulmonary function tests and diffuse interstitial changes of fibrosis on chest radiograph.

  c. Bronchogenic carcinoma: Risk factors of smoking, asbestos exposure, and systemic signs of weight loss and possible hemoptysis.

  d. Bronchial adenoma: Usually no systemic symptoms and possible hemoptysis.

 3. Extrinsic

  a. Thoracic aneurysm: Can cause bronchial or tracheal compression.

  b. Lymphadenopathy: Secondary to sarcoidosis, chronic infection, lymphoma, or cancer. Often there are associated systemic symptoms.

  c. Neuroenteric cysts or pulmonary sequestration: This should be evaluated in the pediatric population on CT scan.

C. Chemical. These cause topical irritation.

 1. Smoke inhalation.

 2. Toxic fumes.

IV. Database

A. Physical Examination Key Points

 1. Vital signs. Measurements of temperature, respiratory rate, and oxygen saturation are useful. Use of accessory respiratory muscles and nasal flaring suggest severe distress.

 2. Pulmonary

  a. Stridor: Represents upper airway obstruction or epiglottitis.

  b. Rhonchi: Seen with bronchitis and inhalation injuries.

  c. Signs of consolidation such as bronchial breath sounds, egobronchophony, and tactile fremitus in pneumonia.

  d. Rales: These are the hallmarks of pulmonary edema.

  e. Localized wheezing/rhonchi: May signify foreign body or obstructing neoplasm.

 3. Cardiac. Signs of cardiac failure (cardiomegaly, S3 gallop).

 4. Skin/extremities. Cyanosis and clubbing are typical in COPD. A rash can be seen in some viral illnesses.

B. Laboratory Data

 1. Hemogram. Leukocytosis and left shift in infectious diseases.

  2. **Calcium.** Hypercalcemia is a paraneoplastic syndrome in some bronchogenic carcinomas.
  3. **Arterial blood gas.** If indicated by dyspnea or cyanosis.
  4. **Arterial carboxyhemoglobin.** In cases of smoke and carbon monoxide inhalation.

C. **Radiologic and Other Studies**
  1. **Chest radiograph.** Look for evidence of pulmonary edema, neoplasm, pneumonia, interstitial lung disease, hilar lymphadenopathy, and in some cases an aspirated foreign body (eg, teeth, coins). Acute aspiration may not be apparent on an initial radiograph.
  2. **Sputum.** Look at gross appearance, noting color, viscosity, odor, and amount. Gram's stain, acid-fast stain, fungal stains, and appropriate cultures are essential. Obtain sputum cytology if pulmonary neoplasm is suspected.
  3. **Purified protein derivative skin test.** If TB is a possibility.
  4. **Pulmonary function tests.** A restrictive pattern (decreased total lung capacity and vital capacity) in interstitial lung disease.
  5. **Bronchoscopy.** To evaluate and biopsy neoplasm, obtain brushings and biopsies for culture. Obtain post-bronchoscopy sputum cultures. May be therapeutic for foreign body aspiration.

V. **Plan.** Attempt to obtain a sputum sample even if told initially that cough is nonproductive and order a chest radiograph. If patient is dyspneic, obtain a room air ABG and begin oxygen therapy.

A. **Infectious Conditions.** (See Section IX for drug dosages).
  1. **Unknown community acquired pneumonia.**
  2. **Community acquired/compromised host (COPD/alcoholic).**
  3. **Hospital acquired.**
    a. **Anaerobic:** Penicillin G or clindamycin.
    b. **Mycoplasma:** Erythromycin or tetracycline.
    c. **Tuberculosis.** Isoniazid and rifampin.
    d. **Immunosuppressed patient** (eg, after transplant).
      i. Requires coverage for *Legionella* (erythromycin) plus an aminoglycoside plus penicillin (PCN) or a cephalosporin.
      ii. When a specific organism is identified by Gram's stain and culture, antibiotic therapy is adjusted appropriately.

        iii. *Pneumocystis carinii* pneumonia is particularly prevalent in AIDS patients and controlled with trimethoprim/sulfamethoxazole or pentamidine.

     e. Coccidioides, blastomycosis, or histoplasmosis: dependent on regional exposures.

B. Pulmonary Edema
  1. Oxygen.
  2. Upright posture.
  3. **Diuretics.** Usual choice is furosemide 20–40 mg IV. If patient is on a chronic oral Furosemide (Lasix) dose, give 1–2 times normal dose intravenously. Follow for hypokalemia.

C. Nonproductive Cough. Associated with viral upper respiratory infection or tracheal irritation.
  1. **Cough suppressant**
    a. Codeine/hydrocodone preparation is most effective.
    b. **Dextromethorphan:** A codeine derivative that acts centrally.
    c. Avoid cough suppressants in patients with a productive cough.
  2. **Expectorants.** There is no clear evidence of value. Best established is guaifenesin (Robitussin etc). Multiple preparations that often combine a cough suppressant, expectorant, and an antihistamine are available.

REFERENCE

Gonzales R. Common symptoms. In: Tierney L, et al, eds. *Current Medical Diagnosis and Treatment.* New York: Lange; 2004, 19–29.

20. CVP (CENTRAL VENOUS LINE) PROBLEMS

(Central venous catheterization techniques are discussed in Section III, page 340.)

  I. Problem. The CVP catheter placed in a patient who is to undergo total hip replacement in the morning is not functioning.

  II. Immediate Questions
    A. What is the appearance of the tracing? A CVP should have a slowly undulating waveform when transduced, which varies with the patient's respirations if properly positioned in the chest. Absence of a waveform may indicate that the catheter is clotted.

    B. Can blood be aspirated from the line? Inability to aspirate blood does not imply that the catheter cannot be used for fluid infusions. It may indicate that the tip of the catheter is against the vessel or that the line is kinked or clotted.

C. **How long has the line been in place?** The longer a line is in place, the higher the incidence of infection. Also look for skin reaction at the catheter entrance site.

D. **Is the line in the correct position?** This must be evaluated on a chest radiograph. The tip should be in the superior vena cava. If there is any question, get a new film and compare it with the post-placement radiograph.

E. **Is there bleeding from the site?** This may represent a local problem or a diffuse coagulopathy.

III. **Differential Diagnosis**

A. **Clotted Catheter.** This happens more frequently with slowly running lines.

B. **Catheter in Incorrect Position.** Evaluated by chest radiograph. Subclavian lines occasionally go up into the neck and will not fluctuate with respiration.

C. **Kinked Catheter.** These include kinking of the line at the skin entry site or kinking under the clavicle. This can usually be seen as an acute bend on radiograph.

D. **Other Mechanical Problems.** Cracking of the catheter at the hub or a loose connection.

E. **Flush Line or Transducer Malfunction.** Easily ruled out by checking the system.

F. **Infected Catheter.** Using antibiotic-coated catheters help decrease the rate of catheter related infection. Any question of sepsis originating in a central venous line requires expeditious evaluation. The best technique involves drawing cultures through the catheter, removing the line, and culturing the tip.

IV. **Database**

A. **Physical Examination Key Points**

1. **Vital signs.** Fever signifies infection, whereas tachycardia and hypotension may represent excessive bleeding, tension pneumothorax, or hemothorax.

2. **HEENT.** Tracheal deviation may indicate tension pneumothorax or an expanding hematoma, especially immediately after CVP line placement.

3. **Lung.** Diminished breath sounds may indicate a pneumothorax, hemothorax, or hydrothorax.

4. **Check line site.** Inspect for evidence of cellulitis, bleeding, catheter kinking, or leakage from a cracked hub.

B. Laboratory Data
  1. Draw blood cultures if sepsis must be evaluated. Obtain cultures from the catheter and peripherally (see Subsection V-E below).
  2. CBC count or coagulation profile if bleeding is present.

V. Plan. In general, replacing the line will usually solve problems associated with the line itself. Unless the line is infected, it can be changed over a guidewire. Be sure to carefully suture it in place. All line manipulations should be performed using sterile technique and with the patient in the Trendelenburg (head down) position to prevent air embolus.

A. Clotted Catheter. Antithrombolytic agents can be used to declot a line, but side effects can limit their use.

B. Kinked Catheter. Inspection of the site may demonstrate a kinked catheter that can be corrected by repositioning skin sutures using sterile technique.

C. Misdirected Catheter. Usually requires removal and replacement, often to another site. Rarely, fluoroscopy may be needed to direct a difficult catheter.

D. Bleeding. Site bleeding can usually be controlled with direct pressure.

E. Workup of the Infected Catheter. Draw 2 blood cultures from the line and 2 blood cultures from a peripheral site. Positive cultures from the line and peripheral blood confirm that the catheter is infected and mandate its removal.

F. Hints for Catheter Insertion. (See Section III, page 340). There are many "tricks" to inserting a central venous catheter, most of which are personal preferences rather than proven helpful tools.
  1. The most common locations are subclavian and internal jugular (IJ). The problem with IJ lines is fixing them to the patient for long periods. Subclavian lines are easier to fix to the skin. Femoral lines are acceptable when there is no upper body alternative and when rapid access is needed during CPR.
  2. Most commonly for subclavian lines, the patient in a Trendelenburg position is placed with a roll between the scapulae. This presumably makes the vein more prominent and simplifies puncture. Recent evidence in the literature contradicts this commonly held view. The needle is passed below the clavicle and aimed toward the sternal notch. After obtaining a good blood return (make sure it is venous), the syringe is removed, carefully holding the needle still. Watch for spontaneous blood return. The guidewire is passed through the nee-

dle and the needle removed. The guidewire should pass easily. Remember that if the guidewire goes to the right ventricle, arrhythmias may be induced. The skin is nicked with a scalpel, and the catheter is passed over the guidewire. After removing the guidewire, it should be nearly straight. Affix the catheter at the hub to the skin.

3. The IJ vein is approached with the patient turning the head away from the side approached. The needle is inserted 2 fingerbreadths above the clavicle, in the V-shaped area between the 2 heads of the sternocleidomastoid muscle. Aim for the ipsilateral nipple. Identifying the vein with a small needle (eg, 20 gauge) before using the large needle to pass the guidewire is strongly recommended. Many institutions require the use of ultrasound during line placement to decrease the incidence of errant line placement.

4. In placing a central venous line, there are 4 signs of successful placement:
   a. Easy aspiration of blood through the syringe.
   b. Easy passing of the guidewire.
   c. After removal, the guidewire should be nearly straight.
   d. Blood should aspirate easily through the catheter after placement.

REFERENCE

McGee D, Gould M. Current concepts: preventing complications of central venous catheterization. *N Engl J Med* 348:1123–33, 2003.

21. DEATH

I. **Problem.** On a cold night a homeless man is brought to the emergency room unresponsive and pulseless after being found on a park bench.

II. **Immediate Questions**

   A. **Is the patient responsive?** See Problem 11, page 44 and Problem 17, page 77.

   B. **Is the patient cold from exposure?** If the core body temperature is <32.2°C, the patient is hypothermic. Warm air ventilation, warming blanket, warm bladder, gastric lavage, and warm intravenous fluids are effective. More effective is cardiac bypass, which is generally not indicated with a core temperature >30°C.

C. **What medications or drugs has the patient taken?** Narcotics, alcohol, or overdose may cause coma and cardiac arrhythmias.

D. **Does the patient have a declaration of agreement regarding organ donation?** If unavailable, next of kin can allow procurement if the patient is an acceptable candidate. Respiration and cardiac function must be supported until procurement.

E. **Are family or close friends available?** Family should be notified when a patient's hospital course changes markedly. In the acute setting, it is suggested that families not be informed of unexpected death by telephone but instead be asked to come to the hospital immediately. However, for chronically ill patients, it may be appropriate to inform the family of the patient's death by telephone.

F. **Is rigor mortis present?** Resuscitation is not appropriate.

III. **Differential Diagnosis.** History from family, witnesses, and emergency medical services personnel may assist in diagnosis.

A. See Problem 11, page 44 and Problem 17, page 77 for a complete list of acute causes.

B. Intoxications and metabolic disorders are common causes of coma and cardiopulmonary arrest that can be reversible if corrected in time. CPR must continue (according to ACLS protocol) unsuccessfully for 20 minutes before pronouncing the patient dead.

C. **Hypothermia.** Core temperature <32°C is protective against hypoxic neurologic damage. Death cannot be pronounced until the patient has been warmed to ≥32.2°C and a full 20 minutes of ACLS protocol CPR has been provided (see page 45).

IV. **Database**

A. **Physical Examination Key Points**
   1. **Evaluate Brainstem Function.** Presence of brainstem function is incompatible with brain death.
      a. **Pupillary light reflex.**
      b. **Corneal reflex:** corneal sensation
      c. **Oculocephalic reflex** (doll's eyes): Tested by holding the upper eyelids open and flexing and then quickly extending the neck. If the eyes move in a direction opposite to the movement of the head, the brainstem is intact. This should not be done unless

a cervical spine fracture has been definitively ruled out.

   d. **Oculovestibular reflex** (cold calorics). Can be done without risk of cervical spine injury. A tympanic membrane perforation must be ruled out before beginning. The head of the patient's bed is set at 30 degrees 60–100 mL is injected into 1 ear. If the brainstem is intact, conjugate deviation of the eyes toward the irrigated ear is seen. This may take up to 5 minutes to occur. An attempt to test the contralateral ear can be made after 15 minutes.

   e. **Apnea test.** This test should only be done if the diagnosis of brain death is reasonably assured because hypercarbia can lead to an increase in intracranial pressure and precipitate herniation. Proceed by administering 100% oxygen for 15 minutes and a tracheal suction catheter with oxygen 6 L/min, which is placed into the lungs during the procedure to prevent hypoxia. The ventilator should be set to keep the P_{CO_2} >40 to decrease time without support. Begin the test by disconnecting the ventilator and obtaining an ABG. Do not stop until the patient breathes, becomes hypotensive, develops arrhythmias, or the Sa_{O_2} decreases <80 mm Hg. If no spontaneous respirations occur after the P_{CO_2} increases >60 mm Hg, apnea can be attributed to brain death.

   f. **Oropharyngeal reflex** (gag reflex).

2. `**Motor response to deep central pain.** Decerebrate and decorticate posturings are not consistent with brain death, although spinal reflexes may remain intact.

3. **Chest.** Confirm and document absence of apical pulse and spontaneous respirations.

4. **Skin.** Any patient arriving at the emergency department with livor or rigor mortis is considered dead and CPR does not need to be initiated.

B. **Laboratory Data.** As needed in diagnosis of inciting cause of death.

   1. **Hemogram.** Sepsis, anemia.

   2. **Serum electrolytes.** Arrhythmogenic abnormalities, uremia, glucose.

   3. **Drug screen.** Alcohol, barbiturates, opiates, or benzodiazepines

   4. **Arterial and venous blood gases.** Acid-base abnormalities.

C. **Radiologic and Other Studies.** As needed in the diagnosis of inciting cause of death.

1. **Chest radiograph**. Pneumothorax, hemothorax, etc.
2. **Head CT**. For all comatose patients.
3. **Electrocardiogram.**   Arrhythmia,   electromechanical dissociation.
4. **Electroencephalogram**. Blood flow study, brain scintigram, or cerebral angiogram.

V. Plan

A. **Resuscitation.** See Problem 17, page 77 and Problem 11, page 44. After full resuscitation and thorough investigation of possible causes and their management, if the patient has no response to CPR after 20 minutes of ACLS protocol, they can be pronounced dead. Make sure temperature, intoxicant, and brain death criteria are met. Do not electrically cardiovert a hypothermic patient. Allow a longer period of observation in children because they are more resilient to hypoxic injury.

B. **Pronouncing Death.** Confirm death and note time.

C. Maintain support of ventilation and circulation if the patient is a potential organ donor.

D. **Notification**
   1. **Attending physician, chief of service, etc.**
   2. **Next of kin.**
   3. **Transplant coordinator.** Coordinators should be made aware of a potential donor before the declaration of death. The coordinator generally makes arrangements with the family. Transplant coordinators and then the physician should approach the family for consent.
   4. **Morgue.** Transfer is arranged by nursing staff. Allow time for family to view the body before transfer.
   5. **Coroner.** Laws regarding definition of "coroner's cases" differ across states. The medical examiner will investigate all traumatic, perioperative, and suspicious deaths.

E. **Preparation.** Most institutions have standard "mortuary packs" that contain a plastic shroud and state death certificate. All IV lines, chest and endotracheal tubes, and other invasive devices are left in place. The endotracheal tube (ETT) is disconnected and IV lines are tied off or capped.

F. **Documentation**
   1. **Discharge summary.** The patient needs to be formally discharged.
   2. **Death certificate.** Do *not* list cardiopulmonary arrest as the cause of death because this is how everyone dies. Give the main reason for hospitalization as the primary cause of death. Other events that contributed to death can be listed secondarily.

G. **Reflection.** As the physician, the families view you with authority. However, be sensitive to the emotional state of those grieving.

REFERENCES

Wijdicks EF. Brain death worldwide: accepted fact but no global consensus in diagnostic criteria. *Neurology* 58:20–5, 2002.
Wijdicks EFM. The diagnosis of brain death. *N Engl J Med* 344:1215–21, 2001.

22. DIARRHEA

I. **Problem.** A 56-year-old man develops diarrhea 2 days after an aortobifemoral vascular graft is placed.

II. **Immediate Questions**

A. **What are the patient's vital signs?** Tachycardia may indicate volume depletion. Hypotension and fever may indicate sepsis. Tachypnea can be found in sepsis and is a response to significant metabolic acidosis as may be found in ischemic injuries such as bowel infarction.

B. **What are the characteristics of the stool? Is the diarrhea bloody?** Bloody diarrhea may be seen after ischemic injury to the bowel, with colonic neoplasms (carcinoma and villous adenoma), and infection (*Shigella, Clostridium difficile*) and other inflammatory states.

C. **Is this an acute or chronic problem?** Acute diarrhea is usually infectious in origin, medication induced, or from mesenteric ischemia. Chronic diarrhea usually does not require urgent management.

D. **What medication is the patient taking?** Many medicines cause diarrhea. Antibiotics can cause diarrhea by altering colonic flora that leads to malabsorption or *Clostridium difficile* overgrowth and pseudomembranous colitis, a toxin-induced diarrhea.

E. **Is there a history of pelvic radiation therapy?** Radiation therapy for malignancies (cervix, prostate, rectal) can cause chronic diarrhea.

III. **Differential Diagnosis**

A. **Acute Diarrhea**

1. **Infectious.** Rare causes of acute diarrhea in the surgical patient include viral and bacterial infections and parasitic infestations (*Salmonella, Shigella, Campylobacter, Yersinia*).

    2. Ischemic. A catastrophic cause of diarrhea, mesenteric ischemia is a surgical emergency. Abdominal distention and severe pain, loss of bowel sounds, and bloody diarrhea in the critically ill, hypotensive patient, or the vascular surgery patient after aortic cross clamping and ligation of the inferior mesenteric artery are suspicious for mesenteric ischemia and bowel necrosis.

    3. GI hemorrhage. Blood acts as a cathartic agent (see Problem 10, page 39).

    4. Drug induced.

        a. Quinidine, digoxin, colchicine, antacids (magnesium based), chemotherapeutic agents (methotrexate, Adriamycin), and laxatives. Opioid withdrawal

        b. Many antibiotics may cause pseudomembranous colitis; most frequently implicated are clindamycin, cephalosporins, and ampicillin parenteral aminoglycosides.

B. Chronic Diarrhea

    1. Inflammatory. Regional enteritis (Crohn's disease) and ulcerative colitis cause diarrhea as can radiation injury to the bowel.

    2. Neoplastic. Colon cancer can cause diarrhea. Classically, villous adenoma causes copious watery diarrhea, often associated with hypokalemia.

    3. Endocrine. Diarrhea can be found with carcinoid syndrome, hyperthyroidism, and in the islet-cell tumors (gastrinoma, Zollinger-Ellison syndrome, vasoactive-intestinal polypeptide hormone-secreting tumors).

    4. Postoperative. Diarrhea can be seen after gastrectomy (dumping), significant small and large bowel resections, and pancreatic resection.

    5. Pancreatic. Exocrine pancreatic dysfunction results in steatorrhea and malabsorption.

    6. Paradoxic. Fecal impaction may result in diarrhea because only liquid stool can be expelled past the point of impaction.

    7. Other. Psychogenic, irritable bowel syndrome, lactose intolerance, radiation induced.

IV. Database

    A. History. Diarrheal episodes, quality and quantity of loose stools, associated abdominal pain, and use of medicines and laxatives may aid in the diagnosis.

    B. Physical Examination Key Points

        1. Vital signs. Irregular pulse may indicate atrial fibrillation, a possible source of embolus and mesenteric ischemia.

2. **Abdominal examination.** Pain is rarely seen with diarrhea. When present, bacterial infections, such as *Shigella* and *Yersinia,* and mesenteric ischemia must be considered. Distention is seen with bowel ischemia. Bowel sounds vary, but absent sounds may indicate ischemic injury.

3. **Rectal examination.** Must always be performed to rule out neoplasm and impaction and to check for occult blood.

4. **Skin.** Jaundice, spider angiomata, and palmar erythema should be looked for to determine possible liver and, secondarily, pancreatic disease from alcohol abuse.

C. **Laboratory Data**

1. Stool for occult blood using a Hemoccult or other test kit. Serial examinations increase sensitivity.

2. Stool culture for enteric pathogens, examine for ova and parasites, fecal leukocytes (see page 320), *Clostridium difficile* toxin assay.

3. **Hemogram.** Monitor hematocrit, especially if there is evidence of GI bleeding. Look for leukocytosis as evidence of infection or perforation.

4. **Electrolytes.** Severe diarrhea may derange serum electrolytes. Hypokalemia and bicarbonate loss may lead to metabolic acidosis with a normal anion gap (see page 275). Hypokalemia can be a result of the diarrhea caused by villous adenomas. Also, a patient with vasoactive-intestinal polypeptide (VIP) hormone-secreting tumors may have watery diarrhea, hypokalemia, and achlorhydria (WDHA syndrome).

5. **Arterial blood gas.** Assess metabolic acidosis, especially if mesenteric ischemia is suspected.

6. **Stool electrolytes.** Potassium, sodium, and bicarbonate determinations make fluid replacement more physiologic in severe cases. See Section IV, page 390 to guide replacement.

D. **Radiologic and Other Studies**

1. **Sigmoidoscopy/colonoscopy.** Performed in patients with suspected pseudomembranous colitis and severe diarrhea. Classic findings are whitish green plaques or confluent pseudomembranes. Patients with a mass on rectal examination should undergo sigmoidoscopy and biopsy of the suspicious area. Ischemic injury in the left colon can often be seen through a sigmoidoscope or colonoscope.

2. **NG aspiration.** An NG tube should be placed to rule out UGI bleeding if diarrhea is grossly bloody or melanotic.

3. **Abdominal and chest radiographs.** Look for evidence of obstruction or ileus (dilated loops and air-fluid levels) or perforation (free air, best appreciated on an upright chest film), air in the portal system (ischemic bowel necrosis), pancreatic calcifications.
4. Diagnostic laparoscopy should be considered in a patient with a history and physical examination suspicious for ischemic bowel as should exploratory laparotomy if required.
5. **Arteriogram.** Considered when ischemic bowel injury is first recognized, although most patients can be diagnosed by colonoscopy or require surgery more urgently.
6. **Electrocardiogram.** Rarely, mesenteric embolization can occur from atrial thrombus in atrial fibrillation or after MI.

V. Plan

A. Fluid and Electrolytes

1. Significant dehydration can occur with acute diarrhea; shock requires rehydration with a central venous catheter and, rarely, with a pulmonary artery catheter. α-Adrenergic agents will worsen mesenteric ischemia but may be unavoidable in severe cases.
2. Frequent loose stools of toxic or endocrine origin (carcinoid) require fluid replacement with additives, eg, bicarbonate. See Section IV, page 385.

B. Stop Possible Causative Medications and Antibiotics

C. Control Agents. (Medication doses can be found in Section IX, page 447).

1. **Narcotics.** Tincture of opium, diphenoxylate with atropine (Lomotil), loperamide (Imodium), codeine, and paregoric can be used carefully to control diarrhea. These agents rarely prolong infection diarrhea, making the illness worse. They should not be used in cases of impaction or low lying neoplasms.
2. **Bismuth subsalicylate (Pepto-Bismol).** Controls some types of diarrhea by inhibiting prostaglandin synthesis.
3. Kaolin and pectin do not work in most cases.
4. Dietary changes.
   a. Avoid lactose-containing foods.
   b. Clear liquid diet for 24–48 hours.
   c. Advance diet slowly.

D. Antibiotics

1. **Bacterial diarrhea.** Trimethoprim-sulfamethoxazole covers most infections, but therapy should be based on

bacteriologic results. With the exception of shigellosis, antibiotics are not necessary and are indicted in the immunocompromised patient only.

2. **Pseudomembranous colitis.** Can be manageed with vancomycin (125 mg PO) every 6 hours or metronidazole (500 mg PO) every 6 hours, usually for 7 days. IV metronidazole or vancomycin may be used, although oral is preferred. If pseudomembranous colitis is suspected, empiric therapy can be initiated before the results of the clostridium toxin assay.

E. **Operation.** Embolectomy, bowel resection, and mesenteric artery bypass for mesenteric ischemia. Resection is required for colonic malignancies, villous adenoma, and some complicated cases of inflammatory bowel disease. Tumor localization and resection should be performed for carcinoid and islet-cell tumors.

F. **Other**
1. **Control GI bleeding.** See Problems 10 and 34, pages 39 and 130.
2. **Disimpaction.** Manual with a gloved finger and adequate lubrication.
3. **Pancreatic insufficiency.** Administer large doses of replacement enzymes (Pancrease, Viokase, etc).
4. **Control thyrotoxicosis.** Propylthiouracil or methimazole, iodide, β blockers, dexamethasone.
5. Steroids or sulfasalazine for inflammatory bowel disease.
6. Proton pump inhibitors for diarrhea caused by gastrinoma.

REFERENCES

Gore JI. Severe acute diarrhea. *Gastroenterol Clin North Am* 32:1249–67, 2003.

Turgeon DK. Laboratory approaches to infectious diarrhea. *Gastroenterol Clin North Am* 30:693–707, 2001.

23. DRAIN OUTPUT—CHANGING AMOUNT

I. **Problem.** You are notified that a patient, 2 days after a hepatic lobectomy, has a 3-fold increase in volume from a Jackson-Pratt drain over the prior 8 hours.

II. **Immediate Questions**

A. **Exactly where is the drain and what operative procedure was performed?** To manage problems with drains, you must know the location of the drain and the expected character and volume of output. Review the operative note and talk to the operating surgeon, if necessary.

B. What is the nature of the drain fluid? Transudates, exudates blood, pus, lymph (chyle), bile, pancreatic juice, intestinal contents, urine, or cerebrospinal fluid (CSF). Some of these fluids can be identified by gross visual inspection and others by laboratory analysis. For example, to evaluate drainage from a drain placed next to the bladder, you can obtain a creatinine level on the fluid to determine whether it is urine.

C. Are there any new symptoms associated with the change in drain output? Ask specifically about pain, signs of infection, hypotension, and abdominal distention.

D. What is the pattern of postoperative drainage? Variations in drain output reflect a change in drain function or a change in the amount of fluid produced. A change in the output from 1 drain may affect the output from other drains in the same area.

E. Has there been any change in the patient's activities coincident with changing drain output? A patient started on oral intake might have increased drainage of pancreatic secretions, thoracic duct flow, or T-tube output. If a patient has increased physical activity such as ambulation or physical therapy, then extremity/lymph node dissection drains may increase. A change in position may result in an increase in chest tube output from dependent accumulated fluid.

III. Differential Diagnosis. Drains may be categorized by the location and type of drain. Below are the more commonly used surgical drains, the purpose of the drain, and specific problems to be expected.

A. Extremity/Lymph Node Dissection (Axillary, Inguinal) Drains
   1. Prevents accumulation of lymph and serous fluids so wound healing is facilitated.
   2. Increased output is usually lymph and associated with increased motion. Immobilize the affected area.

B. Mediastinal Tubes
   1. Identifies excessive bleeding and prevents cardiac tamponade, when functioning properly.
   2. Increased output is bloody and may be due to a specific bleeding point.
   3. A sudden decrease in output may be due to an obstructed tube and may precede tamponade.

C. Chest Tubes (Pleural). (See also Problem 13, page 63.)

1. Drains blood, pus, air, or fluid from pleural cavities.
2. Increased drainage associated with oral intake may indicate fluid from injured thoracic duct.

D. Hepatic/Biliary Tube

1. **Hepatectomy.**
   a. Drains lymph, bile, and blood from cut surface of the liver and any bile leak from the ligated hepatic duct.
   b. **Examine for bile:** When multiple drains are present, be aware of total output.
2. **Cholecystectomy** (often not drained).
   a. Drain identifying leak from ligated cystic duct or excessive bleeding.
   b. Examine drain output for bile.
3. **Common duct exploration.**
   a. T-tubes are used to stent a choledochotomy, prevent bile leaks, and provide a path for further diagnostic or therapeutic studies (cholangiogram or extraction of retained stones).
   b. Increased output may signify distal obstruction from a retained stone, edema, or the start of oral intake.

E. Pancreatic Procedures

1. Used when pancreatic parenchyma is violated (islet-cell tumor resection, trauma) or when ductal system is opened (external drainage of pseudocyst) to prevent the accumulation of pancreatic fluid.
2. Drain output increases with feeding or with distal duct obstruction.

F. Esophageal Procedures

1. Identify leaks and evacuate irritating or infectious fluid.
2. **Output increased with anastomotic leak.** Examine for appearance of saliva or refluxed GI contents.

G. Urinary Tract Procedures

1. After radical cystectomy and urinary diversion, radical prostatectomy or other procedures where the collecting system or bladder had been opened. Prevents urinoma formation and, in the case of a concomitant node dissection, lymphocele formation.
2. Increased output may represent increased lymph leakage or urinary leakage from an anastomotic site.

IV. Database

A. Physical Examination Key Points

1. Examine drainage fluid for blood, pus, and bile. Look at the tube for clots or other obstructing materials.
2. **Lungs.** Changes or absent breath sounds in chest tube.

3. **Cardiac.** Physical signs of tamponade such as increased jugular venous pressure, pulsus paradoxus, or quiet heart sound.
4. **Abdomen.** Pain, abdominal distention, or a fluid wave
5. **Extremities.** Examine for collections of undrained fluid under surgical site.

B. **Laboratory Data**
   1. **Hemogram.** Infection or excess bleeding may be present.
   2. **Hematocrit of drainage fluid.** Grossly bloody fluid is mostly serum or lymph. Compare the drainage hematocrit with the blood hematocrit.
   3. **Gram's stain.** Culture the drainage if any question of infection.
   4. **Chemistries.** Performed to help identify specific types of fluids being drained.
      a. **Amylase:** Markedly high in pancreatic secretions, also present in saliva.
      b. **Triglycerides:** High in thoracic duct lymph.
      c. **Creatinine:** If the drained fluid is urine, creatinine in the fluid will be markedly high.
      d. **pH:** Pleural fluid pH <7.2 may be associated with an empyema.
      e. **Lactate dehydrogenase and protein:** See Section III for discussion of ascitic fluid (paracentesis) and pleural fluid (thoracentesis).

C. **Radiologic and Other Studies**
   1. **Chest radiograph.** Especially if changing amount in pleural or mediastinal tube to determine whether there is an increasing fluid collection.
   2. **Plain films.** Drains are marked with a radiopaque stripe so the drain position can be verified with plain films.
   3. **Contrast studies.** Routine with T-tube after common duct exploration. Contrast studies identify fistulas, leaks, or cavities of accumulated fluid.

V. **Plan.** Identify type of drain, location, and type of fluid draining; formulate ideas about the likely source of fluid.

   A. **Emergent Management.** Drain management rarely requires urgent action with the exception of mediastinal tubes on the cardiac surgery service.
      1. **Increased output.** Usually blood. Document rate of bleeding by noting output every 30–60 minutes and after serial hematocrit determinations. Measure coagulation parameters and correct as necessary with FFP and platelets. Notify senior staff and operating team

about rate of bleeding when possibility of returning to the operating room exists.

2. **Decreased output.** A sudden decrease in output may be a result of a clot in the tube and may lead to an episode of cardiac tamponade. If blood pressure decreases, open the lower portion of the wound and evacuate blood and clot from the retrosternal space.

B. **Routine Management**
   1. Record the amount, characteristics, and laboratory analysis of increased drain output.
   2. Replace high output with appropriate fluids
      a. **Pancreatic, biliary, and small bowel:** See Section IV.
      b. **Mediastinal bloody drainage:** Use blood.
   3. Suction on a drain will encourage persistent drainage. Put drains on "passive" (gravity) drainage to decrease volume.
   4. Never pull a drain unless it is appropriate and the surgeon in charge wants it pulled.

REFERENCE

Memon MA,et al. The uses and abuses of drains in abdominal surgery. *Hosp Med* 63:282–8, 2002.

24. DRAIN OUTPUT—CHANGING CHARACTER

I. **Problem.** A 45-year-old man, 2 days after cholecystectomy, has bilious drainage from a right flank drain.

II. **Immediate Questions**

A. **What are the characteristics of the drainage?** Bloody, bilious, serous, serosanguineous, purulent, or urine-like

B. **What kind of drainage was there previously?** A previously serous fluid that currently looks like urine, stool, or bile may indicate a new fistula or anastomotic leak.

C. **What volume of drainage is present?** This volume must often be replaced and is addressed in Problem 23, page 97.

D. **What was the operation and where was the drain placed?** These questions must be answered to assess the nature of new drainage. This may require discussion with the operating surgeon.

III. **Differential Diagnosis.** Depends on the characteristics of the drainage and the location of the drain. See Problem 23, page 97.

A. Bloody Drainage. Read the operative note to see if there is any mention of a "generalized ooze" of blood at the end of the procedure.

B. Serous Drainage. Usually of no concern a few days after surgery. An increased volume of drainage may be a result of irritation from the drain.

C. Purulent Drainage. Usually indicates infection.

D. Bilious Drainage. May indicate an anastomotic leak after a duodenal, pancreatic, biliary, or gastric procedure. If noted after a cholecystectomy, the source may be a duct of Luschka or a loose tie or clip from the cystic duct stump.

E. Intestinal Drainage. May be a fistula to the skin wound.

F. Urine Drainage. A fistula may have developed.

G. Chylous Drainage. Indicates injury to the thoracic duct.

IV. Database

A. Physical Examination Key Points

1. **Vital signs.** Signs of infection (tachycardia, fever) and volume loss.
2. **Abdomen.** Check for signs of peritonitis.
3. **Wound.** Examine for signs of infection or fluid collection.

B. Laboratory Data

1. **Hemogram.** Check WBC count and hematocrit. WBC counts may be high 24 hours after surgery, but this is common and may not represent an infection.
2. **Coagulation profile.** PT/PTT, platelets, fibrin split products if bleeding is excessive.
3. **Send drain fluid for chemistry as appropriate.** See Problem 23, page 97.

C. Radiologic and Other Studies

1. **Angiogram.** May help localize bleeding site if rate is ≥1 mL/min.
2. **Fistulogram.** Useful to identify origin of cutaneous fistulae.
3. **CT scans and ultrasound.** May localize undrained fluid collections.

V. Plan

A. Supportive care in patients who are bleeding. Administer fluids or blood to maintain blood pressure. Determine the bleeding site and control by angiogram, reoperation, or correction of coagulopathy.

    B. Antibiotics. Indicated if purulent fluid is noted and in certain fistulae such as colovesical fistulae.

    C. Reoperation. Needed if biliary drainage from an abdominal wound or drain is present.

    D. Drain Abscess. Purulent drainage from within a body cavity always mandates continuous drainage until the abscess is cleared. If the abscess remains, ultrasound or CT localization can be performed. If loculated, operative intervention may be required.

    E. Replace fluids as needed (see Section VI, page 385).

REFERENCES

Foster CE, Lefor AT. Gastrocutaneous fistulas: initial management. *Surg Clin North Am* 76:1019–33, 1996.

O'Connor TW, Hugh TB. Abdominal drainage: a clinical review. *Aust N Z J Surg* 49:253–60, 1979.

25. DT'S (DELIRIUM TREMENS)

  I. Problem. A 55-year-old intoxicated man is admitted with abdominal pain and high amylase level. Narcotic analgesia is initiated. On the third hospital day, he is found talking to the walls and shaking violently.

  II. Immediate Questions

    A. What is the patient's airway status? Any patient with an altered level of consciousness is at increased risk of aspiration. Always assess the airway first (ABCs).

    B. What are the patient's vital signs? Hypertension, tachycardia, and fever may represent signs of autonomic overactivity.

    C. What is the patient's mental status? Specifically, look for altered levels of consciousness, impaired cognitive function, hallucinations, confusion with autonomic hyperactivity, and unresponsiveness. Visual hallucinations are more commonly associated with toxic psychosis (EtOH, etc), and auditory hallucinations with psychiatric illness.

    D. What medication is the patient taking? Pay particular attention to addictive substances.

    E. Is there a history of drug or alcohol abuse? This is central to the accurate diagnosis.

  III. Differential Diagnosis. Delirium is a manifestation of diffuse cerebral dysfunction. Focal neurologic deficits indicate a structural abnormality. The differential diagnosis of delirium is more extensive than the following list indicates and includes any source of diffuse cerebral dysfunction (see also Problem 14, page 66). The patient presenting may be have a very wide range of problems and may be delirious based on any of the following diagnoses.

A. Withdrawal Syndromes
  1. **Delirium tremens.** A form of alcohol withdrawal that must be considered in any patient known to be a heavy drinker who developed delirium 3–4 days after hospitalization. In the patient not known to be a drinker, other causes must be investigated.
  2. **Barbiturate withdrawal.** Clinically indistinguishable from delirium tremens.
  3. **Opioid withdrawal.** Occurs up to 48 hours after cessation of agent (most rapid with heroin) and symptoms include restlessness, rhinorrheal lacrimation, nausea, diarrhea, and hypertension.

B. Metabolic Abnormalities
  1. **Electrolyte abnormalities.** Chronic vomiting, pancreatitis, renal failure, and severe liver disease can cause electrolyte and metabolic abnormalities, which can manifest as delirium.
  2. **Hypoxia.** Congestive heart failure can produce hypoxia and delirium.
  3. **Drug intoxication.** Check urine for presence of suspected drugs (opiates, benzodiazepines, cocaine).

C. Endocrine Abnormalities. Abnormal thyroid and adrenal cortical functions can cause delirium. Hypoglycemia from an insulin-secreting tumor or from intentional or accidental insulin overdose should be considered. Diabetic ketoacidosis and hyperosmolar coma should also be considered.

D. CNS Infections. Meningitis and encephalitis can cause delirium.

E. ICU Psychosis. A special, rather common form called "post pump psychosis" or "post pericardiotomy syndrome" or ICU psychosis is associated with patients having undergone coronary bypass procedures.

F. Sepsis. Any cause of sepsis can lead to altered mental status.

IV. **Database**
  A. Physical Examination Key Points
    1. **Vital signs.** Tachycardia is a common manifestation of withdrawal states.
    2. **Neck.** Look for jugular venous distention, which suggests CHF and thyroid masses (hyperthyroidism).

3. **Chest examination.** Look for signs of CHF and other causes of pulmonary edema and hypoxia.
4. **Abdomen.** Check for bladder distention.
5. **Skin.** Profuse sweating is typical.
6. **Neurologic examination.** Mental status changes, hallucinations, confusion, and disorientation are typical. Reflexes will be exaggerated but symmetrical. Pupils are reactive. Any focal findings on motor, sensory, deep tendon or cranial nerve examination point to a structural abnormality, either spinal or intracranial.

B. **Laboratory Data**
   1. **Electrolytes and glucose.** Look for hyponatremia, hypoglycemia, and calcium abnormalities.
   2. **Arterial blood gases.** Obtain if hypoxemia is likely.

C. **Radiologic and Other Studies.** History, physical examination, and simple tests provide the diagnosis. Chest radiograph might show cardiomegaly and pulmonary edema. Evaluation of the CNS by head CT scan or lumbar puncture is necessary, especially in the septic patient or one with focal neurologic findings. Electroencephalography is rarely useful.

V. Plan

A. **Prevention.** Patient should be treated while hospitalized with around-the-clock benzodiazepines, most commonly oxazepam (15–30 mg PO every 4–6 hours) or Lorazepam 1 mg PO/IV every 8 hours.

B. **Delirium tremens.** Alcohol abusers typically display electrolyte abnormalities (from vomiting) and hepatic encephalopathy.
   1. Benzodiazepine is given IV initially (diazepam 5–10 mg IV every 4–6 hours) followed by PO treatment with diazepam, chlordiazepoxide, or oxazepam in the nonvomiting patient.
   2. Restraints may be needed in the prone position (to decrease risk of aspiration).
   3. Intravenous fluid replacement for volume and electrolyte abnormality correction. IV fluids are supplemented with ("banana bag") thiamine (100 mg), multivitamins, and folate (1 mg).
   4. Withdrawal seizures are controlled with phenytoin or paraldehyde.

C. **Hypoxia**
   1. **Oxygen therapy.** Supplemental mask. Check pulse oximeter. Always consider intubation when appropriate.
   2. **Morphine sulfate and diuretics (Lasix).** These are used in the setting of pulmonary edema.

3. **Digoxin or dopamine and nitrates.** Used in the situation of pulmonary edema caused by CHF.

D. **Other**
1. **Narcotics withdrawal.** Managed with relatively large doses of minor tranquilizers or with methadone (10–20 mg PO, every 2–6 hours). Clonidine may be used as alternate therapy to combat autonomic symptoms.
2. **Drug intoxication.** Minor or major tranquilizers can be used.
3. **Endocrine abnormalities.** These are managed appropriately.
4. **CNS infections.** Appropriate antibiotics, with or without drainage of abscess, are indicated.
5. **ICU psychosis.** Attempt to keep the patient oriented. Agitation can be controlled with oral or parenteral haloperidol (Haldol). Avoid benzodiazepines.
6. **Thiamine prophylaxis** should be given to patients with a predisposing history (EtOH abuse).
7. **Sepsis.** Control with appropriate antibiotics and fluid resuscitation.

REFERENCES

Bayard M. Alcohol withdrawal syndrome. *Am Fam Phys* 69:1443–50, 2004.
Chang PH. Alcohol withdrawal. *Med Clin North Am* 85:1191–212, 2001.

26. DYSPNEA

I. **Problem.** A patient on the trauma service with a diagnosis of myocardial contusion complains of difficulty breathing.

II. **Immediate Questions**

A. **What was the patient doing when the dyspnea occurred?** Shortness of breath with exertional activity may indicate an underlying problem, depending on the severity of the dyspnea. Dyspnea associated with a reclining position (ie, orthopnea) points to cardiac dysfunction.

B. **Did the dyspnea occur abruptly, or did it have a gradual onset?** The diagnosis for acute dyspnea differs from that for subacute dyspnea and points often to a specific event such as a PE, pneumothorax, or MI.

C. **What is the baseline respiratory status of the patient?** Inquire specifically about current work and recreational physical activities.

D. **Are there other symptoms such as chest pain coincident with the dyspnea?** Ask if chest pain or pressure is occurring. Dyspnea may be the sole presenting symptom of an acute MI.

E. Is there wheezing or stridor? Acute asthma attacks and anaphylactic reactions are controllable if identified quickly.

F. Is there a history of asthma or other pulmonary condition?

III. **Differential Diagnosis.** Within each category, the underlying mechanism is predominantly pulmonary or cardiac.

   A. **Acute**
   1. **Pulmonary**
      a. **Pneumothorax:** Can be caused by trauma-associated with rib fractures and a hemothorax and may progress over hours. Usually spontaneous in males with tall thin bodies.
      b. **Pulmonary embolus:** Risk factors of immobilization, recent surgery, neoplastic disease, and estrogen use.
      c. **Asthma or allergic reactions:** Asthma is clearly identified by wheezing. Anaphylactic reactions are identified by stridor, atopic history, hives, and facial edema (see Problem 5, page 22).
      d. **Aspirated foreign body.** In young or mentally impaired patients, rely on physical examination and radiologic studies.
      e. **Reflux with aspiration:** See Problem 8, page 31.
   2. **Acute MI.** Be sure to consider this if cardiac risk factors are present. This is usually but not always associated with chest pain or pressure.
   3. **Anxiety attack.** Not a common cause of shortness of breath and is frequently associated with chest pain. Tachypnea often cycles with a period of normal breathing and may resolve when patients are not aware of being observed.

   B. **Subacute/Chronic**
   1. **Pulmonary**
      a. **COPD:** These patients usually have a smoking history with baseline dyspnea on exertion. Look for evidence of infectious process.
      b. **Pneumonia:** Often associated with leukocytosis, fever, productive sputum, and chest radiographic changes (infiltrates).
      c. **Interstitial lung disease:** Chest radiograph and pulmonary function tests are diagnostic.
   2. **Cardiac**

   a. **Congestive heart failure:** Physical examination
      shows high jugular venous pressure, rales, periph-
      eral edema, cardiac gallop, and displacement of left
      ventricular impulse. Dyspnea is associated with
      lying down (orthopnea).

IV. Database
A. Physical Examination Key Points
   1. **Vital signs.** Fever may signify infection but may also be
      seen with a PE. Tachypnea may accompany hypoxia,
      embolus, or a pneumothorax. Check oxygen saturation
      as soon as possible.
   2. **Lung.** Observe respiratory rate, work of breathing, and
      use of accessory muscles. Listen for wheezes, stridor,
      rales, evidence of consolidation, and decreased breath
      sounds. Tracheal shift may indicate pneumothorax.
   3. **Cardiac.** High jugular venous pressure, displacement
      of left ventricular impulse, new murmur of mitral regurgi-
      tation. Check for pulsus paradoxus.
   4. **Extremities.** Leg swelling is evidence for deep venous
      thrombosis. Evaluate for evidence of cyanosis.
   5. **Neurologic.** Confusion and drowsiness may signify se-
      vere hypoxia.

B. Laboratory Data
   1. **Hemogram.** Leukocytosis may be present with infec-
      tion. Anemia greatly decreases oxygen delivery to tis-
      sues
   2. **Arterial blood gas.** Documents level of respiratory
      compromise and guides therapeutic decisions. Look for
      A-a gradient in PE.
   3. **Sputum Gram's stain/culture.** In patients with pneu-
      monia or tracheobronchitis.
   4. **Blood chemistries.** May reveal evidence of renal fail-
      ure. Tachypnea may be a manifestation of respiratory
      compensation for metabolic acidosis.

C. Radiologic and Other Studies
   1. **Chest radiograph.** If the patient is in distress, obtain
      immediate portable chest radiograph (upright if possi-
      ble). Look for pulmonary edema, pneumothorax, effu-
      sion, or pneumonia.
   2. **Electrocardiogram.** Always obtain ECG if there is any
      question of cardiac cause.
   3. **Pulmonary function tests.** Not applicable to acute sit-
      uations but helpful in patients with obstructive or restric-
      tive chronic lung disease.
   4. **V/Q scan.** V/Q scan will evaluate for PE.

5. **CT angiogram**. Very sensitive for PE and may be more easily obtained on an urgent basis.
6. **Pulmonary angiogram.** Especially with an equivocal V/Q scan in the diagnosis of PE.
7. **Radionuclide angiogram.** This documents left ventricular ejection fraction and level of CHF.
8. **Exercise tolerance test.** Useful if episode of dyspnea is related to ischemic heart disease.
9. **Echocardiogram.** To evaluate for valvular disease, akinesis, failure, etc.

V. Plan

A. Emergent Therapy

1. **Oxygen supplementation.** If the patient is short of breath, institute oxygen therapy. Acutely use 100%, with adjustments made to keep arterial oxygen at ≥60–80 mm Hg or oxygen saturation <90% based on blood gas measurements or pulse oximetry. Long-term oxygen therapy at this level can cause toxicity. Do not worry about suppression of hypoxic drive (chronic lung disease) in the acute situation. Patients with a history of COPD and CO_2 retention may be at increased risk to lose their "hypoxic drive" to breathe.
2. Stat portable chest radiograph, ECG, and ABGs are indicated if the cause is not immediately obvious.

B. Specific Urgent/Immediate Therapies

1. **Asthma/COPD exacerbation.** Order an immediate therapy of Alupent nebulizer 0.3 mL in 2–3 mL NS by a respiratory therapist and Atrovent 0.5 mL in 3 mL NS.
2. **Anaphylaxis.** Refer to Problem 5, page 22.
3. **Myocardial ischemia.** If immediate evaluation is consistent with myocardial ischemia, administer sublingual nitroglycerin. Refer to Problem 12, page 54.
4. **Acute CHF.** Control with oxygen, diuretics (IV Lasix 10–40 mg dependent on previous exposure), and nitroglycerin and sit the patient upright if blood pressure allows.
5. **Pneumonia.** Control with antibiotics and pulmonary toilet.
6. **Pneumothorax.** Place a chest tube as outlined in Section III, page 347. Needle decompression may be necessary first for *tension* pneumothorax.

REFERENCES

Campbell M. Terminal dyspnea and respiratory distress. *Crit Care Clin* 20:403–9, 2004.

Thomas JR. Clinical management of dyspnoea. *Lancet Oncol* 3:223–8, 2002.

27. DYSURIA

I. **Problem.** A patient complains of dysuria 4 days after an uncomplicated radical neck dissection.

II. **Immediate Questions**

   A. **How long has this symptom been present?** If the illness
   is chronic, check previous urinalysis.

   B. **What is the patient's urologic history; specifically, is
   there any history of infections or stone disease?** Females are especially prone to recurrent urinary infections.
   Urethritis or prostatitis may be present in males.

   C. **Are there any associated voiding symptoms?** Fever,
   chills, and back pain are signs of upper urinary tract infection (pyelonephritis). Frequency, urgency, and pain on uri-
   nation suggest lower urinary tract infection (cystitis,
   prostatitis, urethritis).

   D. **Has the patient recently had a Foley catheter removed?**
   A catheter may result in an infection. Mild urethral irritation
   usually resolves shortly after the catheter is removed.

III. **Differential Diagnosis**

   A. **Urinary Tract Infection**
      1. **Upper.** Pyelonephritis may occasionally cause dysuria.
      2. **Lower.** Cystitis is often associated with urgency and
      frequency. Urethritis may be gonococcal or nongono-
      coccal, often caused by *Chlamydia*. Prostatitis may be
      acute (associated with fever, chills, signs of sepsis) or
      chronic (associated with voiding symptoms or recurrent
      urinary tract infections).

   B. **Vaginitis.** Can present with initial complaints of dysuria.
   Can be due to *Candida*, *Trichomonas*, and *Gardnerella* organisms. Atrophic vaginitis in postmenopausal women.

   C. **Genital Infections.** Herpes or condylomata.

   D. **Chemical Irritants.** Allergic reaction to a variety of agents
   (deodorant, douches).

   E. **Postprocedure.** A frequent complaint after bladder
   catheterization or cystoscopy; usually resolves spontaneously if no infection intervenes

   F. **Urethral Syndrome.** Frequent in women with dysuria and
   voiding complaints without evidence of urinary tract infection.

   G. **Miscellaneous.** Urethral stricture, bladder tumor, urolithiasis, and interstitial cystitis.

IV. Database

A. Physical Examination Key Points

1. **Abdominal examination.** Look for signs of suprapubic tenderness or costovertebral angle tenderness.
2. **Genitalia.** Including urethral meatus, urethra, testicles, and epididymis in men. Vaginal discharge suggests vaginitis. Women may require a formal pelvic examination if the cause is not readily obvious.
3. **Rectal examination.** Including prostate. Be aware that vigorous exam of an acutely inflamed prostate can induce bacteremia and may be contraindicated in the presence of high fever and chills.

B. Laboratory Data

1. **Urinalysis and culture.** Pyuria (0.5 WBC/high-power field), presence of leukocyte esterase or nitrites, and positive culture.
2. **Hemogram.** Leukocytosis and a left shift will be seen with acute pyelonephritis and acute prostatitis and not normally seen in urethritis, chronic prostatitis, or cystitis.
3. **Urethral discharge culture and Gram's stain.** Thayer-Martin media should be used if gonorrhea is suspected. *Neisseria gonorrhea* can be seen as gram-negative intracellular diplococci on Gram's stain.
4. **Urine cytology.** Dysuria may be a subtle manifestation of transitional cell carcinoma.

C. Radiologic and Other Studies.
Full urologic evaluation may be required for definitive diagnosis.

V. Plan

A. Positive Urinalysis.
Start antibiotic therapy. If the patient is healthy and not systemically septic, then oral antibiotics may be started.

B. Systemic Sepsis.
A patient with signs of fever, chills, nausea, malaise, or hypotension (often associated with acute pyelonephritis or prostatitis) should be evaluated with appropriate cultures. Start systemic antibiotics. Use a third-generation cephalosporin (cefoperazone, ceftazidime) or ampicillin with an aminoglycoside until culture and sensitivities are available.

C. Chronic Prostatitis.
Positive urine culture with findings of prostatitis but are not septic. Therapy is a 3–week course of trimethoprim/sulfa or quinolone.

D. Vaginitis.
Controlled with nystatin vaginal cream or suppositories for *Candida,* oral metronidazole for *Trichomonas,* or dienestrol (AVC) cream for atrophic vaginitis.

   E. **Other Infections.**
      1. **Gonococcal urethritis.** Procaine penicillin G 4.8 mil-
         lion units IM plus probenecid 1 g PO, ceftriaxone 250
         mg IM, ampicillin 3 g PO, followed by a 7–day course of
         tetracycline.
      2. **Nongonococcal urethritis (***Chlamydia***).** Doxycycline
         100 mg PO twice daily, tetracycline 500 mg PO daily for
         7–10 days.
   F. **Symptomatic Relief.** Achieved with phenazopyridine
      (Pyridium) 100–200 mg PO 3 times daily (turns urine or-
      ange) while workup or treatment is in progress. A small
      subset is sensitive to excessively alkaline or acidic urine.

REFERENCE

Bremnor JD. Evaluation of dysuria in adults. *Am Fam Phys* 65:1589–96,
   2002.

28. EPISTAXIS

 I. **Problem.** A 45-year-old hypertensive patient, 1 day after a la-
    paroscopic cholecystectomy, complains of a nosebleed that
    has lasted for 2 hours.

 II. **Immediate Questions**
    A. **What are the patient's vital signs?** Hypertension is a re-
       sponse to rather than a cause of epistaxis. Tachycardia
       represents agitation of the patient but rarely indicates sig-
       nificant blood loss. Check for orthostatic hypotension.
    B. **Is there a history of nosebleed or any recent trauma?**
       New onset of epistaxis should alert to intranasal pathology.
       Recurrent epistaxis is usually traumatic, especially in the
       younger patient.

 III. **Differential Diagnosis.** Epistaxis has multiple causes such
      as hematologic malignancies and coagulation disorders.
      Ninety percent of epistaxis has its origin in the anterior portion
      of the nasopharynx.
    A. **Trauma.** Blunt trauma to the nose often causes epistaxis
       that ceases spontaneously. Digital trauma (nose-picking)
       is a major cause of epistaxis. The source is almost always
       an anterior site called the Kiesselbach's triangle, a submu-
       cosal mat of blood vessels located on the anteriormost as-
       pect of the nasal septum.
    B. **Hypertension.** Hypertension may make control of bleed-
       ing more difficult but is rarely a cause of bleeding.

C. **Intranasal Pathology.** The adult patient who presents with new epistaxis in the absence of trauma may have an intranasal lesion. These include polyps and benign and malignant tumors. Typically, no anterior source of bleeding is apparent. Local infections may also be an underlying condition. Juvenile angiofibroma, a locally aggressive tumor that presents as a purple polypoid mass, must be ruled out in pubescent males.

D. **Systemic Illnesses and Medications.** Patients who take anticoagulants or have end-stage liver disease can develop epistaxis when PT is overly prolonged. Renal failure and aspirin interfere with platelet function. Obscure causes of epistaxis include leukemia, hemophilia, and chemotherapy-induced thrombocytopenia. Arteriosclerosis commonly predisposes to posterior epistaxis in the elderly.

IV. **Database**
  A. **Physical Examination Key Points**
    1. **Vital signs.** Hypertension often decreases as the patient relaxes. Chronic hypertension can be controlled. Orthostatic hypotension can be found after significant nasal hemorrhage.
    2. **Skin.** Look for petechiae and ecchymoses to suggest a systemic problem.
    3. **Nose.** Examine the nasal cavity with a headlamp or mirror and a nasal speculum. Examine as much of the mucosa as possible for a bleeding site. Briefly examine the contralateral nasal cavity. Topical cocaine controls bleeding in most cases if examination is difficult.

  B. **Laboratory Data**
    1. **Coagulation studies.** May reveal over-anticoagulation.
    2. **Hemogram.** The hematocrit will not accurately reflect blood loss in the acute period. Look for unsuspected thrombocytopenia.

V. **Plan**
  A. **Initial Control of Bleeding.** With the patient in an upright position, apply bilateral alar pressure and 5% cocaine locally. Cocaine acts as a vasoconstrictor and anesthetic.

  B. **Cauterization and Anterior Packing**
    1. **Silver nitrate sticks.** If examination reveals a likely bleeding source after initial control is achieved, silver nitrate sticks cauterize the site.
    2. **Anterior nasal packing.** An anterior pack can be placed if cauterization is not successful. A piece of Gelfoam can be placed over the bleeding site, and then

bacitracin impregnated Nu-Gauz can be layered into the nose. Tape a drip pad to the nose. Start on antibiotics (ampicillin or erythromycin). Packing can usually be removed in 2–4 days.

C. Posterior Packing. Persistent bleeding with no localized anterior site requires posterior packing and admission to the otolaryngology service. These patients require antibiotics (as above), oxygen, and analgesia, usually with narcotic. Three methods are commonly used to place posterior packs.

  1. A 14F Foley catheter can be passed into the nasopharynx, inflated with saline, and gently drawn into choanae.

  2. Specialized nasal balloons (Nasal-Stat).

  3. A pack made of 434 cotton gauze. Three 434-gauze sponges are rolled and tied with 3 large silk ties. A rubber catheter is passed into the nose and pulled out the mouth with a clamp. Two sutures from the pack are tied to the catheter and then pulled up into the nasal pharynx under guidance with a finger. An anterior pack is then placed and the posterior pack sutures are tied. The remaining pack suture comes out the mouth and is taped to the face. This allows removal of the pack in 4–5 days.

D. Recurrent Bleeding. Recurrent bleeding after removal of a posterior pack is an indication for angiography and embolization of the causative vessel or endoscopic cauterization. If this fails, surgery will be needed to ligate the internal maxillary artery with or without the anterior and posterior ethmoid arteries.

REFERENCES

Huang CL. Epistaxis: a review of hospitalized patients. *Zhonghua Yi Xue Za Zhi* 65:74–81, 2002.
Kassutto Z. Clinical and laboratory features of 178 children with recurrent epistaxis. *Ann Emerg Med* 41:283–9, 2003.

29. EPIDURAL CATHETER PROBLEMS

I. Problem. A nurse reports the inadvertent dislodgement of an epidural catheter in a patient 1 day after a radical nephrectomy.

II. Immediate Questions. Lumbar epidural catheters, usually placed for intraoperative anesthesia, are also used for postoperative analgesia by the injection of narcotics or local anesthetics into the extradural space through a soft catheter.

A. **When was the last dose of epidural narcotic?** Long-acting narcotics injected into the extradural space can provide reliable analgesia for 12–18 hours after each dose.

B. **Is the patient in pain?** If yes, then supplemental intravenous or intramuscular narcotics will be required.

C. **Is the patient otherwise stable?** Delayed respiratory depression can occur from systemic absorption of the narcotic.

D. **Is the catheter tip intact?** A retained epidural catheter tip can lead to infectious complications, such as epidural abscess. The tip of the catheter is marked by a black dot.

III. Database

A. **Physical Examination Key Points**
1. **Vital signs.** Hypotension and respiratory depression can occur with unintentional intravascular injection even up to several hours later. Cardiopulmonary collapse occurs if epidural doses of narcotics or anesthetics are given into the subarachnoid space, usually 15–30 minutes after injection.
2. **Chest.** Check breath sounds for depth and rate.
3. **Neurologic.** Check mental status, determine level of anesthesia (if still present), and motor and sensory functions. Patients should be able to move their feet and feel you touch them. Rarely, epidural hematomas can occur, causing symptoms of an epidural mass that requires immediate neurosurgical decompression.
4. **Catheter exit site.** Examine for bleeding and signs of infection.
5. **Catheter tip.** Examine the tip to make sure the entire catheter has been removed.

B. **Laboratory Data.** Generally of little value unless coagulopathy or cardiopulmonary complications arise.

C. **Radiologic and Other Studies.** Usually not necessary.

IV. Plan

A. **Ensure that no complications of epidural anesthesia have occurred.**
1. **Overmedication.** Contact anesthesia staff and provide adequate monitoring and support for the patient. Overmedication is the primary reason that patients who receive epidural anesthesia should remain monitored.
2. **Hematoma.** Diagnose and correct any coagulopathy and contact the neurosurgical service immediately.

3. **Inadvertent subarachnoid puncture.** Causes a severe frontal or occipital headache that is exacerbated by sitting up. Initial therapy includes bedrest, caffeine, and analgesics. If the headache lasts >24 hours, a "blood patch" procedure can be performed by the anesthesiologist. This generally provides relief within 30 minutes and can be repeated if no improvement is noted. If pain persists, an alternate explanation for the headache must be sought (migraine, meningitis, cortical vein thrombosis, intracranial hemorrhage).

4. **Urinary retention.** Infrequently seen with epidural anesthesia; use an indwelling catheter to drain the bladder.

5. **Itching.** Commonly seen. Control with Benadryl 25–50 mg IM or PO.

B. **Analgesia.** Supplement pain relief with additional IV, IM, or PO analgesics. Make sure you know the last dose given through the catheter to avoid overmedication.

C. **Wound care.** Cover site with a sterile, dry dressing and inspect daily for signs of infection.

D. **Positioning.** Patients should remain recumbent for a few hours after catheter removal to decrease "spinal headache."

REFERENCES

Liu SS. Current issues in spinal anesthesia. *Anesthesiology* 94:888–906, 2001.
Steffen P. Bacterial contamination of epidural catheters: microbiological examination of 502 epidural catheters used for postoperative analgesia. *J Clin Anesth* 16:92–7, 2004.

30. FALL FROM BED

I. **Problem.** The day after an open reduction and internal fixation of a humeral fracture, a 60-year-old man fell from bed while trying to go to the bathroom. He has a laceration on his forehead.

II. **Immediate Questions.** Most falls from bed are not associated with serious injury. However, they are extremely upsetting to the patient and the patient's family. Every fall from bed warrants a complete evaluation, documentation of the incident, and thorough search for injury. Pay attention to the ABCs.

A. **Is the patient able to speak?** Quickly assess the airway and mental status by having the patient answer the question, "What happened?"

B. **Is the patient back in bed?** To avoid further injury, log roll the patient onto a backboard, or use in-line traction or cervical immobilization before placing the patient back in bed. Assume cervical spine injury and place the patient in a soft cervical collar.

C. **Is the patient in pain?** Perform a thorough physical examination.

III. **Differential Diagnosis.** History obtained from the patient, visitors, and staff may be helpful in determining the reason for the fall. Head injury, skeletal fractures, and dislocations lead the list. Review medication list and any recent medications the patient may have received.

A. **Delirium.** See Problem 25, page 103 for a complete list.

B. **Dementia.** Pre-existing risk factor for falling and should be recognized for prevention.

C. **Acute Change in Neurologic Status.** See Problem 14, page 66 and Problem 17, page 77.

D. Delayed recovery from anesthesia.

E. Musculoskeletal weakness in postoperative period.

IV. **Database**

A. **Physical Examination Key Points**

1. **Vital signs.** Fever can cloud the sensorium; hypotension, a factor for septic or cardiogenic shock; arrhythmias; respiratory rate and pattern.

2. **HEENT.** Closely examine the scalp and face for signs of head injury, cranial nerves, and teeth.

3. **Neck.** JVD, C-spine tenderness, nuchal rigidity.

4. **Chest.** Bilateral breath sounds, wheezing, consolidation, cardiac murmurs, palpate ribs.

5. **Abdomen.** Tenderness, bowel sounds to screen for abdominal injury.

6. **Skin.** Bruising, lacerations.

7. **Extremities.** Tenderness, obvious fractures, check IV lines.

B. **Laboratory Data**

1. **Hemogram.** Anemia, infection.

2. **Serum electrolytes.** Hypo- and hyperglycemia, kalemia, calcemia, natremia, and magnesemia; uremia, ammonia.

3. **Cardiac enzymes.** If MI suspected.

4. **Toxic drug screen.** If clinically indicated.

5. **ABG and venous blood gas.** Acid-base disorders, hypoxia.

      6. Cultures. Blood, urine, sputum, if infection is suspected.

  C. Radiologic and Other Studies

    1. Electrocardiogram. If MI is suspected or arrhythmia is noted.

    2. Chest radiograph. If respiratory or infectious source likely and to check for fractures. Rib detail films may be needed to evaluate for fractures.

    3. Head CT. For change in mental status.

    4. Plain radiographs. Tender extremities and joints to check for fracture or dislocation.

    5. Lumbar puncture. If indicated (check for nuchal rigidity)

    6. Electroencephalogram. If indicated.

    7. Pulse oximetry. Noninvasive means of checking for hypoxia.

V. Plan. Overall, an underlying cause for the fall must be sought and managed. See Problem 17, page 77 and Problem 14, page 66 for specific treatment plans.

  A. Fractures and dislocations should be splinted and the orthopedic service contacted for definitive care and follow-up. Always check for distal pulses before and after splinting.

  B. Lacerations should be cleaned and sutured. Use local wound care for abrasions.

  C. If C-spine injury is suspected, immobilize the neck and keep the patient flat until the spine can be evaluated radiographically.

  D. Prevention of Further Injury. Mild sedation if warranted (perform a brief GCS examination before sedation). Make sure bed side rails are up and that the patient is properly oriented to and can reach the nurse call button. Use restraints, if necessary, according to protocol. A bedside commode may be useful for the weak or elderly and for physical therapy for reconditioning.

  E. Incident Report. Risk management includes completion of the report and documentation of the incident in the chart.

REFERENCES

Hitcho EB, et al. Characteristics and circumstances of falls in a hospital setting. *J Gen Intern Med* 19:732–9, 2004.

Kerzman H, et al. Characteristics of falls in hospitalized patients. *J Adv Nurs* 47:223–9, 2004.

31. FEVER

I. **Problem.** You are notified that a patient on another service who had a gastrectomy for cancer has a fever of 38.9°C.

II. **Immediate Questions**

   A. **How many days postop is the patient?** Most medical students know the mnemonic: "The Five W's of postop infection: wind, water, walk, wound, wonder drugs" for postoperative fever. These 5 causes, in order from the mnemonic, are pneumonia, urinary tract, thrombophlebitis, wound infection, and drug reaction.

   B. **What is the fever pattern?** Check the chart for the previous 2–3 days to see any emerging or changing fever patterns. Spiking fevers are often associated with infections in a closed space (ie, abscesses). Continuing fevers are often found in cases of vascular involvement such as infected prosthetic grafts or septic phlebitis.

   C. **Does the patient have chills/rigors with the fever?** Often rigors are associated with more serious fevers and indicate an episode of bacteremia. Fevers associated with drug reactions or atelectasis usually do not have associated rigors.

   D. **Did the patient have fevers before the operation?** A patient may have a chronic disease associated with fever (lymphoma, etc). Even if the patient does not have one of these diagnoses, keep them in mind when no other source of fever is identifiable.

   E. **Has the patient recently stopped taking an antipyretic agent?** Occasionally a new fever is the realization of a suppressed fever in patients who take aspirin, acetaminophen, or NSAID. Noting this may be important to diagnose fever in certain cases.

   F. **Has the patient recently been taking antibiotics?** Find out why, which drug, and the time of the last dose.

   G. **Are there any associated complaints such as cough, dysuria, diarrhea, abdominal pain, or pain around any IV sites or incisions?** These may point to the cause of the fever if present.

   H. **Is the patient immunocompromised?** This could be a neutropenic fever.

III. **Differential Diagnosis.** Usually the febrile patient seen in an emergency room or outpatient setting has an acute infection that is readily diagnosed from associated complaints. This type of febrile patient will not be discussed. The common febrile patient on a surgical service is one who has postoperative fever. However, other patients (postoperative or otherwise) may have a fever of unknown origin, defined as a temperature ≥38.5°C daily for ≥3 weeks and no diagnosis after 1 week of in-hospital investigation. The differential diagnosis of postoperative fevers and fever of unknown origin is given below.

A. Postoperative Fever
   1. **Atelectasis.** Fever is usually <39°C and occurs in first 12–48 hours postoperatively.
   2. **Urinary tract infection.** Typically occurs 3–5 days postoperatively in the hospitalized patient and usually follows urinary tract manipulation such as placement of a Foley catheter.
   3. **IV catheter infection.** The longer a catheter is left in, the greater the risk of infection.
      a. **Peripheral:** The site will often appear infected.
      b. **Central:** Diagnosed on high degree of clinical suspicion and usually by positive blood cultures drawn through the line.
   4. **Deep venous thrombosis.** The fever is usually low grade (37.5–38.5°C). Pulmonary embolus may also have an associated low grade fever.
   5. **Wound infection**
      a. **Early:** Organisms are often *Clostridium* or *Streptococcus* in first 12–36 hours postoperatively. These are often characterized by drainage that appears like "dirty dishwater," with thin, serous drainage. Treatment consists of rapid surgical debridement and appropriate antibiotics.
      b. **Late:** More common 5–8 days postoperatively, commonly because of *Staphylococcus, Pseudomonas,* etc.
   6. **Drug reaction.** Most commonly antibiotics (penicillins, cephalosporins).
   7. **CNS origin.** Central fever in trauma patient with head injuries or meningitis in spinal anesthetic complication. This is a diagnosis of exclusion.
   8. **Thyroid storm.** After thyroidectomy for Grave's disease.
   9. **Blood transfusion.** See Problem 68, page 234.
  10. **Postpericardiotomy syndrome.** Usually seen 5–7 days postoperatively.
  11. **Anastomotic bowel leak.** Usually seen 7–10 days postoperatively and usually associated with peritoneal irritation.

12. **Otitis, sialadenitis, sinusitis.** Especially in patients with long-term NG tubes.
13. **Addisonian crisis.**
14. **Acalculous cholecystitis.** May be seen with prolonged periods of being NPO, associated with trauma and other severe illnesses.
15. **Pancreatitis.**
16. ***Clostridium difficile*** enterocolitis. Typically diffuse green, watery, foul-smelling, or bloody diarrhea.
17. **Diabetic ketoacidosis.** Infection is a frequent trigger.

B. **Fever of Unknown Origin**
   1. **Infections**
      a. **Granulomatous:** Caused by *Mycobacterium* or fungal agents.
      b. **Endocarditis:** Especially with valvular heart disease.
      c. **Abscess:** Hepatic, subphrenic renal, or pelvic.
      d. **Parasites:** May have frequent high temperatures and often diagnosed by eosinophilia.
   2. **Neoplastic.** Fevers can be a part of "paraneoplastic syndromes."
      a. Lymphoma.
      b. Renal cell carcinoma.
      c. Hepatic metastatic disease.
   3. **Connective tissue disease**
      a. Systemic lupus erythematosus.
      b. Rheumatoid arthritis (usually juvenile).
      c. Polymyalgia rheumatica.
   4. **Miscellaneous**
      a. Drug reaction.
      b. Recurrent pulmonary emboli/pelvic or deep vein thrombosis.
      c. Inflammatory bowel disease.

IV. **Database**

A. **Physical Examination Key Points**
   1. **Vital signs.** Check how temperature was taken (oral, rectal, etc).
   2. **Skin.** Examine wound and all past and current IV sites.
   3. **HEENT.** Check for sialadenitis, otitis, and pharyngitis.
   4. **Pulmonary.** Listen for rhonchi, evidence of consolidation.
   5. **Abdomen.** Right upper quadrant tenderness, peritoneal signs.
   6. **Trunk.** Costovertebral angle tenderness.
   7. **Extremities.** Evidence for DVT (pain, swelling, etc).

8. **Wound.** Check the wound for erythema, fluid collection, subcutaneous air, crepitation, and tenderness. If the wound is relatively recent, remember to use strict aseptic technique. Culture any drainage.

B. Laboratory Data
1. **Hemogram.** Leukocytosis, left shift with infection. Anemia may be seen with endocarditis.
2. **Electrolytes.** Hyponatremia and hyperkalemia in addisonian crisis.
3. Thyroid hormone levels, T_3 and T_4.
4. Urinalysis and urine culture.
5. Throat culture if indicated.
6. Wound culture if indicated.
7. Blood cultures, ≥ 2 peripheral. Drawback cultures from central line if present. Line exit site cultures are minimally helpful. Multiple cultures on different days may be best for endocarditis.
8. Sputum Gram's stain and culture if indicated.
9. Stool for fecal leukocytes and *Clostridium difficile* toxin assay.

C. Radiologic and Other Studies
1. **Chest radiograph.** Linear densities with atelectasis; infiltrates with pneumonia; occasional wedge-shaped infarction with pulmonary emboli.
2. **Electrocardiogram.** ST elevations in postpericardiotomy syndrome.
3. **Venous Doppler/venogram.** If DVT is suspected.
4. **Abdominal CT.** This is very useful for the evaluation of intra-abdominal abscess.
5. **Abdominal ultrasound.** In acalculous cholecystitis can demonstrate sludge or pericholecystic fluid and may demonstrate abscesses (subphrenic or hepatic).
6. **HIDA scan.** Useful in establishing the diagnosis of acute acalculous cholecystitis.
7. **Gallium scan.** Using labeled WBCs may help identify an otherwise elusive abscess.

V. Plan. The primary goal is to diagnose and control the underlying cause. A second goal is to control the fever. Antipyretics can be given with caution after cultures are obtained. Some preventive measurements for postoperative fever are discussed.

A. Management of Specific Causes
1. **Atelectasis and pneumonia**
   a. Incentive spirometry, ambulation, and coughing are general measures to control and help prevent atelectasis and pneumonia.

    b. For pneumonia, antibiotics are empirically started, based on results of the Gram's stain, and then tailored based on culture results. These are frequently nosocomial so be familiar with antibiotic susceptibility patterns of the particular hospital.

  2. Urinary tract infection. See Problem 27, page 110.

  3. IV catheter sepsis

    a. Peripheral: Remove all suspicious catheters and apply local heat to area. Use cefazolin or dicloxacillin as antibiotic if required. Observe for suppurative phlebitis, which usually requires vein excision.

    b. Central: The best option is to remove the line and culture tip. Manage with antibiotics (cephalosporin or vancomycin) for 1–2 days before using a wire (see Problem 20, page 86). Using peripheral cultures and cultures drawn through the line, obtained in Isolator (Dupont) tubes, one can compare the number of colonies. If the number of colonies in the line culture is <5 times that in the peripherally obtained culture, the line is not the source of sepsis.

  4. Thyroid storm. Control with propylthiouracil 400 mg every 6 hours, sodium iodide 250 mg PO/IV every 6 hours, propranolol 1 mg/min IV for 2.8 minutes, and hydrocortisone 100 mg IV.

  5. Postpericardiotomy. Indomethacin 25–50 mg 3 times daily with food or antacids.

  6. Addisonian crisis. 100 mg hydrocortisone IV every 8 hours.

  7. Wound infection. Open wound carefully, culture drainage, and pack with saline-moistened gauze. Dress with dry gauze and secure to patient. Change 3 times daily. Remember that early rapid surgical debridement is mandatory.

  8. *Clostridium difficile* colitis (see page 93).

B. Management of Fever

  1. Antipyretics. Acetaminophen 650 mg PO/rectally every 4–6 hours is preferred because aspirin inhibits platelet action.

  2. Maintain adequate hydration. Fever increases baseline fluid requirements by 500 mL/24 hours for each degree centigrade >38.3°C (101°F).

  3. Cooling blanket. Useful in decreasing body temperature.

C. Preventive Measures

  1. Atelectasis. Have smokers quit for a few weeks before an elective operation. Teach all patients incentive spirometry preoperatively.

2. **Intravenous catheters.** Change peripheral IVs routinely every 2–3 days or sooner if needed.
3. Deep venous thrombosis
   a. Early ambulation should be encouraged.
   b. For high-risk patients (obesity, prior DVT, neoplasia), consider heparin SC.
   c. Sequential compression devices are frequently used postoperatively until the patient is ambulatory.
4. **Blood transfusion.** Acetaminophen 650 mg and diphenhydramine (Benadryl) 25–50 mg IV/PO about 30 minutes before transfusion in patients with a history of transfusion reaction may blunt the febrile response.
5. **Thyroid storm.** Use saturated solution of potassium iodide 2 drops 3 times daily and propranolol 20–40 mg PO daily for 7–10 days before surgery.

REFERENCES

Galicier C, Richet H. A prospective study of postoperative fever in a general surgery department. *Infect Control* 6:487, 1985.
Garibaldi RA, et al. Evidence for the non-infectious etiology of early postoperative fever. *Infect Control* 6:273, 1985.
Mourad O, et al. A comprehensive evidence-based approach to fever of unknown origin. *Arch Intern Med* 163:545, 2003.

32. FIRE IN THE OPERATING ROOM

I. **Problem**: A 14-year-old boy is undergoing excision of a dermoid cyst on his face under local anesthesia and intravenous sedation. In the middle of the procedure, use of electrocautery results in a fire that engulfs the area around the patient's head.

II. **Immediate questions:**

A. **What is on fire?** (patient's hair, drapes, respiratory apparatus, sponges, etc). Quickly remove burning materials (drapes, towels, sponges, etc) from the operative field.

B. **What gas is the anesthesiologist using?** (oxygen, nitrous oxide). Be sure the oxygen is turned off immediately.

C. **Where is the fire activation system?** (electrocautery, laser, fiberoptic lights, argon beam coagulator). Turn off any system still in use.

D. **Where is the nearest fire extinguisher?** (alarm pull station). Bring directly to the operating room.

III. **Differential diagnosis:**

A. **Fire, which is an exothermic reaction, requires the combination of an oxidizing agent, ignition, and fuel.** It is the lethal combination of these 3 things (often referred to as the "fire triangle") that leads to an operating room fire. In the operating room, these 3 elements commonly come into intimate contact, which leads to a fire. Therefore, once a fire starts, the goal is to separate these 3 factors.

1. **Oxidizing agents** include oxygen and nitrous oxide. Nitric oxide will support combustion as well as oxygen does. An oxygen-rich environment exists, such as oxygen trapped under drapes or towels.
2. **Ignition sources** include electrosurgical units, lasers, headlights, endoscopic lights, argon beam coagulators, microscopes, endoscopes and burrs.
3. **Fuels** include lanugo (fine hair), hair, gowns, masks, ointments, surgical drapes, dry sponges, prepping agents, large bowel gas, respiratory apparatus (endotracheal tubes, cannulas, face masks), and other surgical equipment.

IV. **Database.** Prevention is primary: "the best way to avoid a problem is not to get into it in the first place."

A. **Prevention**
1. Minimize oxygen concentration as tolerated by the patient.
2. Allow flammable preparations to dry (usually 2–3 minutes) before draping.
3. Avoid use of flammable preparations near the airway.
4. Adjust head draping to prevent oxygen accumulation. This is especially important in head and neck cases in which the surgeon works near the oxygen source, often with drapes that lead to collections of oxygen.
5. Avoid accidental activation of electrocautery or laser.
   a. Keep cautery stick in holster when not in use.
   b. Minimize voltage as necessary.
   c. Keep laser device on standby when not in use.
   d. Protect endotracheal tube if lasers are used nearby.
6. Use water-based lubricant to coat hair before use of cautery in that area.
7. Moisten sponges for airway or oropharyngeal surgery.
8. Communication between surgeon, anesthesiologist, and nursing staff is paramount.
9. Be sure that sponges used in body cavities (eg, intrathoracic cases) are moist to minimize flammability.

B. **Before surgery, identify fire plan of facility.**
1. Review fire prevention policy.
2. Review fire response policy.
3. Identify locations of fire alarm activation pull stations and fire extinguisher.

    4. Regular participation in fire drills

  C. Exercise care in the use of electrosurgical units, argon beam coagulators, and lasers.
    1. If possible, halt use of supplemental oxygen for 1 minute before using these devices.
    2. Activate the unit only when the tip is in view, especially when looking through a microscope.
    3. Deactivate the unit before the tip leaves the field.
    4. Place lasers in standby mode when not in active use. Place electrosurgical electrodes in holsters when not in use.
    5. Avoid the use of rubber catheter sleeves over electrosurgical electrodes.
    6. Be sure that sterile water or saline is available on the back table to douse a fire if necessary.

  D. Fiberoptic light sources.
    1. Fiberoptic light sources can start fires.
    2. Be sure that all connections are tight before activating the light source.
    3. Be sure the unit is in standby mode or turned off when disconnecting the cables.
    4. Never leave an illuminated cord on top of the drapes.

V. Plan
  A. Remove all burning materials (fuels) from the patient's body.
  B. Turn off the oxygen or nitrous oxide valve.
  C. Activate the fire alarm system.
  D. Fire extinguishers of choice in an operating room setting include halon and CO_2 extinguishers.
  E. Use sterile water or saline to douse the patient.
  F. Initiate standard care: think ABCs.
    1. Restore adequate ventilation, which may require intubation. (If previously intubated and the fire involved the endotracheal tube, this would have to be replaced.)
    2. Assess circulation.
    3. Manage initial pain if the patient is awake by a deeper sedation/general anesthesia.
  G. General evaluation survey of the extent of the burn. If the head and neck are involved, evaluate ocular or airway injury appropriately.
  H. Complete necessary portion of surgery.
  I. Resume standard care according to extent of burn injury; transfer to ICU or burn unit.

REFERENCES

Demos JE. Fire in the operating room. *Plast Reconstr Surg* 95:419–20, 1995.

ECRI. A clinician's guide to surgical fires: how they occur, how to prevent them, how to put them out [guidance article]. *Health Devices* 32:5–24, 2003.

JCAHO. Sentinel event alert. *JCAHO* 29, 2003.

33. FOLEY CATHETER PROBLEMS

(Bladder catheterization is discussed in Section III, Bedside Procedures.)

I. **Problem.** The Foley catheter in a patient, 2 days after undergoing a sigmoid colon resection, is not draining.

II. **Immediate Questions**

A. **What has the urine output been?** If the urine output has slowly tapered off, then the problem may be oliguria rather than a nonfunctioning Foley catheter. A Foley catheter that has never put out urine may not be in the bladder.

B. **Is the urine grossly bloody; are there any clots in the tubing or collection bag?** Clots or tissue fragments can obstruct the flow of urine in a Foley catheter.

C. **Is the patient complaining of any pain?** Bladder distention often causes severe lower abdominal pain; bladder spasms are painful and may cause urine to leak out around the catheter rather than through the catheter.

D. **Was any difficulty encountered in catheter insertion?** Problematic urethral catheterization should raise the possibility that the catheter is not in the bladder.

E. **How is the catheter secured in place?** Sometimes a suture or wire may restrict the flow or the catheter may have been damaged during placement.

G. **Has anyone tried to flush the catheter?** Flushing often helps relieve any obstruction due to clot or debris in the catheter lumen.

III. **Differential Diagnosis**

A. **Low Urine Output.** This may be a result of dehydration, hemorrhage, acute renal failure, and a host of other causes (see Problem 57, page 205).

B. **Obstructed Foley Catheter**
   1. Kinking of catheter or tubing.

2. **Clots, tissue fragments.** Most common after transurethral resection of the prostate or bladder. Grossly bloody urine suggests a clot has formed. "Tea"-colored or "rusty" urine suggests that an organized clot may be present even though the urine is no longer grossly bloody. Bleeding will often accompany "accidental" catheter removal with the balloon still inflated and with coagulopathy.

3. **Sediment/stones.** Chronically indwelling catheters can become encrusted and obstructed. Calculi can lodge in the catheter.

C. **Improperly Positioned Foley Catheter.** These problems are much more common in males. In traumatic urethral disruption the catheter can pass into the periurethral tissues. Strictures or prostatic hypertrophy may cause the end of the catheter to be positioned in the urethra and not in the bladder.

D. **Bladder Spasms.** The patient may complain of severe suprapubic pain or pain radiating to the end of the penis. With a spasm, urine may leak around the sides of the catheter. Spasms are common after bladder or prostate surgery or surgery around the bladder. Spasms may be the only catheter complaint or may be so severe as to obstruct the flow of urine.

E. **Bladder Disruption.** Resulting from blunt abdominal trauma or operative complication or caused by severe distention secondary to a blocked catheter.

F. **Inability to Deflate Foley Balloon.** Always test the catheter balloon before insertion.

IV. **Database**

A. **Physical Examination Key Points**
1. **Vital signs.** Check for tachycardia or hypotension, which is characteristic of hypovolemia.
2. **Abdominal examination.** Determine if the bladder is distended (suprapubic dullness to percussion with or without tenderness); may be indicative of an obstructed Foley catheter. Percuss the bladder to help identify distention.
3. **Genital examination.** Bleeding at the meatus suggests urethral trauma or partial removal of the catheter with the balloon inflated.
4. **Rectal examination.** A "floating prostate" suggests urethral disruption. This is of particular importance in the post-trauma patient. Palpation of a "floating prostate" usually accompanies a pelvic fracture secondary to blunt trauma.

     5. General. Look for signs of hypovolemia causing low urine output such as skin turgor, mucous membrane appearance, etc.

B. Laboratory Data. Most problems are usually mechanical in nature so that laboratory data are somewhat limited in this setting.

     1. BUN, serum creatinine. Increases may be seen with cases of renal insufficiency.

     2. Coagulation studies. Especially if severe bleeding is present.

C. Radiologic and Other Studies. In the acute setting of a Foley catheter problem, usually not needed. Ultrasound may demonstrate hydronephrosis in cases of obstructive uropathy.

V. Plan

A. First, be sure the catheter is functioning. A rule of thumb is that a catheter will not irrigate if it is in the urethra and not in the bladder. Start by gently irrigating the catheter by an using aseptic technique with a catheter-tipped 60-mL syringe and sterile NS. If sterile saline cannot be satisfactorily instilled and aspirated, the catheter should be replaced. Catheter irrigation or change in any patient who has undergone bladder or prostate surgery must be done with extreme care.

B. If the catheter irrigates freely, consider the workup for anuria. See Problem 57, page 205.

C. Bladder spasms can be controlled with oxybutynin (Ditropan), propantheline (Pro-Banthine), or belladonna and opium (B&O) suppositories (see dosage in Section IX, page 447). Be *sure* to discontinue these medications before removing the catheter to allow normal bladder function.

D. Bladder scan. If ultrasound shows fluid in bladder with a Foley catheter in place, it is not draining. Not as useful in large patients or patients with ascites.

E. Techniques to deflate a balloon that will not empty include:

     1. Injection of mineral oil 5–10 mL into the inflation port will cause balloon rupture in latex catheters in 5–10 minutes. Follow-up cystoscopy is recommended to make sure there are no retained fragments.

     2. Threading a 16F central venous catheter or 0.38–inch guidewire into the inflation channel (after the valve is removed) may bypass the obstruction.

     3. As a last resort, ultrasound-directed transvesical needle puncture of the balloon may be needed.

REFERENCES

Hollingsworth M, et al. The management of retained Foley catheters. *Can J Urol* 11:2163–6, 2004.
McGee S, et al. Is this patient hypovolemic? *JAMA* 281:1022, 1999.
Stickler D, et al. Why are Foley catheters so vulnerable to encrustation and blockage by crystalline bacterial biofilm? *Urol Res* 31:306–11, 2003.

34. HEADACHE

I. **Problem.** A 42-year-old man complaining of a headache presents to the clinic 4 days after inguinal hernia repair under spinal anesthesia.

II. **Immediate Questions**

   A. **What does the headache feel like?** Is it similar to previous headaches? A patient who complains that this is the worst headache of his life and is associated with vomiting and stiff neck may have a subarachnoid bleed or meningitis. Most other causes of headache require less immediate attention.

   B. **What makes the headache better or worse?** Spinal headaches typically increase as the patient sits up and decrease when the patient lies flat.

III. **Differential Diagnosis**

   A. **Spinal Headache.** Relatively common after spinal anesthesia or lumbar puncture because of a slow leak of cerebrospinal fluid. The use of smaller spinal needles has decreased the incidence of such headaches.

   B. **Sinusitis.** Often associated with specific areas of facial pain that can be reproduced by percussion over the sinus.

   C. **Vascular**
      1. **Cluster headaches and migraine headaches.** These are usually recurrent and unilateral.
      2. **Subarachnoid hemorrhage.** Often leads to severe headache and nuchal rigidity.
      3. **Others.** Giant cell arteritis, and sub- or epidural hematoma may cause headaches.

   D. **Tension.** This is by far the most common cause of headache in any patient population. This tension is usually a constant, band-like pressure, often occipital, and frequently associated with muscular tension in the neck.

   E. **Neoplastic.** Rarely does neoplasm result in headache in the absence of other focal neurologic abnormalities.

F. **Meningitis.** Nausea, vomiting, headache, fevers, and a stiff neck are hallmarks of this disease.

G. **Other.** Fever, dehydration, trauma, hypertension, and systemic viral illnesses can cause headache.

IV. Database

A. **History.** Determine whether the patient had a recent operation under spinal anesthesia. Determine history of similar headache and associated symptoms (eg, scotomata or nausea and vomiting).

B. **Physical Examination**
   1. **Vital signs.** Check temperature and blood pressure.
   2. **Head and neck.**
      a. Nuchal rigidity may indicate subarachnoid irritation or meningitis.
      b. Injected conjunctiva and excessive tearing are common with migraine.
      c. Percuss sinuses looking for tenderness.
      d. Tenderness in the temporal area can be associated with temporal arteritis.
      e. Papilledema suggests increased intracranial pressure.
      f. Tight trapezius muscles are associated with tension headaches.

C. **Laboratory Data.**
   1. **Hemogram.** A high WBC count may indicate infection.
   2. **Erythrocyte sedimentation rate.** A nonspecific test, but often high in temporal arteritis.

D. **Radiologic and Other Studies**
   1. **Head CT scan.** A scan of the head can be performed if subarachnoid hemorrhage is suspected or in new onset severe headache to rule out intracranial mass. Sinusitis can also be detected by CT scan. It should also be performed if neurologic examination reveals focal findings. If the headaches are recurrent and suspicious for migraines or cluster headaches, a CT scan is usually not immediately necessary.
   2. **Temporal arteritis**. Although a rare cause of headache, the diagnosis is confirmed by arterial biopsy, which requires a 1.5- to 2-cm segment of the temporal artery.

V. Plan.
Careful examination and history reveal the benign nature of headache in most cases. Most can be managed without narcotics.

A. **Spinal Headaches.** Headaches after lumbar puncture for spinal anesthesia should not be ignored. They can be very persistent and often require rest in a supine position, analgesics, and IV hydration. Refractory spinal headaches can be managed by injecting an autologous blood "patch" into the epidural space to seal the dural leak.

B. Migraine.
   1. Acute therapy for a mild-moderate migraine. Standard analgesics are usually effective, eg, NSAIDs, Fiorinal, Midrin, and butorphanol nasal spray (once in each nostril, repeat in 3–5 hours).
   2. Acute therapy for a severe migraine. Sumatriptan (Imitrex) 6 mg SC or dihydroergotamine (DHE 45) 1 mg IM, repeat 2 times at 1-hour intervals if needed.
   3. Some migraine patients require chronic prophylaxis with β blockers, tricyclic antidepressants (amitriptyline), or methysergide.

C. Intracranial Tumor or Subarachnoid Hemorrhage. Requires neurosurgical intervention.

D. Infections. Acute sinusitis can be controlled with PO antibiotics such as trimethoprim-sulfamethoxazole. Frontal sinusitis may need to be drained by the otolaryngology service. Meningitis requires urgent therapy with large-dose antibiotics.

REFERENCES

Dumas MD, et al. Computed tomography evaluation of patients with chronic headache. *CMAJ* 151:1447, 1994.
Lipton RB, et al. Efficacy and safety of acetaminophen in the treatment of migraine. Results of a randomized, double-blind, placebo-controlled, population-based study. *Arch Intern Med* 160:3486, 2000.
Smetana GW. The diagnostic value of historical features in primary headache syndromes. A comprehensive review. *Arch Intern Med* 160:2729, 2000.

35. HEMATEMESIS

Treat these patients like trauma patients!

Immediate Actions

1. Assess Airway, Breathing, and Circulation.
2. Obtain vital signs.
3. Intubate if necessary.
4. Ensure large-bore IV access and begin IV fluid or blood resuscitation. Send specimen for "type and cross."
5. Place NG tube.

I. Problem. A patient admitted for an elective LeVeen shunt suddenly begins vomiting blood.

II. Immediate Questions

A. **What are the blood pressure and orthostatic signs?** Initial management focuses on maintaining intravascular volume and perfusion pressure.

B. **Any bleeding tendencies?** Review available history, physical examination, and laboratory data regarding any correctable coagulation problem (PT, PTT, platelet count).

C. **Any stigmata of liver disease?** Look for ascites or signs of portal hypertension (caput medusae, etc).

D. **Did the patient retch or vomit before hematemesis?** A Mallory-Weiss tear is the fourth most common cause of hematemesis and is associated with severe substernal pain after an episode of *violent* vomiting.

E. **Does the patient have any history of aortic disease or a previous aortic vascular procedure?** Although rare, an aortoduodenal fistula should always be included in the initial differential diagnosis of UGI bleed, especially if the patient has a history of aortic surgery. Aortoduodenal fistula is extremely rare without previous aortic surgery.

III. Differential Diagnosis.
Hematemesis is virtually always associated with bleeding proximal to the ligament of Treitz. Ulcer disease, gastritis, esophageal varices, and Mallory-Weiss tears account for 90–95% of episodes of hematemesis. Esophageal varices are the most common cause of UGI bleeding.

A. **Esophagus**

1. **Esophageal varices.** Associated with cirrhosis and portal hypertension.

2. **Mallory-Weiss tear.** Usually a mucosal tear at the gastroesophageal junction that is associated with severe retching with or without vomiting.

3. **Esophagitis.** Classic history of heartburn, waking up with an acidic taste or food in the mouth, and increasing of symptoms with recumbency.

4. **Esophageal tumors.** Squamous or adenocarcinomas occasionally present with bleeding.

B. **Stomach**

1. **Gastritis.** Significant hematemesis may occur with alcoholic or ICU stress-induced gastritis.

2. **Gastric ulcer.** Symptoms can include severe pain, abdominal distention, nausea, and vomiting.

3. **Gastric tumors.** Rarely can present with bleeding. Associated with weight loss and inability to tolerate food.

4. **Gastric varices.** Almost always present with esophageal varices.

C. Duodenum
  1. **Duodenal ulcer.**
  2. **Aortoduodenal fistula.** Almost exclusively in cases of aortic reconstruction.
  3. **Postendoscopic sphincterotomy.**

D. Hemobilia. Usually secondary to tumor, liver, or biliary trauma or iatrogenic causes.

E. Systemic Causes
  1. **Coagulopathy** (DIC, leukemia, etc).
  2. **Osler-Weber-Rendu.** Associated with multiple telangiectases.
  3. **Peutz-Jeghers.** Associated with multiple hamartomas.

F. Non-GI source. Nasopharyngeal bleeding (see Problem 28, page 112).

IV. Database

A. Physical Examination Key Points
  1. **Vital signs.** Check orthostatic blood pressure measurements. Tachycardia or hypotension also suggests hypovolemia.
  2. **Skin.** Cool, moist, pale skin indicates volume loss; evidence of liver disease such as spider angiomata or palmar erythema; signs of systemic disease such as multiple bruises, telangiectases, or hamartomas of lips or oral mucosa.
  3. **HEENT.** Evidence of epistaxis or other nasopharyngeal source.
  4. **Abdomen.** Scars from previous surgery (ulcer, vascular, etc). Pain or evidence of peritonitis. Signs of portal hypertension (hepatosplenomegaly, caput medusa, or ascites).
  5. **Rectal.** Check for gross blood or melena. Check stool for occult blood (guaiac).
  6. **Genitourinary.** Check for testicular atrophy or gynecomastia as evidence for alcohol abuse.

B. Laboratory Data
  1. **Hemogram.** Obtain serial hematocrits (about every 4 hours) and document time drawn and relation to transfusions.
  2. **Platelet count.** Keep count >40,000.
  3. **PT/PTT.** Helps identify coagulopathies.
  4. **Renal function.** Should be determined as a baseline.
  5. **Liver function tests.** To document liver disease.
  6. **Blood bank specimen.** Remember with the initial blood draw to type and crossmatch for packed RBCs up to 6–10 U.

C. **Radiologic and Other Studies**
1. **Chest radiograph.** Look for mediastinal air, evidence of aspiration, free air under the diaphragm.
2. **Upper endoscopy.** This is the diagnostic and therapeutic procedure of choice. The endoscopist should be contacted immediately for urgent EGD.
3. **UGI series.** May be used if endoscopy is unavailable and if bleeding has stopped. It interferes with endoscopy and angiography so it is not usually a first-line study.
4. **Angiogram.** Rarely used unless endoscopy does not identify source.

V. **Plan.** In general, the treatment algorithm is to control volume loss, establish a diagnosis, and then implement specific therapies. Continued bleeding in any of these conditions requires the appropriate surgical intervention. However, about 85% of cases of UGI bleeding resolve without operative intervention.

A. **Initial Management**
1. Large-bore IVs (≥18 gauge) or central venous access to begin crystalloid boluses.
2. Type and crossmatch for packed RBCs (≥6 U).
3. **Place NG tube.** This documents ongoing bleeding and clears the stomach for endoscopy. Irrigate the stomach free of clots.
4. **Monitor volume replacement.**
a. Always chart serial hematocrits, timing, and amount of transfusions because this measures the rate of bleeding, which is the major criterion to decide if surgery is needed in many instances.
b. **Foley catheter.** Keep urine output >30 mL/h.
c. Central line and Swan-Ganz catheters may be needed especially in patients with cardiac/respiratory disease. Remember that rapid volume infusion is more efficient through a large peripheral line than through a central venous catheter.
5. Correct coagulopathy with platelets or FFP.
6. Consider intubation to protect the airway from aspiration.

B. **Specific Treatment.** After acute bleed has stabilized.
1. **Duodenal ulcer.**
a. **Antacids** through NG tube every 1–2 hours.
b. **IV H$_2$-receptor blockers** (cimetidine, ranitidine). May prevent rebleeding but probably does not stop ongoing bleeding. May be used with antibiotics.
c. **Endoscopic coagulation or heater probe.** If this fails, the patient will need surgical intervention. Note

that a posterior duodenal ulcer or massive bleeding will almost always require surgical intervention. The presence of a "visible vessel" also is associated with a higher incidence of rebleeding after endoscopic management and requires surgical intervention.

2. **Stress gastritis.**
   a. Antacids and IV H_2-receptor blockers.
   b. Endoscopic coagulation. If this fails, the patient may require urgent surgical resection.

3. **Esophageal varices.**
   a. Injection sclerotherapy by endoscopy.
   b. IV octreotide.
   c. Balloon tamponade (Sengstaken-Blakemore or Minnesota Tube) if endoscopy is unsuccessful. Should be placed only if you are experienced with these devices. Before placement, be sure to read the instruction manual that accompanies the device.
   d. Consider emergency portocaval shunt or radiologic transjugular intrahepatic portocaval shunting.

4. **Mallory-Weiss tear**
   a. Usually stops spontaneously.
   b. Endoscopic coagulation, surgical oversewing, and angiographic embolization are accepted therapies.

REFERENCES

Aljebreen AM, et al. Nasogastric aspirate predicts high-risk endoscopic lesions in patients with acute upper-GI bleeding. *Gastrointest Endosc* 59:172, 2004.

Antinori CH, et al. The many faces of aortoenteric fistulas. *Am Surg* 62:344, 1996.

Baradarian R, et al. Early intensive resuscitation of patients with upper gastrointestinal bleeding decreases mortality. *Am J Gastroenterol* 99:619, 2004.

36. HEMATURIA

I. **Problem.** A 51–year-old patient has blood in his urine 3 days after undergoing vagotomy and pyloroplasty.

II. **Immediate Questions**

A. **Is it gross or microscopic hematuria?** Microscopic hematuria may have been present for a long time, suggesting a chronic process, whereas gross hematuria usually will not have gone unnoticed in the past.

B. **Does the patient have a Foley catheter or ureteral stents in place?** Irritation of bladder mucosa by a Foley catheter is a common cause of hematuria in the hospitalized patient. Stents placed perioperatively by cystoscopy for difficult pelvic cases can cause minor bleeding.

C. Has the patient recently undergone abdominal surgery? Recent abdominal surgery (especially the night after surgery) may implicate intragenic ureteral, renal, or bladder injury.

D. Does the patient have abdominal pain or fever? Abdominal pain may suggest an inflammatory or infectious process. Infection would often be accompanied by fever. Renal colic typically radiates from the flank into the groin and suggests a stone.

E. Has the urine output remained adequate? Urine output is one of the best indicators of adequate renal function and perfusion. A sudden decrease in urine output may be indicative of rapid changes in renal function or a mechanical blockage due to clots.

F. Does the patient have symptoms of urinary tract infection? Dysuria, frequency, and urgency are common symptoms associated with urinary tract infections.

G. What is the history? A history of recent transurethral resection of the prostate (TURP) or resection of bladder tumor may explain the bleeding (microhematuria may persist 2–3 months after TURP). A remote history of bladder tumor may suggest a recurrent tumor. Chemotherapy with agents such as Cytoxan may cause acute hemorrhagic cystitis.

H. If female, when was the last period? Menses will often contaminate the urinalysis.

III. Differential Diagnosis

A. Foley Catheter Irritation/Trauma. This must be considered a diagnosis of exclusion in a patient with a Foley catheter. Be sure to complete the evaluation before attributing hematuria to this cause (see Problem 33, page 127.)

B. Stone. A calculus anywhere in the urinary tract from the kidney to the urethra can cause hematuria. It is usually associated with severe abdominal pain, especially when the stone is in the ureter.

C. Infection. An infection in the urinary tract can cause hematuria. It is important to obtain a clean-catch specimen for culture.

D. Tumor. Painless hematuria is the sine qua non of bladder tumors and can occur with renal cell carcinoma or prostatic carcinoma.

E. **Trauma.** Post-traumatic hematuria can be caused by a variety of lesions, such as renal parenchymal injury, or urethral injury secondary to pelvic fracture. A Foley catheter should *not* be inserted in any patient with suspected urethral injury (ie, blood at the urethral meatus) until a retrograde urethrogram has been performed to rule out urethral tear. Also consider an iatrogenic injury if the patient has undergone surgery adjacent to the urinary tract.

F. **Excessive Anticoagulation.** A common cause of hematuria in anticoagulated patients and requires adjustment of drug dosage. But also keep in mind that anticoagulants can cause bleeding from a pathologic lesion.

G. **Structural Abnormalities.** Polycystic kidney and medullary sponge kidney can cause hematuria. It is important to rule out other potential causes of hematuria in patients with known structural abnormalities.

H. **Prostatic Hypertrophy or Cancer.** Benign prostatic hypertrophy or prostatic cancer is a common cause in older males.

I. **Glomerulonephritis.** Red cell casts are often seen on urinalysis.

J. **Enterovesical Fistula.** As with most fistulas to the urinary tract, hematuria usually will not be the first sign. Often pneumaturia or an infection is the first sign.

K. **Vascular.** A variety of vascular lesions such as renal infarction, renal vein thrombosis, and atrioventricular malformations cause hematuria.

L. **Renal Papillary Necrosis.** Predominantly a disease of diabetics.

M. **Drugs.** Especially cyclophosphamide can cause hemorrhagic cystitis.

N. **Radiation Cystitis.** History of rectal or urologic malignancy.

O. **Hemorrhagic Cystitis.** Usually a complication of chemotherapy with Cytoxan and may predispose to transitional cell carcinoma.

P. **Systemic Diseases.** Systemic lupus erythematosus, hemolytic-uremic syndrome, and Goodpasture's syndrome (see Problem 37, page 141).

Q. **Tuberculosis.** Although the lung accounts for most cases of TB in the United States, renal involvement does occur, can cause hematuria, and is associated typically with sterile pyuria.

R. Sickle-Cell Anemia. Black patients with hematuria and no other obvious cause should be evaluated for sickle cell disease.

S. Contamination. Often caused by menstrual period or dysfunctional uterine bleeding. Check a catheterized specimen to exclude this cause.

T. Benign Essential Hematuria. A diagnosis of exclusion when no pathologic evidence of clinical bleeding can be found.

IV. Database

A. Physical Examination Key Points

1. **Abdomen.** Examine for palpable masses and tenderness indicative of tumors, infection, sickle cell disease, or inflammatory processes. Palpate the flanks for tenderness indicating a stone or pyelonephritis.

2. **Urethral meatus.** Look for gross blood at the meatus, especially in post-traumatic patients or in males with a pelvic fracture.

3. **Rectal examination.** Critical in the trauma patient. May reveal a "free-floating prostate" that may signify urethral disruption. Prostatic carcinoma or prostatitis may also be detected.

4. **Pelvic examination.** For evidence of cervical bleeding.

B. Laboratory Data

1. **Urinalysis.** Red cell casts are associated with upper tract bleeding; myoglobinuria (from crush or electrical injury) may be confused with hematuria (this is diagnosed with positive blood on the urinalysis but a 0 RBC count).

2. **Clotting studies** (PT/PTT/platelet count). Especially important to evaluate in the patient taking anticoagulant medication (warfarin, heparin, etc).

3. **Hemoglobin electrophoresis.** If sickle cell disease is suspected.

4. **Hemogram.** Attention to hematocrit and platelet count.

5. **Urine cytology.** May diagnose transitional cell carcinoma but not renal cell or prostate carcinoma. Many clinical laboratories offer "localization" studies in which the site of bleeding can be identified as renal or postrenal based on RBC morphology.

6. **Urine culture.** To rule out bacterial infection. Acid-fast stain checked on several urine specimens will help rule out TB of the urinary tract.

7. **BUN and creatinine.** Baseline renal function should be determined.

C. **Radiologic and Other Studies**
   1. **Abdominal plain radiograph.** Plain radiograph may show a urinary calculus
   2. **Excretory urography (IVP).** Usually the first diagnostic test performed after laboratory studies in patients with a suspected urinary calculus.
   3. **Retrograde urethrogram/cystogram.** In cases of pelvic trauma or clinical suspicion of urethral disruption or bladder rupture.
   4. Further studies that may be indicated include CT of the abdomen (especially in trauma patients or patients with suspected ureteral stone), ultrasound, angiography, and cystoscopy.

V. **Plan.** Therapy depends on the cause, which could take several days to ascertain. The "standard workup" of hematuria in the adult is physical examination, urinalysis, urine culture, urine cytology, IVP, and cystoscopy. Hematuria is rarely a cause for significant acute blood loss, and as long as renal function and urine output are not impaired, the workup of hematuria is generally not an emergency.

A. **Gross Hematuria with Clots.** Most frequently arises from the bladder and usually requires placement of a large irrigating "3-way" Foley catheter (eg, 24–26F, 30-mL balloon). Irrigate out the clots with a 60-mL syringe because clots present in the bladder will perpetuate bleeding. Irrigation with NS will often be necessary to keep urine clear until the source of bleeding is corrected.

B. **Specific Treatments**
   1. **Urinary tract infection.** Controlled with appropriate antibiotics. Follow-up urinalysis is needed to document the resolution of hematuria. Recurrent urinary tract infections need further workup.
   2. **Urolithiasis.** If the stone is expected to pass spontaneously (usually <1 cm), expectant therapy with analgesics and hydration is customary. Strain the urine to find the stone. If the stone does not pass, urologic consultation for ureteroscopy should be obtained.
   3. **Tumors.** Requires complete evaluation, usually with abdominal CT and other studies as indicated by urologic consultation.
   4. **Collecting system abnormality.** Requires further workup, usually retrograde ureteropyelogram and cystoscopy, and then management as indicated.
   5. **Coagulopathy.** Adjust dose of anticoagulant or manage with fresh frozen plasma as indicated.

6. Glomerulonephritis. Medical management as indicated; usually requires a biopsy.

7. Hemorrhagic cystitis. Controlled with saline irrigation and occasionally alum irrigation. Refractory, life-threatening cases may require formalin instillation in the operating room.

REFERENCES

Culclasure TF, et al. The significance of hematuria in the anticoagulated patient. *Arch Intern Med* 154:649, 1994.

Mariani AJ, et al. The significance of adult hematuria: 1000 hematuria evaluations including risk-benefit and cost-effective analysis. *J Urol* 141:350, 1989.

Sutton JM. Evaluation of hematuria in adults. *JAMA* 263:2475, 1990.

37. HEMOPTYSIS

I. **Problem.** A 50-year-old male smoker admitted for elective aortofemoral bypass coughs up bloody sputum.

II. **Immediate Questions**

A. **What are the vital signs?**
1. Fever (pulmonary infection).
2. Orthostasis, hypotension, and tachycardia (significant blood loss).
3. Tachycardia associated with tachypnea and decreased oxygen saturation (PE).

B. **Has this happened before?** Chronic hemoptysis, acute onset, amount of blood, history of epistaxis, and pain on coughing.

C. **Is the patient a smoker?** May suggest a neoplasm or chronic bronchitis.

D. **What volume of blood was coughed up?** Massive hemoptysis is defined as blood loss >500 mL in a 24–hour period.

E. **History of TB or pneumonia?** TB is associated with hemoptysis.

III. **Differential Diagnosis**

A. **Pulmonary Sources**
1. **Neoplastic**
a. **Bronchial carcinoma:**
i. Early: streaked sputum only.

        ii. Advanced: may erode into pulmonary vessels and cause severe hemorrhage or exsanguination.

    b. Bronchial adenoma: Uncommon, often highly vascular lesion.

  2. Infectious

    a. Tuberculosis.

    b. Fungal infections (eg, coccidiomycosis).

    c. Bacterial pneumonia: Rarely results in more than blood-streaked sputum. Exceptions: *Klebsiella* often results in bloody sputum, *Serratia marcescens* results in reddish sputum that is often confused with blood.

    d. Chronic bronchitis (smokers).

    e. Bronchiectasis.

  3. Vascular

    a. Pulmonary infarction from emboli: Hemoptysis accompanied by dyspnea and pleuritic chest pain. Look for DVT.

    b. Vascular aneurysms: Aortic aneurysms rarely erode into the bronchial tree, resulting in rapid exsanguination.

  4. Trauma. Pulmonary contusion after blunt trauma or vessel laceration after penetrating trauma can cause hemoptysis.

  5. Foreign body aspiration.

  6. Mitral stenosis. Rupture of pulmonary vessels due to high left atrial pressures.

B. Nonpulmonary Sources. Consider GI, oral, or nasal bleeding as the source of blood.

C. Systemic Causes. Hemoptysis is rarely the sole site of hemorrhage in a patient with a bleeding diathesis or systemic vasculitis (eg, leukemias, idiopathic thrombocytopenic purpura, Henoch-Schönlein purpura, Goodpasture's syndrome, and lupus erythematosus).

IV. Database

A. Physical Examination Key Points

  1. Vital signs including blood pressure (orthostasis, tachypnea).

  2. HEENT. Consider oral and nasal sources of bleeding.

  3. Chest. Decreased breath sounds (chest trauma), pleural rub (effusion or pulmonary infarction).

  4. Cardiac. Irregular beats (atrial fibrillation, atrial source of emboli) and mitral stenosis (low, rumbling diastolic murmur).

      5. **Abdomen.** Evaluate tenderness associated with peptic ulcer disease, a disease that can be confused with hemoptysis.

      6. **Extremities.** Evidence of DVT or cyanosis may be present.

B. Laboratory Data

    1. Hemogram (hematocrit and platelet counts).

    2. Coagulation studies.

    3. Sputum examination.

      a. **Culture routinely and send for Gram's stain:** A properly collected specimen will have few epithelial cells. Large numbers of epithelial cells suggest a saliva collection rather than sputum.

      b. **Acid fast bacillus (AFB) culture and stain.**

      c. **Sputum cytology.**

    4. **Renal function** (BUN/creatinine). Renal dysfunction usually accompanies hemoptysis in Goodpasture's syndrome.

C. Radiologic and Other Studies

    1. **Chest radiograph is mandatory.** It may show infiltrates, infarct, obstructing lesion, contusion, pneumothorax, rib fracture, or aortic aneurysm.

    2. **Chest CT scan** further defines suspicious lesions seen on routine chest radiograph.

    3. **Bronchoscopy,** although not as readily available as a chest radiograph, often will allow diagnosis of the source of hemoptysis. This should be performed when acute bleeding subsides (rigid bronchoscopy may be helpful).

    4. **Angiogram** can define a possible fistula between the aneurysm (seen on radiograph or CT) and the bronchial tree or visualizes bleeding sources not seen on bronchoscopy. Pulmonary angiogram provides the definitive diagnosis of PE.

    5. **Electrocardiogram** evaluates an irregular pulse or suspected atrial fibrillation.

    6. Purified protein derivative skin test to evaluate for TB infection.

    7. **Nuclear V/Q scan.** Initial evaluation of suspected PE.

V. Plan

A. Immediate Management. With significant hemorrhage, ICU monitoring of the patient is required.

    1. Establish venous access with large-bore ($\geq$16 gauge) IVs. Replace volume as for any patient with blood loss. Type and crossmatch.

2. Protect the airway because these patients are at significant risk for asphyxia. Consider endotracheal intubation.
3. Gastric lavage with an NG tube differentiates between GI and pulmonary hemorrhage.
4. Nurses should collect and quantify all bloody sputa.
5. Pulmonary consultation for urgent bronchoscopy should be obtained if balloon tamponade may be required.

B. Specific Plans

1. **Neoplasm.** Pulmonary resection should be performed when feasible (emergently if there is massive bleeding).
2. **Infection.** Initially start empirical antibiotics and then modify based on culture results. TB or fungal cavities that are bleeding may require urgent surgical excision.
3. **Vascular.**
   a. Pulmonary infarction from embolization is controlled with heparin to prevent further clot propagation. Consider streptokinase or urokinase in the nonoperative patient. Thoracotomy and embolectomy is used in the salvageable critically ill patient. A Greenfield filter may be necessary if anticoagulation fails or is contraindicated.
   b. **Aneurysm:** Sentinel bleeding from eroding aneurysms can precede exsanguinating hemorrhage. Resection with prosthetic replacement should be attempted when possible.
   c. Erosion into the innominate artery from a tracheostomy tube (usually heralded by minor sentinel bleedings) is life threatening. Evaluate all tracheostomy patients who have even minor bleeding. In acute bleeding, apply digital pressure inside the anterior wall of the trachea or with the inflated balloon of an endotracheal.
4. **Trauma.**
   a. Blunt flail chest with underlying pulmonary contusion leading to hemoptysis often results in severe respiratory decompensation. Control with positive pressure mechanical ventilation and aggressive pulmonary toilet.
   b. Penetrating trauma resulting in hemoptysis should be initially managed with tube thoracostomy; persistent bloody drainage or hemoptysis mandates exploratory thoracotomy. Bronchial tree disruption can cause hemoptysis and requires thoracotomy.
5. **Foreign body** is usually successfully retrieved by rigid bronchoscopy.
6. **Massive hemoptysis.**

a. Thoracotomy and resection are sometimes needed in cases of massive hemoptysis.
b. Double lumen endotracheal tubes allow for complete collapse of the affected lung, resulting in shunting of circulation away from this lung. This method of control also allows for localization of the bleeding site to the affected side.
c. Bronchoscopy with balloon tamponade can also be used if available.

REFERENCES

Santiago S, et al. A reappraisal of the causes of hemoptysis. *Arch Intern Med* 151:2449, 1991.
Weinberger SE. *Principles of Pulmonology Medicine,* 3rd ed. Philadelphia: WB Saunders; 1998, p 27–8.
Wiese T, et al, eds. *Pulmonary Diseases,* 7th ed. Philadelphia: Lippincott Williams & Wilkins; 2004, p 89–90.

38. HICCUPS (SINGULTUS)

I. **Problem.** A patient admitted for right upper quadrant pain with possible cholecystitis develops hiccups for 4 hours.

II. **Immediate Questions**

A. **Is there new or increased abdominal pain?** Hiccups may be associated with a variety of significant intra-abdominal diseases. Evaluate associated abdominal symptoms.

B. **Is there shoulder pain or pain with respiration?** Referred pain to the shoulder or pleuritic pain may suggest diaphragmatic irritation (subphrenic abscess, cholecystitis, pneumonia) that is associated with hiccups.

C. **Does the patient have any cardiac history or symptoms?** On rare occasions, ill patients who complain of hiccups may be presenting with a transmural MI.

D. **Are there any emotional problems with the patient?** Anxiety or other psychogenic causes associated with hiccups are prevalent in women. Inquire about previous problems with hiccups.

III. **Differential Diagnosis.** Hiccups are usually a short-term innocuous complaint, often a result of aerophagia caused by rapid eating, drinking, or laughter. Even in chronic situations, no organic cause may be found. The list below presents some organic disorders in which hiccups may be present.

A. **Diaphragmatic/Phrenic Nerve Irritation**
1. Subphrenic abscess

      2. Pneumonia/pleuritis
      3. MI
      4. Pericarditis
      5. Peritonitis
      6. Metastatic implants on the diaphragm
      7. Lung tumors
      8. Postoperative

B. GI Diseases
      1. Gastric dilatation
      2. Hiatal hernia
      3. Pancreatitis

C. Metabolic Diseases
      1. Uremia
      2. Diabetes
      3. Alcohol abuse

D. CNS Dysfunction. "Central hiccups" is often caused by posterior fossa tumor or infarction or encephalitis. In neonates, it may indicate a seizure.

E. Psychogenic. The hallmark is that these stop when the patient is asleep.

IV. Database

A. Physical Examination Key Points
      1. Vital signs. Spiking temperatures (abscess).
      2. Pulmonary. Decreased diaphragmatic excursion (accompanies diaphragmatic irritation). Evidence for an infiltrate or effusion.
      3. Cardiac. Pericardial friction rub.
      4. Abdomen. Distention (ascites or gaseous), pain, peritoneal signs, hepatosplenomegaly, tympany, especially over the gastric area, may suggest a diagnosis. "Punch tenderness" over the lower ribs may suggest diaphragmatic inflammation.

B. Laboratory Data
      1. Hemogram especially with infection.
      2. Renal function tests. Increased BUN and creatinine with uremia.
      3. Glucose. Glucose tolerance test to diagnose diabetes.
      4. Amylase. High in pancreatic disease.

C. Radiologic and Other Studies
      1. Chest radiograph. Elevation of diaphragm, effusion, infiltrate, or tumor.
      2. Abdominal radiograph. Gastric dilatation may be seen on this study or on chest radiograph.

    3. Electrocardiogram. Rule out ischemic changes if clinically indicated.
    4. Ultrasound/CT abdomen. May display subphrenic fluid collections or other pathology.
    5. CT chest. Chest tumors may irritate the phrenic nerve.

V. Plan. Any significant associated condition (MI, gastric dilatation, subphrenic abscess) should be managed in the appropriate manner.

  A. Mechanisms to Interfere with Respiration. Low P_{CO_2} accentuates hiccups, whereas high P_{CO_2} inhibits them. Maneuvers to increase P_{CO_2}:
    1. Breath holding.
    2. Drinking water rapidly.
    3. Rebreathing from a paper bag.

  B. Mechanisms to Alter Afferent Pathways
    1. Stimulate nasopharynx with cotton swab.
    2. Swallow dry granulated sugar 1 teaspoon.

  C. Pharmacologic Management
    1. Chlorpromazine. 25–50 mg PO/IM every 6 hours.
    2. Perphenazine. 4–8 mg PO or 5 mg IM every 8 hours.
    3. Metoclopramide. 10 mg PO every 6 houes for several days.

REFERENCES

Anthoney TR, et al. On temporal structure of human hiccups: etiology and chronobiology. *Int J Chronobiol* 5:477–92, 1978.
Fischer JE, et al. Manifestation of gastrointestinal disease. In: Schwartz SI, et al, eds. *Principles of Surgery.* New York: McGraw-Hill; 1999, p 1046–7.
Kolodzik PW, Eilers MA. Hiccups (singultus): review and approach to management. *Ann Emerg Med* 20:565–73, 1991.

39. HYPERCALCEMIA

I. Problem. A 45-year-old male who is scheduled for surgery in the morning has a serum calcium of 12.5 mg/dL (normal 8.5–10.5 mg/dL).

II. Immediate Questions

  A. Is the patient symptomatic? "Stones, bones, abdominal groans, and psychic overtones" is an often used phrase to describe the symptom complex associated with hypercalcemia. Delirium, confusion, lethargy, nausea and vomiting, abdominal pain, symptoms of kidney stones such as cerebrovascular accident (CVA) tenderness, and bone pain are often seen with calcium levels >12 mg/dL (or ionized level >3.0 mmol/L).

B. Has the patient recently had surgery? In particular, adrenal surgery (hypoadrenalism) or long-term immobilization that can cause excessive bone resorption and hypercalcemia.

C. What IV fluids and medications are currently being given? There may be medications increase calcium levels (lithium, thiazide diuretics, vitamin D) or administration of exogenous calcium.

D. Is there any history of cancer or parathyroid disease? Hypercalcemia can be caused by a paraneoplastic syndrome associated with cancer (secretion of hormone resembling parathyroid hormone [PTH]). Bone metastasis can also cause hypercalcemia.

E. Is there a history of peptic ulcer disease? Milk alkali syndrome is seen when a patient tries to relieve symptoms of peptic ulcers by drinking excessive amounts of milk.

F. Is there a history of granulomatous disease? TB, coccidiomycosis, histoplasmosis, and sarcoidosis can cause hypercalcemia.

III. Differential Diagnosis. (See also Section II, page 279)

A. Hyperparathyroidism. About 20% of patients with hypercalcemia will have associated hyperparathyroidism. Primary hyperparathyroidism is usually diagnosed with high calcium level, low phosphate level, and high PTH level.

B. Malignant Neoplasm. This is the most frequent cause of hypercalcemia, usually caused by bone metastasis or by blood-borne factors secreted by the tumors (multiple myeloma, lung, breast, kidney).

C. Thiazide Diuretics. Increases renal resorption of calcium (eg, hydrochlorothiazide).

D. Granulomatous Diseases. The granulomatous tissue may produce a vitamin D metabolite.

E. Vitamin D Intoxication. Usually chronic ingestion.

F. Milk-Alkali Syndrome. Excessive alkali and calcium in the management of peptic ulcer disease (less frequent today with use of magnesium-containing antacids).

G. Hyperthyroidism.

H. Adrenal Insufficiency.

I. Paget's Disease. Usually with secondary hyperparathyroidism.

J. Acute tubular necrosis (diuretic phase).

K. Acromegaly.

L. Excessive calcium administration.

M. Long-term immobilization.

IV. Database.

A. Physical Examination Key Points

1. **Vital signs.** Hypertension may accompany hypercalcemia.
2. **Cardiac.** Arrhythmias (bradycardia, tachycardia).
3. **Chest.** Breast carcinoma may be suggested by a mass lesion or previous mastectomy.
4. **Abdomen.** Check for masses.
5. **Bones.** Tenderness to palpation (metastatic disease).
6. **Nodes.** Lymphadenopathy (cancer, granulomatous disease).
7. **Neurologic** weakness, hyperactive reflexes, impaired mentation (stupor, delirium).
8. **Skin.** Pruritus.
9. **Rectal examination.** Evidence of prostate cancer (high likelihood of bone metastases).

B. Laboratory Data

1. **Serum calcium and albumin.** Repeat to confirm high levels. **Caution:** Units of calcium measurement may differ across institutions (mg/dL vs mEq/dL). With abnormal albumin, a corrected calcium level must be determined (see page 279).
2. **Phosphorus.** Low in hyperparathyroidism except if renal failure is present.
3. **Potassium, magnesium.** Decreases may be associated with high serum calcium level.
4. **Arterial blood gases.** Acidosis with hyperchlorhydria.
5. **Alkaline phosphatase.** High in hyperparathyroidism with bone disease.
6. **Renal function.** Renal insufficiency will exacerbate hypercalcemia.
7. **PTH level.** Increased in primary or secondary hyperparathyroidism, often decreased in hypercalcemia not caused by hyperparathyroidism.

C. Radiologic and Other Studies

1. **Chest radiograph.** Hilar adenopathy (sarcoidosis, lymphoma).
2. **Abdomen radiograph.** Renal stones (hyperparathyroidism).
3. **Skull.** Punched out lesions (multiple myeloma).

4. **Bones.** Osteolytic lesions (metastatic cancer), osteitis fibrosa cystica (brown cysts in bone), or subperiosteal resorption on radial aspect of second and third phalanges and distal clavicles.

5. **Intravenous pyelogram.** Renal stones (hyperparathyroidism, renal cell carcinoma).

7. **Electrocardiogram.** Shortened QT interval and prolonged PR interval.

8. **Cortisone suppression test.**
   a. No response: hyperparathyroidism.
   b. Decrease in calcium: metastatic cancer, myeloma, sarcoid, vitamin D intoxication, milk-alkali syndrome, adrenal insufficiency.

V. Plan

A. **Initial Management.** Decrease serum calcium (if necessary) and then control underlying cause.
   1. **Levels <12 mg/dL.** Manage underlying cause.
   2. **Moderate increase (12–15 mg/dL).** Hydration and loop diuretics (furosemide).
   3. **Severe hypercalcemia (>15 mg/dL or any symptomatic patient regardless of level).** A life-threatening emergency that requires more rigorous therapy.

B. **Specific Plans**
   1. Restrict calcium intake, encourage mobilization, and control underlying disorder in all cases. Calcium-containing and calcium-increasing medications include calcium carbonate antacids (Tums), vitamins A and D, and thiazide diuretics (hydrochlorothiazide).
   2. **Saline diuresis.** After the patient is adequately hydrated, use IV NS and furosemide (goal: urine 100–200 mL/h). Sodium increases calcium excretion by competing for resorption in distal tubule. Use caution in the presence of renal or cardiac failure. Monitor serum calcium, phosphate, potassium, magnesium, and BUN.
   3. **Furosemide** can be given 20–40 mg IV every 2–4 hours to bring calcium levels <12 mg/dL after hydration. Monitor serum potassium during diuresis and replace as necessary.
   4. **Corticosteroids.** Ineffective against primary hyperparathyroidism and may take 1–2 weeks to see effect; used with malignancies. Prednisone 5–15 mg PO daily is fairly typical dosing.
   5. **Bisphosphonates.** Pamidronate (preferred bisphosphonate) 90 mg over 24 hours or etidronate 7.5 mg/g IV daily for 3 days followed by 5–20 mg/kg PO per day. Potent inhibitors of bone resorption due to cancer. Do

not use in renal failure. Onset of action is delayed by
4–5 days.

6. **Calcitonin** inhibits bone resorption and works quickly,
but only minimally decreases the amount of hypercalcemia (maximum decrease is 0.5 mmol/L). Administer 4
U/kg every 12 hours.

7. **Dialysis.** As a last resort if extremely high levels cannot
be decreased.

8. **Other agents.** Mithramycin is used as a last resort in
the management of hypercalcemia due to the severe
complication of aplastic anemia (25 µg/kg over 4
hours).

REFERENCES

Bilezikian JP. Management of acute hypercalcemia. *N Engl J Med*
326):1196–203, 1992.
Bourke E, Delaney V. Assessment of hypocalcemia and hypercalcemia.
Clin Lab Med 13:157–81, 1993.
Greenfield LJ, et al. *Surgery: Scientific Principles and Practice,* 2nd ed.
Philadelphia: Lippincott-Raven; 1997, p 257–8.

40. HYPERGLYCEMIA

I. **Problem.** An elderly woman who has just undergone hemi-
colectomy has a high urine output and is complaining of thirst.
A stat serum glucose is 285 mg/dL (normal 70–105 mg/dL).

II. **Immediate Questions**

A. **Is there a history of diabetes?** Patients with insulin-dependent diabetes require a portion of their daily insulin
dose even while NPO (usually 50% of their morning dose
before surgery). Surgical stress may temporarily create insulin requirements in the patient with non-insulin-dependent diabetes. No history of diabetes suggests other
problems: over-alimentation, sepsis, side effects of glucocorticoid use, etc.

B. **What are the vital signs?** Fever may represent a septic
episode, which can cause glucose intolerance. New onset
or sudden hyperglycemia in a patient with diabetes can be
the first sign of infection.

III. **Differential Diagnosis.** (See also Section II, page 299.)

A. **Diabetes**
1. **Insulin-dependent (type I; formerly called juvenile
diabetes).** Requires insulin even when NPO.
2. **Non-insulin-dependent (type II; formerly called
adult onset diabetes).** Surgical stress often aggra-

vates diabetes. Thus, patients whose diabetes is controlled with diet or oral hypoglycemic agents may develop a worsening of their diabetes that requires therapy with insulin.

B. Hyperosmolar Coma (nonketotic hyperglycemic). Syndrome characterized by impaired consciousness, extreme dehydration, sometimes seizures, and extreme hyperglycemia that is not accompanied by ketoacidosis. It is a complication of non-insulin-dependent diabetes mellitus and has a >50% mortality rate.

C. Sepsis. Glucose intolerance is often an early sign of sepsis in the critically ill patient.

D. Hyperalimentation. Typical central parenteral nutrition solutions contain up to 35% glucose solution. Advancing too quickly or receiving amounts above nutritional requirements may cause hyperglycemia.

E. Gestational Diabetes. Some women develop hyperglycemia during pregnancy.

F. Other Causes
  1. Medication. Insulin resistance can result from steroid use or oral contraceptives.
  2. Cushing's syndrome.
  3. Pancreatic disease or resection.

IV. Database

A. Physical Examination Key Points
  1. Vital signs. Fever and tachycardia suggest infection, and hypotension suggests sepsis. Kussmaul respiration (deep, rapid respiratory pattern) may be seen with severe ketoacidosis.
  2. HEENT. Fruity odor on the breath may signify ketoacidosis.
  3. Lungs. Listen for evidence of pneumonia.
  4. Abdomen. Exclude intra-abdominal causes of sepsis.
  5. Neurologic. Obtundation may indicate deterioration of a diabetic condition and the development of ketoacidosis.

B. Laboratory Data.
Significantly increased chemstick results should be confirmed with a serum glucose determination and electrolytes to rule out ketoacidosis.
  1. Serum electrolytes. Potassium and phosphorus must be monitored closely in DKA.
  2. Arterial blood gas. Any suspicion of sepsis or DKA should be followed-up with a determination of serum pH and partial pressure of oxygen (PO_2).

3. Serial serum ketones and anion gap are useful in following therapy for DKA.
4. **Hemogram.** High leukocyte count (infection).
5. Culture blood, urine, central lines, etc, if infection is suspected.
6. **Urine glucose.** Thresholds for spilling glucose in the
urine can vary widely; confirm with serum glucose if any
doubt exists.

C. **Radiologic and Other Studies.** Studies should be selected based on clinical impression. For example, infection
in the postoperative hyperglycemic patient may be evaluated with a chest radiograph if a pulmonary source is suspected or an abdominal CT scan if an intra-abdominal
abscess is considered.

V. Plan

A. **Initial Management.** Controlling serum glucose quickly
and safely and managing predisposing infection appropriately.

B. **Specific Plans**
1. **Sliding scale insulin.** Small doses of regular insulin
SC can be given every 6 hours based on rapid, automated evaluation of blood sugars using chemsticks.
This is the best way to achieve good control of sugars
in the patient on NPO therapy. Typically, a serum glucose level <200 mg/dL is considered adequate control.
A typical sliding scale is as follows: for glucose <80
mg/dL, call physician; 81–150 mg/dL, no units;
151–200 mg/dL, regular human insulin 2 U SC;
201–250 mf/dL, 4 U; 251–300 mg/dL, 6 U; 301–350
mg/dL, 8 U; >350 mg/dL, call physician. Any chemstick
level >400 mg/dL should be confirmed with a stat
serum measurement from the laboratory. It is safer to
start with a low dosing scale because patients with
more resistant diabetes may need larger doses.
2. **Diet.** Modification is needed in diabetic patients, with
caloric restriction in the obese patient being important.
Usual diet ordered is 1800 cal/day of diet as recommended by the American Diabetes Association for females and 2000 cal/day for males.
3. **Oral hypoglycemic agents.** Many patients with type II
diabetes who are admitted on these medications require insulin supplements after an operation but are
usually discharged on the same agent.
4. **Severe glucose intolerance due to sepsis and DKA**.
Requires aggressive therapy in an ICU setting. DKA is
usually manifested as tachypnea, dehydration, ketones

on the breath, abdominal pain, with hyperglycemia, hyperketonemia, and metabolic acidosis.

  a. **Precipitating factors:** In the surgical patient, infection precipitates severe glucose intolerance. It should be appropriately controlled.

  b. **Dehydration:** Patients become volume depleted, often because of severe glycosuria. Rehydrate initially with dextrose-free saline. Increased urine output may be a result of osmotic diuresis and may not be a reflection of the true volume status. Assess volume status by other means (eg, Swan-Ganz catheter).

  c. **Potassium:** As DKA decreases, serum potassium levels decrease (ions become intracellular). Total body potassium is also depleted. Start replacing potassium with the second bag of IV solution.

  d. **Bicarbonate:** Correction of severe acidosis with bicarbonate is sometimes needed. Continue insulin until the bicarbonate normalizes. This may require insulin and glucose intravenously.

  e. **Insulin:** Start with a 10- to 20-U IV bolus followed by a continuous drip. Infusion rate will vary (2–5 U/h initially and adjust as needed). Fingerstick glucose should be checked frequently (every 2 hours) while using an insulin drip.

  f. **Dextrose:** Change IV fluids to those containing D5 when serum glucose levels decrease to 300 mg/dL.

  g. **Maintenance insulin:** Once IV therapy has controlled severe hyperglycemia, maintenance insulin is needed. To achieve better control, administer NPH plus regular insulin SC twice daily. Calculate starting dose by adding daily insulin requirements (total of sliding scale insulin administered previous day) and giving two-thirds in the morning and one-third in the afternoon (two-thirds NPH and one-third regular insulin). Patients on hyperalimentation receive maintenance insulin by adding it directly to the solution.

REFERENCES

Alberti KG, Zimmet PZ. Definition, diagnosis and classification of diabetes mellitus and its complications. Part 1: diagnosis and classification of diabetes mellitus. Provisional report of a WHO consultation. *Diabet Med* 15:539–45, 1998.

Greenfield LJ, et al. *Surgery: Scientific Principles and Practice,* 2nd ed. Philadelphia: Lippincott-Raven; 1997, p 54–9.

Rose BD, Post TW. *Clinical Physiology of Acid-Base and Electrolyte Disorders,* 5th ed. New York: McGraw-Hill; 2001, p 809–15.

41. HYPERKALEMIA

I. **Problem.** A patient with a crush injury has a serum potassium level of 7.1 mmol/L on the second hospital day (normal 3.5–5.1 mEq/L).

II. **Immediate Questions**

A. **What are the vital signs?** Cardiac effects of hyperkalemia can result in life-threatening arrhythmias.

B. **What is the patient's urine output?** Inability to excrete endogenous or exogenous potassium load is the most common cause of acute hyperkalemia on a surgical service. Evaluate urine output and recent renal function chemistries. Ensure there is no obstruction to urinary flow.

C. **Is the patient receiving potassium in an IV solution?** A bag of IV solution may contain potassium 20–40 mEq/L and hyperalimentation solutions may contain more. Stop all exogenous potassium until the problem is resolved.

D. **Is the laboratory result accurate?** Abnormally high potassium levels are often entirely unexpected or inconsistent. Inquire about hemolysis of the specimen, which can falsely increase potassium.

E. **Is the patient on any medication that could increase potassium?** If the patient is receiving spironolactone, triamterene, or indomethacin, stop these medications immediately.

III. **Differential Diagnosis.** The measured laboratory value of extracellular potassium concentration is the level that correlates with the harmful consequences of hyperkalemia. This extracellular level can be increased by redistribution of potassium from intracellular stores (where 98% of the total body potassium is located) or by a real increase in total body potassium.

A. **Redistribution**
   1. **Acidosis.**
   2. **Insulin deficiency.**
   3. **Digoxin overdose.**
   4. **Succinylcholine.** Increased risk in chronically debilitated or burn patients.
   5. **Cellular breakdown.**
      a. **Crush injury** (rhabdomyolysis).
      b. **Hemolysis.**

B. **Increased Total Body Potassium**
   1. **Renal causes.**
      a. **Acute renal failure.**

      b. Chronic renal failure: Potassium will not usually be high until end-stage disease, typically with creatinine clearance <20 mL/s.

      c. Renal tubular dysfunction: Associated with renal transplantation, lupus erythematosus, sickle cell disease, or myeloma.

  2. Mineralocorticoid deficiency.

      a. Addison's disease.

      b. Hypoaldosteronism (hyporeninemic).

  3. Drug-induced. Common causes:

      a. Spironolactone.

      b. Triamterene.

      c. Indomethacin: Interferes with renal prostaglandin levels.

      d. Cyclosporine.

      e. Excess potassium supplementation.

      f. Heparin: Decreases aldosterone synthesis.

C. Pseudohyperkalemia

  1. Hemolysis of the specimen.

  2. Prolonged period of tourniquet occlusion before drawing blood.

  3. Thrombocytosis/leukocytosis: WBCs and platelets release potassium as the clot forms.

IV. Database

A. Physical Examination Key Points

  1. Cardiac. Bradycardia, ventricular fibrillation, and asystole with markedly high potassium levels.

  2. Neuromuscular. Tingling, weakness, flaccid paralysis, and hyperactive deep tendon reflexes. Cardiac arrest often precedes these symptoms.

B. Laboratory Data

  1. Electrolytes, BUN, and creatinine. Hyperkalemia usually diagnosed by this study, and renal failure may be detected.

  2. Arterial blood gas. Non-anion gap acidosis associated with hyperkalemia.

  3. Platelet count, WBC count. Increases may yield factitious hyperkalemia. With significant platelet and WBC increases, order a plasma potassium level.

  4. Cortisol levels or corticotropin stimulation test.

  5. Digoxin level if indicated.

  6. Myoglobin level in serum/urine. Useful in crush injury.

C. Radiologic and Other Studies

  1. Electrocardiogram. The second most important test other than potassium level. Can separate pseudohyperkalemia from actual increases in potassium. Changes seen as potassium increases include peaked T waves, flat P waves, prolonged PR interval, and a widened QRS complex progressing to a sine wave and arrest (Figure I–15). A simple way to remember this is to think of the "T wave" as a potassium reservoir.

2. **Ultrasound.** Especially based on renal insufficiency. May show obstructed kidneys or bladder or small kidneys owing to chronic renal disease.

V. **Plan.** Severity of hyperkalemia as judged by serum level and ECG dictate therapy. In general, aggressive therapy of hyperkalemia is indicated for a serum potassium level >6.5–7 mmol/L or if ECG changes are present. Therapeutic methods ranked by the rapidity of the response are mechanisms that counteract membrane effects of hyperkalemia, move potassium into cells, and remove potassium from the body.

A. **Immediate Actions**
   1. Severe hyperkalemia (>6.5 mEq/L) necessitates immediate ECG monitoring.
   2. Administer 10% calcium gluconate 10–20 mL IV (protects the heart from dysrhythmias).
   3. Begin maneuvers to decrease potassium levels as noted below.

B. **Specific Plans**
   1. **Counteract membrane effects.** Counteract membrane effects and protect the heart by using 10% calcium gluconate 10–20 mL IV over 3–5 minutes while on a cardiac monitor. Use with close monitoring in patients on digitalis because arrhythmia may occur.
   2. **Transfer Potassium to the Intracellular Compartment.**

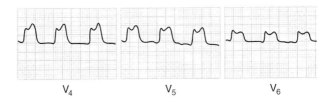

Figure I–15. Diffuse tall T waves in leads V4, V8, and aVF with widened QRS complex and junctional rhythm (loss of P waves), representing hyperkalemia. *(Reproduced, with permission, from Lefor AT. Critical Care On Call. Copyright (c) 2002 by The McGraw-Hill Companies, Inc.)*

a. **Sodium bicarbonate 1 ampule (44 mEq) IV.** May repeat 1–2 times every 20–30 minutes. Works best in patients with acidosis but also has effects in those with normal pH.

b. **Insulin/glucose.** 50% dextrose in water (D50W) 1 ampule and regular insulin 10 U IV given over 5 minutes.

c. A combination therapy of the above 2 methods consists of D10W 1 L mixed with sodium bicarbonate 3 ampules. Administer over 2–4 hours with regular insulin 10 U SC every 4–6 hours.

3. **β-Agonists.** Albuterol nebulizer every 4 hours will drive potassium intracellularly.

C. **Removal of Potassium from the Body**
   1. **Kayexalate (exchange resin).**
      i. **Oral:** 30 g in 70% sorbitol 30–70 mL every 4–6 hours.
      ii. **Rectal:** 50–100 g in water 200 mL given as a retention enema for 30 minutes every 2–4 hours.
   a. **Dialysis:** Peritoneal or hemodialysis.
   b. **Furosemide:** Monitor urine output and volume status carefully. Administer furosemide IV.
   2. **Remove all potassium from IV fluids.**

D. Any ECG changes should incite prompt transfer to a monitored bed (see Figure I–15).

E. Consider Foley catheter insertion to aid in assessing urine output and eliminate sources of lower urinary tract obstruction.

F. **Long-term Therapy.** For diseases such as chronic renal failure, use potassium-restricted diet (40–60 mEq/day). Addison's disease usually requires glucocorticoid and mineralocorticoid therapy.

REFERENCES

Berne RM, Levy MN. *Cardiovascular Physiology,* 4th ed. St Louis: Mosby; 1981, p 7–17.
Greenfield LJ, et al. *Surgery: Scientific Principles and Practice,* 2nd ed. Philadelphia: Lippincott-Raven; 1997, p 236–7, 255–6.
Rose BD, Post TW. *Clinical Physiology of Acid-Base and Electrolyte Disorders,* 5th ed. New York: McGraw-Hill; 2001, p 383–96, 898–910, 913–9.

42. HYPERNATREMIA

I. **Problem.** The laboratory calls to tell you that an 85–year-old female patient has a serum sodium level of 155 mmol/L (normal 136–145 mmol/L).

II. Immediate Questions

  A **Is the patient alert and oriented, or seizing?** Symptoms of hypernatremia usually occur once the level is >160 mmol/L (irritability, ataxia, anorexia, cramping). Levels >180 mmol/L may result in confusion, stupor, or seizure.

  B. **Is this an acute or chronic problem?** Look at the trends of the patient's laboratory values.

  C. **What medication is the patient taking?** Look for diuretics.

  D. **What are the intake/output values for the past few days?** A loss of total body water by fluid deprivation can cause hypernatremia.

  E. **Are there underlying conditions?** Diabetes insipidus (after pituitary surgery, head injury, or nephrogenic) is associated with hypernatremia. Any patient with cerebral edema may be on mannitol, which promotes fluid loss. Patients after coronary artery bypass grafting can have hypernatremia due to water loss secondary to antidiuretic hormone (ADH) inhibition.

  F. **Is the laboratory value accurate?** Check previous sodium levels and trends. If this is an acute change, a redraw may be indicated.

  G. **What is the composition of IV fluids administered?** Is the patient receiving free water? If so, is the amount adequate (usually 35 mL/kg over 24 hours)?

III. Differential Diagnosis. Hypernatremia occurs when there is a deficit of water in relation to sodium in the body.

  A. **Inadequate Fluid Intake.** Water deprivation (renal patients, neurosurgical or cardiac patients with fluid restrictions, postoperative patients with minimal intake).

  B. **Increased Water Loss**
    1. **Nonrenal losses.**
       a. **GI losses:** NG suction, diarrhea, fistulas.
       b. **Pulmonary losses:** Insensible losses in intubated patients.
       c. **Cutaneous losses:** Insensible losses increase in the febrile patient. Air-filled or heated beds also increase cutaneous losses.
    2. **Renal losses.**
       a. **Diuretics.**
       b. **Hypercalcemic nephropathy.**
       c. **Hypokalemic nephropathy.**
       d. **Diabetes insipidus.**
       e. **Acute tubular necrosis:** Polyuric phase.

      f. Postobstructive diuresis: Usually caused by relief of longstanding bilateral renal obstruction.

      g. Diabetes mellitus: Water loss caused by osmotic diuresis.

      h. ADH inhibition (water loss) by baroreceptor activation.

C. Iatrogenic

    1. Medications. Lithium, ethanol, phenytoin, colchicine, sodium bicarbonate, amphotericin B, demeclocycline, and mannitol.

    2. Administration of hypertonic parenteral nutrition, hypertonic saline, or bowel preparation before an operation/procedure.

D. Increased Mineralocorticoids or Glucocorticoids

    1. Primary aldosteronism.

    2. Cushing's syndrome.

    3. Ectopic corticotropin production.

    4. Over-administration of exogenous steroids.

IV. Database

A. Physical Examination Key Points

    1. Vital signs. Look for orthostatic blood pressure changes, tachycardia, and decreased weight.

    2. Skin. Check turgor and mucous membranes. Note any "cushingoid" features.

    3. Neurologic examination. Look for irritability, weakness, twitches, or seizures.

B. Laboratory Data

    1. Serum electrolytes. Often electrolyte disorders involve >1 extracellular ion. High BUN level may indicate dehydration.

    2. Serum osmolality. Increased with volume loss.

    3. Urine osmolality. Hypertonic urine suggests extrarenal fluid loss, whereas isotonic or hypotonic urine suggests renal losses.

    4. Spot urine sodium. A level <20 mEq/L suggests extrarenal volume losses.

    5. Hematocrit. May be high because of hemoconcentration.

V. Plan. Control the underlying cause and administer free water. The existing deficit and on going losses must be replaced. Rate of correction should not exceed 0.5 mmol/L per hour or 10 mmol/L per 24 hours. Overly rapid correction may result in cerebral edema.

A. **Determine volume of free water needed TBW (total body water):**

$$\text{Water Deficit} = (0.6 \times \text{weight in kg}) - \text{TBW}$$

$$\text{TBW} = \frac{140}{\text{Serum Na}} \times (0.6 \times \text{weight in kg})$$

Administer the fluids over a 24-hour period as D5W.

B. **Identify and control the underlying cause of hypernatremia**
   1. Replace unusually large nonrenal losses of free water due to fistula or NG tube output.
   2. Manage diabetes mellitus with insulin.
   3. Manage diabetes insipidus with adequate free water and desmopressin (DDAVP) (2–4 µg/day IV or SC in 2 divided doses).

REFERENCES

Adrogue HJ, Madias NE. Hypernatremia. *N Engl J Med* 342:1493–9, 2000.
Kapoor M, Chan GZ. Fluid and electrolyte abnormalities. *Crit Care Clin* 17:503–29, 2001.
Verbalis JG. Diabetes insipidus. *Rev Endocr Metab Disord* 4:177–85, 2003.

43. HYPERTENSION

I. **Problem.** After vagotomy and antrectomy, a 45-year-old man has a blood pressure of 190/110 mm Hg in the recovery room.

II. **Immediate Questions**
   A. **What is the pulse and respiratory rate?** Postoperative pain is often manifested by tachycardia and hypertension; the addition of tachypnea should alert you to the possibility of postoperative hypoxia, especially in the presence of agitation. Bradycardia and hypertension suggest increased intracranial pressure (Cushing's sign).

   B. **Is there a history of hypertension?** *Mild* blood pressure increases are often seen in hypertensive patients after large intraoperative fluid infusions; this is rarely worrisome in the absence of other findings.

   C. **Is the patient having chest pain?** Patients with a history of coronary artery disease need rapid control of severe hypertension to prevent cardiac strain and ischemia. Aortic dissection presents with back and chest pain.

   D. **What medication is the patient taking?** Sympathomimetic agents at incorrect doses can cause hypertension. Check dilutions and rates of all IV infusions. Steroids and oral contraceptives can increase blood pressure. To prevent postoperative hypertension, most cardiac medications and antihypertensives with the exception of diuretics should be administered in their usual doses with a small sip of water the morning of the operation.

III. **Differential Diagnosis.** There are 6 surgically correctable causes of hypertension: coarctation of the aorta, pheochromocytoma, Cushing's syndrome, primary hyperaldosteronism, unilateral renal parenchymal disease, and renovascular hypertension.

A. **Postoperative**
   1. **Pain induced.**
   2. **Fluid overload.**
   3. **Hypoxia.**
   4. **Vasospasm.** Decreased body temperature frequently takes place during surgery, resulting in the patient "clamping down" to preserve body heat. This may also be seen after aortic cross-clamping.
   5. **Carotid sinus reflex disturbance.** May augment postoperative hypertension after CVA and can lead to intracerebral hemorrhage.

B. **Essential Hypertension.** There is no specific cause found in 90–95% of patients with chronic hypertension.

C. **Secondary Hypertension**
   1. **Renal.** Vascular or parenchymal disease.
   2. **Endocrine.** Pheochromocytoma, Cushing's syndrome.
   3. **Drug-induced.** Oral contraceptives, amphetamines, ketamine, other sympathomimetic causes.
   4. **Pregnancy.** Preeclampsia or eclampsia.
   5. **Coarctation of the aorta.**
   6. **Increased intracranial pressure.** Usually associated with bradycardia.
   7. **Polycythemia vera.**
   8. **Baroreceptor stimulation.**

D. **Factitious.** Using too small a blood pressure cuff on an obese arm may falsely increase readings.

IV. **Database**

A. **History.** Check for history of hypertension and type of therapy.

B. **Physical Examination Key Points**
   1. **Vital signs.** Measure pressure in both arms. Check cuff size in relation to arm.
   2. **HEENT.** Papilledema (representative of high intracranial pressure), retinal hemorrhages, or exudates may be present.

3. **Lungs.** Rales may indicate pulmonary edema and possible heart failure.
4. **Abdomen.** Pulsatile mass with aneurysm or bruit with renovascular hypertension.
5. **Neurologic examination.** Focal changes may represent cerebral ischemia.

C. **Laboratory Data**
1. **Arterial blood gas.** Should be performed if concerned about hypoxemia.
2. **Urinalysis, BUN, serum creatinine.** Indicate level of renal function.
3. **Serum catecholamines, urinary vanillylmandelic acid (VMA), and metanephrine.** If pheochromocytoma is suspected.
4. **Dexamethasone suppression test** may be needed to rule out Cushing's syndrome.
5. **Toxicology screen.** Indicated to evaluate use of illicit drugs.

D. **Radiologic and Other Studies**
1. **Electrocardiogram.** May show ischemic changes in the absence of symptoms.
2. **Pulmonary artery catheter.** Determination of cardiac output and pulmonary capillary wedge pressure facilitates evaluation of cardiac function. Its use is not indicated in the vast majority of cases.
3. New onset hypertension in patients <30 years and >60 years or hypertension refractory to medical treatment should prompt thorough evaluation for secondary causes of hypertension. This often includes renal arteriography, selective renal vein renin measurements, and renal ultrasonography.

V. **Plan**

A. **Emergent Management.** A "hypertensive emergency" is defined as severely increased blood pressure with signs or symptoms of acute target organ damage. Severe hypertension is usually managed emergently with sodium nitroprusside. Other agents can be used to control acute hypertension (diazoxide, labetalol, hydralazine) but do not offer the advantage of titration as nitroprusside does. Hydralazine can cause reflex tachycardia in patients taking non-β blockers. With evidence of myocardial ischemia, use IV nitroglycerin. In neurologic hypertensive emergencies, a short-acting IV drug should be given, and the patient examined frequently. Some say decreasing blood pressure in these patients can threaten watershed areas of the brain and may worsen the final neurologic deficit.

1. **Sodium nitroprusside 0.5–10 µg/kg per minute IV infusion.** Titrate to effect. Monitor for thiocyanate toxicity and methemoglobinemia.
2. **Nitroglycerin 5–100 µg/min.** Titrate to effect.
3. **Nifedipine 10–20 mg PO/sublingually.** Often a useful oral adjunct to immediately decrease blood pressure.
4. **Fenoldopam 0.03–0.1 µg/kg per minute IV infusion.** Titrate to effect.

B. **Preoperative Management.** The goal is to obtain good control of blood pressure before performing elective procedures.
   1. Check ECG for signs of ischemia or failure.
   2. All blood pressure and cardiac medications (except diuretics) can be given on the morning of the operation.
   3. Weight loss and a low-salt diet should be encouraged as the first step.
   4. Typical staged therapy includes starting with a β blocker or thiazide diuretic. If a second agent is needed, add the first-line agent that was not used. Check for contraindications. Third-line drugs include hydralazine, prazosin, and angiotensin-converting enzyme inhibitors (captopril). Calcium channel blockers are also frequently used.

C. **Postoperative Management**
   1. Ensure adequate oxygenation and pain relief and warm the patient with blankets or heating blanket if necessary.
   2. **Sedatives and pain control are often all that are needed to control mild hypertension.** Mild hypertension can be controlled with different agents. In the immediate postoperative period, sublingual nifedipine (10–20 mg) is useful but watch for hypotension. Hydralazine 5–10 mg IV/IM, sublingual captopril (12.5 mg), and sublingual clonidine (0.1 mg) are also good choices postoperatively. Hypertension in a pregnant patient is controlled with methyldopa, which is safe for the fetus. Always exclude eclampsia before managing hypertension in pregnancy.
   3. Newly diagnosed hypertensive patients need appropriate follow-up after discharge.

REFERENCES

Elliot WJ. Hypertensive emergencies. *Crit Care Clin* 17:435–51, 2001.

Gifford RW Jr. Management of hypertensive crises. *JAMA* 266:829–35, 1991.

Post JB IV, Frishman WH. Fenoldopam: a new dopamine agonist for the treatment of hypertensive urgencies and emergencies. *J Clin Pharmacol* 54:295–8, 1998.

44. HYPOCALCEMIA

(See also Section II, page 268)

I. **Problem.** A patient admitted to the trauma service with blunt
trauma in a motor vehicle accident has a serum calcium level
of 7.7 mg/dL (normal 8.5–10.5 mg/dL).

II. **Immediate Questions**

   A. Are there any symptoms relevant to hypocalcemia?
Asymptomatic hypocalcemia usually does not require
emergency treatment. Signs and symptoms of hypocalcemia include peripheral and perioral paresthesias,
Trousseau's sign (carpopedal spasm), Chvostek's sign
(fascial nerve twitching with percussion of the facial nerve),
confusion, muscle twitching, tetany, or seizures.

   B. Is there a history of neck surgery? Look for scars from a
previous neck operation.

   **C. Does the low calcium level represent the true ionized
calcium?** Obtain serum albumin values and correct for the
total calcium level or determine the ionized calcium.

    Corrected Ca = [(normal albumin – patient's albumin) × 0.8]
+ patient's measured serum Ca

III. **Differential Diagnosis.**

   A. PTH Deficits. Can be due to surgical excision (can occur
12 hours to 5 days postoperatively), injury, or irradiation of
the parathyroids.

   B. Pseudohypoparathyroidism. Resistance to PTH at the
tissue level.

   C. Vitamin D Deficiency

     1. **Malnutrition.**

     2. **Malabsorption.**

       a. Pancreatitis.

       b. Postgastrectomy.

       c. Short-gut syndrome.

       d. Laxative abuse.

       e. Sprue.

       f. Hepatobiliary disease with bile salt deficiency.

     3. **Defective metabolism.**

       a. Liver disease: Failure to synthesize 25(OH) vitamin
D.

       b. Renal disease: Failure to synthesize 1–25 dihy-
droxy vitamin D.

   c. Anticonvulsive treatment: Phenobarbital and
   phenytoin produce inactive metabolites of vitamin D.

D. Magnesium Deficiency. Correcting the magnesium deficit
will often correct the calcium level.

E. Calcium Loss/Displacement
   1. Hyperphosphatemia. Increases bone deposition of
   calcium.
      a. Acute phosphate ingestion.
      b. Acute phosphate release by rhabdomyolysis, tumor
      lysis.
   2. Acute pancreatitis.
   3. Blood transfusions. Citrate in stored blood binds calcium.
   4. Osteoblastic metastases. Especially breast and
   prostate cancers.
   5. Medullary carcinoma of the thyroid. Resulting from
   increased thyrocalcitonin.
   6. Decreased bone resorption. Agents such as actino-
   mycin, calcitonin, and mithramycin.
   7. Alkalosis causes increased binding of calcium to
   plasma proteins.

IV. Database

A. Physical Examination Key Points
   1. Skin. Dermatitis, eczema with chronic hypocalcemia.
   2. HEENT. Cataracts may be present; laryngospasm is
   rare but life threatening. Look for surgical scars on the
   neck.
   3. Neuromuscular. Confusion, spasm, twitching, facial
   grimacing, hyperactive deep tendon reflexes, and depression.
   4. Specific tests for tetany of hypocalcemia.
      a. Chvostek's sign: Tap on facial nerve near the zy-
      goma of patient's jaw and observe for twitch.
      b. Trousseau's sign: Inflate a blood pressure cuff
      higher than systolic pressure for 3 minutes and ob-
      serve for carpal spasm.

B. Laboratory Data
   1. Serum electrolytes. In particular calcium, phosphate,
   potassium and magnesium Check serum albumin level
   and correct appropriately. Hypomagnesemia and hyperkalemia may potentiate symptoms of hypocalcemia.
   2. Renal function tests. Look for chronic renal insufficiency.
   3. PTH levels.

      4. Vitamin D levels. 25–hydroxy and 1,25–dihydroxy vitamin D levels.

      5. Urinary cyclic adenosine monophosphate levels. This is increased with increased PTH levels.

    C. Radiologic and Other Tests

      1. Electrocardiogram. Prolonged QT interval.

      2. Bone films. Bone changes in renal failure or osteoblastic metastases.

V. Plan. Once the diagnosis is established, treatment depends on symptomatic or asymptomatic hypocalcemia. Symptomatic hypocalcemia should be managed as soon as it is diagnosed. Patients with asymptomatic hypocalcemia may be followed with serial laboratory values or treated depending on the underlying etiology.

    A. Acute Treatment. Give elemental calcium 200–300 mg rapidly.

      1. 10% calcium gluconate. One 10-mL ampule contains calcium 90 mg. Give 20–30 mL total IV.

      2. 10% calcium chloride. One 10-mL ampule contains calcium 360 mg. Give 10 mL IV. Should be given through a central line.

    B. Long-term Treatment. With primary PTH deficiency, give calcium 2–4 g PO daily and then add vitamin D if necessary. In vitamin D disorder, supplement with vitamin D. The use of aluminum phosphate gels will limit phosphate absorption.

      1. Calcium carbonate. Calcium 240 mg per 600-mg tablet.

      2. Os-Cal-500. A 1.25–g calcium carbonate tablet provides elemental calcium 500 mg.

      3. Dihydrotachysterol vitamin D2. 0.25–1.0 µg/day.

    C. Magnesium Deficiency

      1. 10% magnesium sulfate 1–2 g IV over 20 minutes or $MgSO_4$ 40–80 mEq/L IV fluid.

      2. Long-term replacement with magnesium oxide 600 mg 1–2 tablets daily.

REFERENCES

Ariyan CE, Sosa JA. Assessment and management of patients with abnormal calcium. *Crit Care Med* 32(suppl):S146–54, 2004.

Kapor M, Chan GZ. Fluid and electrolyte abnormalities. *Crit Care Clin* 17:503–29, 2001.

Mittendorf EA, et al. Post-parathyroidectomy hypocalcemia: incidence, risk factors, and management. *Am Surg* 70:114–20, 2004.

45. HYPOGLYCEMIA

I. Problem. The nurses tell you that a 40-year-old man with a history of type I diabetes mellitus has a serum glucose level of 40 mg/dL (normal fasting level 70–105 mg/dL).

II. Immediate Questions

A. Is the patient diabetic and on insulin? A common cause of hypoglycemia is the inadvertent over-administration of insulin.

B. What medication is the patient taking? Are there any oral hypoglycemic medications being given?

C. What IV fluids are running? Has the patient recently been discontinued from hyperalimentation? This can cause a reactive hypoglycemia, although it is quite rare. If still receiving hyperalimentation, is insulin in the formulation? Is the patient receiving IV fluids containing dextrose?

D. What is the patient's diagnosis? There are certain disease states associated with hypoglycemia, such as retroperitoneal sarcoma, insulinoma, and paraneoplastic syndromes (especially squamous cell carcinoma of the lung). Pancreatic transplant recipients can have hypoglycemia secondary to dysfunctional autoregulation postoperatively. Patients who are in the postoperative period after liver resection commonly have hypoglycemia because the liver is the site of stored glycogen.

E. What is the patient's clinical state? Is the patient awake, alert, comatose, or diaphoretic? Diaphoresis and tremulousness are usually a manifestation of catecholamine discharge.

III. Differential Diagnosis

A. Medications
1. **Insulin.** Inadvertent administration.
2. **Oral hypoglycemic agents.** Tolbutamide, chlorpropamide, acetohexamide, and others.
3. **Others.** Pentamidine, ethanol, and monoamine oxidase inhibitors are infrequent causes.

B. Severe Liver Failure/Resection Extensive Hepatic Destruction

C. Insulinoma. These present with Whipple's triad: symptoms of hypoglycemia, documented serum glucose level <50 mg/dL, and relief of symptoms with administration of glucose.

D. **Sudden Discontinuation of Total Parenteral Nutrition.** Rare problem. Most patients easily tolerate sudden discontinuation of total parenteral nutrition.

E. **Retroperitoneal Sarcoma.** These tumors can cause hypoglycemia.

F. **Paraneoplastic Syndrome.** Hypoglycemia can be caused by secretion of insulin or insulin-like substances by tumors.

G. **Surreptitious Insulin/Oral Hypoglycemic Administration**

H. **Reactive Functional Hypoglycemia**

I. **Alimentary Hypoglycemia.** Found in 5–10% of patients who have undergone partial to complete gastrectomies and resulting from rapid gastric emptying time.

J. **Factitious Hypoglycemia.** A rare but possibly confounding diagnosis, it is caused by the use of glucose in the red top tube by leukocytes and is found in patients with WBC counts >40,000. These patients will have asymptomatic hypoglycemia. Thus, any patients with very high WBC counts should have serum glucose determinations from blood collected in tubes that contain sodium fluoride (gray top), which inhibits WBC metabolism.

K. **Hormone Deficiencies.** Glucocorticoids, growth hormone, thyroid hormone, glucagon, or panhypopituitarism.

L. **Miscellaneous.** Sepsis, alcoholism, or severe malnutrition.

IV. **Database**

A. **Physical Examination Key Points**

1. **Vital signs.** Tachycardia may be caused by adrenergic response to decreasing glucose levels.

2. **Skin.** Diaphoresis is also an adrenergic response.

3. **Neurologic examination.** Orientation and level of consciousness may be altered.

B. **Laboratory Data**

1. **Serum glucose.** The most important diagnostic test is serum glucose level. Levels <50 mg/dL are diagnostic in the presence of symptoms. Rapid glucose measurements should be confirmed with a serum level.

2. **Urine glucose levels.** Of little help in this setting.

3. **Serum insulin levels.** If insulinoma is suspected or to detect surreptitious insulin administration.

4. **C peptide levels.** Detects endogenous insulin production. High levels of C peptide and serum insulin suggest insulinoma. If serum insulin is increased and C peptide

level is decreased, insulin overdosage or surreptitious insulin administration is likely.

C. Radiologic and Other Studies. May be indicated to diagnose tumors as suspected from the clinical picture.

V. Plan. In acute cases, increase serum glucose and eliminate symptoms and then identify the cause.

A. Administer Glucose. Do not await results of serum glucose (drawn before treatment) if you strongly suspect the diagnosis. The mainstay of initial therapy is glucose, given PO if the patient is awake, alert, and able to take fluids or IV otherwise.

1. **Oral.** Give orange juice with or without additional sugar.
2. **Parenteral.** Administer 1 ampule of D50 IV push. If there is no change, repeat the ampule of D50. A lack of response at this point should lead the clinician to question the diagnosis,
3. When IV access is not possible, glucagon 0.5–1 mg IM or SC may be given immediately. Vomiting may occur.
4. Start maintenance IV of D5W at 50–100 mL/h to help prevent recurrence and follow-up with serial glucose measurements.

B. Adjust Medications. Reevaluate the current dosing schedule of insulin or other hypoglycemic agents.

C. Workup of Hypoglycemia. After controlling the acute episode, diagnostic tests are required to evaluate the patient for the cause of the hypoglycemia. Serum insulin levels, C-peptide levels, liver function tests, glucose tolerance tests, and appropriate radiographic tests are to be considered.

D. Liver Resection. Patients after liver resection should be maintained on IV fluids containing 10% dextrose with frequent serum glucose determinations.

REFERENCES

Bolli GB. Treatment and prevention of hypoglycemia and its unawareness in type 1 diabetes mellitus. *Rev Endocr Metab Disord* 4):335–41, 2003.
Hypoglycemia in diabetes: common, often unrecognized. *Clevel Clin J Med* 71:335–42, 2004.
Service FJ. Hypoglycemia. *Med Clin North Am* 79:1–8, 1995.

46. HYPOKALEMIA

I. Problem. A 72-year-old man on long-term diuretics for heart failure develops abdominal distention and an ileus. His serum potassium level is 2.5 mEq/L (normal 3.5–5.1 mEq/L).

II. Immediate Questions

A. What medication is the patient taking? Loop diuretics are kaliuretic and cause significant renal potassium wasting. Thiazide diuretics can cause hypokalemia, but the level is rarely dangerous, except when digoxin is used concomitantly. Hypokalemia will potentiate digitalis toxicity. Amphotericin B causes potassium wasting by direct renal toxic effects.

B. Is there a history of vomiting, NG suction, or diarrhea? These are common causes of hypokalemia in the surgical patient.

C. What are the vital signs? Look for irregular pulse, which could represent new premature atrial or ventricular contractions due to increased myocardial irritability.

D. Is the patient symptomatic? Symptoms of hypokalemia include weakness, nausea, vomiting, and abdominal tenderness.

III. Differential Diagnosis

A. Potassium Losses

1. **Gastrointestinal.**
   a. Prolonged NG suction without replacement can cause hypokalemia through direct losses, induced renal losses, and through potassium shifts due to the development of metabolic alkalosis. This is the most common electrolyte abnormality in surgical patients.
   b. Intractable vomiting (same mechanism as NG suction).
   c. Bowel obstruction can result in hypokalemia through the pooling of secretions and inefficient potassium absorption.
   d. Diarrhea, fistula, villous adenoma.

2. **Renal.**
   a. **Diuretics:** Especially loop diuretics, such as furosemide.
   b. Renal tubular acidosis results in hypokalemia when K^+ is secreted and H^+ is absorbed.
   c. **Antibiotics:** Carbenicillin, others. Amphotericin B may also cause magnesium wasting.
   d. Postobstructive diuresis or the diuretic phase of acute tubular necrosis.

B. Potassium Redistribution

1. **Alkalosis.** Cation balance requires that, as H^+ moves out of cells to correct alkalosis, K^+ moves in.
2. **Insulin.** Insulin administration results in glucose and potassium transport into cells.

C. **Inadequate Intake.** Most often iatrogenic (administration of potassium-free IV fluids over a prolonged period). In the absence of other losses, normal daily potassium requirements with normal renal function are 40–60 mEq/24 hours.

IV. **Database.** Because potassium is the principal intracellular cation, hypokalemia usually represents a significant loss of body potassium. Thus, serum levels of 3.0 mEq/L (mmol/L) often represent total deficits of 100–200 mEq in the adult.

A. **Physical Examination Key Points**
1. **Cardiac.** Irregular pulse may represent new arrhythmias (premature atrial contraction, premature ventricular contraction) or digoxin toxicity.
2. **Abdomen.** Look for evidence of distention and listen for bowel sounds. Obstruction can cause hypokalemia; rarely, ileus results from hypokalemia and thus exacerbates the condition. Vomiting may cause hypokalemia or indicate digitalis toxicity.
3. **Neurologic examination.** Severe hypokalemia can cause blunting of reflexes, paresthesias, and paralysis.

B. **Laboratory Data**
1. **Serum electrolytes.** Hypocalcemia and hypomagnesemia may coexist.
2. **Arterial blood gas.** Severe electrolyte abnormalities often have accompanying acid-base defects. Renal tubular acidosis and metabolic alkalosis often result in hypokalemia.
3. **Urine electrolytes.** Useful only in the patient not taking diuretics; renal wasting can be evaluated by simple "spot" determinations of urine K^+, Na^+, and osmolality.
4. **Digoxin level** if appropriate.

C. **Radiologic and Other Studies.** ECG and rhythm strip should be done on the patient with evidence of digitalis toxicity, new premature atrial contractions, and new premature ventricular contractions as manifested by a new irregular pulse. T-wave flattening, U waves, and ST-segment changes also occur with hypokalemia.

V. **Plan.** More severe cases of hypokalemia, usually levels <3.0 mmol/L, or those cases associated with ECG abnormalities should be controlled aggressively because of the potential for life-threatening arrhythmias. Good renal function should be established before replacement.

A. **Parenteral Replacement**
1. **Indications.** Should be considered in the following patients: digoxin toxicity or significant arrhythmia, severe

hypokalemia (<3.0 mmol/L), and those who cannot take oral replacement (NPO, ileus, nausea, and vomiting). Parenteral administration is ideally given through a central venous catheter.

2. **Replacement.** Maximum concentrations of KCl used in peripheral veins should generally not exceed 40 mEq/L because of damaging effects on the veins (although in an emergent situation 60 mEq/L can be attempted). KCl 10–20 mEq diluted in D5W or NS 50–100 mL can be infused over 1 hour through a central line safely, and doses can be repeated as needed when severe depletion is present. Special care must be taken to ensure slow infusion of these large doses. For lesser degrees of hypokalemia that require parenteral replacement, 10–40 mEq/h can be infused peripherally.

3. **Monitoring.** Check serum levels frequently to avoid, every 2–4 hours depending on clinical response. ECG/ICU monitoring is required for arrhythmias or for rapid infusions of KCl.

B. **Oral Replacement**. Generally indicated for asymptomatic, mild levels of potassium repletion (K usually <3.0 mEq/L). Oral replacements include liquids and powders. Slow-release pills typically contain >10 mEq/tablet and thus are not usually appropriate for repletion therapy. Replacement doses should be 40–120 mEq/day in divided doses depending on the patient's weight and level of hypokalemia. Maintenance therapy, if needed, should be given in doses of 20–40 mEq daily using the preparation best tolerated by the patient. In patients with normal renal function, it is difficult to induce hyperkalemia by PO administration of potassium. Avoid the use of potassium supplements in patients on potassium-sparing diuretics to prevent hyperkalemia.

C. **Replace Ongoing Losses.** Large amounts of NG aspirate should be replaced milliliter for milliliter with D5 1/2 NS with 20 mEq/L KCl every 4–6 hours.

D. **Refractory Cases.** Rarely, hypokalemia may not be correctable because of concomitant hypomagnesemia or hypocalcemia. Replace calcium and magnesium accordingly.

REFERENCES

Kapor M, Chan GZ. Fluid and electrolyte abnormalities. *Crit Care Clin* 17:503–29, 2001.

Mandal AK. Hypokalemia and hyperkalemia. *Med Clin North Am* 81:611–39, 1997.

Robertson JI. Treatment of hypokalemia. *N Engl J Med* 340:155–62, 1999.

47. HYPONATREMIA

(See also Section II, page 318)

I. **Problem.** An elderly woman admitted for a mastectomy has a serum sodium level of 119 mEq/L on routine admission laboratory tests (normal 136–145 mEq/L).

II. **Immediate Questions**

A. **Does the patient have any CNS symptoms relevant to the hyponatremia?** Symptomatic hyponatremia manifests primarily CNS symptoms as brain cells become edematous in a hypo-osmotic state. Inquire about lethargy, agitation, disorientation, or obtundation. Usual neurologic manifestations are evident when the sodium level is ≤120 mEq/L.

B. **Are there any recent prior sodium levels to document the chronicity of the hyponatremia?** The rate of development of hyponatremia correlates directly with the severity of symptoms it produces. Acute changes in serum sodium concentration are more likely to produce severe symptoms.

C. **Does the patient take diuretics?** A common single cause of hyponatremia is long-term diuretic use.

D. **Is the hyponatremia real, or is it a laboratory artifact?** Osmotic agents and space-occupying compounds at high concentrations can alter the reported laboratory value of sodium. This is also known as pseudohyponatremia. Note the concentration of glucose and triglycerides.

E. **Is the patient receiving IV fluids?** Overhydration with excess free water is the most common cause of hyponatremia in the surgical patient.

F. **Has the patient had recent surgery?** Surgery and anesthesia often result in temporary inappropriate ADH secretion and transient hyponatremia.

III. **Differential Diagnosis.** The initial differentiation is between true hyponatremia and laboratory artifact. Hyponatremia may be classified according to the volume status of the patient: hypovolemic, euvolemic, or hypervolemic. Hypovolemic hyponatremia may be further classified by serum and urine chemistries.

A. **Laboratory Artifact (Pseudohyponatremia)**
1. **Osmotic agents.** Hyperglycemia is most common. Adjust the serum sodium up 1.6 mEq/L for every excess 100 mg/dL of glucose over the normal value of 100 mg/dL.

    2. Space-occupying compounds. Lipids (hyperlipidemia) are the most common. The laboratory can ultracentrifuge the specimen to find the corrected plasma level.

B. Hypovolemic Hyponatremia
  1. Spot urinary sodium <10 mEq/L.
    a. GI fluid losses: Vomiting or diarrhea. In surreptitious vomiting or bulimia, urinary chloride level is usually <10 mEq/L.
    b. Third-space fluid loss: Such as pancreatitis or peritonitis.
    c. Burns.
  2. Urinary sodium level >10 mEq/L.
    a. Diuretic usage: Caused by thiazides (eg, hydrochlorothiazide) and loop (furosemide) diuretics and often associated with hypokalemia and alkalosis; with surreptitious diuretic use, urinary chloride is >20 mEq/L.
    b. Renal disorders: Medullary cystic disease, polycystic disease, and chronic interstitial nephritis can result in hyponatremia.
    c. Addison's disease: Hyperkalemia and low urinary potassium are also found.
    d. Osmotic diuresis: Most commonly due to glucose, mannitol, or ketones (as in DKA).

C. Euvolemic Hyponatremia
  1. SIADH. The diagnosis of syndrome of inappropriate ADH (SIADH) is based on the finding of low serum osmolality, increased urine sodium, and slightly concentrated urine (osmolality near serum).
    a. Postoperative: Anesthesia and surgical procedures increase ADH. The TURP syndrome is caused by excessive fluid absorption during transurethral surgery.
    b. Tumors: Small-cell lung cancer most common.
    c. Pulmonary infections: Such as TB and other bacterial pneumonia.
    d. CNS disorders: Trauma, tumors, and infections.
    e. Stress: Including perioperative stress.
    f. Drugs: PO hypoglycemics, chemotherapeutics (cyclophosphamide, vincristine), psychiatric drugs (haloperidol, tricyclic antidepressants), and clofibrate.
  2. Hypothyroidism.
  3. Hypopituitarism.

D. Hypervolemic Hyponatremia
  1. CHF.
  2. Cirrhosis.

      3. Renal disease.
         a. Chronic renal failure.
         b. Nephrotic syndrome.
      4. Psychogenic polydipsia.

IV. Database

  A. Physical Examination Key Points. Close attention should be paid to the assessment of volume status.

    1. Vital signs. Evaluate for orthostatic blood pressure changes. A decrease in blood pressure >10 mm Hg or a pulse increase >10 beats/min is highly suggestive of volume depletion. Tachypnea may suggest volume overload and pulmonary edema.

    2. Skin. Tissue turgor will be diminished and mucous membranes dry with dehydration. Edema suggests volume overload. Evidence of cirrhosis includes jaundice and caput medusae.

    3. HEENT. Evaluate the IJ vein with the bed up at 45 degrees (veins are flat with volume depletion and markedly engorged with volume overload).

    4. Lungs. Rales may be heard with volume overload.

    5. Heart. An S_3 gallop murmur suggests volume overload.

    6. Abdomen. Evidence of hepatosplenomegaly, ascites, or other evidence of liver disease should be carefully sought on examination. A hepatojugular reflex may be present in CHF.

    7. Neurologic examination. Hyperactive deep tendon reflexes, altered mental status, confusion, coma, or seizures usually indicate a sodium level <120 mmol/L.

  B. Laboratory Data

    1. Serum electrolytes.

    2. Spot urine electrolytes and creatinine. Obtain before any diuretic therapy.

    3. Urine and serum osmolality. Serum osmolality will be normal in cases of laboratory artifact but decreased in true hyponatremia.

    4. Liver function tests. To detect liver disease.

    5. Arterial blood gases. Acidosis/alkalosis may be present.

    6. Thyroid function.

    7. Cortisol levels, corticotropin stimulation test.

    8. Cultures (blood and sputum).

  C. Radiologic and Other Studies

    1. Chest radiograph. Evidence of CHF or a lung tumor.

    2. Head CT scan if indicated.

    3. Water load test. Bring the serum sodium to a safe level by fluid restriction, challenge with water 20 mL/kg PO, and collect urine hourly for 5 hours. If <75% of intake volume is excreted or if urine osmolarity fails to decrease to <200 mL/kg, then SIADH is present.

V. Plan. The underlying cause of the hyponatremia and the presence and severity of symptoms guide therapy.

A. Acute Therapy

1. **NS and furosemide 1 mg/kg IV.** Use the combination of NS and diuretics to achieve a net negative volume balance. Carefully document volume in and volume out. Supplement fluids with potassium as needed.

2. **Hypertonic saline (3%) is rarely, if ever, needed.** Most institutions have banned its use entirely because of possible serious complications.

B. Specific Therapies

1. **Hypovolemic hyponatremia.**
   a. For almost all causes, manage by repleting volume and sodium (NS IV infusion).
   b. For diuretic abuse, repletion of lost body potassium is also needed.

2. **Euvolemic hyponatremia.**
   a. **SIADH:** Water restriction to 800–1000 mL daily. Demeclocycline for increased urine sodium or urine osmolarity.
   b. **Hypothyroidism:** Manage with thyroid replacement.
   c. **Hypopituitary:** Manage with hormone replacement.

3. **Hypervolemic hyponatremia.** Restrict IV and PO fluids. Check urine sodium (low is <10 mEq/L).
   a. **CHF:** Manage with digoxin, diuretics, water restriction.
   b. **Nephrotic syndrome:** Steroids, water restriction, and increased protein intake commonly used.
   c. **Cirrhosis:** Water restriction, diuretics, and portosystemic shunt if indicated. Urine sodium >20 mEq/L.
   d. **Renal failure:** Managed with water restriction and dialysis if indicated.

REFERENCES

Adrogue HJ, Madias ME. Hyponatremia. *N Engl J Med* 342:1581–9, 2000.

Milionis HJ, et al. The hyponatremic patient: a systematic approach to laboratory diagnosis. *CMAJ* 166:1056–62, 2002.

Vachharajani TJ, et al. Hyponatremia in critically ill patients. *J Intensive Care Med* 18:3–8, 2003.

Yeates KE, et al. Salt and water: a simple approach to hyponatremia. *CMAJ* 170:365–9, 2004.

48. HYPOTENSION (SHOCK)

Immediate Actions

1. Assess airway and breathing. Intubate if necessary.
2. Ensure large-bore IV access and begin 500-mL Ringer's lactate (LR) bolus.
3. Control external hemorrhage (if present) with direct pressure.
4. Trendelenburg position.
5. See Figure I–12, page 56.

I. **Problem.** A 40-year-old woman who underwent total abdominal hysterectomy earlier that day has a blood pressure of 80/50 mm Hg.

II. **Immediate Questions**

   A. **What is the patient's pulse?** A high pulse rate indicates cardiovascular response to hypovolemia, whereas a normal pulse is less suggestive of a hypovolemic state.

   B. **What have been the blood pressure readings preoperatively?** Always double check any arterial line blood pressure readings with a careful cuff determination.

   C. **When was the patient's surgery?** If this is the first postoperative night, then hypovolemia or active bleeding is especially likely.

   D. **What is the cardiac rhythm?** Abnormal rhythms can cause hypotension, especially atrial fibrillation or flutter. Hypotension with bradycardia suggests heart block.

   E. **What is the patient's mental status?** Determine whether the hypotension is affecting critical organ perfusion.

   F. **What medication is the patient taking?** A patient on β blockers can have a lower pulse, which will worsen hypotension by blunting reflex tachycardia. Narcotics and some sedatives can induce hypotension. Anaphylactic reactions may be caused by medications or IV contrast agents (see Problem 5, page 22). Epidural anesthesia may occasionally cause hypotension.

   G. **What is the fluid balance?** Urine output provides a clue to the volume status of the patient. A decreasing urine output with hypotension suggests poor renal perfusion. Be sure that the patient has been adequately hydrated and that excessive losses (eg, NG tube drainage) are being replaced.

H. Is there any obvious bleeding source? Inquire about blood on the dressings, bloody NG drainage, increased chest tube, or mediastinal tube output.

I. Addisonian crisis (adrenal insufficiency). This is especially important to consider after adrenal surgery or radical nephrectomy. Any patient who has taken steroids over the previous year may have blunted adrenal response to the stress of surgery.

J. Is there underlying sepsis? There may be bouts of hypotension throughout the septic episode.

III. Differential Diagnosis. As a rule of thumb, a systolic blood pressure of 90 mm Hg in an adult is considered hypotension. Hypotension may cause shock, a state characterized by inadequate tissue perfusion. Shock can be classified as hypovolemic, neurogenic, vasogenic, and cardiogenic. Each type is presented below.

A. Hypovolemia. This etiology of shock is often seen in surgical patients.
  1. Hemorrhagic.
   a. Traumatic: Significant blood loss may not be readily apparent (chest, abdomen, retroperitoneal; into fracture sites such as the pelvis, long bones; or into soft tissues) or obvious external bleeding.
   b. Postoperative: Internal hemorrhage postoperatively or direct exsanguination through surgically placed drains, etc.
   c. Others: DIC, GI tract bleeding, ruptured aneurysms. Ruptured ovarian cyst or ectopic pregnancy should be suspected in female patients.
  2. Fluid losses. Severe vomiting, diarrhea, sweating, extensive burns, and "third-space losses" (eg, pancreatitis, bowel obstruction). It can also be a result of inadequate hydration during surgery.

B. Neurogenic Shock. Typically seen in patients with spinal cord trauma that is characterized by hypotension and a normal or low pulse rate. These patients will usually have normal urine output after fluid administration. They may require large amounts of fluid or Neo-Synephrine due to loss of sympathetic tone.

C. Vasogenic Shock. Septic shock, anaphylactic reactions, or adrenocortical insufficiency may cause decreased vascular tone (low systemic vascular resistance, see page 379). These patients are usually in a hyperdynamic state with high cardiac output and low peripheral vascular resistance.

D. Cardiogenic Shock. "Pump failure" (usually due to MI or cardiomyopathy), arrhythmia (atrial fibrillation, complete heart block), tension pneumothorax, or PE can lead to cardiogenic shock. Lesions such as pericardial tamponade, aortic valve disease (late), and septal rupture can also present with hypotension.

IV. Database

A. Physical Examination Key Points

1. **Vital signs.** Tachycardia is the usual response to hypotension, with bradycardia suggesting heart block. Irregularity of the pulse suggests an arrhythmia. Tachypnea may indicate hypoxia or acidosis resulting from poor perfusion or early sepsis. Fever or hypothermia might suggest sepsis; however, elderly or immunosuppressed patients may be afebrile in the face of sepsis.

2. **Skin.** Cool, clammy skin may indicate shock.

3. **Neck.** Check for jugular venous distention. Bulging neck veins are compatible with congestive failure, pericardial tamponade, or tension pneumothorax.

4. **Chest.** Rales suggest CHF; wheezing and stridor are consistent with anaphylaxis; decreased breath sounds may indicate hemothorax or pneumothorax.

5. **Cardiac.** Check for new murmurs, arrhythmias, or rubs. Heart sounds may be muffled with cardiac tamponade.

6. **Abdomen.** Distention, pulsatile mass, flank ecchymoses, or active bleeding at drain sites or wound dressings may suggest the cause.

7. **Rectal examination.** Gross (hematochezia) or occult blood.

8. **Pelvic examination.** Pelvic fractures can result in a large amount of blood loss. Pelvic examination in females may reveal a gynecologic cause.

9. **Extremities.** Absent or "thready" pulses are consistent with shock; long bone fractures (especially femur) may result in significant bleeding into soft tissues. Examine IV sites for evidence of infection. Edema is often seen with CHF.

10. **Neurologic examination.** Mental status alterations suggest poor central perfusion. Loss of motor and sensation functions suggest spinal cord trauma.

B. Laboratory Data

1. **Blood.** Should be set up immediately. Type and crossmatch for appropriate number of units of blood.

2. **Hemogram.** Serial hematocrit determinations are essential because the hematocrit may not decrease for some time after an acute bleed.
3. **Serum electrolytes.** Addisonian crisis causes hyperkalemia with hyponatremia.
4. **Coagulation panel (PT, PTT, platelet count).** If excessive bleeding due to DIC is suspected, use fibrinogen and fibrin split products.
5. **Arterial blood gases.** Early sepsis may result in respiratory alkalosis; acidosis may indicate inadequate tissue perfusion; hypoxia may require ventilatory support.
6. **Cardiac injury panel.** Troponin levels may demonstrate evidence of myocardial injury (see Section II, page 323).
7. **Pregnancy test.** Especially if a ruptured ectopic pregnancy is suspected.

C. **Radiologic and Other Studies**
   1. **Chest radiograph.** Look for evidence of CHF, cardiac enlargement, pneumothorax, or hemothorax.
   2. **Electrocardiogram.** Myocardial ischemia may show flipped T waves or ST-segment depression; arrhythmias may be noted.
   3. **Pulmonary artery (PA) catheter.** A PA catheter is helpful in managing the patient in whom fluid overload would be particularly dangerous. By using a PA catheter, filling pressures are measured directly, thus avoiding iatrogenic pulmonary edema. Can also help differentiate cardiogenic from hypovolemic or vasogenic causes. For diagnostic and insertion details, see Section III, page 375.
   4. **Angiogram.** May help identify bleeding sites (especially for GI tract bleeding).
   5. **Nuclear V/Q scan.** To diagnose PE.
   6. **Echocardiogram.** To examine valves (mitral stenosis, aortic insufficiency, etc), pericardial fluid, and intracardiac thrombi.
   7. **Blood, sputum, urine cultures.** In cases of suspected sepsis.
   8. Peritoneal tap, thoracentesis, or culdocentesis if indicated (see Section III, page 323).

V. **Plan.** Re-establish adequate tissue perfusion as soon as possible if the patient is in shock. In general, a blood pressure >90 mm Hg and urine output ≥0.5 mL/kg per minute are acceptable goals.

A. **Initial Emergency Management.** For all forms of shock. See Figure I–12 page 56 for a useful algorithm.

1. Control external hemorrhage with direct pressure.
2. Establish good venous access and closely monitor the patient in shock. Two large-bore IVs (≥18 gauge) or a central venous line. The large-bore peripheral IV lines are superior for rapid administration of large volumes of IV fluid.
3. Trendelenburg position (supine with feet higher than head) may improve cerebral perfusion and blood pressure immediately. Tightly wrapping the pelvis with a sheet or placement of a C-clamp may help control bleeding in a patient with a pelvic fracture, when appropriate.
4. Except for cardiogenic shock, replace volume immediately with IV crystalloid (NS, lactated Ringer's solution, etc).
5. Foley catheter to monitor urinary output.
6. Supplemental oxygen or ventilatory support if needed.
7. CVP line or PA catheter to better manage volume replacement and accurately diagnose the cause of the shock.

B. Hypovolemic Shock. Restore intravascular volume.
1. **Administer fluids.** Use blood if the hematocrit is low or crystalloids (NS or lactated Ringer's solution) if blood is not available or if hematocrit is "acceptable" (ie, >30%).
2. Titrate fluids by following blood pressure and urine output.
3. Initial resuscitation goals should aim to replace fluid losses. Do not use pressor agents (eg, dopamine) unless there is persistent hypotension despite adequate cardiac filling pressures ("a full tank," wedge pressure >12 mm Hg). Hypotension with low filling pressures (wedge pressure <6 mm Hg) are initially managed with IC fluids. A PA catheter is necessary for monitoring when using pressor agents.
4. With good filling pressures and adequate cardiac output, the next step is peripheral vasoconstrictors such as dopamine or Neo-Synephrine in a patient who is still hypotensive.

C. Neurogenic Shock
1. Use moderate IV fluids to avoid volume overload.
2. Small-dose vasopressors (Neo-Synephrine or dopamine) may help support blood pressure.
3. A major neurologic injury may not be obvious at the time of presentation in an unconscious trauma patient.

D. Vasogenic Shock
1. **Septic shock.** Therapy is directed at the underlying sepsis.

    a. Measure cardiac output and systemic vascular resistance (typically high cardiac output with low systemic resistance) with a PA catheter (see Section III, page 375).

    b. Administer IV fluids to support pressure and urine output.

    c. Culture aggressively to identify source.

    d. Control the underlying cause of sepsis. Initiate appropriate antibiotics and consider laparotomy or percutaneous drainage of an abscess if indicated.

    e. Use pressors as needed. First line is often dopamine. Dopamine is discussed in Section IX, page 481. The smallest effective dose of dopamine to maintain blood pressure and urine output should be used. Physiologic effects of dopamine are as follows:

        i. 3–5 µg/kg per minute: Renal and splanchnic vasodilatation through dopamine receptors.

        ii. 5–10 µg/kg per minute: Positive inotrope through β_1-receptors.

        iii. >10 µg/kg per minute: Peripheral vasoconstriction through α-receptors.

  2. Anaphylactic shock; see Problem 5, page 22.

E. Cardiogenic Shock

  1. Cardiac output is maximized by the judicious use of inotropic (dopamine or dobutamine) agents. Dobutamine is the drug of choice for pump failure. Severe pulmonary edema is managed with diuretics (eg, furosemide) and vasodilators (eg, nitrates).

  2. Myocardial ischemia is managed with oxygen, pain relief (morphine), aspirin, and nitrates acutely.

  3. Arrhythmia is identified and controlled appropriately to return to normal sinus rhythm.

  4. Pulmonary embolus (see Problem 26, page 106).

REFERENCES

Dellinger RP. Cardiovascular management of septic shock. *Crit Care Med* 31:946–55, 2003.

Holmes CL, Walley KR. The evaluation and management of shock. *Clin Chest Med* 24:775–89, 2003.

Marvin RG, et al. Critical care. In: Townsend CL, ed. Sabiston *Textbook of Surgery,* 16th ed. Philadelphia: WB Saunders; 2001, p 375–93.

49. HYPOXIA

  I. Problem. An intubated patient has become hypoxic after the morning chest radiograph and is not responding to 100% fraction of inspired oxygen (F_{IO_2}).

II. Immediate Questions

A. Are the monitoring devices accurately connected? Cardiac monitor and continuous pulse oximeter should be applied correctly.

B. Is the airway secure? With repositioning the patient for chest radiograph, the endotracheal tube may have been advanced into the right mainstem bronchus, or the cuff may have been ruptured or above the vocal cords, necessitating repositioning or replacing the endotracheal tube.

C. Are the breath sounds equal? Absence of breath sounds indicates lung collapse, pneumothorax, or mucous plug.

D. Is the chest moving symmetrically? Pain from rib fracture, lung injury, or incision can cause splinting and decreased air movement.

E. Does the patient have a history of pulmonary disease or CHF?

F. Is the patient alert? Severe hypoxia will alter mental functions. Opioid overdose may cause hypoventilation.

III. Differential Diagnosis.
Alveolar-arterial (A-a or A-aDO$_2$) gradient is useful to determine the cause and severity of the oxygenation defect (see following section, "Database"). It is of greatest use in the ventilated patient.

A. Low Inspired Oxygen Tension. Seen in high altitude situations such as mountain climbing or improper ventilator settings. Normal A-a gradient.

B. Hypoventilation. CNS depression from drug overdose, CVA, or spinal cord injury, chest wall failure from circumferential burns, splinting, neuromuscular disease, compensation for metabolic alkalosis, airway obstruction. Normal A-a gradient.

C. Diffusion Impairment. Carbon monoxide poisoning, pulmonary fibrosis. Increased A-a gradient.

D. Ventilation. Perfusion imbalance. There is perfusion of nonventilated alveoli in PE, fat emboli, pneumonia, COPD, ARDS, pulmonary contusion, asthma, atelectasis, TB, and pneumothorax. Increased A-a gradient.

E. Right to Left Shunt. Pulmonary edema, nitroglycerin, cardiac anomalies (patent ductus arteriosus, patient foramen ovale, arterial septal defect, ventricular septal defect). Increased A-a gradient.

IV. Database

A. Physical Examination Key Points

1. **Vital signs.** Tachypnea, tachycardia, and hypertension are common early indicators of respiratory distress.
2. **Chest.** Careful auscultation for equal breath sounds to identify pneumothorax, intubation of right mainstem bronchus, consolidation, or mucus plugging. Poor air movement and wheezing with asthma. Palpate for rib fractures.
3 **Heart.** Murmur suggesting valvular disease, signs of CHF.
4. **Skin and nailbeds.** Look for cyanosis, signs of emboli.
5. **CNS.** Confusion and agitation are signs of inadequate CNS perfusion.
6. **Respiratory equipment.** Inspect for loose connections, incorrect settings.

B. **Laboratory Data**
   1. **ABG** and mixed venous blood gas.
   2. **Hematocrit.** Check for anemia.
   3. **Cardiac enzymes** if MI suspected.
   4. A-a or A-aDO$_2$ is a useful calculated value that determines the difference in the alveolar oxygen and the arterial oxygen content in the pulmonary capillary bed. Normal is 20–65 mm Hg on 100% O$_2$.
      a. Place patient on 100% O$_2$ (FiO$_2$ 1.0) for 20 minutes.
      b. Obtain peripheral ABG.
      c. A-a gradient (mm Hg) = atmospheric pressure (760 mm Hg) minus partial pressure of H$_2$O (47 at 37°C) minus arterial PCO$_2$ minus arterial PO$_2$.
      d. The larger the gradient, the more severe the defect. Gradients >400 mm Hg are severe.

C. **Radiologic and Other Studies**
   1. **Chest radiograph.** To evaluate pneumothorax, pleural effusion, and pulmonary edema and to check position of endotracheal tube.
   2. **Electrocardiogram.** Acute MI will decrease cardiac output, and right heart strain may indicate PE.
   3. **Nuclear V/Q scan,** followed by pulmonary angiography if PE is suspected.
   4. **Chest CT.** If indicated, after initial evaluation and stabilization of the patient.

V. **Plan.** Overall, the underlying cause should be ascertained while improving patient oxygenation. The patient should be in a monitored setting.

A. **Increase FiO$_2$.** Use nasal cannula, Ventimask, or face tent as needed. If there is any question about the patient's ability to protect the airway or maintain sufficient ventilation without aid, the patient should be intubated and mechanical ventilation begun. When an acceptable level of oxygenation has been achieved, wean the FIO$_2$ back as tolerated. Remember that oxygen at high concentrations can lead to atelectasis (by eliminating nitrogen from alveoli) and oxygen toxicity.

B. Pneumothorax or other mechanical problems should be diagnosed and managed as rapidly as possible. Chest tube and endotracheal tube insertion or manipulation should be followed by a chest radiograph to ensure proper position.

C. Airway Care. Suctioning, postural drainage.

D. Manage Atelectasis. Chest physiotherapy, incentive spirometry, increase tidal volume, and positive end-expiratory pressure (PEEP).

E. Bronchodilators. Relieve bronchospasm and increase clearance of secretions. Inhalational metaproterenol, IV theophylline, and PO or SC terbutaline are the most commonly used agents. Asthma refractory to these may require steroids.

F. Other Medications. Antibiotics, inotropic agents, or anticoagulation as indicated.

REFERENCES

Marvin RG, et al. Critical care. In: Townsend CL, ed. *Sabiston Textbook of Surgery,* 16th ed. Philadelphia: WB Saunders; 2001, p 375–93.
Sigillito RL, DeBlieux PM. Evaluation and initial management of the patient in respiratory distress. *Emerg Med Clin North Am* 21:239–58, 2003.
Summer WR. Respiratory failure. In: Goldman L, Bennett JC, eds. *Cecil Textbook of Medicine,* 21st ed. Philadelphia: WB Saunders; 2000, p 466–75.

50. INABILITY TO VOID (URINARY RETENTION)

I. Problem. A 66–year-old man with severe suprapubic pain presents to the emergency room after not being able to void for almost 24 hours.

II. Immediate Questions

A. What are the patient's vital signs? Fever and tachycardia may be signs of acute bacterial prostatitis.

B. What medication is the patient taking? Pharmacologic causes of acute urinary retention are common and discussed further below.

C. Is there any history of voiding problems, such as hesitancy, urgency, frequency, or nocturia? These symptoms are suggestive of bladder outlet obstruction in males (prostatic hypertrophy, stricture). Gross hematuria may suggest clot retention.

D. Has the patient had recent surgery? Patients with recent prostate or bladder surgery may rebleed and develop clot retention; patients who have had abdominoperineal resection can develop a neurogenic bladder. In general, after any surgical procedure the patient may develop retention due to pain and increased sympathetic outflow (closes bladder neck) in the immediate postoperative period.

E. Is there a history of neurologic problems? Disk herniation, spinal cord injury, and stroke can affect bladder function.

III. Differential Diagnosis

A. Pharmacologic. Tranquilizers (phenothiazine), antihypertensives (ganglionic blockers, methyldopa), anticholinergic agents (cold preparations), and narcotics can cause urinary retention.

B. Neurologic. Pelvic or lumbar spine trauma can result in urinary retention (detrusor contraction is dysfunctional and bladder sensation is intact). Pelvic surgery, abdominoperineal resection (APR), and neuromuscular diseases commonly cause urinary retention and often resolve with time. Temporary acute urinary retention is also seen after spinal anesthesia and after operative procedures performed in the inguinal or genital region.

C. Anatomic. In the elderly man with acute retention, prostatic enlargement, either benign or malignant, should be immediately considered. Other anatomic causes include acute prostatitis (obtain history of perineal pain and fever) and urethral stricture (history of episodes of sexually transmitted diseases or instrumentation), especially in young patients. A psychiatric patient may present with foreign body obstruction. With a history consistent with urolithiasis (flank pain radiating to the groin, nausea and vomiting), consider an obstructing calculus at the bladder neck. Gross hematuria can result in clot retention. Urethral disruption (eg, blood at the meatus, "floating prostate") may cause retention in the trauma patient.

IV. Database. History should include medications, infections, previous operative and urologic procedures, psychiatric history, and recent trauma or injury.

A. Physical Examination Key Points

1. Rectal examination. Specifically determine the presence of focal or generalized prostatic enlargement.

Tenderness may indicate prostatitis. Note quality of anal sphincter tone as an indicator of pelvic nerve function. A high riding "floating" prostate may indicate urethral disruption.

2. **Genital examination.** Look for purulent (infectious) or bloody (traumatic) meatal discharge.
3. **Abdomen.** Gentle palpation and percussion of the lower abdomen will demonstrate bladder distention.
4. **Neurologic.** Determine presence of normal deep tendon reflexes, cremasteric reflex, normal local sensation, and presence of the "anal wink" (squeezing the glans penis will result in involuntary contraction of the anal sphincter, indicating an intact pelvic reflex arc).

B. **Laboratory Data**
   1. **Hemogram.** High WBC count may indicate infection (prostatitis).
   2. **Serum electrolytes, BUN, creatinine.** Longstanding and acute retention can lead to renal dysfunction.
   3. **Urinalysis and urine culture.** Note presence of blood or crystals. A positive urine culture is almost always seen in acute bacterial prostatitis.
   4. **Culture** urethral discharge.

C. **Radiologic and Other Studies**
   1. **Excretory urography/voiding cystourethrogram (VCUG).** Especially if blood is found on urinalysis or if urolithiasis is suspected. If creatinine level is high, ultrasound is a better test to evaluate for upper tract obstruction.
   2. **Retrograde urethrogram.** Indicated to evaluate for urethral stricture or urethral disruption.
   3. **Cystoscopy.** Indicated in most patients with anatomic and neurologic causes for retention. Usually performed after Foley catheter decompression.

V. **Plan**

A. **Catheterization (see page 338).** First, attempt decompression by passing a 16F–18F Foley catheter gently. If this fails, a coude tip (elbow tip) catheter sometimes passes more readily in males. Injection of water-soluble jelly 30 mL into the urethra may also help pass the catheter. Rarely will filiform and followers or a suprapubic cystostomy be required. Complete decompression should be performed gradually. Catheterization must not be performed in the trauma patient unless urethral disruption has been ruled out with a retrograde urethrogram.

B. **Antibiotics.** Urinary tract infections or sepsis and acute prostatitis will require treatment with appropriate antibiotics. Cultures should be obtained before initiating treatment. Recently, fluoroquinolones have been the empiric choice for urinary tract infections.

C. **Fluid and Electrolyte Management.** Care should be taken to monitor serum electrolytes, especially if postobstructive diuresis follows decompression of the urinary tract obstruction. This is commonly encountered in the setting of chronic obstruction resulting from prostatic hypertrophy. Patients with high BUN and creatinine levels are more prone to this problem. The diuresis is due to impaired concentrating ability of the chronically obstructed kidneys and the osmotic diuresis caused by chronic retention of waste products. Uncontrolled postobstructive diuresis can result in vascular collapse due to hypovolemia. After the bladder is decompressed, monitor urine output and vital signs closely. Initially, use maintenance IV fluids without potassium. Physiologic diuresis is common, but significant urine output associated with hypotension suggests a postobstructive problem. Check electrolytes and replace milliliter for milliliter with IV fluid similar to the urine electrolyte profile. Then gradually change to half milliliter for milliliter and taper IV from there.

D. **Postoperative.** Once ambulatory, many patients will be able to void without difficulty. Limiting pain medications may help. α Blockers (terazosin, doxazosin) may help relax the bladder neck and help restore the voiding pattern.

E. **Cystoscopy.** Cystoscopic and urodynamic studies are usually performed in this setting but rarely needed in acute cases.

REFERENCES

Curtis LA, et al. Acute urinary retention and urinary incontinence. *Emerg Med Clin North Am* 19:591–619, 2001.
Rosenstein D, McAninch JW. Urologic emergencies. *Med Clin North Am* 88:495–518, 2004.
Thomas K, Chow K, Kirby RS. Acute urinary retention: a review of the aetiology and management. *Prostate Cancer Prostatic Dis* 2004;7:32–7.

51. INSOMNIA

I. **Problem.** A patient hospitalized for 14 days of IV antibiotics for fasciitis complains of lying awake for hours at night.

II. **Immediate Questions**

A. **Is the patient bothered by pain?** Most surgical patients experience some degree of pain postoperatively or due to the admission diagnosis.

B. What are the patient's sleep habits during the day? If a patient sleeps for extended periods during the day, he or she will not be able to drop off to sleep at night.

C. Does the patient routinely take sleeping medications? Virtually all sleeping medications show a tolerance effect and a disruption of the sleep patterns that can lead to less restful sleep with constant usage.

D. Does the patient have difficulty lying down? Ask specifically about shortness of breath (orthopnea) and calf pain (ischemic rest pain) as causes for disrupted sleep.

E. What is the patient's sleep pattern? Early morning awakening is associated commonly with depression. Anxiety usually causes difficulty in getting to sleep.

F. Does the patient use recreational drugs or abuse alcohol? Withdrawal may lead to insomnia and hallucinations.

III. Differential Diagnosis

A. Medical Causes
1. **Pain.** Inadequate control is often correctable.
2. **Congestive heart failure.** Orthopnea is the hallmark of this condition.
3. **Peripheral vascular disease.** Ischemic rest pain indicates advanced disease.
4. **Hyperthyroidism.**
5. **Sleep apnea syndrome.** Most often seen with morbid obesity. Patients often awaken with a sense of panic and complain of chronic lethargy.

B. Drug/Toxin
1. **Tolerance** to sleeping medications or tranquilizers.
2. **Alcohol abuse.** With secondary chronic disruption of appropriate sleep patterns.

C. Psychiatric
1. **Depressive illness.** Bipolar or unipolar.
2. **Anxiety.**

D. Situational
1. **Noise.** Close to nursing station or a noisy roommate.
2. **Anger.** Unexpressed anger toward staff or family.
3. **Anxiety.** About medical condition, possible operation, or discharge from the hospital.

IV. Database. Most important is the history, including an evaluation of the mental status of the patient.

A. Physical Examination Key Points
1. **Neurologic examination.** Mental status. Evaluation for anxiety or depression.

   2. **Cardiopulmonary.** Rales, displaced PMI or gallop rhythm to suggest CHF.
   3. **Extremities.** Decreased or absent pulses, pallor on elevation, dependent rubor.
 B. **Laboratory Data.** Many times the cause of insomnia will be determined without the use of laboratory tests.
   1. **Screening chemistries.** Include hepatic and renal function.
   2. **Thyroid hormone levels.** If clinically indicated.
 C. **Radiologic and Other Studies**
   1. Chest radiograph if indicated for cough or CHF.
   2. Ankle/brachial blood pressure or other vascular studies if indicated.
   3. Sleep laboratory for chronic sleeping difficulty and to rule out sleep apnea.

V. **Plan**

 A. **Etiology.** Attempt to determine the cause of the insomnia. Most cases will be secondary to a situational cause or just being in the hospital. For this reason it is wise to include a prn sleeping medication order with all admission and post-operative orders unless specifically contraindicated. Any specific medical problem should be managed and pain should be adequately controlled.
 B. **Specific Treatments**
   1. **Oral sleeping medication.** Frequently used agents are:
     a. Diphenhydramine (Benadryl) 25–50 mg.
     b. Temazepam (Restoril) 15–30 mg.
     c. Zolpidem (Ambien) 5 or 10 mg. Nonbenzodiazepine agent that does not distort the natural sleep cycle.
     d. Lorazepam (Ativan) 0.5–1 mg.
     e. Chloral hydrate 500–1000 mg.
     f. Triazolam (Halcion) 0.125 or 0.25 mg. Use 0.125 mg for elderly.
   2. **Nonoral sleeping medications**
     a. Diphenhydramine 25–50 mg IV.
     b. Ativan 0.5–1 mg IV.
     c. Chloral hydrate 500–1000 mg per rectum.
     d. Nembutal 100 mg per rectum.
   3. **Nonmedical treatments.** Often as effective and may include discussing apprehensions, having the patient's room changed, or providing activities during the day to normalize sleep habits.
   4. **Sleep apnea** is usually managed by night-time nasal continuous positive airway pressure (CPAP) support.

REFERENCES

Holbrook AM, et al. The diagnosis and management of insomnia in clinical practice: a practical evidence-based approach. *CMAJ* 2:210–6, 2000.

Holbrook AM, et al. The role of benzodiazepines in the treatment of insomnia. *J Am Geriatr Soc* 49:824–6, 2001.

Schenck CH, et al. Assessment and Management of Insomnia. *JAMA* 19:2475–9, 2003.

52. IRREGULAR PULSE

Immediate Actions

1. Assess Airway, Breathing, Circulation. Intubate if necessary. Check vital signs. Administer O_2.
2. Assess effect on hemodynamic stability. Hypotension associated with arrhythmia requires rapid action.
3. Ensure IV access.
4. Assess mental status for a baseline before proceeding further.

I. **Problem.** On routine check of vital signs, a nurse discovers that a 75-year-old man, status post below-the-knee amputation, has an irregular pulse.

II. **Immediate Questions**

A. **What is the pulse rate?** For instance, the ventricular rate in atrial fibrillation is rarely >150 beats/min, whereas supraventricular tachycardias are usually >150 beats/min.

B. **What are the other vital signs?** You must know if the irregular pulse is associated with hemodynamic instability (hypotension).

C. **What medication is the patient taking?** Be especially careful to note cardiac medications or diuretics, which can induce hypokalemia.

D. **Is there a history of cardiac disease?** Check for history or previous documentation of irregular rhythm. Postoperative arrhythmias are rare in individuals <40–45 years.

E. **Is the rhythm regular, irregular, irregularly irregular?** The rhythm can provide a clue about the nature of the problem. Although an ECG is necessary to formally evaluate rhythm, a quick check of the pulse is helpful. Obtain the old chart and compare with a previous ECG/rhythm strips.

    F. What are the laboratory results? Chemistry, CBC count, thyroid-stimulating hormone. Electrolyte abnormalities, anemia, and hypo-/hyperthyroidism may lead to arrhythmias.

III. Differential Diagnosis. Remember that an irregular pulse is a result of a disease process, not a diagnosis.

    A. Impulse Formation Disorders

        1. Premature atrial and ventricular contractions.

        2. Sinus arrhythmia. A benign variation of pulse.

        3. Escape beats. Seen especially in bradycardias.

        4. Extra systoles. Has a constant interval between a sinus beat and the extrasystole. Usually abolished by exercise.

        5. Atrial fibrillation. Commonly associated with many types of underlying heart disease (ischemic, valvular). Absent P waves on the cardiogram and an irregularly irregular ventricular rate. Flutter waves may also be seen.

        6. Pacemaker malfunction.

        7. Sick sinus syndrome.

        8. Paroxysmal atrial tachycardia with variable block. The atrial rate is 140–250 beats/min with a variable ventricular response.

    B. Conduction Disorders

        1. Sinoatrial block. Can be associated with ischemia or caused by digoxin.

        2. Partial AV block. Mobitz type I (Wenckebach) or type II second-degree block.

        3. Pulsus alternans. Regular rhythm with alternation in amplitude of equally spaced beats.

    C. Myocardial Ischemia. The first evidence of asymptomatic ischemic myocardium (or infarction) is often an arrhythmia.

    D. Pulmonary Disease. Pulmonary embolus can present as atrial fibrillation or other arrhythmia. Supraventricular arrhythmias often occur after thoracic/pulmonary surgical procedures.

    E. Pericardial Disease. Constrictive pericarditis and tamponade can cause irregular pulse.

IV. Database

    A. Physical Examination Key Points

        1. Vital signs. Pulse regularity and rate; tachypnea may suggest PE.

        2. Heart. A rub is associated with pericarditis or a transmural infarction; murmurs suggest valvular disease.

        3. Neck. Look for jugular atrial waves, venous distention.

    4. Blood pressure. Check for pulsus paradoxus-associated with constrictive pericarditis, pericardial tamponade, or severe asthma. A positive test shows >10 mm Hg decrease in blood pressure with inspiration.

B. Laboratory Data
    1. Electrolytes. Electrolyte abnormalities, especially potassium, can cause a variety of arrhythmias.
    2. Arterial blood gases. Hypoxia can cause arrhythmias and may be associated with PE.
    3. Cardiac panel (troponin I, CPK, lactate dehydrogenase, isoenzymes, aspartate aminotransferase). To look for evidence of myocardial ischemia.
    4. Digoxin level. In the patient already on digoxin.
    5. Thyroid hormone levels. Hyperthyroidism can lead to arrhythmias.

C. Radiologic and Other Studies
    1. 12-Lead ECG/rhythm strip. Atrial fibrillation will be an obvious diagnosis on ECG. Look for signs of acute ischemia. Compare with old ECGs.
    2. Chest radiograph. Look for signs of CHF, cardiomegaly, primary pulmonary disease, and pneumothorax. The tip of a central line may cause irritation and arrhythmia if advanced too distally.
    3. Ultrasound. Identify intracardiac mural thrombus in a patient with chronic atrial fibrillation, valvular disease, or pericardial effusion.
    4. Nuclear V/Q scan and/or CT angiogram. If PE is suspected.

V. Plan

A. Overall Plan. Eliminate the arrhythmia by controlling the underlying cause. It is imperative to rapidly treat any patient who is hemodynamically compromised (hypotensive) or symptomatic (shortness of breath or chest pain) from the arrhythmia. An otherwise stable patient can be treated more conservatively.
    1. Start O_2 in any patient with an arrhythmia.
    2. IV access should be established if not already present.

B. Specific Plans. Drug dosages are discussed in detail in Section IX, page 447.
    1. Sinus arrhythmia. No treatment needed.
    2. Atrial fibrillation
        a. Control underlying electrolyte imbalance or hypoxia.
        b. If the patient is hemodynamically stable, treatment options include IV diltiazem, verapamil, digoxin, or propranolol.

    d. Amiodarone is the preferred agent in patients with low ejection fraction (<35%) or structural heart disease.

    e. A patient with hemodynamic compromise should be electrically cardioverted.

3. Pulmonary embolus

    a. Diagnosed by nuclear V/Q scan or CT angiogram.

    b. Treat with heparin (bolus followed by constant drip to maintain PTT >1.5–2 times control) or streptokinase.

    c. If contraindications to anticoagulation exist, insert a Greenfield filter.

4. Myocardial infarction. The usual supportive therapy is indicated: monitor, oxygen, pain relief (morphine), nitrates, and β blocker.

REFERENCES

Braunwald E. *Heart Disease: A Textbook of Cardiovascular Medicine,* 6th ed. Philadelphia: WB Saunders; 2001, p 833–5.

Falk RH. Atrial fibrillation. *N Engl J Med* 344:1067–78, 2001.

Roy D, et al. Amiodarone to prevent recurrence of atrial fibrillation. *N Engl J Med* 342:913–20, 2000.

53. IV (INTRAVENOUS) ACCESS PROBLEMS

  I. Problem. A 40-year-old IV drug abuser enters the hospital with abdominal pain and protracted vomiting. No arm veins are usable for rehydration due to scarring.

  II. Immediate Questions

    A. What is the nature of the patient's illness? Patients who require immediate IV access (eg, hypotension with shock) should undergo percutaneous central line placement or cutdown in the absence of large peripheral veins. Consider bleeding diatheses or coagulopathies before placing a central venous line. Remember that bleeding from the subclavian artery during a misadventure in placement is impossible to manually tamponade.

    B. Is there a history of IV drug abuse or of prolonged hospitalization and loss of venous access? What routes of access were used on other occasions? Chronically hospitalized patients often lose usable peripheral veins because of multiple IV and venipunctures.

  III. Differential Diagnosis. Peripheral IV access may be poor in the following situations:

    A. Intravenous Drug Abuse.

    B. Obesity.

    C. Prior Chemotherapy.

    D. Prolonged Hospitalization. Numerous previous IV lines.

    E. Lymphedema. After mastectomy or axillary lymphadenectomy.

    F. Anasarca.

    G. Hypotension and Hypovolemia.

IV. Database

    A. Physical Examination Key Points

        1. Upper extremities. Look for needle marks indicating previous IV access. Look for antecubital vein.

        2. Vital signs. Hypotension or other signs of shock often cause peripheral veins to collapse.

    B. Laboratory Data. Consider a hematocrit and platelet count in children because even a small amount of blood loss can be significant in a child.

V. Plan. IV access should be approached in the following order in elective and emergent situations. In emergencies, evaluation should be undertaken quickly to provide rapid access (see also Section III, pages 357, 340, 336).

    A. Peripheral (Arm). Start distally and work proximally. Catheters 14–16 gauge are the lines of choice in trauma situations because they allow for massive fluid repletion, more so than central lines. Lower extremity lines should be avoided because they do not last long in ambulatory patients and have a higher incidence of thrombophlebitis.

    B. External Jugular. Simple 1– to 2-inch angiocatheters can be placed in the external jugular vein without difficulty and with little or no patient risk. Placing the patient in the Trendelenburg (head down) position and gently occluding the vein just above the clavicle will usually dilate it.

    C. Central Lines. Include IJ, subclavian, and femoral. Experience with a particular route of access is an important determinant for which route to access. IJ and subclavian lines are useful for measuring CVP. Many people believe that femoral lines should be used rarely because of the increased risk of infection; these lines are adequate for short-term use for fluid resuscitation. The literature does not support the concern about increased rates of infection.

    D. Cutdowns. Three veins are readily accessible by cutdown techniques.

    E. Other. In children with no IV access, tibial puncture with a large needle (interosseous line) allows infusion of fluid and medication. This clearly represents a technique of last resort in pediatric patients near death. The incidence of osteomyelitis in survivors is relatively high.

G. Clotted Catheter. Occasionally, clotted catheters can be cleared by gentle irrigation with agents such as urokinase (see page 530).

REFERENCES

Roberts R. *Clinical Procedures in Emergency Medicine,* 4th ed. New York: Elsevier; 2004, p 450–3.

Ross AK. Pediatric trauma. Anesthesia management. *Anesthesiol Clin North Am* 19:309–37, 2001.

Sweeney MN. vascular access in trauma: options, risks, benefits, complications. *Semin Anesth* 20:47–50, 2001.

54. NAUSEA/VOMITING

I. Problem. A patient complains of nausea and then vomits repeatedly 1 week after a colectomy for diverticulitis.

II. Immediate Questions

A. Are there any associated symptoms, in particular GI? Nausea and vomiting may accompany a wide spectrum of illnesses covering most body systems. Inquire about related concurrent symptoms to focus the differential diagnosis. Ask about abdominal pain, distention, diarrhea, or constipation/obstipation associated with the nausea and vomiting.

B. What is the appearance and odor of vomitus? The vomited material can give clues to the nature of the underlying dysfunction. First, look and test for blood (see Problem 35, page 132). Feculent vomitus indicates stasis or distal obstruction. Bilious vomit merely implies a patent pyloric channel. A change in the vomit from bilious to bloody may indicate a Mallory-Weiss tear.

C. How is the vomiting related to eating or specific medications? In the postoperative setting, note if the vomiting correlates with beginning or advancing an enteral diet. Vomiting 1–2 hours after eating (especially if the vomit is partially digested food) points to gastric stasis or gastric outlet obstruction. Vomiting concurrent or immediately after eating is often psychogenic. Certain medications can cause vomiting, such as narcotics or NSAIDs. Does the patient have antiemetics prescribed to accompany the narcotic medications?

D. **Is the vomiting projectile?** Projectile vomiting is often associated with CNS dysfunction. However, it may also occur with certain types of food poisoning.

E. **Does the patient have an NG drainage tube in place?** Confirm proper functioning and positioning. Check the blue sump for a sucking sound. If not functioning, inject air with a syringe and confirm sucking sound.

III. **Differential Diagnosis.** The following differential list is structured around the primary system involved in the underlying cause of nausea and vomiting.

A. **Gastrointestinal**
   1. **General**
      a. Peritonitis.
      b. Postoperative ileus.
      c. Mechanical obstruction at any level.
      d. Gastroenteritis.
   2. **Stomach**
      a. Gastric outlet obstruction.
      b. Peptic ulcer disease.
      c. Gastric atony.
   3. **Hepatobiliary/pancreas**
      a. Biliary colic or acute cholecystitis.
      b. Pancreatitis.
      c. Hepatitis.
   4. **Colon**
      a. Diverticulitis.
      b. Malignant obstruction from colorectal cancer.
      c. Appendicitis.

B. **Metabolic**
   1. Uremia.
   2. Hepatic failure.
   3. Metabolic acidosis.
   4. Electrolyte abnormalities.
      a. Hypercalcemia.
      b. Hyperkalemia.

C. **Endocrine**
   1. **Diabetes.** Gastroparesis.
   2. Adrenal insufficiency.
   3. Hypothyroidism.

D. **Drug/Toxin**
   1. Alcohol abuse.
   2. Botulism.
   3. Food poisoning (eg, staphylococcal).
   4. Food or drug allergy.

  5. Narcotics, especially codeine.
  6. NSAIDs (eg, ibuprofen).
  7. Chemotherapeutic agents.

E. Cardiopulmonary
 1. Acute MI. Particularly inferior MI.
 2. CHF.

F. Genitourinary
 1. Renal colic.
 2. Pelvic inflammatory disease.
 3. Pregnancy.

G. Nervous System
 1. Space-occupying CNS lesion; increased intracranial pressure.
 2. Migraine headache.
 3. Labyrinthitis.

H. Acute Febrile Illnesses. Particularly in pediatric patients.

IV. Database

A. Physical Examination Key Points
 1. Vital signs. Orthostatic signs, fever, tachycardia.
 2. HEENT. Pharyngitis, otitis, or other evidence of acute infections, papilledema.
 3. Skin. Turgor, mucus membranes to estimate volume status. Jaundice.
 4. Abdomen. Evaluate for bowel sounds, abdominal distention, peritoneal signs, and areas of tenderness. Pain out of proportion to physical findings may indicate ischemic bowel.
 5. Rectal examination. Evidence of impaction, positive fecal occult blood, mass, or fluctuance (suggestive of abscess).
 6. Neurologic examination. Mental status changes may signify CNS lesion or severe electrolyte disorder.
 7. Pelvic examination. Consider if pelvic inflammatory disease is suspected.

B. Laboratory Data
 1. Hemogram. For signs of infection or blood loss.
 2. Urinalysis and urine culture. May reveal infection or blood seen with stones.
 3. Chemistries. General screening includes electrolytes, BUN/creatinine, liver function tests. Calcium levels.
 4. Amylase.
 5. ABGs if indicated.
 6. Urinary human chorionic gonadotropin (HLG) to diagnose pregnancy.

C. **Radiologic and Other Studies**
   1. **Kidneys, ureter, bladder and upright abdominal films.** Obtain abdominal films in most patients with vomiting and in all patients with abdominal distention.
   2. **Chest radiograph.** To aid in the diagnosis of pneumonia, CHF, and evidence of aspiration. Pleural effusion can be seen with pancreatitis. Look for free air on upright film.
   3. **Electrocardiogram.** If possibility of ischemic heart disease.
   4. **Abdominal ultrasound/HIDA scan.** If possibility of biliary colic.
   5. **UGI series/upper endoscopy.** If significant obstruction is likely, use water-soluble contrast (Gastrografin) instead of barium.
   6. **Barium enema/colonoscopy.** If evidence of colonic pathology or obstruction. Be careful when using barium in patients with suspected obstruction.
   7. **CT of the head.** Obtain this study if an intracranial lesion is suspected.
   8. **CT of abdomen/pelvis.** If a mass lesion or extrinsic compression is suspected (ie, gastric outlet obstruction requires a saline load test).

V. **Plan**

   A. **Overall Plan.** Assess the patient for level of hypovolemia and begin appropriate fluid resuscitation. Make the patient NPO. Screen for drug allergies/reactions. Narcotics are common offenders in the postoperative surgical patient. Control electrolyte abnormalities.

   B. **Abdominal Causes.** Always make the patient NPO and treat with IV fluids. Place NG tube if there is persistent vomiting, mechanical obstruction, or abdominal distention. Proceed with diagnostic workup.

   C. **Nonabdominal causes**, such as metabolic disorders, labyrinthitis, minor infections (eg, acute viral gastroenteritis). Assess volume status, administer IV fluids if indicated, control the underlying disorder, and manage vomiting with antiemetics. Frequently used antiemetics include:
   1. Compazine 10 mg IM/PO every 6 hours.
   2. Tigan 250 mg PO every 6–8 hours, 200 mg IM/rectally every 6–8 hours.
   3. Phenergan 12.5–25 mg PO every 8 hours, or 25 mg IM every 8 hours.
   4. Antivert 25–50 mg PO every 8–12 hours. Useful for nausea in labyrinthitis or vertigo.

5. Reglan 10 mg IV/PO every 6 hours. Useful in diabetics or other situations with poor gastric emptying not due to obstruction.
6. Kytril 10 µg/kg IV over 5 minutes before chemotherapy.

REFERENCES

Quigley EM. AGA technical review on nausea and vomiting. *Gastroenterology* 120:263–86, 2001.
Stadler M. Difference in risk factors for postoperative nausea and vomiting. *Anesthesiology* 98:46–52, 2003.
Watcha M. Postoperative nausea and emesis. *Anesthesiol Clin North Am* 20:471–9, 2002.

55. NASOGASTRIC TUBE MANAGEMENT—BLOODY DRAINAGE

I. **Problem.** A 43-year-old male has bloody output from his NG tube 2 days after a small bowel resection for a Meckel's diverticulum.

II. **Immediate Questions**

A. **How long has the NG tube been in place?** A tube that has been placed recently may have bloody drainage from the trauma of insertion or gastric surgery. An old tube may show blood from local mucosal irritation.

B. **How much bloody drainage has there been?** A tube that passes large amounts of bright red blood is obviously a more critical situation than one that passes a few red streaks.

C. **Has the patient had recent or remote UGI surgery?** If the surgery is recent, there may be bleeding at a newly formed anastomotic site, or there may be a marginal ulcer at an old anastomotic site.

D. **Is the patient receiving antacids? What is the pH of the fluid?** The presence of acidic gastric secretions increases the likelihood of the development of gastritis.

E. **Evaluate the patient's blood pressure and pulse**. Hypotension and tachycardia are indicative of volume loss.

III. **Differential Diagnosis**

A. **Insertion Trauma.** Usually in the nasopharynx.

B. **Mucosal Irritation.** Often from a tube that has been in place for some time. There is usually an associated acidic pH.

    C. Suture Line Disruption or Hemorrhage. Especially in a patient who recently underwent an operation.

    D. Swallowed Pharyngeal Blood. From an upper source of bleeding perhaps unrelated to the NG tube.

    E. Ulceration (Curling, Cushing, Pre-existing). Look for associated conditions: burns, head injury, etc.

    F. Gastric Erosion/Gastritis/Esophagitis/Variceal Bleed.

    G. Coagulopathy. Physiologic or pharmacologic.

IV. Database

    A. Physical Examiantion Key Points
        1. Vital signs. Look for tachycardia and hypotension as evidence of sepsis or excessive blood loss.
        2. Abdomen. Look for peritoneal signs, epigastric tenderness, or gastric distention.
        3. HEENT. Evidence of pharyngeal bleeding.

    B. Laboratory Data
        1. CBC count. To check for excessive blood loss.
        2. PT/PTT and platelet count. To rule out coagulopathy.

    C. Radiologic and Other Studies
        1. Upright chest radiograph. To look for free intra-abdominal air. Look at the mediastinum and both lung fields for air that may be a result of esophageal perforation after forceful vomiting (Boerhaave's syndrome).
        2. pH. Check the pH of the gastric fluid. Is it <4.0?

V. Plan

    A. Overall Plan. To determine whether the cause of bleeding is serious enough to require specific aggressive therapy.

    B. Specific Plans
        1. For life-threatening UGI bleeding, establish venous access and begin fluids. Hypotensive patients will require vigorous blood and fluid replacement. Transfer the patient to the ICU. See Problem 48, page 178.
        2. Begin antacid therapy. Start IV H_2-receptor blockers or proton pump inhibitors. Sucralfate can also be helpful.
        3. Irrigate the NG tube with saline. Irrigation enables diagnosis of further bleeding. It also serves as a therapeutic maneuver of removing clots from the stomach, which lead to distention and persistent bleeding.
        4. The presence of peritoneal signs or new free intra-abdominal air requires emergency laparotomy.
        5. Perform UGI endoscopy if bleeding persists (see Problem 35, page 132).

REFERENCES

Aljebreen AM. Nasogastric aspirate predicts high-risk endoscopic lesions in patients with acute upper-GI bleeding. *Gastrointest Endosc* 59:172–8, 2004.

Bini EJ. Endoscopic treatment compared with medical therapy for the prevention of recurrent ulcer hemorrhage in patients with adherent clots. *Gastrointest Endosc* 58:707–14, 2003.

Lefkovitz Z. Radiologic diagnosis and treatment of gastrointestinal hemorrhage and ischemia. *Med Clin North Am* 86:1357–99, 2002.

56. NASOGASTRIC TUBE MANAGEMENT— CHANGE IN AMOUNT OF OUTPUT

I. **Problem.** A 56-year-old woman with pancreatitis has a sudden increase in the amount of NG tube aspirate on the fifth hospital day. Another patient has minimal NG aspirate after small bowel resection 3 days previously.

II. **Immediate Questions**

A. **Is there associated abdominal distress?** If the patient developed a generalized ileus or a distal obstruction, the amount of aspirate will increase.

B. **Is the output bilious?** Bilious NG output indicates a more distal problem with bile reflux into the stomach or an NG tube placed distal to the pylorus.

C. **Is the tube functioning?** Tubes often become obstructed with mucous or antacids. Listen for whistle from the sump tube, which indicates patency.

D. **Is the patient passing flatus or stool?** Often decreased NG output correlates with return of bowel function.

E. **Is an NPO patient surreptitiously taking in fluid?** Often ice chips given to patients with NG tubes can be excessive and cause high NG tube outputs.

III. **Differential Diagnosis**

A. **Increased Output**
   1. Tip of tube distal to pylorus.
   2. Distal bowel obstruction or gastric outlet obstruction.
   3. Return to higher secretory state after discontinuation of H_2-receptor blockers, eg, cimetidine.
   4. Surreptitious ingestion.

B. **Decreased Output**
   1. Return of normal bowel motility and function.
   2. Obstructed/kinked tube.
   3. Use of H_2-receptor blocker, which decreases gastric secretion, or agents that improve motility and gastric emptying.

   4. Tip of tube above gastroesophageal junction or coiled
      in the oropharynx.

IV. Database
A. Physical Examination Key Points
   1. Abdomen. Listen for bowel sounds and their quality.
      No sounds may indicate ileus or far advanced obstruc-
      tion. High-pitched, hollow sounds indicate obstruction.
      Distention may mean obstruction or ileus.
   2. Mouth. Look for tube coiled or kinked in mouth or
      throat.
   3. Rectal examination. Determine presence or absence
      of stool.
   4. Tube. Check patency and function by flushing with air
      or saline.

B. Laboratory Data
   1. Serum electrolytes. Carefully monitor hydration status,
      potassium, and bicarbonate levels during NG suction.
   2. Nasogastric aspirate. A pH >6 indicates use of
      antacids or that the catheter tip is distal to the pylorus.

C. Radiologic and Other Studies
   1. Upright chest radiograph. Look for a large stomach
      bubble, indicating poor gastric emptying. Check posi-
      tion of the tube tip.
   2. Upright and flat abdominal radiographs. Show dis-
      tended bowel indicating ileus or obstruction.
   3. Contrast swallow. Order a Gastrografin swallow study.
      Serial radiographs will show normal or delayed empty-
      ing and passage of contrast. Contrast should *not* be
      used in the presence of ileus or complete obstruction.

V. Plan.
The first priority is to determine that the NG tube is functioning properly and in a proper position.

A. Position.
Based on radiograph and acidic aspirate.

B. Function.
Sump tubes should whistle continuously on low
suction. Flush with saline (30 mL) every 3–4 hours to
maintain patency.

C. Increased Output
   1. Poor gastric emptying (no obstruction). Try metoclo-
      pramide 10 mg IV every 6 hours.
   2. Distal obstruction. Continue NG suction; consider fur-
      ther workup and operation to relieve obstruction.
   3. Ileus. Patience and observation are necessary, espe-
      cially if immediately postoperative. Correct electrolyte
      abnormalities, especially hypokalemia. Continue NG

suction. Prolonged ileus may indicate intra-abdominal sepsis.

D. Decreased Output
1. Often indicates return of bowel function. Correlate with physical examination and passage of flatus or stool. Remove the tube if appropriate.
2. Irrigate tube to clear it, or advance tube into stomach if it is not positioned correctly.

REFERENCES

Bass BL. What's new in general surgery: gastrointestinal conditions. *J Am Coll Surg* 195:835–54, 2002.

Leung FW. The venerable nasogastric tube. *Gastrointest Endosc* 59:255–60, 2004.

Maglinte DD. Current concepts in imaging of small bowel obstruction. *Radiol Clin North Am* 41:263–83, 2003.

57. OLIGURIA/ANURIA

I. **Problem.** A patient has sequential hourly urine outputs of 22, 15, 9, and 4 mL through an indwelling Foley catheter 1 day after an aortic aneurysm repair.

II. **Immediate Questions**

A. What is the patient's volume status? The most common cause of oliguria in the postoperative setting is hypovolemia. The most important and most frequent differential diagnosis is acute tubular necrosis (usually secondary to ischemia). Assess the volume status by left-sided pressures from a pulmonary artery catheter, weight change, and physical examination. Be sure that hypovolemia is not a result of hemorrhage.

B. Did the patient develop any periods of documented hypotension? Ischemic acute tubular necrosis is a cause of oliguria on the surgical service. Review the operative record of the anesthesiologist and note any episodes of intraoperative hypotension.

C. What is the baseline renal function? Look at the admission BUN and creatinine and any subsequent electrolyte studies. Any insult to the kidneys will be amplified by any pre-existing chronic renal dysfunction.

D. Is the patient taking any renal toxic drugs? Aminoglycosides are a major cause of renal toxicity. Obtain appropriate drug levels and hold the next dose until the results are evaluated. Also consider IV contrast dye as a potential nephrotoxin.

E. Is the patient taking any medication that is excreted by the kidneys? Digoxin and antibiotics are the most important medications in this category. Modify or hold the dose until renal function improves or drug levels become available.

F. Is the Foley catheter patent? Flush the catheter at least once to make sure the oliguria is a reflection of renal function (see Problem 33, page 127).

III. Differential Diagnosis. The differential diagnosis for acute oliguria as with acute renal failure may be viewed as prerenal, renal, or postrenal.

A. Prerenal (Renal Hypoperfusion)
  1. **Shock/hypovolemia.**
     a. **Hemorrhage:** Traumatic or as a postoperative complication.
     b. Inadequate fluid administration.
     c. Sepsis.
  2. Apparent intravascular hypovolemia, a relative decrease in the effective circulating volume.
     a. **"Third-space" losses:** Very common in the initial postoperative period after major operations or with major burns. Prolonged exposure of bowels during a lengthy operative procedure may account for insensible losses of 4–6 mL/kg per hour of operative time.
     b. CHF.
     c. Cirrhosis may have associated hepatorenal syndrome.
     d. Nephrotic syndrome.
  3. **Vascular.**
     a. Renal artery occlusion (acute or chronic).
     b. Aortic dissection.
     c. Emboli (eg, cholesterol).

B. Renal
  1. **Acute tubular necrosis.**
     a. **Ischemic:** Secondary to shock, sepsis.
     b. **Toxins:** Medications (aminoglycosides), contrast media, heavy metals.
  2. **Acute interstitial nephritis.**
     a. **Drugs:** β-lactamase-resistant penicillins, NSAIDs.
     b. **Hypercalcemia:** Can cause nephrocalcinosis.
  3. **Acute glomerular disease.**
     a. Malignant hypertension.
     b. Immune complexes.
     c. Systemic diseases (Wegener's, thrombotic thrombocytopenic purpura, systemic lupus erythematosus, Goodpasture's syndrome).

C. Postrenal

1. Urethral obstruction (prostatic hypertrophy, catheter obstruction).
2. Bilateral ureteral obstruction (carcinoma or retroperitoneal fibrosis).

IV. Database

A. Physical Examination Key Points

1. **Vital signs.** Weight change, orthostatic signs to document fluid loss.
2. **Skin.** Tissue turgor, mucus membranes, or edema.
3. **Cardiopulmonary.** Rales, high venous pressure, cardiac gallop, or JVD.
4. **Abdomen.** Determine if there is ascites, or if the bladder is distended.
5. **Extremities.** Assess perfusion by color and temperature.

B. Laboratory Data

1. **Electrolytes, BUN, and creatinine.** If BUN/creatinine >20:1, then the cause is likely prerenal; if BUN/creatinine <15:1, then the cause is likely renal. Hyperkalemia can be life threatening and may accompany acute renal insufficiency.
2. **Urinalysis.** Protein, RBC casts support glomerular disease. Eosinophils are associated with hypersensitivity reactions. WBC casts may indicate glomerulonephritis.
3. **Spot or random urine electrolytes and creatinine.** Obtain before giving diuretics. Urinary sodium <20 mEq/L indicates prerenal cause; urinary sodium >20 mEq/L is suggestive of renal cause. Calculate renal function index as urinary sodium multiplied by plasma creatinine divided by the urine creatinine. If the index is >1, it is likely a renal cause; if the index is <1, it is likely prerenal (see also Section II, page 318).
4. **CBC count.** For evidence of infection or anemia.
5. **Drug levels.** Evaluate for any renal toxic drugs.

C. Radiologic and Other Studies

1. **Chest radiograph.** May reveal CHF.
2. **PA catheter.** Will provide useful information about volume status.
3. **Kidneys, ureter, bladder.** May reveal obstructing renal calculi.
4. **IV pyelogram.** A combination of ultrasound, renal scan, and retrograde studies will provide equivalent information without renal toxic contrast media.
5. **Ultrasound.** Examines the bladder and upper urinary tract for signs of obstruction.

6. **Renal scan.** Technetium-labeled diethylenetriamine penta-acetic acid or MAG-3 nuclear medicine study to assess blood flow to the kidneys, especially if embolus is a concern.
7. **Angiogram.** To visualize vascular anatomy.
8. **Renal biopsy.** Occasionally needed to determine specific diagnosis of renal cause of oliguria.

V. Plan

A. **Overall Plan.** As a general rule, the minimal acceptable urine output in an adult is 0.5 mL/kg per hour. Oliguria in most surgical patients results from hypovolemia. In almost every case it is appropriate to give the patient a volume challenge (eg, NS 500 mL). In patients with fragile cardiorespiratory status, smaller boluses and central venous catheters should be used to monitor volume status. Also stop or alter all nephrotoxic or renally excreted drugs and remove potassium from the IV fluids.

B. **Prerenal**
   1. Treat with volume boluses to increase urinary output and increase maintenance IV rate.
   2. Monitor volume replacement with central lines, if needed.
   3. **Follow hourly urine output.**

C. **Renal**
   1. Monitor volume status with central lines.
   2. Remove potassium from IV solutions unless it is abnormally low.
   3. Attempt to increase urine output once volume status is corrected.
      a. **Furosemide:** Use escalating doses to obtain response of increased urine output. Review patient's previous creatinine levels; if high, then fluid challenge may be warranted before administration of Lasix.
      b. **Mannitol:** 12.5–25 g (25% solution 50–100 mL) to induce an osmotic diuresis.
   4. **Review medications.** Adjust doses or stop nephrotoxic drugs.
   5. **Monitor electrolytes.**

D. **Postrenal.** Usually requires urologic consultation. Ureteral stents or percutaneous nephrostomy may be needed. A blocked Foley catheter can be unblocked as outlined in Problem 32, page 127.

REFERENCES

Cuhaci B. Oliguria: fluid deprivation or furosemide deficiency? *Crit Care Med* 30:1402–12, 2002.

Mehta RL. Acute renal failure definitions and classification: time for change? *J Am Soc Nephrol* 14:2178–87, 2003.

Wilson WC. Oliguria. A sign of renal success or impending renal failure? *Anesthesiol Clin North Am* 19:841–83, 2001.

58. PARESTHESIAS

I. **Problem.** A 62-year-old male patient is complaining of paresthesias (tingling or "pins and needles") 1 day after undergoing a right radical neck dissection.

II. **Immediate Questions**

  A. **Where are the paresthesias?** A patient with paresthesias in an extremity and with known or likely peripheral vascular occlusive disease presents a different clinical dilemma than one with circumoral paresthesias.

  B. **Does the patient have peripheral vascular disease?** Paresthesias are 1 of the "5 Ps" of peripheral vascular occlusive disease; the others are pain, pallor, pulselessness, and paralysis.

  C. **Has the patient had these symptoms before?** It is important to determine if the condition was present preoperatively or as a consequence of the recent surgical procedure.

  D. **Did the paresthesia appear suddenly or gradually?** Find out if they can be linked to a particular event. Was there any unusual positioning during the surgical procedure?

  E. **What does the operative wound look like?** Is there a hematoma or a mass causing compression in the neck?

III. **Differential Diagnosis.** Paresthesias may be reported as tingling, "pins and needles," or numbness.

  A. **Vascular Insufficiency.** Paresthesias may be one of the early symptoms of vascular compromise, and early action may be necessary to save the affected extremity.

  B. **Hypocalcemia.** Paresthesias primarily involve the lips, tongue, fingers, and feet and are an especially significant symptom after thyroid or parathyroid surgery (see Problem 44, page 165).

  C. **Operating Room Causes.** Surgeons leaning on the patient for prolonged periods in the operating room may lead to postoperative paresthesias in a peripheral nerve distribution. Improper positioning and padding of extremities during a case is another preventable cause.

   D. Hyperventilation. Results in bilateral hand and finger tip numbness, thereby reproducing the symptoms. Anxiety may result in hyperventilation.
   E. Transient Ischemic Attack. Often bilateral extremity numbness that may accompany speech and sight difficulties.
   F. Peripheral Neuropathy. Often classic "glove and stocking" distribution seen in patients with diabetes, alcoholism, or chronic renal insufficiency.
   G. Nerve Compression. Such as carpal tunnel syndrome or a dressing that is applied too tightly.
   H. CNS Tumors, Neurosyphilis.

IV. **Database**
   A. Physical Examination Key Points
      1. **Vital signs.** Tachypnea associated with hyperventilation.
      2. **Peripheral pulses.** Especially in an affected extremity.
      3. **Look for causes of pressure in the area.** Dressings, casts, etc.
      4. **Check for physical signs of hypocalcemia.** Chvostek's and Trousseau's signs (see Problem 44, page 165).
      5. Carotid bruit may be present to suggest transient ischemic attacks.
      6. **Neurologic examination.** Signs of peripheral neuropathy include symmetric loss of pinprick sensation. Reflexes are decreased with nerve compression.
   B. Laboratory Data
      1. **Serum electrolytes and calcium.** To rule out hypocalcemia, renal failure, and diabetes.
   C. Radiologic and Other Studies
      1. **Electrocardiogram.** Look for atrial fibrillation, which predisposes to thrombus and embolization.
      2. **Nerve conduction velocities.** Assist with the diagnosis of nerve compression.
      3. Doppler blood flow determination may reveal blood flow in an extremity with a nonpalpable pulse.

V. **Plan**
   A. Vascular Insufficiency with Paresthesias. Requires rapid therapy to save the extremity. Reoperating on a clotted graft or angiographic study of an acutely obstructed vessel is indicated (see Problem 63, page 220).
   B. Hypocalcemia. In the patient with paresthesias after thyroidectomy, repletion of serum calcium is indicated with PO or IV calcium (see Problem 44, page 165).

C. **Transient Ischemic Attacks.** Transient ischemic attacks are often managed surgically to remove carotid plaques.

D. **Peripheral Neuropathies.** For example, alcoholism and diabetes are most often chronic and irreversible.

E. **Dressings and Casts.** Should be revised as appropriate.

REFERENCES

Casati A. Paresthesia but no motor response: what's going on? *Anesthesiology* 98:586–8, 2003.

Pascuzzi RM. Peripheral neuropathies in clinical practice. *Med Clin North Am* 87:697–724, 2003.

Shapiro BE. Entrapment and compressive neuropathies. *Med Clin North Am* 87:663–96, 2003.

59. PHLEBITIS

I. **Problem.** A 32-year-old woman had an exploratory laparotomy for ovarian cancer. An IV in her arm has not been changed for 5 days and the site is now red and painful.

II. **Immediate Questions**

A. **What are the patient's vital signs?** Fever can develop from superficial thrombophlebitis and DVT.

B. **Can pus be expressed from the site?** Pus indicates a local infection, and sepsis with pus may indicate suppurative thrombophlebitis. Look for red streaks proximal to the IV site.

C. **What medications are being administered through the line?** Agents such as potassium and calcium can cause phlebitis. Peripheral parenteral nutrition may also cause phlebitis.

III. **Differential Diagnosis.** Acute venous inflammation or occlusion can occur in superficial or deep veins. DVT usually does not have a significant inflammatory component and rarely is infected.

A. **Superficial Thrombophlebitis.** Acute inflammation without infection is the most common presentation.
  1. Site of IV catheter, especially in upper extremities.
  2. Extravasation of irritant medications, such as chemotherapeutic agents.
  3. Unknown cause, especially in lower extremities.

B. **Suppurative Thrombophlebitis.** Persistent fever, sepsis, and positive blood cultures indicate significant infection. Pus is expressed, and there may be daily increases in the length of vein involved despite local therapy. This occurs rarely at upper extremity IV sites and is slightly more common at emergent cutdown sites.

C. Other
1. DVT (see Problem 66, page 229).
2. Septic thrombophlebitis of subclavian vein.

IV. Database
A. Physical Examination Key Points
1. **Vital signs.** Pay close attention to signs of sepsis.
2. **Extremities.** Old intravenous sites should be examined in the febrile patient. Palpate the calves for tenderness. Gently squeeze erythematous IV sites in an attempt to express pus.

B. Laboratory Data
1. **Hemogram.** Leukocytosis is present in suppurative superficial thrombophlebitis.
2. Culture and Gram's stain of pus from old IV site.

C. Radiologic and Other Studies.
Venography is rarely indicated if central vein infection or DVT is suspected in the septic patient.

V. Plan.
Prevention of thrombophlebitis by frequent rotation of IV sites.

A. Superficial Thrombophlebitis
1. Local heat, dry or moist.
2. Limb elevation.
3. NSAIDs.
4. Consider administering heparin if patient has no contraindications.

B. Suppurative Thrombophlebitis
1. Local care.
2. Analgesics and anti-inflammatory agents.
3. **IV antibiotics.** Broad spectrum with good anti-staphylococcal coverage (nafcillin, etc).
4. Persistent or progressing infection mandates exploratory venotomy and venectomy of the entire involved segment of vein. Segments of vein should be sent to pathology and microbiology, and the wound should be left open and packed.
5. Consider administering heparin if patient has no contraindications.

C. Other.
Suppurative thrombophlebitis of a subclavian vein requires resection in the operating room and IV antibiotics.

REFERENCES

Kagel EM. Intravenous catheter complications in the hand and forearm. *J Trauma* 56:123–7, 2004.

O'Grady NP. Guidelines for the prevention of intravascular catheter-related infections. Centers for Disease Control and Prevention. *MMWR Recomm Rep* 51(RR-10):1–29, 2002.

Tagalakis V. The epidemiology of peripheral vein infusion thrombophlebitis: a critical review. *Am J Med* 113:146–51, 2002.

60. POSTOPERATIVE PAIN MANAGEMENT

I. **Problem.** The night after an open lung biopsy the patient threatens to pull out his chest tube and leave the hospital because of severe incisional pain.

II. **Immediate Questions**

A. **Is there any evidence of a wound infection, hematoma, or other problem?** Early wound infections (*Clostridium*, *Streptococcus*) may be a factor in early postoperative pain. Also, a wound hematoma may amplify expected postoperative pain.

B. **What is the current pain medication regimen—what drug, what dose, and how often has it been given?** Titrate the dose to relieve pain, make certain the frequency is appropriate, and ensure the nurses are administering the medication appropriately. If patient has an epidural, discuss the case with the anesthesiologist before adding pain medications. One may also consider patient-controlled analgesia in the awake patient.

C. **Is there any history of narcotic use or abuse?** Tolerance to narcotics is a real phenomenon and these patients need their doses increased sometimes to alarmingly high levels to achieve pain control.

III. **Differential Diagnosis.** Discussions of postoperative pain almost always indicate incisional pain.

A. **Inadequate Analgesic Regimen**
1. **Too small a dose.**
2. **Too long between doses.**
3. **Patient-controlled analgesia.** Dosing may be too low or lockout too long.

B. **Wound Complications**
1. **Infections.** Be alert for aggressive life-threatening infections (*Clostridium*, *Streptococcus*, necrotizing fasciitis) that may only initially present with pain.
2. **Hematoma.**

3. Dehiscence.
4. Nerve entrapment or excessive pressure from a dressing.
5. Compartment syndrome developing in an extremity.

C. **Drug-Seeking Behavior.** A patient's complaint of pain should be attended to in the immediate postoperative period. However, if reported pain persists or increases as time passes, a contributing factor, including drug-seeking behavior, should be considered.

IV. Database

A. Physical Examination Key Points
1. **Vital signs.** Fever and tachycardia suggest an infection. Early postoperative tachycardia with hypertension suggests pain.
2. **Wound.** Look for signs of infection (erythema, purulence, crepitation, margination, drainage) or developing hematoma. Make sure the dressing is not the cause of the pain.
3. **Neurologic examination.** Observe for posturing, grimacing, splinting, and other body movements consistent with pain. Disorientation or obtundation is consistent with narcotic overdose or sepsis.

B. Laboratory Data
1. CBC count if infection is suspected.
2. Wound culture if it is the suspected source.

C. Radiologic and Other Studies. Chest radiograph if indicated.

V. Plan

A. Overall Plan. Realize that pain management is part of the complete care of the surgical patient.

B. Pain Medications. Medications are discussed in detail in Section IX, page 447.
1. **Morphine sulfate.** Gold standard for postoperative pain. Dose is 2–10 mg SC every 3–4 hours in most cases.
2. **Demerol.** 50–75 mg IM every 3 hours.
3. **Dilaudid.** 1–2 mg IM every 3–4 hours.
4. **Percocet, Percodan, or Tylenol with codeine.** Given as 1 or 2 tablets PO every 4–6 hours as needed.
5. **Hydroxyzine (Atarax, Vistaril).** Use as adjunct to parenteral narcotics 25–50 mg every 8 hours. It is useful to potentiate the pain-relieving action and minimize nausea associated with narcotics.

C. **Alternative Methods of Pain Control**
   1. **Epidural narcotics.** An epidural catheter is left in place by the anesthesia team and is usually managed by the anesthesiologists.
   2. **Patient-controlled analgesia.** Infuses boluses, continuous IV morphine, or both and is controlled to some extent by the patient.
   3. **Nerve blocks.** For certain incisions (thorax, flank) that can be extremely painful especially in the first few hours postoperatively; infiltration with a long-acting anesthetic in the operating room at the end of the case can be helpful.

REFERENCES

Dirks J. Mechanisms of postoperative pain: clinical indications for a contribution of central neuronal sensitization. *Anesthesiology* 97(6):1591–6, 2002.

Doyle D. Patient-controlled analgesia. *CMAJ* 164:620A-620, 2001.

Weaver M. Abuse liability in opioid therapy for pain treatment in patients with an addiction history. *Clin J Pain* 18(suppl):S61–9, 2002.

61. PRURITUS

I. **Problem.** Three days after a low anterior resection, a 49-year-old male is complaining of severe pruritus (itching) of both legs.

II. **Immediate Questions**
   A. **What is the duration of the symptom?** An acute condition can more often be related to an exact cause, such as a change in laundry soap, new medication, etc.

   B. **Has the patient recently started taking any new medications, eating different foods, wearing different clothing, using new detergents or soaps?**

   C. **Is there an associated rash or lesions?**

   D. **Does the patient have any allergies?**

III. **Differential Diagnosis**
   A. **Skin Disorders.** Pruritus associated with visible skin lesions.
   1. Papulosquamous skin diseases.
   2. Vesicobullous diseases.
   3. Allergic reactions, eg, contact dermatitis.
   4. Infestations, eg, scabies.
   5. Infection, eg, viral exanthemas.

   B. Systemic. Itching can be associated with a variety of systemic conditions without an associated rash.

      1. Dry skin. Especially in the elderly, may be related to cold weather.

      2. Liver disease. Often with jaundice and cholestasis.

      3. Uremia. May be unrelated to BUN.

      4. Hypothyroidism.

      5. Hyperparathyroidism.

      6. Diabetes mellitus.

      7. Gout.

      8. Hodgkin's disease, leukemias.

      9. Intestinal parasites, eg, pinworms or hookworms.

      10. Drug reactions.

      11. Pregnancy.

      12. Polycythemia vera.

      13. Blood-borne neoplasms.

   C. Psychosomatic Pruritus.

   D. Neurologic and Circulatory Disturbances.

IV. Database

   A. Physical Examination Key Points. Check the patient's skin (not just the affected area); examine the distribution of rash and any skin lesions. What looks like a rash may be a skin breakdown secondary to severe scratching of the pruritic area. Examine skin carefully near IV sites.

   B. Laboratory Data

      1. Liver function tests. To help rule out liver disease.

      2. BUN and creatinine. May reveal renal insufficiency and uremia.

V. Plan

   A. Overall Plan. Pruritus does not require immediate therapy unless caused by a significant systemic disease or early anaphylaxis. The primary goal is to enhance the patient's comfort until the definitive diagnosis is available to dictate therapy.

   B. Specific Measures

      1. Dry skin. Skin hydration by daily bathing in warm water, followed immediately by applying skin moisturizer cream.

      2. Uremic pruritus. Ultraviolet light and lidocaine IV may help.

      3. Cholestasis. Cholestyramine may help in pruritus secondary to hepatic disease.

      4. Medical treatment. There are 3 oral medications useful in the management of symptomatic pruritus.

   a. **Diphenhydramine (Benadryl)** 25–50 mg PO or IV
      every 8 hours.
   b. **Cyproheptadine (Periactin)** 4 mg PO 3 times daily.
   c. **Hydroxyzine (Atarax)** 25 mg PO daily or 3 times
      daily.
   d. **Topical steroids** range from mild (hydrocortisone),
      to mid potency (triamcinolone [Kenalog]), high po-
      tency (halcinonide [Halog]), and the highest potency
      (betamethasone dipropionate [Diprolene]).
5. **Discontinuation of medication** that is causing pruritus, if possible.

REFERENCES

Bergasa N. An approach to the management of the pruritus of cholestasis
   Clin Liver Dis 8:55, 2004.
Etter L. Pruritus in systemic disease: mechanisms and management. *Dermatol Clin* 20:459–72, vI–vii, 2002.
Moses S. Pruritus. *Am Fam Phys* 68:1135–42, 2003.

62. PULMONARY ARTERY
CATHETER PROBLEMS

(Technique of pulmonary artery catheterization is discussed in
Section III, Bedside Procedures, page 375)

I. **Problem.** A PA catheter inserted into a septic patient will not
   "wedge."

II. **Immediate Questions**

   A **Has the catheter ever been in good "wedge" position?**
      Make sure the catheter worked before. Check the tip posi-
      tion on radiograph, which may reveal that the catheter is
      not in proper position.

   B. **Is the balloon working properly, or is there any prob-
      lem with the monitor or transducer system?** Balloons
      occasionally rupture. A PA pressure tracing suggests that
      the transducer system is otherwise intact.

   C. **Flush all ports thoroughly and check transducer be-
      fore insertion.** Be certain that all the air has been evacu-
      ated from the lines.

III. **Differential Diagnosis**

   A. **Placement Problem.** The most frequent sites of catheteri-
      zation are the IJ and subclavian veins. Fluoroscopically
      and ultrasound-guided techniques can help in certain
      cases, such as in patients who have undergone pneu-

monectomy where careful placement is mandatory. Placement problems include:
1. Passage into the IJ vein or out the contralateral subclavian vein.
2. Looping in the right ventricle.
3. Knotting of catheter.

B. Functional Problems. Functional problems develop relatively frequently after successful placement of a PA catheter.
  1. **No waveform.** A thrombus may occlude the catheter.
  2. **Cannot "wedge" catheter.** Repositioning is usually enough to restore function and is particularly easy if the flexible plastic sheath was used at the time of original placement.
  3. **Balloon rupture.** Never use >1.5 mL of air to inflate the balloon. Make sure the waveform changes from a PA tracing to a wedge as the balloon is inflated.

C. Complications
  1. Pneumothorax/hemothorax.
  2. Infection.
  3. PA perforation.
  4. **Arrhythmias.** Usually ventricular as the catheter passes through the ventricle.
  5. Pulmonary infarction, most often caused by a catheter tip that remains in a small pulmonary artery with the balloon inflated.

IV. Database

A. Physical Examination Key Points
  1. **Look at the catheter and check all connections.** Make sure the patient's heart is level with the measuring apparatus.
  2. **Check how much of catheter is in the patient.** Even in large patients, a wedge waveform will be present by the time 60 cm is used. If much more is used (for a subclavian approach), the catheter is likely not proceeding as desired. **Do not proceed beyond 60 cm.**

B. Laboratory Data. Usually not needed.

C. Radiologic and Other Studies
  1. **Check catheter position on chest radiograph.** The tip usually is in the right main PA. There should be a gentle curve as the catheter passes from the right atrium, through tricuspid valve into ventricle, and out into the pulmonary artery. The catheter should lie in a smooth curve and be no farther than 5 cm from the mid-

line. There is a greater incidence of PA perforation when the catheter tip is in the left main PA.

V. Plan. Placement of a PA catheter should be done with careful monitoring by someone experienced in the technique. The catheter should be flushed and tested before placement. The balloon should be inflated with air 1 mL and then deflated. The catheter should be connected to the transducer before placement to test the electronic aspects of the entire system. Once connected, the tip of the catheter should be briskly tapped, which produces high frequency waves on the monitor.

A. Placement
1. Inflate the balloon in the superior vena cava to allow blood flow to carry the catheter out the right ventricular outflow tract. This is usually at about 20 cm through the subclavian approach. Plan to use the right IJ or left subclavian veins to facilitate the natural curve of the catheter.
2. Be sure that the balloon is **deflated** whenever the catheter is being withdrawn and **inflated** when advancing the catheter.
3. As the catheter passes into the right ventricle, ventricular arrhythmias may develop and should be controlled if persistent or associated with hemodynamic compromise. Some clinicians think it is safest to withdraw the catheter into the right atrium and bolus the patient with lidocaine before replacing the catheter. These rhythm abnormalities are usually short-lived and rarely persist after placement of the catheter into the PA.

B. Functional Problems. These typically occur after a variable period of catheter use. If still needed, a nonfunctioning catheter should be replaced after certain maneuvers have been performed, even if the catheter has just been placed. Most functional problems develop because of thrombosis at the catheter tip or at other ports.
1. Flush nonfunctional ports frequently.
2. **Test balloon.** If the balloon is intact you should be able to remove the same volume of air carefully placed into the balloon. During use, however, passive deflation is safest.
3. Reposition the catheter farther distally with the balloon inflated if unable to "wedge" the balloon. If unable to position the catheter, use fluoroscopy(C-arm).

C. Complications
1. Pneumothorax requires tube thoracostomy.
2. Infected catheter should be immediately removed. Antibiotics may be required with positive blood cultures.

3. Arrhythmias are controlled with lidocaine 1 mg/kg bolus. Withdraw the catheter into the right atrium until the drug is given.

REFERENCES

Cholley BP, et al. Pulmonary artery catheters in high risk surgical patients. *N Engl J Med* 348:66–8, 2003.

Marino PL. The pulmonary artery catheter. In: *The ICU Book*, 2nd ed. Philadelphia: Lippincott Williams & Wilkins; 1998, p 154–65.

Waxman K, et al. Intensive care monitoring. In: Bongard FS, Sue DY, eds. *Current Critical Care Diagnosis and Treatment,* 2nd ed. New York: McGraw-Hill; 2003, p 516–27.

63. PULSELESS EXTREMITY

I. **Problem.** Two days after a coronary artery bypass, a nurse examines an elderly patient and reports that he has no pulses in his right leg.

II. **Immediate Questions**

A. **Is this an acute change for the patient?** Look at admission history and physical for prior documentation of pulses. Unfortunately, a complete vascular examination (at a minimum femoral and pedal pulses) is often a neglected portion of the admit note. Ask the patient if he noted any acute changes in the extremity.

B. **Are there any associated symptoms of pain or numbness in the involved extremity?** Pain, pallor, pulselessness, paresthesias, and paralysis are the "5 Ps" of diagnosis of an acute arterial occlusion. Most patients have pain and pallor. Paresthesias are an early sign, and paralysis is a late sign of ischemic injury to the leg. Ask if these symptoms are new, and if so, how rapidly they developed (see also Problem 58, page 209).

C. **Is there any history of claudication or any previous vascular surgery?** Significant peripheral vascular atherosclerosis may be the underlying cause of an acute arterial occlusion. Also, the degree of chronic obstruction determines the amount of collateral circulation developed in the affected extremity. This may have an effect on how well an acute occlusion is tolerated.

D. **What are the pulses in the other leg?** Chronic peripheral vascular occlusive disease is usually bilateral, and comparison of pulses between the extremities may indicate baseline status of the extremity in question. Some acute events may also be bilateral (eg, saddle embolus).

   E. Any history of palpitations or atrial fibrillation? Atrial
   fibrillation is one of the leading causes of embolic arterial
   occlusion. Even if a patient is found to be in a sinus
   rhythm, ask about any history of arrhythmias or digoxin
   use. A recent conversion to sinus rhythm may be the
   cause of an acute embolic event.

III. Differential Diagnosis. Most acute arterial occlusions occur
in the lower extremity and usually are due to embolic phenomenon. However, thrombosis, vasculitis, and even venous disease may cause an acute occlusion. Review operative note
for any intraoperative complications.

   A. Embolic Causes
      1. Cardiac sources
         a. Coronary artery disease. Prior MI with mural
            thrombi.
         b. Atrial fibrillation.
         c. Rheumatic heart disease. Usually mitral stenosis
            with atrial fibrillation.
         d. Prosthetic cardiac valves.
         e. Endocarditis.
         f. Atrial myxoma.
      2. Peripheral sources
         a. Aortic. Aneurysm with mural thrombi.
         b. Atheroemboli. Often associated with invasive pro-
            cedures (cardiac catheterization) or from peripheral
            sources (aortic, iliac, popliteal); this phenomenon is
            known as blue toe syndrome or "trash foot."
         c. Paradoxical emboli through a patent foramen ovale
            or other type of right-to-left shunt.

   B. Thrombotic Causes. Almost always some degree of atherosclerotic occlusive disease with contributing factors of
   hypovolemia/low flow and hypercoagulable states.
      1. Arterial occlusive disease.
      2. Diabetes.
      3. Hypovolemia/low flow
         a. Trauma and resultant shock.
         b. Dehydration.
         c. Fever.
         d. Sepsis.
      4. Hypercoagulable
         a. Malignancy.
         b. Polycythemia.
         c. Estrogen use.
         d. Heparin-induced thrombosis.

   C. Arterial Dissection.
   D. Trauma. Blunt or penetrating.

  E. Vasculitis
    1. Takayasu's disease. Often causes upper extremity occlusions.
    2. Thromboangiitis obliterans. In young smokers (Buerger's disease).
  F. Acute Femoral/Iliac Vein Occlusion. Phlegmasia cerulea dolens.

IV. Database
  A. Physical Examination Key Points
    1. Vital signs. Look for orthostatic hypotension, hypovolemia, irregular pulse of atrial fibrillation.
    2. Cardiac. Murmur of valvular diseases or endocarditis, rhythm disturbances.
    3. Abdomen. Abdominal bruits, palpable aneurysm.
    4. Extremity examination. Pulses and temperature at all levels compared with the contralateral side. Examine for skin pallor or mottling, and look for a cutoff for the level of ischemia. Look for changes of chronic ischemia, such as hair loss or skin atrophy. Look also for areas of well-demarcated ecchymoses in feet suggesting "trash foot." Do not forget to feel for popliteal and femoral artery aneurysms. Use a Doppler probe if pulses are not readily palpable.
    5. Neurologic examination. Focal signs and paresthesias indicate significant ischemia. Paralysis indicates likely limb loss.

  B. Laboratory Data
    1. Chemistries. Hyperkalemia may be associated with ischemia.
    2. Hemogram.
    3. PT/PTT. Especially if a patient is on anticoagulant therapy (see pages 312 and 315).
    4. Arterial blood gas. Acidosis may be seen with poor perfusion.
    5. Urinalysis. Hemoglobin in absence of RBCs suggests myoglobinuria.
    6. Myoglobin level for rhabdomyolysis suggests tissue loss.

  C. Radiologic and Other Studies
    1. Chest radiograph.
    2. ECG and rhythm strip. To rule out arrhythmia.
    3. Noninvasive vascular study. Always check nonpalpable pulses with Doppler.
    4. Echocardiogram. Looking for valvular disease, ventricular aneurysm, mural thrombi, or akinesis.
    5. Cardiac thallium scan. Evaluate for prior infarct.
    6. Angiogram. This documents level of obstruction, collaterals, occasionally shows aneurysms and other un-

recognized visceral emboli. May show a source of peripheral emboli.

7. **Abdominal ultrasound.** To evaluate for abdominal aneurysmal disease. Ultrasonography is also useful for peripheral aneurysms.

V. Plan

A. Overall Plan. An acute arterial occlusion is a surgical emergency that requires prompt diagnosis and early management to save the extremity. Evaluate for evidence of paresthesias and paralysis as signs of advancing ischemia and impending limb loss. Control with anticoagulation, volume as needed, and prepare for the operating room. An angiogram is usually obtained, but in some cases the diagnosis and the level of obstruction are obvious and the patient may go directly to the operating room.

B. Correct Volume Deficit. Correct with IV fluid boluses to avoid hypovolemia. Monitor urine output and central filling pressures to guide therapy.

C. Anticoagulation. If there is any delay before surgery or an angiogram, load with heparin 10,000 U IV and then give a continuous infusion of 10 U/kg per hour to prevent thrombus progression. Follow with PT/PTT (see Section II, pages 312 and 315). Some centers may use thrombolytic therapy (streptokinase, tissue plasminogen activator) as a first line of treatment. Some debilitated patients who are judged to have significant operative risk may be managed conservatively with anticoagulation only.

D. Antibiotics. Especially if the patient has prosthetic graft material in place.

E. Protection of the Ischemic Extremity. Position the limb in a mildly dependent position. Protect it from trauma.

F. Operation. Alert the appropriate senior staff, anesthesia, and patient's family because most acute occlusions will be managed by embolectomy or some type of reconstruction.

G. Postoperatively, observe for acidosis, hyperkalemia, myoglobinuria, compartment syndrome, which may develop after extremity reperfusion. Also, monitor pulses and neurologic examination every 2 hours.

REFERENCES

Belkin M, et al. Peripheral Arterial Occlusive Disease. In: Townsend CM Jr, ed. *Sabiston Textbook of Surgery*, 16th ed. Philadelphia: WB Saunders; 2001, p 1989–2030.

Krupski WC. Arteries. In: Way LW, Doherty GM, eds. *Current Surgical Diagnosis and Treatment,* 11th ed. New York: McGraw-Hill; 2003, p 813–58.

Ouriel K, Green RM. Acute arterial occlusion. In: Schwartz ST, et al, eds. *Principles of Surgery,* 7th ed. New York: McGraw-Hill; 1999, p 931–1004.

64. SEIZURES

Immediate Actions

1. Ensure Airway, Breathing, and Circulation. Do not force anything into the mouth of a seizing patient.
2. Prevent self-inflicted injuries.
3. Obtain IV access.
4. Single seizures usually end before therapy can be started. A patient in status epilepticus needs therapy. Start with Diazepam (Valium) 10 mg slow IV push.

I. **Problem.** A 25-year-old male is found seizing in bed 1 day after appendectomy.

II. **Immediate Questions**

A. **Has the patient ever had seizures before?** Patients with history of seizures are often on antiseizure medication. A common cause of seizures is the failure to take their medication.

B. **Has the patient been put back on all medications he was taking before admission?** If the patient is NPO, be sure that an appropriate parenteral form is given. Check for other medications because some of these can affect blood levels of antiseizure medication, in particular diphenylhydantoin (Dilantin).

C. **Does the patient have a history of alcohol abuse or diabetes?** This may be confused with alcoholic withdrawal or severe hypoglycemia.

D. **Was the seizure generalized or focal?** Focal seizures suggest a CNS cause.

E. **What are the results of the most recent laboratory tests?** These may reveal obvious electrolyte abnormalities. Make sure the serum levels of antiseizure medications are therapeutic.

F. **Were there any witnesses?** Observers may indicate a prodrome or report whether the patient developed any specific injury or fall.

III. Differential Diagnosis. The hallmark of the seizure is rigid stiffening of the muscles, loss of bladder control, and cyanosis with a postictal phase consisting of confusion, myalgia, lethargy, and headache.

    A. Idiopathic Epilepsy. The most common cause of seizures but must be a diagnosis of exclusion in the acute situation.

    B. Tumors. Primary brain tumors or metastatic lesions can be responsible. Frequent lesions include carcinoma of the breast, lung, or kidney, melanoma or lymphoma.

    C. Infection. In adults, intracranial infection can cause seizures; in children, any infectious process with systemic reaction (fever) can cause seizures.

    D. Trauma. A careful history must be obtained. Was the patient found on the floor? Are there signs of skull fracture?

    E. Alcohol/Drug Withdrawal. This is common in patients who are hospitalized, causing sudden withdrawal (see Problem 25, page xxx).

    F. Chronic Renal Failure. With uremia.

    G. Anoxia. Evaluate ABGs.

    H. Electrolyte Abnormalities. Including hypoglycemia, hypomagnesemia, hypocalcemia, and hyponatremia with rapid correction.

    I. Collagen Vascular Disease.

    J. Hallucinations.

    K. Hypothyroidism.

    L. Degenerative Disease (Tay-Sachs).

    M. Vascular Lesions. Infarcts, emboli, hypertensive encephalopathy, carotid sinus disease, subarachnoid hemorrhage.

    N. Syncope. Often what is thought to be a seizure is just a syncopal episode. Get a careful description about the event.

    O. Hysteria. Such as psychiatric pseudo-seizures.

    P. Inadequate Level of Prescribed Anticonvulsants. Especially phenytoin (Dilantin), where the level can be altered by the addition of other drugs (aspirin, others).

IV. Database

    A. Physical Examination Key Points

        1. Vital signs. Fever suggests infection; febrile seizures may be seen in children. Check blood pressure and palpate pulse to be sure the patient is stable.

2. Do not interfere if the patient is spontaneously breathing. Specifically, do not try to force something into the patient's mouth such as a tongue depressor. This can lead to injury to the patient or yourself and is unnecessary.
3. Check for aspiration.
4. **Neurologic examination.** Look for focal signs that may help diagnose the cause. Perform a complete examination including all cranial nerves, sensation, strength, deep tendon reflecter (DTRs), and mental status. There may be transient deficits after the seizure (postictal state).
5. Is there evidence of fecal or urinary incontinence?

B. Laboratory Data
1. Serum electrolytes, calcium, magnesium, creatinine, and glucose to rapidly screen for metabolic causes.
2. **Arterial blood gases.** To rule out hypoxia.
3. **Drug levels** of anticonvulsants being taken.
4. Cerebrospinal fluid analysis, if indicated (see Section III, page 363.)

C. Radiologic and Other Studies
1. **Head CT scan.** New onset seizures with no obvious cause mandate a CT scan of the head. The scan does not need to be done emergently, unless other evidence suggests a space-occupying lesion that may require emergent therapy.
2. Lumbar puncture may help if there is evidence of meningeal irritation.

V. Plan

A. General Plan.
Support life functions (the ABCs of CPR), and prevent self-inflicted injury during the seizure. This is followed by a careful workup to determine the cause and institute appropriate therapy.

B. Specific Measures
(see Section IX, page 447, for a discussion of drugs listed below).
1. Vital functions, especially airway, must be monitored and supported.
2. Establish IV access as soon as possible.
3. A single seizure will usually finish before the onset of action of any IV medication and therefore does not need to be specifically controlled. However, to manage a second seizure or status epilepticus (repeated seizures with no regaining of consciousness between seizures), diazepam (Valium) IV may be given, usually as 5 mg IV push (slowly), repeating at 10- to 15–minute intervals as needed to control seizure activity.

4. Phenytoin (Dilantin) may be used if Valium fails or to prevent recurrence of seizures if Valium has provided temporary control. It must be given as a slow IV push, no faster than 50 mg/min, directly into the vein. Check levels daily after first starting the drug. Levels are best checked after 24 hours of initial dose. Loading dose is 15–18 mg/kg IV.

5. Phenobarbital may also be used. It is given as a slow IV usually with a 120–240 mg (10–20 mg/kg in children) loading dose. Maintenance doses are given IV, IM, or PO to maintain therapeutic levels.

6. Be alert for the complications of aspiration and hyperthermia.

7. Anticonvulsants are not indicated for alcohol withdrawal seizures, but Librium may be useful to control other symptoms of delirium tremens.

8. Refractory seizures that do not respond to the above management may require general anesthesia.

C. Control Underlying Condition. After the acute seizure episode is controlled, control the underlying condition. Manage electrolyte abnormalities as outlined in the specific on-call problem. Treat CNS lesion as appropriate.

REFERENCES

Angood PB, et al. Surgical complications-neurologic. In: Townsend CM Jr, ed. *Sabiston Textbook of Surgery,* 16th ed. Philadelphia: WB Saunders; 2001, p 297–332.

Doherty GM, et al. Postoperative complications-central nervous system. In Way LW, Doherty GM, eds. Current *Surgical Diagnosis and Treatment,* 11th ed. New York: McGraw-Hill; 2003, p 23–37.

Foldvary-Schaefer N, Wyllie E. Epilepsy. In: Goetz CG, ed. *Textbook of Clinical Neurology,* 2nd ed. Philadelphia: WB Saunders; 2003, p 430–57.

65. SUPRAPUBIC CATHETER PROBLEMS

I. Problem. A patient has a suprapubic catheter that has stopped draining.

II. Immediate Questions

A. Does the patient have a full bladder? This is most easily determined by palpating suprapubic fullness with associated tenderness.

B. Is the total urine output adequate? Gradual decrease in urine may suggest oliguria as opposed to an obstructed tube.

C. **Is urine draining around the suprapubic tube, and is there blood or clots?** This suggests that the tube is blocked or pulled out of the bladder.

D. **Why does this patient have a suprapubic catheter?** Suprapubic cystostomy drains are placed surgically or percutaneously for bladder decompression. Temporary tubes placed emergently (ie, Cystocath, Stamey type, which have a small diameter, ie, 12F–14F) can dislodge if not carefully secured. Tubes placed in the operating room intended for long-term use are usually of the Malecot variety and of larger caliber (22F–24F). They are placed for a wide range of indications such as bladder injury, urethral injury and obstruction, transplant neoureterocystostomy obstruction, or stricture.

E. **How long has the catheter been in place?** A longstanding suprapubic tube usually will have a mature tract into the bladder, whereas a recently placed tube may not.

III. **Differential Diagnosis**

A. **Systemic Causes.** For detailed discussion of low urine output (oliguria), see Problem 56, page 203.

B. **Catheter Obstruction.** Can be caused by blood clots or occasionally by debris. Longstanding tubes can become coated with calcium deposits. Examine catheter for kinks.

C. **Catheter Tip Dislodgement.** More of a problem with a recent suprapubic tube because the tract may be immature.

IV. **Database**

A. **Directed History and Physical Examination.** Attention to fluid status, vital signs, temperature, abdominal examination, catheter exit site, and catheter suture.

B. **Laboratory Data.** Laboratory studies usually are not necessary in acute cases.

C. **Radiologic Studies.** Consider bedside ultrasound to assess urine volume in the bladder.

V. **Plan.** The approach to a poorly functioning tube depends primarily on the age of the tube.

A. **Recently Placed Tube.** Attempt to flush the tube. Tube change probably should be done in the operating room because the tract is immature.

B. **Chronically Indwelling Tube.** A new tube of similar size can be placed because the tract is mature. If a tube is no longer needed, and the patient can void via through urethra, the tract will typically close within 48 hours. Long-term tubes are generally replaced every 4–8 weeks to prevent encrustation. Annual radiography of the kidneys, ureter, and bladder is needed in these patients to evaluate for stone formation. Unless symptomatic, the colonization that accompanies a long-term suprapubic tube is generally not controlled. The notable exception is any colonization with stone-forming organisms (eg, proteus), which must be controlled.

REFERENCES

Han M. Urologic procedures. In: Chen H, Sonnenday CJ, eds. *Manual of Common Bedside Surgical Procedures,* 2nd ed. Philadelphia: Lippincott Williams & Wilkins; 2000, p 205–36.

McAninch JW. Injuries to the genitourinary tract. In: Tanagho EA, McAninch JW, eds. *Smith's General Urology,* 15th ed. New York: McGraw-Hill; 2000, p 330–49.

Smith MS. Cystostomy and vesicostomy. In: Glenn JF, ed. *Urologic Surgery,* 4th ed. Philadelphia: Lippincott; 1991, p 1042–9.

66. SWOLLEN EXTREMITY

I. **Problem.** Three days after a knee replacement, a 49–year-old obese woman develops a swollen left calf and right ankle.

II. **Immediate Questions**

A. **What are the vital signs?** Tachycardia and fever may represent infection. Tachycardia and tachypnea may be manifestations of PE.

B. **Is the patient short of breath?** Complaints of not getting enough air in a patient with a swollen extremity should be evaluated for PE or CHF.

C. **Is the extremity or just the joint swollen?** This would limit the diagnostic possibilities. Is there tenderness to palpation?

III. **Differential Diagnosis**

A. **Venous Obstruction.** DVT, which is usually clinically silent, occurs in a large percentage of immobile postoperative patients. Thrombus can form anywhere from the level of the calf to the pelvis. The major risk of DVT is PE and pulmonary infarction, which are significantly life threatening. Superficial thrombophlebitis can also occur in the upper or lower extremity (see Problem 59, page 211).

B. **Lymphatic Obstruction.** Typically a result of tumor involving inguinal nodes. Obstructed lymphatics produce diffuse, nontender swelling of the entire leg.

    2. Destruction. Operative destruction of draining lymph nodes can produce extremity swelling acutely or years later (eg, after axillary node dissection or radiation therapy).

  C. Infection. Cellulitis of the lower extremity, especially "diabetic foot," can produce swelling to any level depending on the extent of the infection. A foreign body with associated infection can also produce leg swelling.

  D. Congenital. This is usually lymphedema, either tarda or praecox.

  E. Other. Causes of edema, such as renal failure, liver disease, and CHF, typically produce bilateral swelling, although early disease may manifest as a unilateral problem. Joint swelling may be a result of infectious or inflammatory arthritis.

IV. Database

  A. Physical Examination Key Points

    1. Vital signs. Tachypnea is a sign of PE.

    2. Extremities. Check both extremities for swelling. Look for evidence of infection (eg, cellulitis, lymphangitis, or tender superficial veins). Feel for calf tenderness and palpable cords, which are suggestive of DVT. Measure calf and thigh circumferences from a well-marked constant point on both legs as a baseline.

    3. Chest. Listen for rales (CHF).

    4. Abdomen. Look for ascites (liver disease).

    5. Axillary and inguinal nodes. Has a lymphadenectomy been performed? Are nodes palpable (tumor)? Has there been recent breast surgery, or is there a breast mass?

  B. Laboratory Data

    1. Hemogram. Especially if infection is suspected.

    2. Serum electrolytes and glucose. Inflammatory processes can affect the therapy of patients with diabetes and those with chronic renal failure.

    3. Coagulation panel (PT, PTT, platelet count). Obtain baseline values before anticoagulant therapy.

  C. Radiologic and Other Studies

    1. Venogram. The invasive standard for evaluating DVT. Doppler studies are much quicker. CT angiograms are helpful for assessment of PE.

    2. Noninvasive studies such as venous Doppler studies and impedance plethysmography are usually helpful.

    3. Bone radiographs. If "diabetic foot" and cellulitis are suspected. Evaluate for presence of soft tissue air, osteomyelitis, and foreign bodies.

4. CT scan of the abdomen and pelvis to look for a mass that is obstructing the iliac veins or vena cava is recommended.

V. Plan

A. Venous Obstruction

1. Bedrest with elevation of involved extremity.
2. Baseline platelet count and activated PTT should be sent (to check for heparin-induced thrombocytopenia).
3. **Heparin.** 5000–10,000 U IV bolus followed by 1000–1500 U/h continuous infusion to maintain PTT at 2–2.5 times control value.
4. **Coumadin.** Can begin approximately 3–5 days after starting therapeutic heparin and should be continued for 6–12 months or longer for recurrent episodes. PT should be maintained at 1.5–2.5 times control values (international normalized ratio 2–4.5).
5. **Prevention.** Minidose heparin is useful in preventing DVTs when started preoperatively in high-risk patients, eg, those undergoing pelvic or orthopedic procedures, obese patients, or patients with a history of DVT. The dosage is 5000 U SC every 8–12 hours. Pneumatic stockings are available, which intermittently inflate around the calves, presumably reproducing muscle contractions that are effective in preventing DVT. Early ambulation also helps prevent DVT.
6. **Superficial thrombophlebitis.** Typically managed with local heat and NSAIDs (see Problem 58, page 209).

B. Lymphatic Disease.
Local measures, such as heat and elevation, are of little benefit. Custom-made elastic stockings (eg, Jobst) are of some use. Intermittent pneumatic compression may also give some relief.

C. Infection.
Antibiotics should be started, covering for *Staphylococcal* and *Streptococcal* species in the upper extremity and for gram-negative and anaerobic species in the lower extremity. Blood cultures should be obtained in the toxic patient. It may be difficult to differentiate cellulitis from DVT.

D. Pulmonary embolus.
Heparin and Coumadin are therapeutic options. Patients with DVT and contraindications to Coumadin therapy may be best treated with a Greenfield inferior vena cava (IVC) filter.

REFERENCES

Angle N, Freischlag J. Venous disease. In: Townsend CM Jr, ed. *Sabiston Textbook of Surgery*, 16th ed. Philadelphia: WB Saunders; 2001, p 2053–70.

Greenfield LJ. Lymphatic system disorders. In: Greenfiled LJ, ed. *Surgery: Scientific Principles and Practice,* 3rd ed. Philadelphia: Lippincott Williams & Wilkins; 2001, p 1897–902.

Pak LK, Messina LM. Veins and lymphatics. In: Way LW, Doherty GM, eds. *Current Surgical Diagnosis and Treatment,* 11th ed. New York: McGraw-Hill; 2003, p 871–87.

67. SYNCOPE

I. **Problem.** A patient undergoing a preoperative evaluation for a mitral valve replacement has a syncopal episode in the radiology department.

II. **Immediate Questions**

A. **What was the patient doing when the episode occurred?** Vasovagal syncope or fainting from orthostatic hypotension can occur only in a sitting or standing position. Syncope while lying flat is almost always cardiac in origin. Vasovagal attacks have associated factors of heat, anxiety, pain, or closed space. Syncope with exertion is often cardiac. Also ask the patient about coughing, turning or twisting the head, or getting up quickly.

B. **Was the syncope observed, and was there any seizure activity?** In determining the cause of loss of consciousness, a seizure is always in the initial differential diagnosis. Syncopal patients recover quickly, whereas seizure patients have a postictal period. Incontinence is indicative of a seizure.

C. **How did the patient feel immediately before the loss of consciousness?** Patients with vasovagal syncope normally have a presyncopal complex consisting of sweating, lightheadedness, and abdominal queasiness. Cardiac syncope and orthostatic hypotension are usually sudden in onset.

D. **Did anyone take the patient's pulse during the episode?** Vasovagal attacks are associated with bradycardia, orthostatic hypotension with tachycardia, and cardiac syncope with variable heart rates.

E. **Is the patient a diabetic? Insulin dependent?** Hypoglycemic events are an infrequent but readily controllable cause of syncope.

F. **What medications is the patient taking?** Monoamine oxidase inhibitors and antihypertensives can cause orthostatic hypotension if the dose is large enough. Pay close attention to sedatives, especially during and after procedures.

III. Differential Diagnosis

A. Cardiovascular

1. **Reflex syncope.**
   a. Vasovagal (simple faint).
   b. Orthostatic often associated with volume depletion or medications (ie, α blockers such as terazosin).
   c. Carotid sinus syncope.

2. **Cardiac.**
   a. Mechanical.
      i. Aortic stenosis.
      ii. MI.
      iii. Mitral stenosis.
      iv. Cardiomyopathy.
      v. Pulmonary embolism.
   b. Electrical (dysrhythmias).
      i. AV block.
      ii. supraventricular tachycardia (SVT)/ventricular arrhythmias.
      iii. Sick sinus syndrome.
      iv. Pacemaker related.

B. Noncardiovascular

1. **Neurologic.** Subclavian steal, seizure (see Problem 63, page 220).
2. **Metabolic.** Hypoxia, hypoglycemia, hyperventilation.
3. **Psychiatric.** Hysteria, panic.
4. **Pharmacologic.** Review medication list.

IV. Database

A. Physical Examination Key Points

1. **General examination.** Is the patient confused, lethargic, or anxious? Is there any obvious injury? Evidence of incontinence suggests a seizure.
2. **Vital signs.** Orthostatic changes, heart rate, and rhythm. Discrepancy in blood pressure >20 mm Hg between arms is suggestive of subclavian steal syndrome.
3. **Neck.** Carotid bruits, carotid upstroke.
4. **Chest.** Murmurs of aortic stenosis, idiopathic hypertrophic subaortic stenosis (IHSS), rhythm.
5. **Rectal examination.** Heme-positive stools or other evidence of an acute bleed.
6. **Neurologic examination.** Dysarthria, focal signs, mental status.

B. Laboratory Data

1. **Hemogram.** With close attention to the hematocrit.
2. **Chemistry panel.** For electrolytes and glucose.
3. **Blood gas.** Hypoxia or hyperventilation (decreased CO_2, decreased pH) may be present.

C. **Radiologic and Other Studies**
1. **Chest radiograph.** Look for evidence of heart failure or effusion.
2. **ECG with a rhythm strip.** Short PR intervals, delta waves, or any other obvious signs of rhythm disturbance.
3. **Cardiac echo.** May reveal myxoma, valvular lesions, or mural thrombi.
4. Reproduce syncope with maneuvers such as coughing, turning the head, hyperventilation, or carotid massage.
5. **Holter monitor.** Useful for evaluation of dysrhythmias.

V. **Plan**

A. **Overall Plan.** Causes for syncope range from an inconsequential vasovagal attack to the emergency of heart block. Therefore, therapy is dictated by the correct diagnosis. Always assess the patient for injury from a fall during syncope.

B. **Specific Treatments**
1. **Vasovagal.** Instruct the patient to put the head down at the onset of presyncopal symptoms.
2. **Orthostatic hypotension.**
   a. Assess for volume loss (paying close attention for possible GI bleed) and manage accordingly. Patient may need ICU care.
   b. Instruct the patient to change positions slowly.
3. **Cardiac.**
   a. **Control the arrhythmia:** If tachyarrhythmia is causing hypotension, manage as outlined in Problem 68, page 234. Cardiac arrest rhythms are controlled as described in Problem 11, page 44.

C. **Monitor the Patient.** Often, a 24–hour Holter monitor needs to be obtained for diagnosis. Assess patient for hemodynamic stability; if unstable, place patient in the ICU and consider central line placement and Swan-Ganz catheter for fluid status.

REFERENCES

Calkins H, Zipes DP. Hypotension and syncope. In: Braunwald E, et al, eds. *Heart Disease*, 6th ed. Philadelphia: WB Saunders; 2001, p 932–40.

Daroff RB, Carlson MD. Faintness, syncope, dizziness and vertigo. In: Braunwald E, et al, eds. *Harrison's Principles of Internal Medicine*, 16th ed. New York: McGraw-Hill; 2005, p 126–33.

Simon RP. Syncope. In: Goldman L, Bennett JC, eds. *Cecil Textbook of Medicine*, 21st ed. Philadelphia: WB Saunders; 2000, p 2028–9.

68. TACHYCARDIA

I. **Problem.** On a routine check of vital signs, a 68–year-old woman is found to have a pulse of 155 beats/min 2 days after sigmoid colectomy.

II. Immediate Questions

A. What is the patient's normal pulse? Check the chart and obtain appropriate history from the patient.

B. What are the other vital signs? Tachycardia with hypotension in postoperative patients is an important clue to possible hypovolemia. Similarly, fever can cause tachycardia. Rates >150 beats/min with significant symptoms (eg, decreased consciousness, significant hypotension, chest pain, or shortness of breath), may indicate immediate pharmacologic therapy or cardioversion. An ECG with a rhythm strip is necessary before pursuing pharmacologic intervention or cardioversion.

C. Does the patient have underlying heart disease? Is the rhythm regular or irregular (atrial fibrillation)?

D. What medication is the patient taking? If the patient is on an antiarrhythmic, has the patient been receiving the appropriate doses? Diuretics and potassium supplements may cause electrolyte abnormalities and arrhythmias.

III. Differential Diagnosis

A. Sinus Tachycardia

1. **Thyrotoxicosis.** Weight loss, irritability, and tremor are associated symptoms.
2. **Pheochromocytoma.** Associated with headache, abdominal pain, hypertension, and sweating.
3. **Anxiety/pain.** Normal physiologic response related to catecholamine release.
4. **Drug related.** Sympathomimetics, such as epinephrine, can cause tachycardia.
5. **Hypotension.** With associated hypovolemia.
6. **High-output states.** Increase in right atrial pressure from any cause such as thyrotoxicosis, AV fistula, anemia, pregnancy, or severe Paget's disease.
7. **Cardiac failure.** Decreased pulse pressure and increased right atrial pressure lead to tachycardia.
8. **Fever related**.
9. **Sepsis**.
10. **Pneumothorax/pericardial effusion.**

B. Ectopic Tachycardia

1. **Paroxysmal atrial tachycardia.** Often accompanied by palpitations and lightheadedness, with a rate of 140–250 beats/min.
2. **Atrial flutter.** Rates are faster than in atrial or junctional tachycardia (rate 250–350 beats/min; Figure I–16).

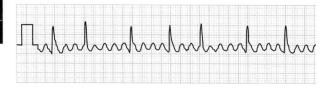

Figure I–16. Atrial flutter with atrioventricular (AV) block (3:1 to 5:1 conduction).
(Reproduced, with permission, from Lefor AT. Critical Care On Call. *Copyright (c) 2002 by The McGraw-Hill Companies, Inc.)*

3. **Ventricular tachycardia.** Usually associated with ischemic heart disease, including acute MI; also can be a forerunner of ventricular fibrillation.

IV. Database

A. Physical Examination Key Points
1. **Vital signs.** Check pulse rate and regularity and for fever.
2. **Cardiac.** Look for evidence of failure, neck vein distention, S_3, etc.
3. **Lungs.** For evidence of cardiac failure, rales, or pneumothorax.
4. **Extremities.** Check for edema or cyanosis.

B. Laboratory Data
1. **Serum electrolytes.** Especially potassium, magnesium, and calcium.
2. **Arterial blood gases.** To rule out hypoxia.
3. **Hemogram.** To evaluate sepsis or anemia.
4. **Thyroid function tests.** If indicated.
5. **Cardiac enzymes.** CK with troponin I

C. Radiologic and Other Studies
1. **Electrocardiogram.** This is the most important piece of information to obtain. This allows correct diagnosis of the particular tachycardia. Be sure to get a formal 12-lead ECG (see Figures I–16 and I–17).
2. **Chest radiograph.** Look for signs of heart failure or primary pulmonary problems.

V. Plan

A. General Plan.
Establish the correct diagnosis. Remember that, even late at night, a medical colleague usually will be glad to help read a confusing ECG. It may be wise to transfer the patient to telemetry or ICU.

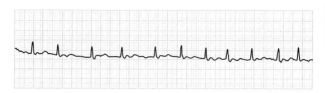

Figure I–17. Atrial fibrillation. *(Reproduced, with permission, from Lefor AT. Critical Care On Call. Copyright (c) 2002 by The McGraw-Hill Companies, Inc.)*

B. Specific Plans
   1. Ventricular tachycardia. This is perhaps the most significant diagnosis because it can rapidly lead to cardiac arrest and death (see Problem 11, page 44 and Figure I–7).
   2. Atrial flutter (Figure I–16) and fibrillation (Figure I–17).
      a. If the patient is hemodynamically compromised, immediate therapy with synchronized electrical cardioversion is indicated (20–50 J) in addition to IV diazepam sedation.
      b. Initially, attempt carotid massage to slow rate and visualize flutter waves.
      c. If the patient is stable, then pharmacologic therapy is indicated.
         i. The first goal is to slow the ventricular response. This is accomplished with IV digoxin or verapamil.
         ii. The second goal is to restore normal sinus rhythm. Quinidine may be used to do this once the ventricular response is lower. Procainamide is an alternative to quinidine (see Problem 52, page 192).
         iii. Digoxin and verapamil should not be used in patients with Wolff-Parkinson-White syndrome.
         iv. Patients with chronic atrial fibrillation may not be convertible to sinus rhythm. Although verapamil acts faster than digoxin, its rapid clearance may require more frequent dosing.
   3. Paroxysmal atrial tachycardia. Can be controlled with:
      a. Vagal maneuvers such as an ice bag on the face, induced vomiting, or carotid massage should be tried first.
      b. Verapamil given IV is also effective, usually starting with 2.5 mg IV push and giving added doses of 2.5 mg every 5 minutes to a total dose of 10 mg.

      c. Combined verapamil with carotid massage is often effective. IV propranolol is also effective.

      d. Synchronized direct current cardioversion is also an effective therapy.

4. Sinus tachycardia., Fever and hypovolemia are the most common causes of this condition in surgical patients. Therapy of sinus tachycardia is based on controlling the underlying condition.

REFERENCES

Doherty GM, et al. Postoperative complications-cardiac. In: Way LW, Doherty GM, eds. *Current Surgical Diagnosis and Treatment,* 11th ed. New York: McGraw-Hill; 2003, p 23–37.

Hastings LA, Balser JR. New treatments for perioperative cardiac arrhythmias. *Anesthesiol Clin North Am* 21:569–86, 2003.

Ommen SR, et al. Atrial arrhythmias after cardiothoracic surgery. *N Engl J Med* 336:1429–34, 1997.

69. TRANSFUSION REACTION

I. Problem. During the transfusion of packed RBCs, a patient's temperature rises to 38.5°C.

II. Immediate Questions

    A. Vital signs. Hypotension should be ruled out. Tachypnea is a sign of a significant reaction. Fever is the most common manifestation of a transfusion reaction.

    B. Does the patient have back or chest pain? Acute coagulopathy can develop from a major transfusion reaction. Chest pain may develop during hemodynamic stress. Other symptoms may include chills, diaphoresis, hypersensitivity reactions (hives, wheezing, pruritus), or exacerbation of CHF, hemoglobinuria, bleeding/DIC, discomfort at infusion site, facial flushing.

    C. Has the transfusion been stopped? If not, do so, and maintain an open IV line with NS.

III. Differential Diagnosis. Differentiating a fever due to a transfusion reaction from other causes of postoperative fever is difficult. Assuming no other source, the following transfusion reactions are possible, in order of decreasing likelihood and increasing severity:

    A. WBC Antigens. Unlike washed RBCs, packed cells contain relatively large numbers of leukocytes. Febrile responses to these cells are usually accompanied by urticaria.

B. **Minor Protein Reactions.** Allergic reactions to transfused serum proteins can cause fever. Sometimes anaphylaxis or acute pulmonary edema can occur.

C. **ABO Incompatibility.** This represents a potentially life-threatening problem, but it occurs rarely. Signs are seen after transfusion of relatively small quantities of blood.

D. **Contaminated Blood.** Bacterial contamination is rare but should be suspected when high fever and hypotension develop early during a transfusion because it is often fatal.

IV. Database

A. Physical Examination Key Points
1. **Lungs.** Listen for rales and wheezing.
2. **Cardiac.** Examine for tachycardia and new flow murmur.
3. **Abdomen.** Evaluate for pain, especially in the flanks.
4. **Skin.** Look for rash or hives.

B. Laboratory Data
1. **Blood bank specimen.** Two freshly drawn clot tubes (red top tubes) should be returned to the blood bank with the remaining untransfused blood. A repeat cross-match will be performed.
2. **Urinalysis.** Hematuria after a transfusion reaction represents hemoglobinuria after hemolysis from a major ABO incompatibility.
3. **Hemogram.** Schistocytes may be present in a transfusion reaction; a worsening anemia may develop in the face of massive RBC destruction.
4. **Serum for free hemoglobin and haptoglobin.** Free hemoglobin will be present with a reaction and haptoglobin will be decreased.
5. **Other laboratory tests.** Coagulation studies and thrombocytopenia may indicate DIC. Monitor renal function by obtaining BUN and creatinine levels and serum electrolytes. ABGs rarely are indicated (cardiovascular collapse).

C. Radiologic and Other Studies. Order if clinically indicated.

V. Plan

A. Immediately Stop Transfusion. Consultation with a blood bank pathologist usually is indicated to evaluate the reaction and to discuss any further transfusions.

B. Maintain IV Access. Monitor urine output and vital signs closely. A patient who is hypotensive may require aggressive fluid resuscitation and ICU monitoring.

C. **Send Blood Bank Appropriate Specimens.** See preceding section, "Laboratory Data." Make sure the bag is returned to the blood bank immediately.

D. **Mild Reactions.** Usually fever without any evidence of more severe symptoms or hemolysis.
   1. Antihistamines (diphenhydramine 25–50 mg IM or IV) and acetaminophen may reverse mild allergic and febrile reactions.
   2. Transfusion can usually be restarted.

E. **Severe Reactions.** Usually signifies that acute hemolysis has taken place. One major goal is to prevent renal failure.
   1. **Circulatory support.** Maintain adequate blood pressure with volume or pressors. Diuresis with furosemide or mannitol, usually with D5W, should be started to prevent renal injury in the setting of marked hemolysis. Also consider alkalinization of the urine with bicarbonate to further protect the kidneys. These steps will usually require immediate transfer to the ICU with monitoring as indicated.
   2. **Antibiotics.** Use if examination of remaining untransfused unit reveals bacterial evidence of bacterial contamination. Organisms are usually gram-negative bacilli.

F. **Known Reactions.** In patients with known febrile reactions to blood products, the patient can be pretreated with antihistamines (Diphenhydramine), antipyretics, or steroids to avoid the reaction. Blood bank products are discussed in Section VI, Blood Component Therapy.

REFERENCES

Fakhry SM, et al. Hematologic principles in surgery. In: Townsend CM Jr, ed. *Sabiston Textbook of Surgery*, 16th ed. Philadelphia: WB Saunders; 2001, p 113–36.

Schwartz SI. Hemostasis, surgical bleeding and transfusion. In: Schwartz SI, et al, eds. *Principles of Surgery*, 7th ed. New York: McGraw-Hill; 1999, p 77–100.

Snyder EL. Transfusion reactions. In: Hoffman R, et al, eds. *Hematology. Basic Principles and Practice*, 3rd ed. Philadelphia: Churchill-Livingstone; 2000, p 2300–9.

70. TRAUMA ASSESSMENT & RESUSCITATION

Immediate Actions

Start with the ABCs of trauma:

1. **Airway.** Check for clear airway. Evaluate C-spine and assume injury until cleared with radiography. Intubate if necessary. Perform cricothyrotomy if needed.

2. Breathing. Administer O_2, ventilate, and check breath sounds.
3. Circulation. Obtain 2 large-bore (14–16 gauge) IVs in the upper extremities and begin crystalloid infusion (LR) as promptly as possible. Draw routine blood work.
4. Evaluate response to initial resuscitation. Begin secondary survey once stabilized.
5. Disability. Rapid neurologic assessment.
6. Examine. Remove all clothing and quickly inspect the patient.
7. Begin ECG monitoring.

I. **Problem.** An 18–year-old female involved in a motor vehicle accident has a blood pressure of 90/50 mm Hg and is combative.

II. **Immediate Questions**

A. **Is the patient able to talk?** Airway obstruction and major chest injuries are rapidly fatal and therefore addressed first. If the patient is unable to talk, but is making ventilatory efforts, sweep the oropharynx with gloved fingers to remove debris. Suction the oropharynx. Grasp the chin and displace it anteriorly. Ventilate with a well-fitting mask and 100% oxygen for 2–3 minutes. If unsuccessful (saturation <90%, no clinical improvement), then intubate with a No. 7 or 8 cuffed endotracheal tube. Rarely patients who present with severe maxillofacial injury cannot be intubated orally and require immediate tracheostomy. A cricothyroidotomy made between the laryngeal cartilage and cricoid is preferred over a formal tracheostomy because it is faster and safer.

B. **Has the patient's ventilatory status improved?** Re-evaluation is essential in trauma management to identify missed injuries. A patient in severe respiratory distress who has not improved with intubation should have chest tubes placed immediately, before chest radiography is performed. Flail chest, tension pneumothorax, and bronchial disruption are lethal but manageable injuries.

C. **How long ago was the injury?** Assessing the degree of shock to plan fluid resuscitation is the next priority. If the injury occurred 2 hours previously and the degree of shock is mild, then massive or ongoing hemorrhage is less likely.

D. **What is the blood pressure?** Blood pressure does not decrease until >20% of intravascular blood volume is lost. Compensatory mechanisms of vasoconstriction and increased heart rate and contractility occur early, allowing blood pressure to be maintained in early shock.

E. What is the heart rate? Tachycardia >120 beats/min should be considered a sign of hypovolemic shock in the trauma setting.

F. Is the skin cool and moist? Vasoconstriction of muscle and skin is an early compensatory mechanism. Epinephrine release causes sweating. Cool, moist skin is a reliable clinical sign of impending shock.

G. What is the urine output? Any patient with serious trauma should have urine output monitored. Visceral vasoconstriction with resulting decreased renal blood flow is reflected in decreased urine output.

H. Are the external jugular veins distended? A trauma patient who appears to be in hypovolemic shock by other parameters but who has distended neck veins most likely has cardiac tamponade.

III. Database

A. Physical Examination Key Points. History and physical examination are performed with the patient fully immobilized and completely exposed. It is particularly important to perform a thorough head-to-toe initial examination to avoid missed injuries such as unsuspected entrance and exit sites in penetrating injuries. Determine the initial GCS before proceeding with the rest of the physical examination.

1. **Lungs.** Evaluate breath sounds while considering the possibility of pneumothorax.
2. **Heart.** Listen for tachycardia and muffled heart sounds.
3. **Abdomen.** Evaluate for distention (possible site of significant bleeding) and peritonitis.

B. Laboratory Data. Send CBC count, coagulation studies, chemistries, toxicology screen, urinalysis, and type and crossmatch sample from blood drain while placing first IV line. Send ABG.

C. Radiologic Studies. Lateral C-spine with collar on, flat pelvis film, upright chest radiograph, and other radiographs as indicated.

IV. Plan

A. Fluid Resuscitation. With moderate to severe hypovolemic shock, therapy is initiated before a complete assessment. Large-bore, peripheral IV lines are started, and ≥2 are required. The upper extremities are used preferably.

1. Cutdowns are placed easily in the saphenous vein at the ankles or the brachial and cephalic veins at the antecubital crease. The use of large-bore lines (No. 8) or cut IV tubing to allow administration of crystalloid 2 L in <15 minutes. Short catheters allow more rapid infusions (thus subclavian CVP lines are not used).

2. Avoid placing percutaneous subclavian or IJ lines. The added risk of iatrogenic pneumothorax is not warranted.

3. Transfusion of RBCs is used to improve oxygen-carrying capacity in patients with hemorrhage. Type-specific blood is preferred, but if unavailable, universal type O should be given. Packed RBCs are more viscid than whole blood. Packed RBCs can be injected into the vein with the crystalloid to increase delivery rate.

B. **Secondary Assessment.** If the initial resuscitation and assessment result in a hemodynamically stable and neurologically intact patient, then a more thorough secondary assessment and re-evaluation occur. If shock persists despite resuscitation, then ongoing hemorrhage is present and immediate operative intervention may be indicated.

C. **Observation.** Once the patient is stabilized, placements of an NG tube and Foley catheter are undertaken. Be careful before placing the Foley catheter if there is any possibility of a urethral injury (eg, pelvic fracture). Observe for blood at the meatus or a free floating prostate on rectal examination. In these cases, urinary catheter placement is performed only after radiographic evaluation of the urethra (retrograde urethrogram and cystogram). FAST scan or peritoneal lavage may be indicated at this time. Temperature monitoring should be started.

D. **Reassess.** Patients who remain in shock despite aggressive resuscitation must be rapidly assessed as to the cause. Hypovolemic shock usually results from blood loss within the chest or abdomen or from a massive pelvic injury. Cardiogenic shock may be due to tension pneumothorax or hemopericardium, both of which are easily controlled once suspected. The detailed secondary survey is begun once the patient is stabilized during the initial resuscitation phase. This includes a comprehensive examination and re-evaluation of the patient.

REFERENCES

American College of Surgeons Committee on Trauma. Initial assessment and management. In: *Advanced Trauma Life Support Student Course Manual (ATLS)*. American College of Surgeons Chicago, IL: 2004, p 11–40.

Burch JM, et al. Trauma. In: Schwartz SI, et al, eds. *Principles of Surgery,* 7th ed. New York: McGraw-Hill; 1999, p 155–222.

Feliciano DV, et al. *Trauma,* 4th ed. New York: McGraw-Hill; 2000, p 153–72.

71. VAGINAL BLEEDING

I. **Problem.** A young woman admitted for observation for possible appendicitis develops vaginal bleeding.

II. **Immediate Questions**

    A. **Is there any evidence of shock?** Vaginal bleeding can be profuse. In some cases visible blood loss may represent only a fraction of the actual blood loss. Assess the patient for hypovolemia or shock.

    B. **Is there any pain associated with the bleeding?** The most serious condition in the differential diagnosis of acute vaginal bleeding is ectopic pregnancy, and pain is always a predominant part of the patient's complaints. Other causes of vaginal bleeding are also associated with pain and other GI symptoms.

    C. **When was the patient's last period, and has she been sexually active since that time?** Inquire about specific details of menstrual history, most recent period, and any abnormal bleeding in the past. Obtain a complete sexual history including contraceptive use and any associated symptoms of early pregnancy (morning sickness, fluid retention, etc).

    D. **Attempt to quantitate the blood loss.** The rate of bleeding has diagnostic and therapeutic implications. If a volume estimate of blood loss cannot be given, ask about number of pads or tampons used and degree of saturation.

III. **Differential Diagnosis**

    A. **Normal Menstrual Period.** This is the most commonly encountered cause.

    B. **Dysfunctional Bleeding (Related to Menstrual Cycle)**
        1. Perimenopausal.
        2. Inadequate luteal phase.
        3. Oral contraceptives.
        4. Endometriosis.

    C. **Pregnancy Related**
        1. Ectopic pregnancy.
        2. Threatened or spontaneous abortion.
        3. Retained products of gestation.

    D. **Neoplasia**

1. Uterine fibroids.
2. Cervical polyps.
3. Carcinoma
   a. Endometrium.
   b. Cervix.
   c. Ovarian.

E. **Infection**
   1. Pelvic inflammatory disease.
   2. Vaginitis.

F. **Trauma**

G. **Bleeding Diathesis.** Bleeding is also usually present at other sites.

IV. **Database**

A. **Physical Examination Key Points**
   1. **Vital signs.** Check orthostatic signs for excessive blood loss; fever is a sign of infection.
   2. **Skin.** Pallor suggests significant blood loss. Bruising and petechiae suggest bleeding diathesis.
   3. **Abdomen.** Observe for peritoneal signs, tenderness, and distention.
   4. **Pelvic examination.** Examine for mass in vagina, cervix, uterus, or adnexa and areas of tenderness including cervical motion pain. Evaluate source and rate of bleeding, and whether the cervical os open or closed, with or without tissue fragments.

B. **Laboratory Data**
   1. **Hemogram.** Check for leukocytosis, hematocrit, or thrombocytopenia.
   2. **PT/PTT.** If coagulopathy is suspected. Check fibrinogen and fibrin split products if DIC is suspected.
   3. **Blood.** Type and crossmatch blood if indicated.
   4. **Serum/urine human chorionic gonadotropin.** A pregnancy test will be positive with an ectopic pregnancy.
   5. Pap smear of cervix.
   6. Cervical culture.

C. **Radiologic and Other Studies**
   1. **Culdocentesis.** This is considered if an ectopic pregnancy is possible.
   2. **Pelvic ultrasound.** Evaluates intrauterine and intratubal lesions and is valuable to check for possible ectopic pregnancy or any pelvic mass.
   3. **CT scan of pelvis.** Good method to detect any mass lesion. Usually not as obtainable in emergencies as an

ultrasound. Be sure there is no salvageable intrauterine pregnancy before obtaining a CT scan.

V. Plan. Most vaginal bleeding does not require specific therapy because it represents normal menstrual bleeding.

A. Overall Plan
1. Resuscitate the patient from the acute blood loss as needed.
2. Establish large-bore IV lines, administer crystalloid, type and crossmatch for blood, monitor urine output, and follow serial hematocrits. Also make the patient NPO because urgent operative procedures may be indicated.

B. Specific Treatment. Virtually all causes of significant vaginal bleeding require evaluation by the gynecology service. Ongoing bleeds require emergency consultation, whereas spotting or a bleeding episode that has resolved can be evaluated as above and seen on an elective basis depending on the diagnosis.

C. Ectopic Pregnancy. If lower abdominal pain is a part of the symptom complex and the patient is of child-bearing age, ectopic pregnancy must be ruled out even if the pregnancy tests are normal. The diagnostic procedure of choice is a pelvic ultrasound; if ultrasound is not available, then use culdocentesis.

REFERENCES

Kawada C. General gynecology. In: DeCherney AH, Nathan L, eds. *Current Obstetric & Gynecologic Diagnosis & Treatment,* 9th ed. New York: Lange/McGraw-Hill; 2003, p 1085–115.

Stenchever MA. Vaginal bleeding. In: Stenchever MA, ed. *Comprehensive Gynecology,* 4th edition. St Louis: Mosby; 2001, p 156–60.

Sutton GP, et al. Gynecology. In: Schwartz SI, et al, eds. *Principles of Surgery,* 7th ed. New York: McGraw-Hill; 1999, p 1838–9.

72. VENTILATOR MANAGEMENT: AGITATION

(Ventilators are discussed in detail in Section VII, page 418)

I. Problem. A patient who is status post craniotomy for a cerebellar lesion is on the ventilator in the ICU. You are notified that he has become agitated and is "bucking" the ventilator.

II. Immediate Questions

A. What are the most recent blood gases? Hypoxia may be evident as may hypocarbia from tachypnea.

B. When was the most recent chest radiograph? Be sure there is a recent chest radiograph. A pneumothorax, dislodged ETT, or an ETT in the right mainstem can cause hypoxia that results in agitation.

C. What is the patient's respiratory rate? Tachypnea may cause "bucking" of the ventilator.

D. What are the ventilator settings (mode, rate, PEEP, FIO_2, tidal volume [TV])?

III. Differential Diagnosis

A. Respiratory Decompensation. This must be ruled out first.
   1. Pneumothorax or tension pneumothorax.
   2. Improper positioning of the endotracheal tube proximally or distally (usually in the right mainstem bronchus).
   3. **Mucous plugging.** Tenacious secretions can obstruct the tube.
   4. **Ventilator malfunction.** Verify with the respiratory therapist that the ventilator is working properly and delivering the preset parameters.
   5. **Aspiration.** Usually around a partially inflated cuff.
   6. **Systemic sepsis.** Can cause agitation.
   7. **Other causes.** CHF, PE, hiccups, pneumothorax.

B. Inadequate Tidal Volume. Is the preset tidal volume sufficient for the patient (5–10 mL/kg)?

C. Insufficient Pain Medication or Sedation.

D. Status Epilepticus.

E. Tetanus.

IV. Database

A. Physical Examination Key Points
   1. **Vital signs.** Blood pressure, respiratory rate, O_2 saturation.
   2. **Neck.** Distended neck veins or tracheal deviation may suggest pneumothorax.
   3. **Lungs.** Examine for bilateral breath sounds, wheezing, or evidence of CHF.
   4. **Chest.** Look for subcutaneous emphysema and symmetric excursion.
   5. Verify that the cuff is inflated properly and listen for any air leaks.

B. Laboratory Data
   1. **Arterial blood gases.** Look for hypoxia, CO_2 retention.
   2. **Serum electrolytes.** To complete acid-base workup.

C. **Radiologic and Other Studies.** Chest radiograph to check endotracheal tube placement, rule out pneumothorax, and effusions, etc. Therapy should not be delayed because of a pending radiograph.

V. Plan

A. **Obtain a STAT ABG and portable chest radiograph.** This should be the first step in any patient on positive pressure ventilation.

B. **Manually ventilate the patient with a bag and 100% O_2.**
   1. If the patient is easily ventilated, check for a mechanical ventilator problem.
   2. If there is increased resistance to ventilation, consider pneumothorax. Be sure to check for bilateral breath sounds, etc. If there is evidence of a pneumothorax, do not wait for the radiograph; place a chest tube immediately if the patient is unstable.
   3. If there is no evidence of pneumothorax, check the ETT for obstruction. Consider replacing the tube if the obstruction cannot be relieved. If there is no obstruction, then consider sepsis, CHF, PE, or aspiration as a cause of decompensation.

C. **Control pain appropriately.** Sedation may also be helpful with diazepam (Valium) IV. Use 2–5 mg IV every 2 hours as a start. Other agents include lorazepam (Ativan), midazolam (Versed), and others. Propofol (Diprivan) may also be used.

D. **Patients "fighting" the ventilator can sometimes be calmed by increasing the tidal volume.**

E. **Remember that IMV mode delivers a fixed tidal volume at preset intervals, regardless of the patient's respiratory rate.** The use of IMV has been beneficial in managing patients with an increased respiratory drive. Assisted control will give a full breath at a preset tidal volume when the patient triggers the ventilator with an inspiration. Therefore, small inspiratory efforts will trigger a full ventilator breath, which can lead to fighting the ventilator. Controlled ventilation should not routinely be used on a conscious patient because it will not allow the patient to initiate any breaths on his own; the use of this modality in the conscious patient may lead to agitation.

F. **Awake patients should be reassured by carefully explaining the mechanical ventilator.** This can often relieve anxiety and assist in ventilator management.

G. **Paralysis must be used with extreme caution, if at all.** This is indicated only in patients with critical respiratory compromise or tetanus. Paralytic agents such as succinyl-choline or pancuronium bromide must be used with adequate sedation and great caution.

REFERENCES

Hogarth DK, Hall J. Management of sedation in mechanically ventilated patients (review). *Curr Opin Crit Care* 10:40–6, 2004.

Grap MJ, et al. Collaborative practice: development, implementation, and evaluation of a weaning protocol for patients receiving mechanical ventilation. *Am J Crit Care* 12:454–60, 2003.

Siegel MD. Management of agitation in the intensive care unit. *Clin Chest Med* 24:713–25, 2003.

73. VENTILATOR MANAGEMENT: HIGH F$_{IO_2}$

(Ventilators are discussed in Section VII, page 418)

I. **Problem.** A mechanically ventilated trauma patient is maintaining a P$_{O_2}$ of only 75 mm Hg on 90% F$_{IO_2}$.

II. **Immediate Questions**

A. **What are the ABG values?** An increased P$_{CO_2}$ indicates hypoventilation. When ventilation is inadequate to maintain a normal P$_{CO_2}$ and there is concomitant lung disease, hypoxemia may result.

B. **What does the chest radiograph show?** Significant atelectasis, pneumonia, pneumothorax, pleural effusion, pulmonary edema, pulmonary contusion, and ARDS can cause hypoxemia and result in high oxygen requirements.

C. **What is the ETT status?** Mucous plugging may occlude the ETT. A cuff leak may prevent adequate inflation. An ETT that is advanced too far may be in the right mainstem bronchus.

D. **What are the ventilator settings?** Poor oxygenation may sometimes be corrected by increasing PEEP but should be done cautiously because it may impede cardiac output or cause barotrauma.

III. **Differential Diagnosis.** Causes of hypoxia can be classified into 2 main categories: problems that cause poor matching between ventilation and perfusion (V/Q mismatch) and pure hypoventilation.

A. **V/Q Mismatches.** This is the most common cause of hypoxemia and high oxygen requirements. The amount of mismatch is referred to as the physiologic shunt.

1. Reactive airways (COPD, asthma).
2. Pneumonia.

   3. Atelectasis.
   4. PE.
   5. Pneumothorax.
   6. Physiologic shunting seen in ARDS and pulmonary edema.
   7. Anatomic shunting seen in congenital heart disease.
   8. Sepsis causing a mild to moderate V/Q mismatch.
   9. Mainstem bronchus ETT. An ETT may migrate down the right mainstem bronchus.
   10. Pulmonary contusion.
B. Hypoventilation. This is a rare cause of hypoxemia.
   1. Inadequate minute ventilation (low tidal volume and/or low rate).
   2. Increased dead space (unavoidable part of mechanical ventilation).
   3. Muscle weakness in nonventilated patient.
   4. Cuff leak.

IV. Database
A. Physical Examination Key Points
   1. Vital signs. Fever, tachycardia, and hypotension may indicate sepsis.
   2. Cardiac. Presence of S_3 and tachycardia may indicate heart failure as cause of pulmonary edema.
   3. Lungs. Careful examination can indicate pulmonary edema (rales), decreased sounds (atelectasis, effusion, pneumothorax), egophony (pneumonia), and wheezing (asthma). Confirm with chest radiograph.
   4. Neck. Look for jugular venous distention.

B. Laboratory Data
   1. Arterial blood gas. Follow serially.
   2. Hemogram. Verify that hemoglobin and hematocrit are adequate.
   3. Cultures. Sputum, blood, urine, drains, and wounds as clinically indicated.
   4. Sputum examination. Tenacious secretions are common in reactive airway disease. Purulent sputum indicates pneumonia, and frothy sputum indicates pulmonary edema. Gram's stain is a quick and useful evaluation of sputum.
   5. Mixed venous oxygen content. Drawn from the PA through a PA catheter, oxygen should normally measure 40 mm Hg (approximately 70% saturated). Lower levels indicate inadequate oxygen delivery to tissues as would be found in major trauma and severe sepsis.
   6. A-a gradient.

C. Radiologic and Other Studies

1. **Chest radiograph.** Careful evaluation of the chest radiograph is critical to understanding the nature of the problem. Look for evidence of:
   a. ARDS.
   b. Pneumonia.
   c. Pulmonary edema.
   d. Atelectasis.
   e. Pneumothorax.
   f. Effusion.
   g. ETT misplacement.
   h. Pulmonary contusion
2. **Electrocardiogram.** Look for dysrhythmias (atrial fibrillation or flutter); ischemic changes may indicate infarction. Be sure to compare with previous ECGs.
3. **V/Q scan or pulmonary angiogram.** These studies are obtained if PE is suspected. More recently, CT angiogram is currently available at many institutions and is more accurate in the diagnosis of PE.
4. **CT scan of abdomen.** If septic focus suspected.
5. **Bronchoscopy.** Use aggressively to clear mucous plugs causing atelectasis; use lavage, biopsy, and brushings as diagnostic aids.
6. **Open lung biopsy.** Rarely indicated; used when hypoxemia and lung disease persist despite aggressive medical therapy and unclear etiology.

V. Plan.
The main objective is to provide adequate tissue oxygenation without causing oxygen toxicity. The goal is to keep F$_{IO_2}$ <60%, especially with long-term oxygen use.

A. Correct Anemia.
Keep hematocrit >30% with transfusions.

B. Correct Pulmonary Disease

1. **Pneumothorax.** Insert tube thoracostomy.
2. **Pneumonia.** Antibiotics and pulmonary toilet, including nebulizer treatments and chest physiotherapy/postural drainage.
3. **Atelectasis.** Ensure adequate tidal volume and frequent suctioning.
4. **Asthma.** Use of bronchodilators, aminophylline, and steroids may help manage reactive airways.
5. **Effusion.** Thoracentesis or tube thoracostomy.
6. **Pulmonary edema.** Diuretics with careful attention to fluid management.

C. Pulmonary Toilet

1. Frequent suctioning.
2. Saline lavage into ETT.

   3. Provide an occasional large tidal volume ("sigh") by bagging before suctioning.
   4. Acetylcysteine (Mucomyst) treatments.
   5. Chest physical therapy.
D. Treat Sepsis. Appropriate antibiotics and surgical drainage as required.
E. Optimize Ventilator Settings
   1. Place radial arterial catheter for frequent ABG measurements.
   2. Maintain normal P_{CO_2}.
   3. Start with 100% F_{IO_2} and wean down to avoid O_2 toxicity.
   4. PEEP should be added slowly. Complications are rare <10–15 mm Hg of PEEP but may include barotrauma and decreased cardiac output (caused by decreased venous return). It may be necessary to increase PEEP to provide adequate oxygenation. This results in higher mean and peak airway pressures. Consider Swan-Ganz catheter for higher PEEP settings (>10 mm Hg).
   5. Sedation or paralysis. Consider in patients "fighting" the ventilator who still require mechanical ventilation. Agitation interferes with adequate function of the ventilator. Pancuronium (Pavulon) should not routinely be used alone. Pavulon induces paralysis but does not provide sedation or pain relief. Use it with morphine or diazepam.
F. Maximize Hemodynamic State. Use of a PA catheter may help in the management of respiratory failure.
   1. Maintain adequate filling pressures (15 mm Hg) with crystalloid or blood products. Give furosemide if the wedge pressure is >20 mm Hg.
   2. Improve cardiac index as needed with dopamine or dobutamine.
G. Heparin. If PE suspected. Heparin 80 U/kg bolus followed by continuous drip at approximately 1000 U/h to maintain activated PTT at 2–2.5 times control values. Some centers use thrombolytic therapy with alteplase.

REFERENCES

Conrad SA, Bidani A. Management of the acute respiratory distress syndrome. *Chest Surg Clin North Am* 12:325–54, 2002.

Tobin MJ. Advances in mechanical ventilation. *N Engl J Med* 344:1986–96, 2001.

Udobi KF, et al. Acute respiratory distress syndrome. *Am Fam Phys* 67:315–22, 2003.

74. VENTILATOR MANAGEMENT: HIGH PEAK PRESSURE

(Ventilators are discussed in Section VII, page 418)

I. **Problem.** An intubated trauma patient with multiple injuries from blunt trauma is continually setting off the peak pressure alarm.

II. **Immediate Questions**

A. **What is the ABG?** A change in peak pressure may represent a ventilator system malfunction, decrease in sedation, or a new pulmonary event or condition. The most important issue is determining if the patient is being adequately ventilated. Send off an ABG immediately.

B. **Has the position of the ETT changed?** An ETT in the right mainstem bronchus can cause the peak pressure to increase. Check the mark on the ETT at the lips and compare with previous positions. Also check chest radiograph.

C. **Are there increased secretions in the ETT?** Find out if increased or thicker secretions are being suctioned from the ETT. The ETT may become partially obstructed with secretions.

D. **Is there any subcutaneous emphysema?** An important cause for increased peak pressure in a patient on a ventilator is a tension pneumothorax, which can be associated with subcutaneous emphysema. Palpate the chest wall and neck for crepitus before obtaining a chest radiograph.

E. **Has there been any change in the ventilator settings?** Make sure that the peak pressure alarm is set correctly. Troubleshoot the ventilator with the respiratory therapist to look for circuit disconnections, etc.

III. **Differential Diagnosis.** If the ventilator's peak pressure alarm is sounded, the problem is with the ventilator or an increased resistance to the delivered tidal volume in the patient. Increased resistance can be a result of intrinsic pulmonary pathology or to resistance to lung expansion from extrinsic compressive forces. Generally speaking, peak inspiratory pressures should be <20–30 cm H_2O.

A. **Ventilator Problems**
1. Lowered peak pressure setting.
2. Incorrect ventilator circuit setup.
3. Shift in position of the ETT.

B. **Intrinsic Pulmonary Problems**

    1. Obstruction of the ETT by secretions.
    2. Pulmonary edema. ARDS and CHF can cause decreased compliance, thus requiring high pressures to ventilate the patient.
    3. Interstitial disease.
        a. Malignancy: Lymphangitic spread.
        b. Fibrosis: Eg, bleomycin induced.
    4. Reactive airway disease. Asthma.

C. Extrinsic Pulmonary Compression
    1. Pneumothorax or tension pneumothorax.
    2. Pleural effusion or hemothorax.
    3. Abdominal distention.
    4. Chest wall/respiratory muscle contraction.
        a. Bucking the ventilator owing to anxiety, pain, or decreased sedation. Agitation may be secondary to hypoventilation and hypoxia, so check the ABG.
        b. Coughing spasm.

IV. Database

A. Physical Examination Key Points
    1. Skin. Look for cyanosis and crepitus.
    2. Lungs. Examine secretions from the ETT noting amount and viscosity. Note decreased or absent breath sounds, rales, and wheezes.
    3. Cardiac. High venous pressure, decreased heart sounds.
    4. Abdomen. Is there marked distention or ascites?

B. Laboratory Data
    1. ABG drawn immediately.
    2. Hemogram. For evidence of decreased hematocrit or leukocytosis.

C. Radiologic and Other Studies
    1. Chest radiograph. Order STAT chest radiograph if the new problem is not due to a technical problem with the ventilator. Look for pleural effusion, pulmonary edema, pneumothorax, or new infiltrate. Check the ETT position (tip should be 2 cm above the carina). If the patient already has a chest tube in place and it is on water seal, placing it on suction may help. Look for a pneumothorax even if the patient has a chest tube.

V. Plan

A. Overall Plan. Initial therapy is to disconnect the patient from the ventilator and bag ventilate by hand. This maneuver allows for immediate hyperventilation, removes the ventilator as the source of the problem, allows manual assessment of

pulmonary compliance, and allows the ETT to be irrigated and suctioned of secretions. At the same time, draw an ABG, call for a portable chest radiograph, and check the ventilator. Decide whether the problem is the patient or the ventilator.

B. Specific Problems

1. **Hemo- or pneumothorax, effusion.** Manage with a tube thoracostomy. In urgent situations a tension pneumothorax can be managed with a 14–gauge IV catheter inserted into the anterior chest at the level of the second or third intercostal space (see page 246).

2. **ETT malposition.** Adjust the tube, retape, and repeat the chest radiograph to document position.

3. Bucking the ventilator.

    a. Administer pain or sedation medications once hypoxia or mechanical problems have been ruled out (see page 246).

    b. Change pattern of ventilation to assist/control. Follow blood gases because patient may hyperventilate on this setting.

4. For cases of fibrosis, infiltrative disease, and ARDS being maximally controlled, higher peak airway pressures may have to be tolerated to ventilate the patient. Adjust the alarm setting and follow closely for pneumothorax resulting from barotrauma.

REFERENCES

Alvarez A, et al. Decelerating flow ventilation effects in acute respiratory failure. *J Crit Care* 13:21–5, 1998.

Hirvela ER. Advances in the management of acute respiratory distress syndrome: protective ventilation. *Arch Surg* 135:126–35, 2000.

Mutlu GM, Factor P. Complications of mechanical ventilation. *Respir Care Clin North Am* 6:213–52, 2000.

75. VENTILATOR MANAGEMENT: LOW Po_2/HIGH Pco_2

(Ventilators are discussed in Section VII, page 418.)

I. **Problem.** An 83–year-old male has an arterial partial pressure of oxygen (Pao_2) of 55 mm Hg 1 day after grafting of a ruptured abdominal aortic aneurysm.

II. **Immediate Questions**

A. **What are the current ventilator settings? Were any recent changes made?** Fio_2, rate (IMV or assisted control), PEEP, and tidal volume? When were the last ventilator changes made, and what was the ABG result before those changes.

B. **What are the most recent ABG results? The prior set? On what ventilator settings?**

C. **What is the patient's respiratory rate?** Tachypnea is an important finding and may indicate inadequate ventilatory support.

D. **What operation has the patient had? Type of incision?** Thoracotomy, flank, and large abdominal incisions are painful and limit patients' ability to breathe on their own.

E. **What are the patient's preoperative blood gases and pulmonary function tests on room air?** This is especially important in the patient with COPD, who often have baseline CO_2 levels in the 50s.

F. **What is the peak pressure?** This allows for the calculation of compliance (by tidal volume/peak pressure) and lung stiffness. A progressively stiffer lung may indicate ARDS as a cause for the low O_2 levels. Normal compliance is >100 mL/cm H_2O.

G. **When was the most recent chest radiograph?** If not within a few hours, repeat chest film immediately.

III. Differential Diagnosis

A. **Mucous Plugging.**

B. **Pulmonary Edema.** Check fluid balance over the past several days. Is the patient fluid overloaded? Hypervolemia may result in a lower Po_2.

C. **Ventilator Leak.** Check for a broken cuff. Be sure the entire tidal volume is delivered.

D. **Pulmonary Parenchymal Disease.** Such as COPD that existed preoperatively.

E. **Inadequate Ventilatory Support.** Such as low tidal volume. Assess by following Pco_2.

F. **Pneumothorax.** Positive pressure ventilation can turn a simple pneumothorax into a tension pneumothorax.

G. **ETT Malposition.** Is the ETT past the carina on chest radiograph?

H. **Aspiration.**

I. **Bronchospasm.** Listen for wheezing.

J. **ARDS.**

K. **Atelectasis/Pneumonia.**

L. **Pulmonary Embolus.** No increase in saturation or Pao_2 may indicate V/Q mismatch.

M. **Circulatory Problems.** Including severe CHF.

N. Low Hemoglobin.

O. Pulmonary Contusion.

IV. Database

A. Physical Examination Key Points

1. **HEENT.** Listen for an air leak.
2. **Neck.** Look for JVD with CHF, volume overload, or pneumothorax.
3. **Lungs.** Evaluate for bronchospasm or pulmonary edema. Check for subcutaneous emphysema (from pneumothorax).
4. Look for equal expansion, tracheal deviation, and adequate breath sounds bilaterally.

B. Laboratory Data

1. **Arterial blood gas.** Follow serial studies.

C. Radiologic and Other Studies

1. **Chest radiograph.** Look for CHF, pneumothorax, ETT position, lobar infiltrate, collapse secondary to mucous plugging, or signs of ARDS.
2. **Nuclear V/Q scan.** If a PE is suspected, then V/Q scan is indicated. An equivocal scan usually necessitates CT scan or pulmonary angiogram.

V. Plan.

The goal is to provide adequate tissue oxygenation. Sudden changes in P_{O_2} and P_{CO_2} in the absence of ventilatory changes are due to such phenomena as altered F_{IO_2}, pneumothorax, mucous plugging, and so on. Consider bronchoscopy for severe mucous plugging.

A. Hypoxemia.

Keep the F_{IO_2} from about 40 to 50% to minimize oxygen toxicity. In general, a $Pa_{O_2} \geq 60$ mm Hg is the goal, because at this level, hemoglobin is about 90% saturated. Measuring cardiac output with a PA catheter is useful. Other indicators of cardiac output (eg, urine output) may be helpful in the absence of a PA catheter. Hypoxemia may be controlled by increasing oxygen delivery or by decreasing oxygen consumption.

1. **Increased delivery**
   a. **Ventilatory**
      i. Increased F_{IO_2}.
      ii. **Decreased shunt:** By increasing PEEP. However, increasing PEEP can significantly affect cardiac output, so that a PA catheter may be needed, especially with PEEP levels >10–15 cm H_2O.
   b. **Circulatory**
      i. Improved cardiac output.

          ii. Management of physical obstruction to circula-
tion such as PE is anticoagulation after diagno-
sis by imaging studies.

    c. Hemoglobin

      i. Transfusion to acceptable range (usually to a
hematocrit >30%).

      ii. Decreased consumption: Sedation, paralysis,
and hypothermia can be combined in critical situations.

B. Hypercarbia. The adequacy of ventilation is indicated by
the PCO_2 and can be affected by changes in the ventilatory
rate or tidal volume.

  1. Rule out mechanical problems such as leaks, plugging
of the ETT, kinking, or malposition of the tube.

  2. Tidal volume should be 5–10 mL/kg body weight. Is the
patient receiving the delivered volume? Hypoventilation
(low minute volume) can increase PCO_2.

  3. Is the PCO_2 increased because of increased CO_2 production or excessive dead-space ventilation?

    a. Increased CO_2 production

      i. Sepsis: Manage appropriately (antibiotics, etc).

      ii. Excessive carbohydrate in hyperalimentation.

    b. Increased dead space: Dead space refers to the
ventilation of areas such as the ventilator tubing,
ETT, nonperfused alveoli, etc, where gas exchange
cannot occur. Correct the following conditions when
possible:

      i. Inadequate cardiac output.

      ii. PEEP causing barotrauma.

      iii. PEs.

      iv. Vasoconstriction of pulmonary vessels by va-
soactive medications.

REFERENCES

Corrado A, et al. Iron lung versus conventional mechanical ventilation in
acute exacerbation of COPD. *Eur Respir J* 23:419–24, 2004.

Perrin F, et al. Clinical decision-making and mechanical ventilation in patients with respiratory failure due to an exacerbation of COPD. *Clin Med*
3:556–9, 2003.

Sin DD, et al. Contemporary management of chronic obstructive pulmonary
disease: scientific review. *JAMA* 290:2301–12, 2003.

76. WHEEZING

I. Problem. A 20-year-old has been admitted for laparoscopic
appendectomy and begins wheezing in the anesthesia holding
area.

II. Immediate Questions

A. What are the vital signs? A respiratory rate of 40 breaths/min may indicate the need for immediate therapy. Associated hypotension may suggest an anaphylactic reaction or an acute MI. Fever may point to an infection or PE.

B. Were any diagnostic tests recently performed or medicines administered? A β blocker given to a stable asthmatic may precipitate acute bronchospasm. Wheezing after administration of a drug, such as penicillin or radiocontrast dye, suggests an anaphylactic reaction.

C. For what condition was the patient admitted? A patient with an MI may have developed acute pulmonary edema, whereas a patient with a gastric ulcer may have gastric outlet obstruction and have aspirated.

D. Is there any history of asthma? Childhood asthma may reactivate at any age.

E. Does the patient have any allergies to medications or other substances, such as shellfish?

III. Differential Diagnosis

A. Diffuse Wheezing

1. **Acute bronchospasm.** Secondary to asthma, exacerbation of COPD, or an anaphylactic reaction.
2. **Aspiration.** This may trigger bronchospasm from mucosal irritation or impacted foreign bodies.
3. **Cardiogenic pulmonary edema.** The primary finding in "cardiac asthma" may be wheezing. Other findings of pulmonary edema should be present and the chest radiograph diagnostic.
4. **Pulmonary embolism.** Mediators may be released that can cause hypoxemia and bronchospasm.

B. Stridor (Upper Airway) Wheezing

1. **Laryngospasm.** This may be part of an anaphylactic reaction or secondary to aspiration.
2. **Laryngeal or tracheal tumor.** History of dysphagia, hoarseness, cough, or weight loss and anorexia may be present.
3. **Epiglottitis.** The patient often will be unable to speak and unable to swallow secretions.
4. **Foreign body aspiration.**
5. **Vocal cord dysfunction.** Bilateral vocal cord paralysis may result in severe stridor and dyspnea. A subgroup of patients recently has been recognized to have "facti-

tious asthma" in which they voluntarily adduct their vocal cords for psychogenic reasons.

C. Localized Wheezing
1. **Tumors.** May obstruct 1 bronchus, leading to localized wheezing.
2. Mucous plugging.
3. Aspirated foreign body.

IV. Database

A. Physical Examination Key Points
1. **Vital signs.** Fever may indicate infection. A pulsus paradoxicum >20 mm Hg indicates severe respiratory distress. Hypotension requires immediate assessment and action.
2. **HEENT.** Check the mouth carefully. Examine the neck for angioneurotic edema. Palpate the sternocleidomastoid muscles for accessory muscle use. Auscultate over the mouth and larynx to localize the wheeze.
3. **Chest.** Listen for bibasilar rales, which may be present in pulmonary edema. Rales, increased fremitus, and egophony suggest pneumonia.
4. **Cardiac.** Check for evidence of an S_3 or S_4 gallop or JVD, which points to pulmonary edema.
5. **Extremities.** Clubbed fingers most likely indicate an underlying lung cancer or severe COPD. Cyanosis indicates underlying hypoxemia. Edema may signify chronic CHF.
6. **Skin.** Urticaria may indicate an allergic reaction. A malar rash may indicate acute systemic lupus erythematosus, which can present with acute pneumonitis.

B. Laboratory Data
1. **Arterial blood gases.** An increased Pco_2 indicates ventilatory failure. Also check for hypoxemia.
2. **CBC count.** An increased WBC count may indicate an underlying infection; however, an increase in WBC count without a left shift can be seen with an acute MI and PE. Eosinophilia suggests an allergic or asthmatic cause to the wheezing.

C. Radiologic and Other Studies
1. **Electrocardiogram.** An ECG may show an acute MI or ischemia. Occasionally, it will be suggestive of a PE, showing an S wave in lead I, Q wave in lead III, and T wave inversion in lead III ($S_1Q_3T_3$), new right bundle branch block and right axis shift, or arrhythmia.
2. **Chest radiograph.** A PE severe enough to cause wheezing usually will be evident on the chest film. Look

for a pleural-based, wedge-shaped lesion. Also, Kerley B lines, bilateral pleural effusions, vascular redistribution, and cardiomegaly may suggest CHF or pulmonary edema. Look for localized infiltrates or masses suggesting other causes.

V. Plan. Therapy depends on the diagnosis.

A. Bronchospasm (Asthma, COPD, Allergic Reaction)

1. Methylprednisolone (Solu-Medrol) 200 mg IV stat dose.
2. Nebulized albuterol (Ventolin) 0.5 mL (2.5 mg) or metaproterenol (Alupent) 0.3 mL of 5% solution in 3.0 mL NS stat and then every 2–4 hours.
3. Aminophylline 6 mg/kg loading dose (assuming the patient is not already on aminophylline) and then a maintenance IV of 0.2–0.6 mg/kg per hour (15–30 mg/h). Aminophylline is now considered to be of only modest benefit and may cause worsening of arrhythmias. Therefore, blood levels need to be monitored closely.

B. Stridor

1. Methylprednisolone 200 mg IV stat dose.
2. Nebulized racemic epinephrine (Micron Ephrine) 0.5 mL in NS 3 mL.
3. Consider intubation or tracheostomy.

C. Pulmonary Edema

1. Furosemide (Lasix) 20–80 mg IV.
2. Nitroglycerin 0.4 mg sublingually; or paste 0.5 inch on skin; or nitroglycerin drip 10–20 μg/min and increase by 5–10 μg every 10 minutes.
3. Afterload reduction with agents such as IV nitroprusside (Nipride) or oral agents such as captopril (Capoten) or enalapril (Vasotec).
4. IV morphine for venodilation and to relieve anxiety. Be prepared to intubate the patient.
5. **Oxygen.** Start with 2 L by nasal cannula.

D. Miscellaneous.
Treatment varies with the disease. Acute allergic reactions may be prevented by pretreatment with Benadryl IV.

REFERENCES

Lung CL, Lung ML. General principles of asthma management: symptom monitoring. *Nurs Clin North Am* 38:585–96, 2003.

Ohta K, et al. Aminophylline is effective on acute exacerbations of asthma in adults-objective improvements in peak flow, spirogram, arterial blood gas measurements and lung sounds. *Clin Exp Allergy* 26(suppl 2):32–7, 1996.

Stoloff SW. Pharmacologic therapy for asthma. *Clin Cornerstone* 1:17–38, 1998.

77. WOUND DEHISCENCE

I. **Problem.** A nurse notifies you that a laparotomy wound in a patient after a bilateral adrenalectomy has opened and there is a piece of fat poking out of the wound.

II. **Immediate Questions**

A. **Is there a wound dehiscence and, if so, to what extent?** Always evaluate the wound yourself as soon as possible. See how much of the wound has opened, how deep it is, and if there is an evisceration. Check the integrity of the fascia with a cotton-tipped applicator. (An "open wound" is not a dehiscence unless the fascia is open. The sine qua non of dehiscence is a gush of fluid from the wound.) **Be sure to differentiate dehiscence from evisceration** (where a part of a viscus pokes through the fascia).

B. **Did any fluid leak from the wound?** Look at the dressing. Serous/serosanguineous fluid is more ominous for a true fascial dehiscence. Grossly bloody or purulent fluid is indicative of a superficial wound infection, a liquefying hematoma, or active bleeding in the superficial tissues.

C. **Are there any predisposing factors to dehiscence?** Sepsis, poor nutrition, diabetes, and steroids predispose to poor wound healing and increase the likelihood of dehiscence.

III. **Differential Diagnosis.** A wound dehiscence is usually the result of a combination of factors including technical problems, local wound problems, poor wound healing, and increased tension on the wound. The following list is not so much a differential diagnosis as a list of contributing factors.

A. **Technical Problems**

1. **Poorly placed sutures.** Failure to take a full-thickness bite or reapproximating muscle instead of fascia.
2. **Inappropriate suture material.** Such as not using a heavy enough gauge suture for an abdominal closure.
3. **Sutures tied too tightly.** This usually induces tissue ischemia that causes the suture to pull out.

B. **Local Wound Problems**

1. **Infection.** Superficial wound infection or intraperitoneal abscess.
2. **Hematoma.** These may predispose a wound to become infected.

C. Poor Wound Healing
1. Poor nutrition.
2. Diabetes.
3. **Steroids.** Endogenous or exogenous.
4. Uremia.
5. Chemotherapy.
6. Advanced malignancy.

D. Decreased Tension on Wound
1. **Abdominal distention.**
   a. Ascites.
   b. Dilated bowel.
2. Vomiting or coughing.
3. **COPD.**

IV. Database

A. Physical Examination Key Points
1. **Incision.** Use sterile gloves, remove all dressings, and examine the entire wound. Look for leakage of fluid when the wound is palpated, and look for signs of infection.

B. Laboratory Data. Wound culture and Gram's stain if indicated.

V. Plan

A. Overall Plan. Determine if there is an evisceration, fascial disruption without evisceration, or a superficial wound separation. In all cases, it is safe to make the patient NPO and start antibiotics (cephalosporins are used frequently) to cover skin organisms until a final plan is formulated.

B. Evisceration/Fascial Dehiscence. Cover the wound with saline-soaked sterile gauze and a large sterile dressing. Prevent insensible losses at all times. Evisceration requires urgent operative repair.

C. Fascial dehiscence without evisceration. If the overlying skin and subcutaneous tissues are intact but there is clearly a fascial defect, it may be managed by operative repair or observation with a resultant ventral hernia. Use an abdominal binder if managing nonoperatively. A binder often compromises respiratory function, especially in the immediate postoperative period.

D. Superficial Wound Separation
1. Healing by secondary intention is mandatory when there is an associated superficial wound infection and it is the safest management in any case. Open the wound

to drain the pus or fluid and then treat with 2–4 wet to dry dressing changes daily.
2. **Closure.** Some surgeons may attempt closure of a superficial wound separation immediately or after a period of wet-to-dry dressing changes. Realize that this carries a substantial risk of developing a superficial infection or spread of the infection to the fascial layer.

REFERENCES

Harlan JW. Treatment of open sternal wounds with the vacuum-assisted closure system: a safe, reliable method. *Plast Reconstr Surg* 109:710–2, 2002.
Sharma R, et al. A modified parasternal wire technique for prevention and treatment of sternal dehiscence. *Ann Thorac Surg* 77:210–3, 2004.

78. WOUND DRAINAGE

I. **Problem.** A patient has new drainage from a midline laparotomy incision 5 days after a small bowel resection for ischemic bowel.

II. **Immediate Questions**

A. **How old is the wound? What was the operative procedure?** The diagnosis can be made partly on the basis of timing of the drainage and the type of surgery.

B. **Was there any prior drainage, and are drains present?** Increase in drainage from a wound may indicate that the drain may not be working.

C. **How was the wound closed? Sutures? Staples? Retention sutures? Packed open?**

D. **What is the character of the drainage? Bloody? Serosanguineous? Purulent? Intestinal contents?**

E. **How much drainage is there?** Quantitation is essential especially to replace GI tract losses in the presence of a fistula. Consider saving and weighing the dressings if volume determination is critical.

III. **Differential Diagnosis**

A. **Wound Infection.** Typically seen 5–7 days postoperatively.
1. **Wound tenderness and fluctuance.** This is often due to *Staphylococcus* or *Streptococcus* and seen 3–5 days postoperatively.
2. **Gas-forming infections** (*Clostridium*, necrotizing fasciitis). **Severe pain and crepitation are typical. This is a surgical emergency and must be promptly**

drained and débrided. May be caused by *Clostridium* or, more commonly, a mixed gram-negative and microaerophilic gram-positive infection. This can present within the first 24 hours after surgery.

B. Impending Dehiscence. Serosanguineous drainage after the first 24 postoperative hours is almost pathognomonic of wound dehiscence.

C. Enterocutaneous Fistula. This is suggested by the obvious drainage of intestinal contents from the wound. Fistulas are categorized as high or low output fistulas. They can be caused by anastomotic breakdown with subsequent fistulization. They are rarely caused by inadvertent suturing of intestine during fascial closure. This usually follows several days of abdominal pain and fevers.

D. Hemorrhage. Excessive bleeding usually exits through a fresh postoperative wound. DIC may manifest as bleeding through the wound and other sites (IV sites, etc).

E. Pancreatic Fistula. Postoperative or post-traumatic.

F. Urinary Fistula. Post-traumatic, neoplasm, postoperative, after radiation therapy, rarely congenital.

G. Ascitic Leak. Often avoided by closing 1 layer in a continuous running suture.

H. Drain Malfunction. If a surgically placed drain is not performing properly, the intended fluid may exit through the wound.

IV. Database

A. Physical Examination Key Points

1. **Vital signs.** Look for fever, tachycardia, and signs of sepsis.
2. **Abdomen.** Look for signs of peritonitis.
3. **Wound.** Examine for surrounding inflammation, dehiscence, or crepitation. If there is any sign of purulent drainage, crepitus, or cellulitis with fluctuance, immediately open the wound and inspect drainage and fascial planes for integrity.

B. Laboratory Data

1. **Hemogram.** Check WBC count for infection or and hematocrit for bleeding. Platelets may be decreased in DIC or in other causes of thrombocytopenia.
2. **Coagulation profile.** PT, PTT, and fibrin split products if DIC is suspected.
3. Send drainage for culture, Gram's stain, and amylase. Amylase may be high in intestinal fistula but markedly high in pancreatic fistula.

4. **Drainage creatinine.** If the drainage is thought to be urine, the creatinine level will be much higher than the serum level.

C. **Radiologic and Other Studies.** Fistulogram may be helpful.

V. Plan

A. **General Plan.** Immediately treat life-threatening complications such as evisceration (see page 263). Effluent from a wound should be sent for Gram's stain and culture. Chemistry determinations on clear fluid for creatinine or amylase may aid in diagnosis.

B. **Specific Plans**

1. **Wound infection.** The wound must be opened and packed with saline-moistened gauze after evacuating pus from the wound. Remove staples or sutures to fully drain the area. Advancing local cellulitis or systemic signs of infection require antibiotics.

   a. **Clostridium.** Early debridement and large-dose IV penicillin.

   b. Gas-forming nonclostridial infections are controlled with broad-spectrum antibiotics.

2. **Dehiscence.** Fascial dehiscence without evisceration can be watched. This results in a ventral hernia, which may require therapy at a later date. However, actual dehiscence with eviscerated abdominal contents (intestine in the bed) requires prompt operative intervention (see Problem 76, page 258).

3. **Enterocutaneous fistula.** Often needs a bag to capture the effluent and protect the skin. Quantitate the drainage. Oral administration of charcoal or dye may be used to confirm the diagnosis. NG suction and keeping the patient NPO are essential. Remember to institute early parenteral nutritional support. Low output fistulas often close spontaneously, whereas high output fistulas will probably require surgical intervention.

4. **Pancreatic fistula.** Skin protection is essential. There can be serious nutritional deficits caused by pancreatic fistulae, especially by high losses of protein. Because alkalinization of intestinal contents is prevented by the fistulous drainage of pancreatic juice, these patients are at high risk for peptic ulcer.

5. **Hemorrhage.** Evaluate the patient's volume status. Remember that a decrease in hematocrit can be late. Replete volume with crystalloid, blood, or both. The decision as whether to reoperate for bleeding depends on the clinical situation and overall status. It may be a

vessel in the skin or subcutaneous fat. If a vessel is seen, it can be cauterized at the bedside with a battery-powered cautery.

REFERENCES

Foster CE, Lefor AT. Gastrocutaneous fistulas: Initial Management. *Surg Clin North Am* 76:1019–33, 1996.

Maykel JA. Fischer JE. Current management of intestinal fistulas. *Adv Surg* 37:283–99, 2003.

Miller PR, et al. Prospective evaluation of vacuum-assisted fascial closure after open abdomen: planned ventral hernia rate is substantially reduced. *Ann Surg* 239:608–16, 2004.

II. Laboratory Tests & Their Interpretation

This section is a selection of the most commonly used laboratory tests on a surgical service. If an increased or decreased value is not clinically useful, it is not listed. Because each laboratory has its own set of "normal" reference values, the normal values given should be used only as a rough guide. The range for common normal values is given in parentheses and, unless specified, reflects normal adult levels.

Acetoacetate (Ketone Bodies, Acetone) (Serum)

- Normal = negative
- Collection: red top tube

Positive: DKA, starvation, emesis, stress, alcoholism, infantile organic acidemias, isopropyl alcohol ingestion

Acid Phosphatase (Prostatic Acid Phosphatase, PAP) (Serum)

- <3.0 ng/mL by radioimmunoassay or <0.8 IU/L by enzymatic assay
- Collection: tiger top tube

Not a useful screening test for cancer; most useful as a marker of response to therapy or in confirming metastatic disease. Prostate-specific antigen (PSA) is more sensitive in diagnosis of cancer.

Increased: Carcinoma of the prostate (usually outside prostate), prostatic surgery or trauma (including prostatic massage), rarely in infiltrative bone disease (Gaucher's disease, myeloid leukemia), prostatitis, or benign prostatic hyperplasia

ACTH (Adrenocorticotropic Hormone) (Serum)

- 8 AM 20–140 pg/mL (Système International [SI] 20–140 ng/L), midnight, approximately 50% of AM value
- Collection: tiger top tube

Increased: Addison's disease (primary adrenal hypofunction), ectopic ACTH production (small [oat] cell lung carcinoma, pancreatic islet cell tumors, thymic tumors, renal cell carcinoma, bronchial carcinoid), Cushing's disease (pituitary adenoma), congenital adrenal hyperplasia (adrenogenital syndrome)

Decreased: Adrenal adenoma or carcinoma, nodular adrenal hyperplasia, pituitary insufficiency, corticosteroid use

ACTH Stimulation Test
(Cortrosyn Stimulation Test) (Serum)

- Collection: tiger top tube

Used to diagnose adrenal insufficiency. Cortrosyn (an ACTH analogue) is given at a dose of 0.25 mg IM or IV in adults or 0.125 mg in children <2 years. Collect blood at 0, 30, and 60 min for cortisol and aldosterone.

Normal Response: Three criteria are required: basal cortisol level ≥5 µg/dL, an incremental increase after cosyntropin (Cortrosyn) injection of ≥7 µg/dL, and a final serum cortisol level ≥16 µg/dL at 30 or 18 mg/dL at 60 min or cortisol increase of >10 µg/dL. Aldosterone increases >5 ng/dL above baseline.

Addison's Disease (Primary Adrenal Insufficiency): Neither cortisol nor aldosterone increases over baseline.

Secondary Adrenal Insufficiency: Caused by pituitary insufficiency or suppression by exogenous steroids, cortisol does not increase, but aldosterone does.

Albumin (Serum)

- Adult 3.5–5.0 g/dL (SI 35–50 g/L), child 3.8–5.4 g/dL (SI 38–54 g/L)
- Collection: tiger top tube; part of SMA-12

Decreased: Malnutrition, overhydration, nephrotic syndrome, cystic fibrosis (CF), multiple myeloma, Hodgkin's disease, leukemia, metastatic cancer, protein-losing enteropathies, chronic glomeru-lonephritis, alcoholic cirrhosis, inflammatory bowel disease, colla-gen-vascular diseases, hyperthyroidism

Albumin/Globulin Ratio (A/G Ratio) (Serum)

- Normal >1

A calculated value (total protein minus albumin = globulins; al-bumin divided by globulins = A/G ratio). Serum protein elec-trophoresis is a more informative test.

Decreased: Cirrhosis, liver diseases, nephrotic syndrome, chronic glomerulonephritis, cachexia, burns, chronic infections and inflammatory states, myeloma

Aldosterone (Serum)

- Serum: supine 3–10 ng/dL (SI 0.083–0.28 nmol/L) early AM, normal sodium intake (3 g sodium/d)
- Upright 5–30 ng/dL (SI 0.138–0.83 nmol/L); urinary 2–16 mg/24 h (SI 5.4–44.3 nmol/d)
- Collection: green or lavender top tube

Discontinue antihypertensives and diuretics 2 weeks before test. Upright samples should be drawn after 2 h. Primarily used to screen hypertensive patients for possible Conn's syndrome (adrenal adenoma producing excess aldosterone).

Increased: Primary hyperaldosteronism, secondary hyperaldos-teronism (CHF, sodium depletion, nephrotic syndrome, cirrhosis with ascites, others), upright posture

Decreased: Adrenal insufficiency, panhypopituitarism, supine posture

Alkaline Phosphatase (Serum)

- Adult 20–70 U/L, child 20–150 U/L
- Collection: tiger top tube; part of SMA-12

A fractionated alkaline phosphatase was formerly used to differ-entiate the origin of the enzyme in the bone from that in the liver. Replaced by the γ-glutamyl transpeptidase (GGT) and 5'-nucleoti-dase determinations.

Increased (highest levels in biliary obstruction and infiltrative liver disease): Increased calcium deposition in bone (hyper-parathyroidism), Paget's disease, osteoblastic bone tumors (metastatic or osteogenic sarcoma), osteomalacia, rickets, pregnancy, childhood, healing fracture, liver disease such as biliary obstruction (masses, drug therapy), hyperthyroidism

Decreased: Malnutrition, excess vitamin D ingestion, pernicious anemia, Wilson's disease, hypothyroidism, zinc deficiency

α-Fetoprotein (AFP) (Serum)

- <16 ng/mL (SI <16 mL)
- Third trimester of pregnancy maximum 550 ng/mL (SI 550 mL)
- Collection: tiger top tube

Increased: Hepatoma (hepatocellular carcinoma), testicular tumor (embryonal carcinoma, malignant teratoma), neural tube defects (in mother's serum [spina bifida, anencephaly, myelomeningocele]), fetal death, multiple gestations, ataxia–telangiectasia, some cases of benign hepatic diseases (alcoholic cirrhosis, hepatitis, necrosis)

Decreased: Trisomy 21 (Down's syndrome) in maternal serum

ALT (Alanine Aminotransferase, ALAT) or SGPT (Serum)

- 0–35 U/L (SI 0–0.58 mkat/L), higher in newborns
- Collection: tiger top tube

Increased: Liver disease, liver metastasis, biliary obstruction, pancreatitis, liver congestion (ALT is higher than AST in viral hepatitis; AST is higher than ALT in alcoholic hepatitis)

Ammonia (Serum)

- Adult 10–80 mg/dL (SI 5–50 mmol/L)
- To convert mg/dL to mmol/L, multiply by 0.5872
- Collection: green top tube, on ice, analyze immediately

Increased: Liver failure, Reye's syndrome, inborn errors of metabolism, normal neonates (normalizes within 48 h of birth)

Amylase (Serum)

- 50–150 Somogyi units/dL (SI 100–300 U/L)
- Collection: tiger top tube

Increased: Acute pancreatitis, pancreatic duct obstruction (stones, stricture, tumor, sphincter spasm secondary to drugs), pancreatic pseudocyst or abscess, alcohol ingestion, mumps, parotiditis, renal disease, macroamylasemia, cholecystitis, peptic ulcers, intestinal obstruction, mesenteric thrombosis, after surgery

Decreased: Pancreatic destruction (pancreatitis, cystic fibrosis), liver damage (hepatitis, cirrhosis), normal newborns in the first year of life

AST (Aspartate Aminotransferase, ASAT) or SGOT (Serum)

- 8–20 U/L (SI 0–0.58 mkat/L)
- Collection: tiger top tube; part of SMA-12

Generally parallels changes in ALT in liver disease.

Increased: Acute myocardial infarction (AMI), liver disease, Reye's syndrome, muscle trauma and injection, pancreatitis, intestinal injury or surgery, factitious increase (erythromycin, opiates), burns, cardiac catheterization, brain damage, renal infarction

Decreased: Beriberi (vitamin B_6 deficiency), severe diabetes with ketoacidosis, liver disease, chronic hemodialysis

Antinuclear Antibody (ANA, FANA) (Serum)

A useful screening test in patients with symptoms suggesting collagen–vascular disease, especially if titer is >1:160; 5% of normal individuals can have positive test.

Positive: Systemic lupus erythematosus (SLE), drug-induced lupus-like syndromes (procainamide, hydralazine, isoniazid, etc), scleroderma, mixed connective tissue disease (MCTD), rheumatoid arthritis (RA), polymyositis, juvenile RA (5–20%). Low titers are also seen in non–collagen-vascular disease.
   Specific Immunofluorescent ANA Patterns *Homogenous:* Nonspecific, from antibodies to deoxyribonucleoproteins (DNP) and native double-stranded DNA. Seen in SLE and a variety of other diseases. Antihistone is consistent with drug-induced lupus.
   Speckled: Pattern seen in many connective tissue disorders. From antibodies to extractable nuclear antigens (ENA), including anti-RNP, anti-Sm, anti–PM-1, and anti-SS. Anti-RNP is positive in MCTD and SLE. Anti-Sm is very sensitive for SLE. Anti–SS-A and anti SS-B are seen in Sjögren's syndrome and subacute cutaneous lupus. The speckled pattern is also seen with scleroderma.
   Peripheral rim pattern: From antibodies to native double-stranded DNA and DNP. Seen in SLE.

Nucleolar pattern: From antibodies to nucleolar RNA. Positive in Sjögren's syndrome and scleroderma

Anticentromere: Scleroderma, Raynaud's disease, CREST syndrome

Anti-DNA (anti–double-stranded DNA): SLE (but negative in drug-induced lupus), chronic active hepatitis, mononucleosis

Antimitochondrial: Primary biliary cirrhosis, autoimmune diseases such as SLE

Antineutrophil Cytoplasmic (ANCA)

c-ANCA: Wegener's granulomatosis (high titers >1:80, very predictive for Wegener's)

p-ANCA: Polyarteritis nodosa, and other vasculitides including Churg-Strauss and microscopic polyarteritis

Anti-SCL 70: Scleroderma

Anti–Smooth Muscle: Low titers are seen in a variety of illnesses; high titers (>1:100) are suggestive of chronic active hepatitis

Sjögren Syndrome Antibody (SS-A): Sjögren syndrome, SLE, RA

Antimicrosomal: Hashimoto's thyroiditis

Base Excess/Deficit (Serum)

- −2 to +2   • See Section I, pages 15 and 19

Bicarbonate (or "Total CO$_2$") (Serum)

- 23–29 mmol/L   • See Carbon Dioxide, page 279

Bilirubin (Serum)

- Total: 0.3–1.0 mg/dL (SI 3.4–17.1 mmol/L)
- Direct: <0.2 mg/dL (SI <3.4 mmol/L)
- Indirect: <0.8 mg/dL (SI <3.4 mmol/L)
- To convert mg/dL to mmol/L, multiply by 17.10
- Collection: tiger top tube

Increased Total: Hepatic damage (hepatitis, toxins, cirrhosis), biliary obstruction (stone or tumor), hemolysis, fasting

Increased Direct (Conjugated): Note: Determination of the direct bilirubin is usually unnecessary with total bilirubin levels <1.2 mg/dL (SI 21 mmol/L) Biliary obstruction/cholestasis (gallstone, tumor, stricture), drug-induced cholestasis, Dubin–Johnson and Rotor's syndromes

Increased Indirect (Unconjugated): Note: This is calculated as total minus direct bilirubin. So-called hemolytic jaundice is caused by any type of hemolytic anemia (transfusion reaction, sickle cell, etc), Gilbert's disease, physiologic jaundice of the newborn, Crigler–Najjar syndrome.

Bilirubin, Neonatal ("Baby Bilirubin")

- Normal levels dependent on prematurity and age in days
- "Panic levels" usually >15–20 mg/dL (SI >257–342 mmol/L in full-term infants)
- Collection: capillary tube

Increased: Erythroblastosis fetalis, physiologic jaundice (may be due to breast-feeding), resorption of hematoma or hemorrhage, obstructive jaundice, others

Bleeding Time

- Duke, Ivy <6 min; template <10 min
- Collection: Specialized bedside test performed by technicians. A small incision is made, and the wound is wicked with filter paper every 30 s until the fluid is clear

In vivo test of hemostasis, tests platelet function, local tissue factors, and clotting factors. Nonsteroidal medications should be stopped 5–7 days before the test because these agents can affect platelet function.

Increased: Thrombocytopenia (DIC, thrombotic thrombocytopenic purpura [TTP], idiopathic thrombocytopenic purpura), von Willebrand's disease, defective platelet function (NSAIDs such as aspirin)

Blood Gases, Arterial & Venous

There is little difference between arterial and venous pH and bicarbonate (except with CHF and shock); therefore, venous blood gas may be occasionally used to assess acid-base status, but venous oxygen levels (PO_2) are significantly lower than arterial levels (Table II–1, page 275).

TABLE II-1. NORMAL BLOOD GAS VALUES.

Measurement	Arterial Blood	Mixed Venous[a]	Venous
pH	7.40	7.36	7.36
(range)	(7.36–7.44)	(7.31–7.41)	(7.31–7.41)
Po_2	80–100 mm Hg	35–40 mm Hg	30–50 mm Hg
(decreases with age)			
Pco_2	35–45 mm Hg	41–51 mm Hg	40–52 mm Hg
O_2 saturation (%)	>95%	60–80%	60–85%
(decreases with age)			
$[HCO_3^-]$	22–26 mEq/L	22–26 mEq/L	22–28 mEq/L
	(mmol/L)	(mmol/L)	(mmol/L)
Base deficit			
(deficit excess)	−2 to +3	−2 to +3	−2 to +3

[a]Obtained from right atrium, usually through a pulmonary artery catheter.

See individual component for differential diagnosis. For acid-base disorders, see the section below and On-Call Problems, Acidosis (Problem 3, page 15) and Alkalosis (Problem 4, page 19).

Metabolic Acidosis: A decrease in plasma HCO_3 followed by a compensatory decrease in PCO_2. Use the anion gap to help establish the diagnosis (Table II–2).
Anion gap = $[Na - (Cl + HCO_3)]$
Normal gap = 8 − 12 mEq/L

Differential Diagnosis: (See also Problem 3, Acidosis).

TABLE II-2. SIMPLE ACID-BASE DISTURBANCES

Acid-Base Disorder	Primary Abnormality	Secondary Abnormality	Expected Degree of Compensatory Response
Metabolic acidosis	↓↓↓$[HCO_3^-]$	↓↓Pco_2	$Pco_2 = (1.5 \times [HCO_3^-]) + 8$
Metabolic alkalosis	↑↑↑$[HCO_3^-]$	↑↑Pco_2	↑ in $Pco_2 = \Delta\ HCO_3^- \times 0.6$
Acute respiratory acidosis	↑↑↑Pco_2	↑$[HCO_3^-]$	↑ in $HCO_3^- = \Delta\ Pco_2/10$
Chronic respiratory acidosis	↑↑↑Pco_2	↑↑$[HCO_3^-]$	↑ in $HCO_3^- = 4 \times \Delta\ Pco_2/10$
Acute respiratory alkalosis	↓↓↓Pco_2	↓$[HCO_3^-]$	↓ in $HCO_3^- = 2 \times \Delta\ Pco_2/10$
Chronic respiratory alkalosis	↓↓↓Pco_2	↓↓$[HCO_3^-]$	↓ in $HCO_3^- = 5 \times \Delta\ Pco_2/10$

Anion gap acidosis ("normochloremic acidosis": gap >12 mEq/L); caused by a decrease in bicarbonate that is balanced by an increase in unmeasured acids. Lactic acidosis, ketoacidosis (diabetic, alcoholic, starvation), uremia, intoxication (salicylate, methanol, paraldehyde, ethylene glycol), hyperalimentation.

Non–anion gap acidosis ("hyperchloremic acidosis": gap 8–12 mEq/L); caused by a decrease in HCO_3 that is balanced by an increase in chloride. Renal bicarbonate losses (renal tubular acidosis, spironolactone, carbonic anhydrase inhibitors), GI tract bicarbonate losses (diarrhea, pancreatic fistulas, biliary tract fistulas, ileal loop, ureterosigmoidostomy.

Low anion gap (gap <8 mEq/L); not seen with acidosis but can be seen with bromide ingestion, hyponatremia, and multiple myeloma.

Metabolic Alkalosis: An increase in plasma HCO_3 followed by a compensatory increase in P_{CO_2}. Spot urine for chloride helps establish the diagnosis (see Table II–2).

Differential Diagnosis: (See also "Alkalosis," page 20)

Urine Chloride <10 mEq/L ("chloride responsive"): Diuretics, GI tract losses (NG suction, vomiting, diarrhea [villous adenoma, congenital chloride wasting diarrhea in children]), iatrogenic (inadequate chloride intake).

Urine Chloride >10 mEq/L ("chloride resistant"): Adrenal diseases (Cushing's syndrome, hyperaldosteronism), exogenous steroid use, Bartter's syndrome, licorice ingestion.

Respiratory Acidosis: A primary increase in P_{CO_2} with a compensatory increase in plasma $HCO_3 \leq 30$ meq/L if acute (see Table II–2).

Differential Diagnosis: (See also "Acidosis," page 15)

Acute: CNS depression (oversedation, narcotics, anesthetic), CNS trauma (CVA, head injury, spinal cord trauma), neuromuscular diseases (myasthenia gravis, Guillain-Barré disease), airway obstruction, laryngospasm, iatrogenic mechanical underventilation, pulmonary lesions (acute pulmonary edema, severe pneumonia), chest trauma (hemothorax, pneumothorax, flail chest)

Chronic: Chronic asthma, emphysema or bronchitis, Pickwickian syndrome

Respiratory Alkalosis: A primary decrease in P_{CO_2} (see Table II–2).

Differential Diagnosis: (See also "Alkalosis," page 19)

CNS causes: Anxiety, hyperventilation syndrome, pain, head trauma, CVA, encephalitis, CNS tumors, salicylates (early toxicity), fever, early sepsis

Peripheral stimulation: Pulmonary embolus, CHF, interstitial lung disease, pneumonia, altitude, hypoxemia of any cause

Miscellaneous: Delirium tremens, cirrhosis, thyrotoxicosis, pregnancy, pregnancy, iatrogenic overventilation

Blood Urea Nitrogen (BUN) (Serum)

- Birth–1 year: 4–16 mg/dL (SI 1.4–5.7 mmol/L)
- 1–40 years: 5–20 mg/dL (SI 1.8–7.1 mmol/L)
- Gradual slight increase with age
- To convert mg/dL to mmol/L, multiply by 0.3570
- Collection: tiger top tube

Less useful measurement of glomerular filtration rate (GFR) than creatinine because BUN is also related to protein metabolism

Increased: Renal failure (including that induced by aminoglycosides, NSAIDs), prerenal azotemia (decreased renal perfusion secondary to CHF, shock, volume depletion), postrenal (obstruction), GI bleeding, stress, drugs (especially aminoglycosides)

Decreased: Starvation, liver failure (hepatitis, drugs), pregnancy, infancy, nephrotic syndrome, overhydration

BUN/Creatinine Ratio (BUN/Cr) (Serum)

- Mean 10, range 6–20; calculated based on serum levels

Increased: Prerenal azotemia (renal hypoperfusion can be due to decreased volume, CHF, cirrhosis/ascites, nephrosis), GI bleed (ratio often >30), high-protein diet, sepsis/hypermetabolic state, ileal conduit, drugs (steroids, tetracycline)

Decreased: Malnutrition, pregnancy, low-protein diet, ketoacidosis, hemodialysis, SIADH, drugs

C-Peptide, Insulin ("Connecting Peptide") (Serum)

- Fasting: <4.0 ng/mL (SI <4.0 mg/L)
- Male >60 years, 1.5–5.0 ng/mL (SI 1.5–5.0 mg/L)
- Female >60 years, 1.4–5.5 ng/mL (SI 1.4–5.5 mg/L)
- Collection: tiger top tube

Differentiates exogenous from endogenous insulin production/ administration; liberated when proinsulin is split to insulin; levels suggest endogenous production of insulin

Decreased: Diabetes (decreased endogenous insulin), insulin administration (factitious or therapeutic), hypoglycemia

CA 15-3 (Serum)

Used to detect breast cancer recurrence in asymptomatic patients and monitor therapy. Levels related to stage of disease.

Increased: Progressive breast cancer, benign breast disease, and liver disease

Decreased: Response to therapy (25% change considered significant)

CA 19-9 (Serum)

- <37 U/mL (SI <37 kU/L)
- Collection: tiger top tube

Primarily used to determine resectability of pancreatic cancers (ie, >1000 U/mL 95% unresectable)

Increased: GI cancers such as pancreas, stomach, liver, colorectal, hepatobiliary, some cases of lung and prostate, and pancreatitis

CA-125 (Serum)

- <35 U/mL (SI <35 kU/L)
- Collection: tiger top tube

Not a useful screening test for ovarian cancer when used alone; best used in conjunction with ultrasound and physical examination. Increasing levels after resection predictive for recurrence.

Increased: Ovarian, endometrial, and colon cancer; endometriosis; inflammatory bowel disease; pelvic inflammatory disease; pregnancy; breast lesions; and benign abdominal masses (teratomas)

Calcitonin (Thyrocalcitonin) (Serum)

- <19 pg/mL (SI <19 ng/L)
- Collection: tiger top tube

Increased: Medullary carcinoma of the thyroid, C-cell hyperplasia (precursor of medullary carcinoma), small (oat) cell carcinoma of the lung, newborns, pregnancy, chronic renal insufficiency, Zollinger–Ellison syndrome, pernicious anemia

Calcium, Serum (Serum)

- Infants to 1 month: 7–11.5 mg/dL (SI 1.75–2.87 mmol/L)
- 1 month to 1 year: 8.6–11.2 mg/dL (SI 2.15–2.79 mmol/L)
- <1 year and adults: 8.2–10.2 mg/dL (SI 2.05–2.54 mmol/L)
- Ionized: 4.75–5.2 mg/dL (SI 1.19–1.30 mmol/L)
- To convert mg/dL to mmol/L, multiply by 0.2495
- Collection: tiger top tube; ionized requires green or red tube

When interpreting a total calcium value, albumin must be known. If it is not within normal limits, a corrected calcium value can be roughly calculated by the following formula. Values for ionized calcium need no special corrections.

Corrected total Ca = 0.8 (normal albumin − measured albumin) + reported Ca

Increased: Note: Levels >12 mg/dL (2.99 mmol/L) may lead to coma and death. Primary hyperparathyroidism, PTH-secreting tumors, vitamin D excess, metastatic bone tumors, osteoporosis, immobilization, milk-alkali syndrome, Paget's disease, idiopathic hypercalcemia of infants, infantile hypophosphatasia, thiazide diuretics, chronic renal failure, sarcoidosis, multiple myeloma

Decreased: Note: Levels <7 mg/dL (>1.75 mmol/L) may lead to tetany and death. Hypoparathyroidism (surgical, idiopathic), pseudo-hypoparathyroidism, insufficient vitamin D, calcium and phosphorus ingestion (pregnancy, osteomalacia, rickets), hypomagnesemia, renal tubular acidosis, hypoalbuminemia (cachexia, nephrotic syndrome, CF), chronic renal failure (phosphate retention), acute pancreatitis, factitious decrease because of low protein and albumin

Carbon Dioxide ("Total CO$_2$" or Bicarbonate) (Serum)

- Adult 23–29 mmol/L, child 20–28 mmol/L
- Collection: tiger top tube; do not expose sample to air

Increased: Compensation for respiratory acidosis (emphysema) and metabolic alkalosis (severe vomiting, primary aldosteronism, volume contraction, Bartter's syndrome)

Decreased: Compensation for respiratory alkalosis and metabolic acidosis (starvation, diabetic ketoacidosis, lactic acidosis, alcoholic ketoacidosis, toxins [methanol, ethylene glycol, paraldehyde], severe diarrhea, renal failure, drugs [salicylates, acetazolamide], dehydration, adrenal insufficiency)

Carboxyhemoglobin (Carbon Monoxide) (Serum)

- Nonsmoker <2%; smoker <9%; toxic >15%
- Collection: gray or lavender top tube; confirm with laboratory

Increased: Smokers, smoke inhalation, automobile exhaust inhalation, normal newborns

Carcinoembryonic Antigen (CEA) (Serum)

- Nonsmoker <3.0 ng/mL (SI <3.0 µg/L)
- Smoker <5.0 ng/mL (SI <5.0 µg/L)
- Collection: tiger top tube

Not a screening test; useful for monitoring response to therapy and tumor recurrence of adenocarcinomas of the GI tract

Increased: Carcinoma (colon, pancreas, lung, stomach), smokers, nonneoplastic liver disease, Crohn's disease, and ulcerative colitis

Catecholamines, Fractionated Serum (Serum)

- Collection: green or lavender tube; check with laboratory

Values depend on the laboratory and method of assay used. Normal levels presented below are based on a high-pressure liquid chromatographic technique. Patient must be supine in a nonstimulating environment with IV access to obtain a sample.

Catecholamine	Plasma (Supine) Levels
Norepinephrine	70–750 pg/mL (SI 414–4435 pmol/L)
Epinephrine	0–100 pg/mL (SI 0–546 pmol/L)
Dopamine	<30 pg/mL (SI 196 pmol/L)

Increased: Pheochromocytoma, neural CREST tumors (neuroblastoma), with extra-adrenal pheochromocytoma, norepinephrine may be markedly high compared with epinephrine.

Chloride, Serum (Serum)

- 97–107 mEq/L (SI 97–107 mmol/L)
- Collection: tiger top tube

Increased: Diarrhea, renal tubular acidosis, mineralocorticoid deficiency, hyperalimentation, medications (acetazolamide, ammonium chloride)

Decreased: Vomiting, diabetes mellitus with ketoacidosis, mineralocorticoid excess, renal disease with sodium loss

Cholesterol (Serum)

- Total
- Normal (Table II–3);
- To convert mg/dL to mmol/L, multiply by 0.02586
- Collection: tiger top tube

Increased: Idiopathic hypercholesterolemia, biliary obstruction, nephrosis, hypothyroidism, pancreatic disease (diabetes), pregnancy, oral contraceptives, hyperlipoproteinemia (types IIb, III, V)

Decreased: Liver disease (hepatitis, etc), hyperthyroidism, malnutrition (cancer, starvation), chronic anemias, steroid therapy, lipoproteinemia, AMI

High-Density Lipoprotein Cholesterol (HDL, HDL-C)
- Fasting male: 30–70 mg/dL (SI 0.8–1.80 mmol/L)
- Fasting female 30–90 mg/dL (SI 0.80–2.35 mmol/L)

HDL-C: Best correlation with the development of coronary artery disease (CAD); decreased HDL-C in males leads to an increased risk. Levels <40 mg/dL are associated with increased risk of CAD. Levels >60 mg/dL are associated with a decreased risk of CAD.

Increased: Estrogen (menstruating females), regular exercise, small ethanol intake, medications (nicotinic acid, gemfibrozil, others)

Decreased: Males, smoking, uremia, obesity, diabetes, liver disease, Tangier disease

Low-Density Lipoprotein Cholesterol (LDL, LDL-C)
- 50–190 mg/dL (SI 1.30–4.90 mmol/L)

TABLE II–3. NORMAL TOTAL CHOLESTEROL LEVELS BY AGE

Age	Standard Units	SI Units
Infant	<65–175 mg/dL	<1.68–4.52 mmol/L
1–19	<120–220 mg/dL	<3.10–5.68 mmol/L
20–29	<200 mg/dL	<5.20 mmol/L
30–39	<225 mg/dL	<5.85 mmol/L
40–49	<245 mg/dL	<6.35 mmol/L
>50	<265 mg/dL	<6.85 mmol/L

Elevated levels correlate with CAD risk

Increased: Excess dietary saturated fats, hyperlipoproteinemia, biliary cirrhosis, endocrine disease (diabetes, hypothyroidism)

Decreased: Malabsorption, severe liver disease, abetalipoproteinemia

Clostridium difficile Toxin Assay, Fecal (Serum)

- Normal = negative

Most patients with pseudomembranous colitis have positive *C difficile*. A positive value is found as follows: >90% of pseudo-membranous colitis, 30–40% antibiotic-associated colitis, and 6–10% cases of antibiotic-associated diarrhea. Falsely positive in some normals and neonates.

Coagulation and Other Hematologic Tests (Blood)

Different coagulation-related and other blood tests follow.

Activated Clotting Time (ACT)

- 114–186 s
- Collection: black top tube from instrument manufacturer

This is a bedside test used in the operating room, dialysis unit, or other facility to document neutralization of heparin (ie, after coronary artery bypass, heparin is reversed)

Increased: Heparin, some platelet disorders, severe clotting factor deficiency

Clotting Time, Lee-White

- 5–15 min
- Collection: draw into plain plastic syringe; clotting time measured in separate tube

Increased: Heparin therapy, plasma-clotting factor deficiency (except factors VII and XIII). *Note:* not a sensitive test, not considered a good screening test.

Mixing study

Used to evaluate prolonged coagulation times. Add normal plasma to patient sample. If problem corrects, a factor deficiency exists (VII, VIII, IX, XI). If not, an inhibitor is present (ie, lupus anticoagulant/antiphospholipid). Prolonged **RVVT (Russell viper venom time)** confirms lupus anticoagulant.

Antithrombin-III (AT-III)
- 17–30 mg/dL or 80–120% of control
- Collection: blue top tube; patient must be off heparin for 6 h

Used in the evaluation of thrombosis. Heparin must interact with AT-III to produce anticoagulation effect.

Decreased: Autosomal-dominant familial AT-III deficiency, PE, severe liver disease, late pregnancy, oral contraceptives, nephrotic syndrome, heparin therapy (>3 days)

Increased: Coumadin, after MI

Complement (Serum)
- Collection: tiger or lavender top tube

Complement describes a series of sequentially reacting serum proteins that participate in pathogenic processes and lead to inflammatory injury.

Complement C3
- 85–155 mg/dL (SI 800–1500 ng/L)

Decreased levels suggest activation of the classic or alternative pathway or both.

Increased: RA (variable finding), rheumatic fever, various neoplasms (GI, prostate, others), acute viral hepatitic, MI, pregnancy, amyloidosis

Decreased: SLE, glomerulonephritis (poststreptococcal and membranoproliferative), sepsis, subacute bacterial endocarditis (SBE), chronic active hepatitis, malnutrition, DIC, gram-negative sepsis

Complement C4
- 20–50 mg/dL (SI 200–500 ng/L)

Increased: RA (variable finding), neoplasia (GI, lung, others)

Decreased: SLE, chronic active hepatitis, cirrhosis, glomerulonephritis, hereditary angioedema (test of choice)

Complement CH50 (Total)
- 33–61 mg/mL (SI 330–610 ng/L)

Tests for complement deficiency in the classic pathway.

Increased: Acute-phase reactants (tissue injury, infections, etc)

Decreased: Hereditary complement deficiencies

Complete Blood Count (CBC): Normal Variations (Blood)

Hemoglobin and hematocrit levels are highest at birth (20 g/100 mL and 60%, respectively). Levels decrease steeply to a minimum at 3 months (9.5 g/100 mL and 32%) and then slowly increase to near adult levels at puberty; thereafter, both values are higher in males. A normal decrease occurs in pregnancy. The WBC count is highest at birth (mean 25,000/mm^3) and slowly decreases to adult levels by puberty. Lymphs predominate (up to 60% from the second week of life until age 5–7 years, when polys begin to predominate). This variation is presented in Table II–4.

The "Left Shift"

The degree of nuclear lobulation of polymorphonuclear neutrophils (PMNs) is thought to provide some indication of cell age. A predominance of immature cells with only 1 or 2 nuclear lobes separated by a thick chromatin band is called a "**shift to the left.**" Conversely, a predominance of cells with 4 nuclear lobes is called a "**shift to the right.**" (Historical note: Left and right designations come from the formerly used manual laboratory counters, in which the keys for entering the stabs were located on the left of the keyboard.) As a general rule, 55–80% of PMNs have 2–4 lobes. More than 20 5-lobed cells/100 WBCs suggest megaloblastic anemia, with a 6- or 7-lobed being poly-diagnostic.

"**Bands**" or "**stabs,**" the more immature forms of PMNs (the more mature forms are called "**segs**"), are identified by the fact that the connections between ends or lobes of a nucleus are greater than one-half the width of the hypothetical round nucleus. The connection between the lobes of the nucleus is by a thick band in bands/stabs and by a thin filament in segs. A band is defined as a connecting strip wide enough to reveal 2 distinct margins with nuclear material in between. A filament is so narrow that no intervening nuclear material is present.

For practical purposes, **a left shift is present in the CBC when more than 10–12% bands are seen or when the total PMN count (segs plus bands) is >80%.**

Left Shift: Bacterial infection, toxemia, hemorrhage

Right Shift: Liver disease, megaloblastic anemia, iron deficiency anemia, glucocorticoid use, stress reaction

Complete Blood Count: Differential Diagnosis (Blood)

Variations in counts of various subsets by age are presented in Table II–5.

TABLE II–4. NORMAL COMPLETE BLOOD COUNT FOR SELECTED AGE RANGES

Age	WBC Count (cells/cu mm) [SI: 10⁹/L]	RBC Count 10⁶/µL [SI: 10¹²/L]	Hemoglobin (gm/dL) [SI: g/L]	Hematocrit (%)	MHC (pg) [SI: pg]	MCHC (g/dL) [SI: g/L]ᵃ	MCV (cu µm) [SI: fl]	RDW
Adult male	4500–11,000 [4.5–11.0]	4.73–5.49 [4.73–5.49]	14.40–16.60 [144–166]	42.9–49.1	27–31	33–37	76–100	11.5–14.5
Adult female	As above	4.15–4.87 [4.15–5.49]	12.2–14.7 [122–147]	37.9–43.9	As above	As above	As above	As above
11–15 years	4500–13,500	4.8	13.4	39	28	34	82	—
6–10 years	5000–14,500	4.7	12.9	37.5	27	34	80	—
4–6 years	5500–15,500	4.6	12.6	37.0	27	34	80	—
2–4 years	6000–17,000	4.5	12.5	35.5	25	32	77	—
4 months–2 years	6000–17,500	4.6	11.2	35.0	25	33	77	—
1 week–4 mo	5500–18,000	4.7 ± 0.9	14.0 ± 3.3	42.0 ± 7.0	30	33	90	—
24 hr–1 week	5000–21,000	5.1	18.3 ± 4.0	52.5	36	35	103	—
First day	9400–34,000	5.1 ± 1.0	19.5 ± 5.0	54.0 ± 10.0	38	36	106	—

ᵃTo convert from standard reference value to SI units, multiply by 10.

TABLE II–5 NORMAL PLATELET AND WHITE BLOOD CELL DIFFERENTIAL FOR SELECTED AGES

Age	Platelet Count (10³ μL) [SI: 10⁹/L]	Lymphocytes Total (% WBC Count)	Neutrophils, Band (% WBC Count)	Neutrophils, Segmented (% WBC Count)	Eosinophils (% WBC Count)	Basophils (% WBC Count)	Monocytes (% WBC Count)
Adult male	238 ± 49	34%	3.0%	56%	2.7%	0.5%	4.0%
Adult female	270 ± 58	As above	As above	As above	As above	As above	As above
11–15 years	282 ± 63	38%	3.0%	51%	2.4%	0.5%	4.3%
6–10 years	351 ± 85	39%	3.0%	50%	2.4%	0.6%	4.2%
4–6 years	357 ± 70	42%	3.0%	39%	2.8%	0.6%	5.0%
2–4 years	357 ± 70	59%	3.0%	30%	2.6%	0.5%	5.0%
4 months–2 years	As above	61%	3.1%	28%	2.6%	0.4%	4.8%
1 week–4 mo	As above	56%	4.5%	30%	2.8%	0.5%	6.5%
24 hr–1 week	240–380	24–41%	6.8–9.2%	39–52%	2.4–4.1%	0.5%	5.8–9.1%
First day	As above	24%	10.2%	58%	2.0%	0.6%	5.8%

Basophils
- 0–1%

Increased: Chronic myeloid leukemia, after splenectomy, polycythemia, Hodgkin's disease, and, rarely, in recovery from infection and from hypothyroidism

Decreased: Acute rheumatic fever, pregnancy, after radiation, steroid therapy, thyrotoxicosis, stress

Eosinophils
- 1–3%

Increased: Allergy, parasites, skin diseases, malignancy, drugs, asthma, Addison's disease, collagen-vascular diseases (handy mnemonic **NAACP: N**eoplasm, **A**llergy/asthma, **A**ddison's disease, **C**ollagen–vascular diseases, **P**arasites), pulmonary diseases including Löffler's syndrome and pulmonary infiltrates with eosinophilia (PIE)

Decreased: Steroids, ACTH, after stress (infection, trauma, burns), Cushing's syndrome

Hematocrit (Male 40–54%, Female 37–47%)

Decreased: Megaloblastic anemia (folate or B_{12} deficiency); iron deficiency anemia; sickle cell anemia or other hemoglobinopathies; acute or chronic blood loss; sideroblastic anemia, hemolysis; anemia due to chronic disease, dilution, alcohol, or drugs

Increased: Primary polycythemia (polycythemia vera), secondary polycythemia (decreased fluid intake or excess fluid loss, congenital and acquired heart disease, lung disease, high altitudes, heavy smoking, tumors [renal cell carcinoma, hepatoma], renal cysts)

Lymphocytes
- 24–44%
- See also Lymphocyte Subsets, page 290

Increased: Viral infection (AIDS, measles, rubella, mumps, whooping cough, smallpox, chickenpox, influenza, hepatitis, infectious mononucleosis), acute infectious lymphocytosis in children, acute and chronic lymphocytic leukemias

Decreased: Normal finding in 22% of population. Stress, burns, trauma, uremia, some viral infections, human immunodeficiency virus (HIV) and AIDS, bone marrow suppression after chemotherapy, steroids, multiple sclerosis

Atypical Lymphocytes

>20%: Infectious mononucleosis, cytomegalovirus infection, infectious hepatitis, toxoplasmosis

<20%: Viral infections (mumps, rubeola, varicella), rickettsial infections, TB

MCH (Mean Cellular [Corpuscular] Hemoglobin)

- 27–31 pg. The weight of hemoglobin of the average red cell. Calculated by:

$$MCH = \frac{Hemoglobin \ (g/L)}{RBC \ (10^6/\mu L)}$$

Increased: Macrocytosis (megaloblastic anemias, high reticulocyte counts)

Decreased: Microcytosis (iron deficiency, sideroblastic anemia, thalassemia)

MCHC (Mean Cellular [Corpuscular] Hemoglobin Concentration)

- 33–37 g/dL (SI 330–370 g/L). The average concentration of hemoglobin in a given volume of RBCs. Calculated by the formula:

$$MCHC = \frac{Hemoglobin \ (g/dL)}{Hematocrit}$$

Increased: Very severe, prolonged dehydration; spherocytosis

Decreased: Iron deficiency anemia, overhydration, thalassemia, an sideroblastic anemia

MCV (Mean Cell [Corpuscular] Volume)

- 78–98 μm^3 The average volume of RBCs. Calculated by the formula:

$$MCV = \frac{Hematocrit \times 1000}{RBC \ (10^6/\mu L)}$$

Increased/Macrocytosis: Megaloblastic anemia (B_{12}, folate deficiency), macrocytic (normoblastic) anemia, reticulocytosis, myelodysplasias, Down's syndrome, chronic liver disease, control of AIDS with azathioprine (AZT), chronic alcoholism, cytotoxic chemotherapy, radiation therapy, Dilantin use, hypothyroidism, newborns

Decreased/Microcytosis: Iron deficiency, thalassemia, some cases of lead poisoning or polycythemia

Monocytes
- 3–7%

Increased: Bacterial infection (TB, SBE, brucellosis, typhoid, recovery from an acute infection), protozoan infections, infectious mononucleosis, leukemia, Hodgkin's disease, ulcerative colitis, regional enteritis

Decreased: Lymphocytic leukemia, aplastic anemia, steroid use

Platelets
- 150–450,000 µL. Platelet counts may be normal in number, but abnormal in function as occurs in aspirin therapy. Abnormalities of platelet function are assessed by bleeding time.

Increased: Sudden exercise, trauma, fracture, after asphyxia, after surgery (especially splenectomy), acute hemorrhage, polycythemia vera, primary thrombocytosis, leukemias, after childbirth, carcinoma, cirrhosis, myeloproliferative disorders, iron deficiency

Decreased: DIC, idiopathic thrombocytopenic purpura, TTP, HUS, congenital disease, marrow suppressants (chemotherapy, alcohol, radiation), burns, snake and insect bites, leukemias, aplastic anemias, hypersplenism, infectious mononucleosis, viral infections, cirrhosis, massive transfusions, HELLP syndrome (a severe form of preeclampsia with microangiopathic **h**emolysis, **e**levated **l**iver function tests, and **l**ow **p**latelet counts), preeclampsia and eclampsia, prosthetic heart valve, >30 different drugs (NSAIDs, cimetidine, aspirins, thiazides, others)

PMNs (Polymorphonuclear Neutrophils) (Neutrophils)
- 40–76%
- See also the "Left Shift," page 284.

Increased
Physiologic (Normal): Severe exercise, last months of pregnancy, labor, surgery, newborns, steroid therapy
Pathologic: Bacterial infections, noninfective tissue damage (MI, pulmonary infarction, pancreatitis, crush injury, burn injury), metabolic disorders (eclampsia, DKA, uremia, acute gout), leukemias

Decreased: Pancytopenia, aplastic anemia, PMN depression (a mild decrease is referred to as **neutropenia,** severe is called **agranulocytosis**), marrow damage (x-rays, poisoning with benzene or antitumor drugs), severe overwhelming infections (disseminated TB, septicemia), acute malaria, severe osteomyelitis, infectious mononucleosis, atypical pneumonias, some viral infections, marrow obliteration (osteosclerosis, myelofibrosis, malignant infiltrate), drugs (>70, including chloramphenicol, phenylbutazone, chlorpromazine, quinine), B12 and folate deficiencies, hypoadrenalism, hypopituitarism, dialysis, familial decrease, idiopathic causes

RDW (Red Cell Distribution Width)

- 11.5–14.5 red cell distribution width is a measurement of the degree of **anisocytosis** (variation in RBC size) and measured by automated hematology counters.

Increased: Many anemias (iron deficiency, pernicious, folate deficiency, thalassemias), liver disease

Lymphocyte Subsets

Specific monoclonal antibodies are used to identify specific T and B cells. Lymphocyte subsets (also called lymphocyte marker assays or T- and B-cell assay) are useful in the diagnosis of AIDS and various leukemias and lymphomas. The designation **CD (clusters of differentiation)** has largely replaced the older antibody designations (eg, Leu 3a or OKT3). Results are most reliable when reported as an absolute number of cells per microliter rather than a percentage of cells. A CD4/CD8 ratio <1 is seen in patients with AIDS. Absolute CD4 count is used to determine when to initiate therapy with antiretrovirals or prophylaxis for certain infections such as *Pneumocystis carinii* pneumonia. The CDC count includes in the category of AIDS any HIV-positive patient with a CD4 count <200.

Normal Lymphocyte Subsets

- Total lymphocytes 0.66–4.60 thousand/μL
- T cell 644–2201 μL (60–88%)
- B cell 82–392 μL (3–20%)
- T-helper/inducer cell (CD4, Leu 3a, OKT4) 493–1191 μL (34–67%)
- Suppressor/cytotoxic T cell (CD8, Leu 2, OKT8) 182–785 μL (10–42%)
- CD4/CD8 ratio >1

Coombs' Test, Direct (Direct Antiglobulin Test)

- Normal = negative
- Collection: Purple top tube

Uses patient's erythrocytes; tests for the presence of antibody on the patient's cells and used in the screening for autoimmune hemolytic anemia.

Positive: Autoimmune hemolytic anemia (leukemia, lymphoma, collagen-vascular diseases), hemolytic transfusion reaction, some drug sensitizations (methyldopa, levodopa, cephalosporins, penicillin, quinidine), hemolytic disease of the newborn (erythroblastosis fetalis)

Coombs' Test, Indirect (Indirect Antiglobulin Test/Autoantibody Test)

- Normal = negative
- Collection: purple top tube

Uses serum that contains antibody, usually from the patient. Used to check crossmatch before blood transfusion in the blood bank.

Positive: Isoimmunization from previous transfusion, incompatible blood due to improper crossmatching or medications such as methyldopa.

Cortisol (Serum)

- 8 AM, 5.0–23.0 mg/dL (SI 138–365 nmol/L)
- 4 PM, 3.0–15.0 mg/dL (SI 83–414 nmol/L)
- Collection: green or red top tube

Increased: Adrenal adenoma, adrenal carcinoma, Cushing's disease, non-pituitary ACTH-producing tumor, steroid therapy, oral contraceptives

Decreased: Primary adrenal insufficiency (Addison's disease), congenital adrenal hyperplasia, Waterhouse-Friderichsen syndrome, ACTH deficiency

Creatine Phosphokinase (Kinase) (CP, CPK) (Serum)

- 25–145 mU/mL (SI 25–145 U/L)
- Collection: tiger top tube

Used in suspected MI or muscle diseases. Heart, skeletal muscle, and brain have high levels.

Increased: Muscle damage (AMI, myocarditis, muscular dystrophy, muscle trauma [including injections], after surgery), brain infarction, defibrillation, cardiac catheterization and surgery, rhabdomyolysis, polymyositis, hypothyroidism

CPK Isoenzymes

MB: (Normal <6%, heart origin). Increased in AMI (begins at 2–12 h, peaks at 12–40 h, returns to normal in 24–72 h), pericarditis with myocarditis, rhabdomyolysis, crush injury, Duchenne's muscular dystrophy, polymyositis, malignant hyperthermia, and cardiac surgery

MM: (Normal 94–100%, skeletal muscle origin). Increased in crush injury, malignant hyperthermia, seizures, IM injections.

BB: (Normal 0%, brain origin). Brain injury (CVA, trauma), metastatic neoplasms (prostate), malignant hyperthermia, colonic infarction.

Creatinine (Serum)

- Adult male <1.2 mg/dL (SI 106 mmol/L)
- Adult female <1.1 mg/dL (SI 97 mmol/L)
- Child 0.5–0.8 mg/dL (SI 44–71 mmol/L)
- To convert mg/dL to μmol/L, multiply by 88.40
- Collection: tiger top tube

A clinically useful estimate of GFR. As a rule of thumb, serum creatinine doubles with each 50% decrease in GFR.

Increased: Renal failure (prerenal, renal, or postrenal obstruction or medication-induced [aminoglycosides, NSAIDs, others]), gigantism, acromegaly, ingestion of roasted meat, falsely positive with DKA

Decreased: Pregnancy, decreased muscle mass, severe liver disease

Creatinine (Urine) and Creatinine Clearance (Urine)

Normal
Adult Male: Total creatinine 1–2 g/24 h (8.8–17.7 mmol/d); clearance 85–125 mL/min per 1.73 m^2

   Adult Female: Total creatinine 0.8–1.8 g/24 h (7.1–15.9 mmol/d); clearance 75–115 mL/min per 1.73 m^2 (1.25–1.92 mL/s per 1.73 m^2)

   Child: Total creatinine (>3 years) 12–30 mg/kg/24 h; clearance 70–140 mL/min per 1.73 m^2 (1.17–2.33 mL/s per 1.73 m^2)

Decreased: A decreased creatinine clearance (CrCl) results in an increase in serum creatinine usually secondary to renal insufficiency.

Increased: Early diabetes mellitus, pregnancy

Creatinine Clearance Determination
CrCl is one of the most sensitive indicators of early renal insufficiency. Clearances are ordered for patients with suspected renal

disease and monitoring patients on nephrotoxic medications (eg, gentamicin). CrCl decreases with age. A CrCl of 10–20 mL/min indicates severe renal failure and usually the need for dialysis. To determine CrCl, order a concurrent serum creatinine and a 24-h urine creatinine. A shorter interval can be used, eg, 12 h, but the formula must be corrected for this change, and a 24-h sample is less prone to collection error.

Example: The following are calculations of (a) CrCl from a 24-h urine sample with a volume of 1000 mL, (b) a urine creatinine level of 108 mg/100 mL, and (c) a serum creatinine level of 1 mg/100 mL (1 mg/dL).

$$\text{Clearance} = \frac{\text{Urine creatinine} \times \text{total urine volume}}{\textit{Plasma creatinine} \times \text{time (1440 min if 24-h collection)}}$$

$$\text{Clearance} = \frac{(108 \text{ mg}/100 \text{ mL})(1000 \text{ mL})}{(1 \text{ mg}/100 \text{ mL})(1440 \text{ min})} = 75 \text{ mL}/\text{min}$$

To determine if the urine sample is valid (ie, a full 24-h collection), the sample should contain 18–25 mg/kg per 24 h of creatinine for adult males or 12–20 mg/kg per 24 h for adult females. If the patient is an adult (150 lb = 1.73 m^2 body surface area), adjustment of clearance for body size is not routinely done. Adjustment for pediatric patients is a necessity.

If the values in the previous example were for a 10-year-old boy who weighed 70 lb (1.1 m^2), the clearance would be:

$$\frac{75 \text{ mL}/\text{min} \times 1.73 \text{ m}^2}{1.1 \text{ m}^2} = 118 \text{ mL}/\text{min}$$

A rapid determination can be made by a formula:

$$\text{CrCl estimate} = \frac{(140 - \text{age}) \times \text{weight (kg) (if female}, \times 0.85)}{\text{Serum creatinine} \times 72}$$

D-Dimer (Serum)

- Negative
- Collection: blue top tube

D-dimers are proteins released when the fibrinolytic system breaks down fibrin; used to evaluate suspected DVTs and PEs; levels return to normal if clot stabilized (ie, therapy with heparin) and the patient is not undergoing any further fibrin deposition or plasmin activation.

Increased: DVT, PE, MI, CVA, sickle cell crisis, cancer, renal failure, CHF, life-threatening infections

Dehydroepiandrosterone (DHEA) (Serum)

- Male 2.0–3.4 ng/mL (SI 5.2–8.7 mmol/L)
- Female, premenopausal 0.8–3.4 ng/mL (SI 2.1–8.8 mmol/L)
- Female, postmenopausal 0.1–0.6 ng/mL (SI 0.3–1.6 mmol/L)
- Collection: tiger top tube

Increased: Anovulation, polycystic ovaries, adrenal hyperplasia, adrenal tumors

Decreased: Menopause

Dehydroepiandrosterone Sulfate (DHEAS) (Serum)

- Male 1.7–4.2 ng/mL (SI 6–15 mmol/L)
- Female 2.0–5.2 ng/mL (SI 7–18 mmol/L)
- Collection: tiger top tube

Increased: Hyperprolactinemia, adrenal hyperplasia, adrenal tumor, polycystic ovaries, lipoid ovarian tumors

Decreased: Menopause

Dexamethasone Suppression Test (Serum)

Used in the differential diagnosis of Cushing's syndrome (high cortisol level)

Overnight Test: In the "rapid" version of this test, a patient takes dexamethasone 1 mg PO at 11 PM and a fasting 8 AM plasma cortisol is obtained. Normally the cortisol level should be <5.0 mg/dL (138 nmol/L). A value >5 mg/dL (138 nmol/L) usually confirms the diagnosis of Cushing's syndrome; however, obesity, alcoholism, or depression may occasionally show the same result. In these patients, the best screening test is a 24-h urine for free cortisol.

Small-Dose Test: After collection of baseline serum cortisol level and 24-h urine-free cortisol level, dexamethasone 0.5 mg is administered PO every 6 h for 8 doses. Serum and urine cortisol measurements are repeated on the second day. Failure to suppress to a serum cortisol level <5.0 mg/dL (138 nmol/L) and a urine-free cortisol level <30 µg/dL (82 nmol/L) confirms Cushing's syndrome

Large-Dose Test: After the small-dose test, dexamethasone 2 mg PO every 6 h for 8 doses will cause a decrease in urinary-free cortisol to 50% of the baseline value in bilateral adrenal hyperplasia (Cushing's disease) but not in adrenal tumors or ectopic ACTH production.

Erythropoietin (EPO) (Serum)

- 5–36 mU/L (5–36 IU/L)
- Collection: tiger top tube

EPO is a renal hormone that stimulates RBC production.

Increased: Pregnancy, secondary polycythemia (high altitude, COPD, etc), tumors (renal cell carcinoma, cerebellar hemangioblastoma, hepatoma, others), PCKD, anemias with bone marrow unresponsiveness (aplastic anemia, iron deficiency, etc)

Decreased: Bilateral nephrectomy, anemia of chronic disease (ie, renal failure, nephrotic syndrome), primary polycythemia (*Note:* The determination of EPO levels before administration of recombinant EPO for renal failure is not usually necessary.)

Estradiol, Serum (Serum)

- Collection: tiger top tube

Serial measurements useful for assessing fetal well-being, especially in high-risk pregnancy. Also useful for evaluation of amenorrhea and gynecomastia in males.

Normal Values

Female
Follicular phase 25–75 pg/mL
Midcycle peak 200–600 pg/mL
Luteal phase 100–300 pg/mL
First-trimester pregnancy 1–5 ng/mL
Second-trimester pregnancy 5–15 ng/mL
Third-trimester pregnancy 10–40 ng/mL
Postmenopause 5–25 pg/mL
Oral contraceptives <50 pg/mL

Male
Prepubertal 2–8 pg/mL
Adult 10–60 pg/mL

Estrogen/Progesterone Receptors (Serum)

These are typically determined on fresh surgical (breast cancer) specimens. The presence of the receptors is associated with a longer disease-free interval, longer survival from breast cancer, and increased likelihood of responding to endocrine therapy. Fifty percent to 75% of breast cancers are positive for estrogen receptors.

Ethanol (Blood Alcohol) (Serum)

- 0 mg/dL (0 mmol/L)
- Collection: tiger top tube; use povidone-iodine, not alcohol, to clean venipuncture site

Physiologic changes can vary with degree of alcohol tolerance of an individual.

- <50 mg/dL (<10.85–mmol/L): Limited muscular incoordination
- 50–100 mmol/L (10.85–21.71 mmol/L): Pronounced incoordination
- 100–150 mmol/L (21.71–32.57 mmol/L): Mood and personality changes; legally intoxicated in most states
- 150–400 mmol/L (32.57–87 mmol/L): Nausea, vomiting, marked ataxia, amnesia, dysarthria
- >400 mmol/L: Coma, respiratory insufficiency, and death

Fecal Fat (Stool)

- 2–6 g/d on an 80–100 g/d fat diet
- 72-h collection time
- Sudan III stain, random <60 droplets fat/high-power field (HPF)

Increased: CF, pancreatic insufficiency, Crohn's disease, chronic pancreatitis, sprue

Ferritin (Serum)

- Male 15–200 ng/mL (SI 15–200 mg/L)
- Female 12–150 ng/mL (SI 12–150 mg/L)
- Collection: tiger top tube

Increased: Hemochromatosis, hemosiderosis, sideroblastic anemia

Decreased: Iron deficiency (earliest and most sensitive test before RBCs show any morphologic change), severe liver disease

Fibrin D-Dimers

- Negative or <0.5 µg/mL
- Collection: blue, green, or purple top tube

Fibrin broken into various D-dimer fragments by plasmin.

Increased: DIC, thromboembolic diseases (PE, arterial or venous thrombosis)

Fibrin Degradation Products (FDP), Fibrin Split Products (FSP) (Blood)

- <10 µg/mL
- Collection: blue top tube

Generally replaced by the fibrin D-dimer as a screen for DIC.

Increased: DIC (usually >40 µg/mL), any thromboembolic condition (DVT, MI, PE), hepatic dysfunction

Fibrinogen
- 123–370 mg/dL (SI 1.23–3.7 g/L) (Panic levels <100 or >500 mg/dL)
- Collection: blue top tube

Most useful in the diagnosis of DIC and congenital hypofibrinogenemia. Fibrinogen is cleaved by thrombin to form insoluble fragments that polymerize to form a stable clot.

Increased: Inflammatory reactions, oral contraceptives, pregnancy, cancer (kidney, stomach, breast)

Decreased: DIC (sepsis, amniotic fluid embolism, abruptio placentae), surgery (prostate, open heart), neoplastic and hematologic conditions, acute severe bleeding, burns, venomous snake bite, congenital

Folic Acid (Serum)

- >2.0 ng/mL (SI >5 nmol/L) (See RBC Folic Acid, below)

Folic Acid, RBC (Blood)

- 125–600 ng/mL (283–1360 nmol/L)
- Collection: lavender top tube

Serum folate can fluctuate with diet. RBC levels are more indicative of tissue stores. Vitamin B12 deficiency can result in RBCs being unable to take up folate despite normal serum folate levels.

Increased: Folic acid administration

Decreased: Malnutrition/malabsorption (folic acid deficiency), massive cellular growth (cancer) or cell turnover, ongoing hemolysis, medications (trimethoprim, some anticonvulsants, oral contraceptives), vitamin B_{12} deficiency (low RBC levels), pregnancy

Follicle-Stimulating Hormone (FSH) (Serum)

- Males <22 IU/L
- Females: non-midcycle <20 IU/L, midcycle surge 40 IU/L (midcycle peak should be 2 times basal level)
- Postmenopausal 40–160 IU/L
- Collection: tiger top tube

Used in the workup of impotence, infertility in men, and amenorrhea in women

Increased: (Hypergonadotropic >40 IU/L.) Postmenopausal, surgical castration, gonadal failure, gonadotropin-secreting pituitary adenoma

Decreased: (Hypogonadotropic <5 IU/L.) Prepubertal, hypothalamic and pituitary dysfunction, pregnancy

FTA-ABS (Fluorescent Treponemal Antibody Absorbed) (Serum)

- Normal = nonreactive
- Collection: tiger top tube

FTA-ABS may be negative in early primary syphilis and remain positive despite adequate therapy.

Positive: Syphilis (test of choice to confirm diagnosis after a reactive Venereal Disease Research Laboratory [VDRL] test), other treponemal infections can cause false-positive (Lyme disease, leprosy, malaria)

Fungal Serologies (Serum)

- Negative <1:8
- Collection: tiger top tube

This is a screening technique for complement-fixed fungal antibodies, which usually detects antibodies to *Histoplasma capsulatum*, *Blastomyces dermatitidis*, *Cryptococcus neoformans*, *Aspergillus* species, *Candida* species, and *Coccidioides immitis.*

Gastrin, Serum (Serum)

- Fasting <100 pg/mL (SI 47.7 pmol/L)
- Postprandial 95–140 pg/mL (SI 45.3–66.7 pmol/L)
- Collection: tiger top tube, freeze immediately

Make sure patient is not on H_2 blockers or antacids.

Increased: Zollinger-Ellison syndrome, medications (antacids, H_2 blockers, and proton pump inhibitors [PPIs]) pyloric stenosis, pernicious anemia, atrophic gastritis, ulcerative colitis, renal insufficiency, and steroid and calcium administration

Decreased: Vagotomy and antrectomy

GGT (Serum γ-Glutamyl Transpeptidase, SGGT) (Serum)

- Male 9–50 U/L
- Female 8–40 U/L
- Collection: tiger top tube

Generally parallels changes in serum alkaline phosphatase and 5′-nucleotidase in liver disease. Sensitive indicator of alcoholic liver disease.

Increased: Liver disease (hepatitis, cirrhosis, obstructive jaundice), pancreatitis.

Glucose (Serum)

- Fasting 70–105 mg/dL (SI 3.89–5.83 nmol/L)
- 2 h postprandial <140 mg/dL (SI <7.8 nmol/L)
- To convert mg/dL to nmol/L, multiply by 0.05551
- Collection: tiger top tube

American Diabetes Association Diagnostic Criterion for Diabetes: normal fasting level <110 mg/dL, impaired fasting level 110–126 mg/dL, diabetes >126 mg/dL, or any random level >200 mg/dL when associated with other symptoms. Confirm with repeat testing.

Increased: Diabetes mellitus, Cushing's syndrome, acromegaly, increased epinephrine (injection, pheochromocytoma, stress, burns, etc), acute and chronic pancreatitis, ACTH administration, spurious increase caused by drawing blood from a site above an IV line containing dextrose, elderly patients, pancreatic glucagonoma, drugs (glucocorticoids, thiazide diuretics)

Decreased: Pancreatic disorders (islet cell tumors), extrapancreatic tumors (carcinoma of the adrenals, stomach), hepatic disease (hepatitis, cirrhosis, tumors), endocrine disorders (early diabetes, hypothyroidism, hypopituitarism), functional disorders (after gastrectomy), pediatric problems (prematurity, infant of a diabetic mother, ketotic hypoglycemia, enzyme diseases), exogenous insulin, oral hypoglycemic agents, malnutrition, sepsis

Glucose Tolerance Test (GTT), Oral (OGTT) (Serum)

A fasting plasma glucose level >126 mg/dL (7.0 mmol/L) or a casual plasma glucose level >200 mg/dL (11.1 mmol/L) meets the threshold for the diagnosis of diabetes, if confirmed on a subsequent day, and precludes the need for any glucose challenge. GTT is usually unnecessary to diagnose asymptomatic diabetes mellitus; it may be useful in gestational diabetes. GTT is unreliable in the presence of severe infection, prolonged fasting, or after injection of insulin. After an overnight fast, a fasting blood glucose sample is drawn, and the patient is given a oral glucose load 75 g (100 g for gestational diabetes screening, 1.75 mg/kg ideal body weight in children up to a dose of 75 g). Plasma glucose is then drawn at 30, 60, 120, and 180 min.

Interpretation of GTT

Adult-Onset Diabetes: Any fasting blood sugar >126 or >200 mg/dL at 120 min and 1 other interval measured

Gestational Diabetes: Any degree or glucose intolerance with onset or first recognition during pregnancy. Diagnosis requires ≥2 abnormal plasma glucose values on a 3-h oral GTT (glucose 100 g). Fasting: 95 mg/dL; 1 h: 180 mg/dL; 2 h: 155 mg/dL; 3 h: 140 mg/dL.

Glycohemoglobin (GHb, Glycated Hemoglobin, Glycohemoglobin, HbA$_{1c}$, HbA$_1$ Hemoglobin A$_{1c}$, Glycosylated Hemoglobin) (Serum)

- 4.6–6.4% or new standard: nondiabetic <6%, near normal 6–7%
- Excellent glucose control <7%
- Good control 7–8%
- Fair control 8–9%
- Poor control >9%
- Collection: lavender top tube

The mean plasm glucose = (HbA1c × 35.6) − 77.3. Useful in long-term monitoring control of blood sugar in diabetics; reflects levels over preceding 3–4 months. Glycated serum protein under study may reflect serum glucose over the preceding 1–2 weeks.

Increased: Diabetes mellitus (uncontrolled), lead intoxication

Decreased: Chronic renal failure, hemolytic anemia, pregnancy, chronic blood loss

Haptoglobin (Serum)

- 40–180 mg/dL (SI 0.4–1.8 g/L)
- Collection: tiger top tube

Increased: Obstructive liver disease, any cause of increased erythrocyte sedimentation rate (ESR; inflammation, collagen-vascular diseases)

Decreased: Any type of hemolysis (transfusion reaction, etc), liver disease, anemia, oral contraceptives, children and infants

Helicobacter pylori Antibody Titers (Serum)

- Immunoglobulin (Ig) G <0.17 = negative

Most patients with gastritis and ulcer disease (gastric or duodenal) have chronic *H pylori* infection that should be controlled. Positive in 35–50% of asymptomatic patients (increases with age). Use in dyspepsia controversial. Four diagnostic methods are available to test for *H pylori,* the organism associated with gastritis and ulcers. These include noninvasive (serology and a carbon 13 breath test) and invasive (gastric mucosal biopsy and the *Campylobacter*-like organism test). The IgG subclass is found in all patient populations; occasionally only IgA antibodies can be detected. Serology most useful in newly diagnosed *H pylori* infection or monitoring response to therapy. IgG levels decrease slowly after therapy and can remain high after clearing infection.

Positive: Active or recent *H pylori* infection, some asymptomatic carriers

Hepatitis Testing (Serum)

Hepatitis tests (collection: tiger top tube; Tables II–6 and II–7)

Hepatitis A
Anti-HAV Antibody: Total antibody to hepatitis A virus; confirms previous exposure to hepatitis A virus, increased for life.

Anti-HAV IgM: IgM antibody to hepatitis A virus; indicative of recent infection with hepatitis A virus; decreases typically 1–6 months after symptoms

Hepatitis B
HBsAg: Hepatitis B surface antigen. Earliest marker of hepatitis B virus (HBV) infection. Indicates chronic or acute infection with HBV. Used by blood banks to screen donors; vaccination does not affect this test.

TABLE II–6. HEPATITIS PANEL TESTING TO GUIDE IN THE ORDERING OF HEPATITIS PROFILES FOR GIVEN CLINICAL SETTINGS

Medical Setting	Test	Purpose
Screening tests		
Pregnancy	• HBsAg	All expectant mothers should be screened during 3rd trimester.
High risk patients on admission (homosexuals, dialysis patients)	• HBsAg	To screen for chronic or active infection
Percutaneous inoculation (donor)	• HBsAg • Anti-HBc IgM • Anti-hepatitis C	To test patient's blood (especially dialysis patients and HIV-infected individuals) for infectivity with HBV and HCV if health care worker exposed.
Percutaneous inoculation (victim)	• HBsAg • Anti-HBc • Anti-hepatitis C	To test exposed health care worker for immunity or chronic infection.
Pre-HBV Vaccine	• Anti-HBc • Anti-HBs	To determine if an individual is infected or has antibodies to HBV.
Screening blood donors	• HBsAg • Anti-HBc • Anti-hepatitis C	Used by blood banks to screen donors for hepatitis B and C.
Diagnostic tests		
Differential diagnosis of acute jaundice, hepatitis, or fulminant liver failure	• HBsAg • Anti-HBc IgM • Anti-HAV IgM • Anti-hepatitis C	To differentiate between HBV, HAV, and HCV in acutely jaundiced patient with hepatitis or fulminant liver failure.
Chronic hepatitis	• HBsAg + HBeAg +Anti-HBe +Anti hepatitis D (total + Ig)	To diagnose HBV infection + If positive for HBsAg to determine infectivity. + If HBsAg patient worsens or is very ill, to diagnose concomitant infection with hepatitis delta virus.
Monitor		
Infant follow-up	• HBsAg • Anti-HBc • Anti-HBs	To monitor the success of vaccination and passive immunization for perinatal transmission of HBV 12–15 months after birth.
Postvaccination screening	• Anti-HBs	To ensure immunity has been achieved after vaccination (CDC mends titer determination, but usually qualitiative assay adequate).
Sexual contact	• HBsAg • Anti-HBc • Anti-hepatitis C	To monitor sexual partners of patient with chronic HBV or HCV.

Source: (Reproduced, with permission, from Gomella LG, (ed.): Diagnosis: Chemistry, Immunology, and Serology. In: Clinician's Pocket Reference, 10/e. McGraw-Hill, 2004).

TABLE II–7. INTERPRETATION OF VIRAL HEPATITIS SEROLOGIC TESTING PATTERNS

Anti-HAV (IgM)	HBsAg	Anti-HBc (IgM)	Anti-HBc (Total)	Anti-HCV (ELISA)	Interpretation
+	—	—	—	—	Acute hepatitis A
+	+	—	+	—	Acute hepatitis A in hepatitis B carrier
—	+	—	+	—	Chronic hepatitis B[a]
—	—	+	+	—	Acute hepatitis B
—	+	+	+	—	Acute hepatitis B
—	—	—	+	—	Past hepatitis B infection
—	—	—	—	+	Hepatitis C[b]
—	—	—	—	—	Early hepatitsis C or other cause (other virus, toxic, etc.)

[a]Patients with chronic hepatitis B (active hepatitis or carrier state) should have HBeAg and Anti-HBe checked to determine activity of infection and relative infectivity. Anti-HBs is used to determine response to hepatitis B vaccination.

[b]Anti-HCV often takes 3–6 months before being positive. Replaced by more sensitive tests, eg, HCV-RNA PCR.

ELISA = enzyme-linked immunosorbent assay.

Source: (Reproduced, with permission, from Gomella LG, ed. Diagnosis: Chemistry, Immunology, and Serology. In: Clinician's Pocket Reference, 10/e. McGraw-Hill, 2004.)

Anti-HBc-Total: IgG and IgM antibody to hepatitis B core antigen; confirms previous exposure to HBV or ongoing infection. Used by blood banks to screen donors.

Anti-HBc IgM: IgM antibody to hepatitis B core antigen. Early and best indicator of acute infection with hepatitis B.

HBeAg: Hepatitis Be antigen; when present, indicates high degree of infectivity. Order only when evaluating for chronic HBV infection.

HBV-DNA: Most sensitive and specific for early evaluation of hepatitis B and may be detected when all other markers are negative.

Anti-HBe: Antibody to hepatitis Be antigen; associated with resolution of active inflammation.

Anti-HBs: Antibody to hepatitis B surface antigen; when present, typically indicates immunity associated with clinical recovery from HBV infection or previous immunization with hepatitis B vaccine. Order only to assess effectiveness of vaccine and request titer levels.

Anti-HDV: Total antibody to delta hepatitis; confirms previous exposure. Order only in patients with known acute or chronic HBV infection.

Anti-HDV IgM: IgM antibody to delta hepatitis; indicates recent infection. Order only in cases of known acute or chronic HBV infection.

Hepatitis C
Anti-HCV: Antibody against hepatitis C virus (HCV). Indicative of active viral replication and infectivity. Used by blood banks to screen donors. Many false-positive results.

HCV-RNA: Nucleic acid probe detection of current HCV infection.

5-HIAA (5-Hydroxyindoleacetic Acid) (Urine)

5–HIAA is a serotonin metabolite useful in diagnosing carcinoid syndrome.

Normal: 2–8 mg (SI 10.4–41.6 mmol) per 24–h urine collection

Increased: Carcinoid tumors (except rectal), certain foods (banana, pineapple, tomato, walnuts, avocado), phenothiazine derivatives

High-Density Lipoprotein Cholesterol (Serum)

• See Cholesterol, page 281.

HLA (Human Leukocyte Antigens; HLA Typing) (Serum)

• Collection: green top tube

This test identifies antigens on the cell surface that comprise the primary determinants of histocompatibility and are useful in assessing transplantation compatibility. Some are associated with specific diseases but are not diagnostic of these diseases.

HLA-B27: Ankylosing spondylitis, psoriatic arthritis, Reiter's syndrome, juvenile RA

HLA-DR4/HLA DR2: Chronic Lyme disease arthritis

HLA-DRw2: Multiple sclerosis

HLA-B8: Addison's disease, juvenile-onset diabetes, Graves' disease, gluten-sensitive enteropathy

Human Chorionic Gonadotropin, Serum (hCG, β-Subunit) (Serum)

- Normal <3.0 mIU/mL
- 10 days after conception, >3 mIU/mL
- 30 days 100–5000 mIU/mL
- 10 weeks 50,000–140,000 mIU/mL
- >16 weeks, 10,000–50,000 mIU/mL
- Thereafter, levels slowly decrease (SI units IU/L equivalent to mIU/mL)
- Collection: tiger top tube

Increased: Pregnancy, some testicular tumors (nonseminomatous germ cell tumors, but not seminoma), trophoblastic disease (hydatidiform mole, choriocarcinoma levels usually >100,000 mIU/mL)

Human Immunodeficiency Virus (HIV) Testing (Serum)

Any HIV-positive person >13 years of age with a CD4+ T-cell level <200/mL or an HIV-positive patient with a CDC-defined indicator conditions (eg, pulmonary candidiasis, disseminated histoplasmosis, HIV wasting, Kaposi's sarcoma, TB, various lymphomas, *P carinii* pneumonia, and others) is considered to have AIDS. (*Note:* HIV testing is regulated by law in regard to confidentiality issues. Most states require that the patients sign a release for HIV testing. Release of HIV information by phone is likewise prohibited in most states and is normally only released in writing to the ordering attending physician on a confidential basis.)

HIV Antibody

- Normal = negative
- Collection: tiger top tube

Assay kits recognize HIV-1 and HIV-2 antibodies. Used in the diagnosis of AIDS and to screen blood for use in transfusion. Antibodies appear in blood 1–4 months after infection in most cases.

HIV Antibody, Enzyme-linked Immunosorbent Assay
- Normal = negative

Initial screen to detect HIV antibody; a positive test is often repeated or confirmed by Western blot.

Positive: AIDS, asymptomatic HIV infection

False-Positive: Flu vaccine within 3 months, hemophilia, rheumatoid factor, alcoholic hepatitis, dialysis

HIV Western Blot
- Normal = negative

The technique is used as the reference procedure for confirming the presence or absence of HIV antibody, usually after a positive result.

HIV Antibody by Enzyme-linked Immunosorbent Assay Determination

Positive: AIDS, asymptomatic HIV infection (if indeterminate, repeat in 1 month or perform polymerase chain reaction [PCR] for HIV-1 DNA or RNA)

False-Positive: Autoimmune or connective tissue diseases, hyperbilirubinemia, HLA antibodies, others

HIV DNA PCR
- Normal = negative

Performed on peripheral blood mononuclear cells. Preferred test to diagnose HIV infection in children <18 months of age

HIV RNA PCR
- Normal = <400 copies/mL

Quantifies "viral load." Establishes diagnosis before antibody production or when HIV antibody is indeterminate. Obtained at baseline, it is an important parameter to initiate or modify HIV therapy (see HIV Viral Load). Not recommended for routine testing of children <18 months.

HIV Viral Load
- Normal <50 copies/mL

Best predictor of progression to AIDS and death among patients with HIV. Used as a baseline and for initiation/modification of HIV therapy, but not for diagnosis (eg, antiretroviral therapy is uniformly initiated when viral load >20,000 copies/mL RNA or reverse transcriptase PCR.)

HIV Antigen (P-24 Antigen)
- Normal = negative

Detects early HIV infection before antibody conversion, used in addition to PCR testing

Iron (Serum)

- Males 65–175 mg/dL (SI 11.64–31.33 mmol/L)
- Females 50–170 mg/dL (SI 8.95–30.43 mmol/L)
- To convert mg/dL to mmol/L, multiply by 0.1791
- Collection: tiger top tube

Increased: Hemochromatosis, hemosiderosis caused by excessive iron intake, excess destruction or decreased production of erythrocytes, liver necrosis

Decreased: Iron deficiency anemia, nephrosis (loss of iron-binding proteins), normochromic anemia of chronic diseases and infections

Iron-Binding Capacity, Total (TIBC) (Serum)

- 250–450 mg/dL (SI 44.75–80.55 mmol/L)
- Collection: tiger top tube

Normal iron/total iron-binding capacity ratio is 20–50%. Decreased ratio (<10%) is almost diagnostic of iron deficiency anemia. Increased ratio is seen with hemochromatosis.

Increased: Acute and chronic blood loss, iron deficiency anemia, hepatitis, oral contraceptives

Decreased: Anemia of chronic diseases, cirrhosis, nephrosis/uremia, hemochromatosis, iron therapy overload, hemolytic anemia, aplastic anemia, thalassemia, megaloblastic anemia

17-Ketogenic Steroids (17-KGS, Corticosteroids) (Urine)

Overall adrenal function test, largely replaced by serum or urine cortisol levels

Normal: Males 5–24 mg/24 h (17–83 mmol/24 h); females 4–15 mg/24 h (14–52 mmol/24 h)

Increased: Adrenal hyperplasia (Cushing's syndrome), adrenogenital syndrome

Decreased: Panhypopituitarism, Addison's disease, acute steroid withdrawal

17-Ketosteroids, Total (17-KS) (Urine)

Measures DHEA, androstenedione (adrenal androgens); largely replaced by assay of individual elements

Normal: Adult males 8–20 mg/24 h (28–69 mmol/L); adult female 6–15 mg/dL (21–52 mmol/L). *Note:* Low values in prepubertal children.

Increased: Adrenal cortex abnormalities (hyperplasia [Cushing's disease], adenoma, carcinoma, adrenogenital syndrome), severe stress, ACTH or pituitary tumor, testicular interstitial tumor and arrhenoblastoma (both produce testosterone)

Decreased: Panhypopituitarism, Addison's disease, castration in men

Lactate Dehydrogenase (LD, LDH) (Serum)

- Adults <230 U/L
- Higher levels in childhood
- Collection: tiger top tube; carefully avoid hemolysis because this can increase LDH levels

Increased: AMI, cardiac surgery, prosthetic valve, hepatitis, pernicious anemia, malignant tumors, pulmonary embolus, hemolysis (anemias or factitious), renal infarction, muscle injury, megaloblastic anemia, liver disease

LDH Isoenzymes (LDH1 to LDH5)

Normally, the LDH1/LDH2 ratio is <0.6–0.7. If the ratio becomes >1 (also termed "flipped"), suspect a recent MI (change in ratio can also be seen in pernicious or hemolytic anemia). With an AMI, the LDH will begin to increase at 12–48 h, peak at 3–6 days, and return to normal at 8–14 days. LDH5 is higher than LDH4 in liver diseases. (Largely replaced by troponin.)

Lactic Acid (Lactate) (Serum)

- 4.5–19.8 mg/dL (SI 0.5–2.2 mmol/L)
- Collection: gray top tube on ice

Suspect lactic acidosis with increased anion gap in the absence of other causes (renal failure, ethanol, or methanol ingestion)

Increased: Lactic acidosis due to hypoxia, hemorrhage, shock, sepsis, cirrhosis, exercise, ethanol, DKA, regional ischemia (extremity, bowel) spurious (prolonged use of a tourniquet)

Lipase (Serum)

- 0–1.5 U/mL (SI 10–150 U/L) by turbidimetric method
- Collection: tiger top tube

Increased: Acute or chronic pancreatitis, pseudo-cyst, pancreatic duct obstruction (stone, stricture, tumor, drug-induced spasm), fat embolus syndrome, renal failure, dialysis (usually normal in mumps) gastric malignancy, intestinal perforation, diabetes (usually in DKA only)

Lipid Profile/Lipoprotein Profile/Lipoprotein Analysis (Serum)

- See also Cholesterol, page 281, and Triglycerides, page 323.

Usually includes cholesterol, HDL-C, LDL-C (calculated), and triglycerides. Useful in the evaluation of CAD and allows classification of dyslipoproteinemias to direct therapy. Initial screening for cardiac risk includes total cholesterol and HDL. The main lipids in the blood are cholesterol and triglycerides. These lipids are carried by lipoproteins. Lipoproteins are further classified by density (least dense to most dense):

- **Chylomicrons** (least dense) rise to surface of unspun serum and are normally found only after a fatty meal is eaten (a "lipemic specimen" on a laboratory report usually refers to these chylomicrons).
- **VLDL** (very LDL) consists mainly of triglycerides. With triglycerides <400 mg/dL, there is 1 cholesterol for each 5 triglycerides in VLDL.
- **LDL** in the fasting state; LDL carries most of the cholesterol.
- **HDL** is the densest and consists of mostly apoproteins and cholesterol.

Low-Density Lipoprotein Cholesterol (LDL, LDL-C) (Serum)

- See Cholesterol, page 281.

Luteinizing Hormone, Serum (LH) (Serum)

- Male 7–24 IU/L
- Female 6–30 IU/L, midcycle peak increase 2- to 3-fold over baseline, postmenopausal >35 IU/L
- Collection: tiger top tube

Increased: (Hypergonadotropic >40 IU/L.) Postmenopausal, surgical or radiation castration, ovarian or testicular failure, polycystic ovaries

Decreased: (Hypogonadotropic <40 IU/L prepubertal.) Hypothalamic, and pituitary dysfunction, Kallmann's syndrome, luteinizing hormone-releasing hormone analogue therapy

Magnesium (Serum)

- 1.6–2.6 mg/dL (SI 0.80–1.20 mmol/L)
- Collection: tiger top tube

Increased: Renal failure, hypothyroidism, magnesium-containing antacids, Addison's disease, diabetic coma, severe dehydration, lithium intoxication

Decreased: Malabsorption, steatorrhea, alcoholism and cirrhosis, hyperthyroidism, aldosteronism, diuretics, acute pancreatitis, hyperparathyroidism, hyperalimentation, NG suctioning, chronic dialysis, renal tubular acidosis, drugs (cisplatin, amphotericin B, aminoglycosides), hungry bone syndrome, hypophosphatemia, intracellular shifts with respiratory or metabolic acidosis

Metanephrines (Urine)

Detects metabolic products of epinephrine and norepinephrine, a primary screening test for pheochromocytoma

Normal: <1.3 mg/24 h (7.1 mmol/L) for adults, but variable in children

Increased: Pheochromocytoma, neuroblastoma (neural crest tumors), false-positive with drugs (phenobarbital, guanethidine, hydrocortisone, monoamine oxidase inhibitors)

MHA-TP (Microhemagglutination, *Treponema pallidum*) (Serum)

- Normal <1:160
- Collection: tiger top tube

Confirmatory test for syphilis, similar to FTA-ABS. Once positive, it remains so, so it cannot be used to judge effects of therapy. False-positive results with other treponemal infections (pinta, yaws, etc), mononucleosis, and SLE.

B$_2$-Microglobulin (Serum)

- 0.1–0.26 mg/dL (SI 1–2.6 mg/L)
- Collection: tiger top tube

A portion of the MHC class I antigen. A useful marker to follow the progression of HIV infections.

Increased: HIV infection, especially during periods of exacerbation, lymphoid malignancies, renal diseases (diabetic nephropathy, pyelonephritis, acute tubular necrosis [ATN], nephrotoxicity from medications), transplant rejection, inflammatory conditions

Decreased: Treatment of HIV with AZT (zidovudine)

Myoglobin (Serum)

- 30–90 ng/ml
- Collection: tiger top tube

Increased: Skeletal muscle injury (crush, injection, surgical procedures), delirium tremens, rhabdomyolysis (burns, seizures, sepsis, hypokalemia, others)

Natriuretic Peptide, B-Type (BNP)

- Normal <100 pg/mL
- Collection: lavender top tube on ice

BNP is released by the ventricular myocardium secondary to volume and pressure overload. BNP increases sodium and water excretion (inhibits sodium reabsorption in the distal nephron). Severity of CHF correlates with level of BNP. Levels <100 pg/mL rule out CHF, levels of 100–400 pg/mL are borderline, and levels >400 pg/mL are highly suggestive of CHF. BNP is very helpful in distinguishing between CHF and other causes of dyspnea (COPD).

Increased: CHF/left ventricular dysfunction

5′-Nucleotidase (Serum)

- 2–15 U/L

Used in the workup of increased alkaline phosphatase and biliary obstruction

Increased: Obstructive or cholestatic liver disease, liver metastasis, biliary cirrhosis

Osmolality, Serum (Serum)

- 278–298 mOsm/kg (SI 278–298 mmol/kg
- Collection: tiger top tube

A rough estimation of osmolality is [2(Na) + BUN/2.8 + glucose/18]. Measured value is usually less than the calculated value. If measured value is 15 mOsm/kg less than calculated, consider methanol, ethanol, or ethylene glycol ingestion or some other unmeasured substance.

Increased: Hyperglycemia; ethanol, methanol, mannitol, or ethylene glycol ingestion; increased sodium because of water loss (diabetes, hypercalcemia, diuresis)

Decreased: Low serum sodium, diuretics, Addison's disease, SIADH (seen in bronchogenic carcinoma, hypothyroidism), iatrogenic causes (poor fluid balance)

P-24 Antigen (HIV Core Antigen) (Serum)

- Normal = negative
- Collection: tiger top tube
- See also Human Immunodeficiency Virus Testing, page 305

Used to diagnose recent acute HIV infection; becomes positive sooner than HIV antibodies. Decreases "window" period. Can be positive as soon as 2–4 weeks but becomes undetectable during antibody seroconversion (periods of latency). With progression of disease, P-24 usually becomes evident again. Used to screen blood donors.

Parathyroid Hormone (PTH) (Serum)

- Normal based on relation to serum calcium, usually provided on the laboratory report
- Also, reference values depend on the laboratory and whether the N-terminal, C-terminal or mid-molecule is measured
- PTH mid-molecule: 0.29–0.85 ng/mL (SI 29–85 pmol/L)
- With calcium: 8.4–10.2 mg/dL (SI 2.1–2.55 mmol/L)
- Collection: tiger top tube

Increased: Primary hyperparathyroidism, secondary hyper-parathyroidism (hypocalcemic states, eg, chronic renal failure, others)

Decreased: Hypercalcemia not due to hyperparathyroidism, hypoparathyroidism

Partial Thromboplastin Time (Activated Partial Thromboplastin Time, PTT, APTT) (Blood)

- 27–38 s
- Collection: blue top tube

Evaluates the intrinsic coagulation system. Most commonly used to monitor heparin therapy

Increased: Heparin and any defect in the **intrinsic coagulation system** (includes factors I, II, V, VIII, IX, X, XI, and XII), prolonged use of a tourniquet before drawing a blood sample, hemophilias A and B

Phosphorus (Serum)

- Adult 2.5–4.5 mg/dL (SI 0.81–1.45 mmol/L)
- Child 4.0–6.0 mg/dL (SI 1.29–1.95 mmol/L)
- To convert mg/dL to mmol/L, multiply by 0.3229
- Collection: tiger top tube

Increased: Hypoparathyroidism (surgical, pseudo-hypoparathyroidism), excess vitamin D, secondary hyperparathyroidism, renal failure, bone disease (healing fractures), Addison's disease, childhood, factitious increase (hemolysis of specimen)

Decreased: Hyperparathyroidism, alcoholism, diabetes, hyperalimentation, acidosis, alkalosis, gout, salicylate poisoning, IV steroid, glucose or insulin administration, hypokalemia, hypomagnesemia, diuretics, vitamin D deficiency, phosphate-binding antacids

Potassium (Serum)

- 3.5–5 mEq/L (SI 3.5–5 mmol/L)
- Collection: tiger top tube

Increased: Factitious increase (hemolysis of specimen, thrombocytosis), renal failure, Addison's disease, acidosis, spironolactone, triamterene, angiotensin-converting enzyme (ACE) inhibitors, dehydration, hemolysis, massive tissue damage, excess intake (PO or IV), potassium-containing medications, acidosis

Decreased: Diuretics, decreased intake, vomiting, nasogastric suctioning, villous adenoma, diarrhea, Zollinger–Ellison syndrome, chronic pyelonephritis, renal tubular acidosis, metabolic alkalosis (primary aldosteronism, Cushing's syndrome)

Progesterone (Serum)

- Collection: tiger top tube

Used to confirm ovulation and corpus luteum function

Sample Collection	Normal Values (female)
Follicular phase	<1 ng/mL
Luteal phase	5–20 ng/mL
Pregnancy	
1st trimester	10–30 ng/mL
2nd trimester	50–100 ng/mL
3rd trimester	100–400 ng/mL
Postmenopause	<1 ng/mL

Prolactin (Serum)

- Males 1–20 ng/mL (SI 1–20 mg/L)
- Females 1–25 ng/mL (SI 1–25 mg/L)
- Collection: tiger top tube

Used in the workup of infertility, impotence, hirsutism, amenorrhea, and pituitary neoplasm

Increased: Pregnancy, nursing after pregnancy, prolactinoma, hypothalamic tumors, sarcoidosis or granulomatous disease of the hypothalamus, hypothyroidism, renal failure, Addison's disease, phenothiazine, haloperidol

Prostate-Specific Antigen (PSA) (Serum)

- <4 ng/dL by monoclonal, eg, Hybritech assay

Most useful as a measurement of response to therapy of prostate cancer; approved for screening for prostate cancer. Although any elevation increases suspicion of prostate cancer, levels >10.0 ng/dL are frequently associated with carcinoma. Popular age-corrected levels: 40–50 years, 2.5 ng/dL; 50–60 years, 3.5 ng/dL; 60–70 years, 4.5 ng/dL; >70 years, 6.5 ng/dL.

Increased: Prostate cancer, acute prostatitis, some cases of benign prostatic hyperplasia, prostatic infarction, prostate surgery (biopsy, resection), vigorous prostatic massage (routine rectal examination does not increase levels), rarely after ejaculation

Decreased: Radical prostatectomy, response to therapy of prostatic carcinoma (radiation or hormonal therapy)

PSA Velocity
A rate of increase in PSA ≥0.75 ng/mL per year is suspicious for prostate cancer based on ≥3 separate assays 6 months apart.

PSA Free and Total
Patients with prostate cancer tend to have lower free PSA levels in proportion to total PSA. Measurement of the free/total PSA can improve the specificity of PSA in the range of total PSA from 2.0–10.0 ng/mL. Some recommend prostate biopsy only if the free PSA percentage is low. Threshold for biopsy is controversial, ranging from a ratio <15% to <25%, with a higher threshold having improved sensitivity and a lower threshold having improved specificity.

Protein (Urine)

Normal: <150 mg/24 h (<0.15 g/d)

Increased: Nephrotic syndrome usually associated with >3.5 g/1.73 m^2 per 24 h

Protein (Serum)

- 6.0–8.0 g/dL
- Collection: tiger top tube

Increased: Multiple myeloma, Waldenström's macroglobulinemia, benign monoclonal gammopathy, lymphoma, chronic inflammatory disease, sarcoidosis, viral illnesses

Decreased: Malnutrition, inflammatory bowel disease, Hodgkin's disease, leukemias, any cause of decreased albumin

Prothrombin Time (PT) (Blood)

- 11.5–13.5 s (INR, normal = 0.8–1.4)
- Collection: Blue top tube PT

Evaluates the **extrinsic coagulation system** that includes factors I, II, V, VII, and X.

The use of **international normalized ratio (INR)** instead of the patient/control ratio to guide anticoagulant (Coumadin) therapy is the current standard. **INR provides a more universal and standardized result because it measures the control against a World Health Organization standard reference reagent.** Therapeutic INR levels are 2–3 for DVT, PE, transient ischemic attacks, and atrial fibrillation. Mechanical heart valves require an INR of 2.5–3.5

Increased: Drugs (sodium warfarin [Coumadin]), vitamin K deficiency, fat malabsorption, liver disease, prolonged use of a tourniquet before drawing a blood sample, DIC

Red Blood Cell Morphology: Differential Diagnosis (Blood)

The following lists some erythrocyte abnormalities and the associated conditions. General terms include **poikilocytosis** (irregular RBC shape such as sickle or burr) and **anisocytosis** (irregular RBC size such as microcytes and macrocytes).

- *Basophilic Stippling:* Lead or heavy-metal poisoning, thalassemia, severe anemia
- *Blister Cell:* DIC, microangiopathic anemia, sickle cell, hemolysis
- *Burr Cells (Acanthocytes):* Severe liver disease; high levels of bile, fatty acids, or toxins
- *Heinz bodies:* Drug-induced hemolysis
- *Helmet Cells (Schistocytes):* Microangiopathic hemolysis, hemolytic transfusion reaction, transplant rejection, other severe anemias, TTP
- *Howell–Jolly Bodies:* After splenectomy, some severe hemolytic anemias, pernicious anemia, leukemia, thalassemia

- *Nucleated RBCs:* Severe bone marrow stress (hemorrhage, hemolysis, etc), marrow replacement by tumor, extramedullary hematopoiesis
- *Polychromasia (Basophilia):* A bluish-gray RBC on routine Wright's stain suggests reticulocytes.
- *Sickling:* Sickle cell disease and trait
- *Spherocytes:* Hereditary spherocytosis, immune or microangiopathic hemolysis, severe burns, ABO transfusion reactions
- *Target Cells (Leptocytes):* Thalassemia, hemoglobinopathies, obstructive jaundice, any hypochromic anemia, after splenectomy

Renin (Serum)

Plasma (Plasma Renin Activity [PRA])

- Adults, normal sodium diet, upright 1–6 ng/mL per hour (SI 0.77–4.6 nmol/L per hour)
- Renal vein renin (left and right should be equal)

Useful in the diagnosis of hypertension associated with hypokalemia. Values highly dependent on salt intake and position. Stop diuretics, estrogens for 2–4 weeks before testing.

Increased: Medications (ACE inhibitors, diuretics, oral contraceptives, estrogens), pregnancy, dehydration, renal artery stenosis, adrenal insufficiency, chronic hypokalemia, upright posture, salt-restricted diet, edematous conditions (CHF, nephrotic syndrome), secondary hyperaldosteronism

Decreased: Primary aldosteronism (renin will not increase with relative volume depletion, upright posture)

Renal Vein Renins
- Normal (left and right should be equal)

A ratio >1.5 (affected/unaffected) suggests renovascular hypertension

Reticulocyte Count (Blood)

- Collection: lavender top tube

The reticulocyte count is not a part of the routine CBC count. The count is used in the initial workup of anemia (especially unexplained) and in monitoring the effect of hematinic or erythropoietin therapy, monitoring recovery from myelosuppression or engraftment after bone marrow transplant. Reticulocytes are juvenile RBCs with remnants of cytoplasmic basophilic RNA. These are suggested by **basophilia** of the RBC cytoplasm on Wright's stain;

however, confirmation requires a special reticulocyte stain. The result is reported as a percentage, and one should calculate the **corrected reticulocyte count** for interpretation of the results: corrected reticulocyte count = reported count × patient's hematocrit ÷ normal hematocrit.

This corrected count is an excellent indicator of erythropoietic activity. The **normal corrected reticulocyte count is <1.5.**

Normal bone marrow responds to a decrease in erythrocytes (shown by decreased hematocrit) with an increase in the production of reticulocytes. Lack of increase in a reticulocyte count with anemia suggests a chronic disease, a deficiency disease, marrow replacement, or marrow failure.

Rheumatoid Factor (RA Latex Test) (Serum)

- <15 IU by Microscan kit or >1:40
- Collection: tiger top tube

Increased: Collagen-vascular diseases (RA, SLE, scleroderma, polyarteritis nodosa, others), infections (TB, syphilis, viral hepatitis), chronic inflammation, SBE, some lung diseases, MI (*note:* 15% of patients with RA are negative for rheumatoid factor)

Sedimentation Rate (Erythrocyte Sedimentation Rate, ESR) (Blood)

- Collection: lavender top tube

A nonspecific test with a high sensitivity and a low specificity. Most useful in serial measurements to follow the course of disease (eg, polymyalgia rheumatica or temporal arteritis). ZETA rate is not affected by anemia. ESR correlates well with C-reactive protein levels.

Wintrobe Scale: Males 0–9 mm/h, females 0–20 mm/h

ZETA Scale: 40–54% normal, 55–59% mildly increased, 60–64% moderately increase, >65% markedly increased

Westergren Scale: Males <50 years, 15 mm/h; males >50 years, 20 mm/h; females <50 years, 20 mm/h; females >50 years, 30 mm/h

Increased: Any type of infection, inflammation, rheumatic fever, endocarditis, neoplasm, AMI

SGGT (Serum γ-Glutamyl Transpeptidase) (Serum)

- See GGT, page 299.

SGOT (Serum Glutamic-Oxaloacetic Transaminase) (Serum)

- See AST, page 272.

SGPT Serum (Glutamic-Pyruvic Transaminase) (Serum)

- See ALT, page 271.

Sodium, Serum (Serum)

- 136–145 mmol/L
- Collection: tiger top tube

In factitious hyponatremia due to hyperglycemia, for every 100 mmol/L blood glucose above normal, serum sodium decreases 2.4 mmol/L. For example, a blood glucose level of 800 mmol/L and a sodium level of 125 mmol/L would factitiously lower the sodium value: $(800 - 100) \div 100 = 7 \times 2.4$, or 16.8. Corrected serum sodium would therefore be 125 + 17 = 142.

Increased: Associated with low total body sodium (glycosuria, mannitol, or lactulose use, urea, excess sweating), normal total body sodium (diabetes insipidus [central and nephrogenic], respiratory losses, and sweating), and increased total body sodium (administration of hypertonic sodium bicarbonate, Cushing's syndrome, hyperaldosteronism)

Decreased: Associated with excess total body sodium and water (nephrotic syndrome, CHF, cirrhosis, renal failure), excess body water (SIADH [small cell lung cancer, pulmonary disease including TB, lung cancer, pneumonia, CNS disease including trauma, tumors, and infections, perioperative stress, drugs including selective serotonin reuptake inhibitors and ACE inhibitors and after colonoscopy], hypothyroidism, adrenal insufficiency, psychogenic polydipsia, beer potomania), decreased total body water and sodium (diuretic use, renal tubular acidosis, use of mannitol or urea, mineralocorticoid deficiency, cerebral salt wasting, vomiting, diarrhea, pancreatitis), and pseudo-hyponatremia (hyperlipidemia, hyperglycemia, and multiple myeloma)

Spot Urine Studies

The so-called spot urine, which is often ordered to aid in diagnosing various conditions, relies on only a small sample (10–20 mL) of urine.

Spot Urine for β_2-Microglobulin

- <0.3 mg/L is a marker for renal tubular injury

Increased: Diseases of the proximal tubule (ATN, interstitial nephritis, pyelonephritis), drug-induced nephropathy (aminoglycosides), diabetes, trauma, sepsis, HIV, lymphoproliferative and lymphodestructive diseases

Spot Urine for Electrolytes

The usefulness of this assay is limited because of large variations in daily fluid and salt intake, and the results are usually indeterminate if a diuretic has been given.

1. **Sodium <10 mEq/L (mmol/L):** Volume depletion, hyponatremic states, prerenal azotemia (CHF, shock, etc), hepatorenal syndrome, glucocorticoid excess
2. **Sodium >20 mEq/L (mmol/L):** SIADH, ATN (usually >40 mEq/L), postobstructive diuresis, high salt intake, Addison's disease, hypothyroidism, interstitial nephritis
3. **Chloride <10 mEq/L (mmol/L):** Chloride-sensitive metabolic alkalosis (vomiting, excessive diuretic use), volume depletion
4. **Potassium <10 mEq/L (mmol/L):** Hypokalemia, potassium depletion, extrarenal loss

Spot Urine for Microalbumin
- Normal <30 µg albumin/mg creatinine (timed collection <20 µg/min)

To determine which patients with diabetes are at risk for nephropathy. Clinical albuminuria occurs at >300 µg albumin/mg creatinine. Repeat 2–3 separate determinations over 6 months. Diabetics with levels of 30–300 µg have microalbuminuria and are usually initiated on ACE inhibitor or angiotensin receptor blocker.

Spot Urine for Myoglobin
- Qualitatively negative

Positive: Skeletal muscle conditions (crush injury, electrical burns, carbon monoxide poisoning, delirium tremens, surgical procedures, malignant hyperthermia), polymyositis

Spot Urine for Osmolality
- 75–300 mOsm/kg (mmol/kg), varies with water intake. Patients with normal renal function should concentrate >800 mOsm/kg (mmol/kg) after a 14-h fluid restriction; <400 mOsm/kg (mmol/kg) is a sign of renal impairment.

Increased: Dehydration, SIADH, adrenal insufficiency, glycosuria, high-protein diet

Decreased: Excessive fluid intake, diabetes insipidus, acute renal failure, medications (acetohexamide, glyburide, lithium)

Spot Urine for Protein
- Normal <10 mg/dL (0.1 g/L) or <20 mg/dL (0.2 g/L) for a sample taken in the early AM

Stool for Occult Blood (Fecal Occult Blood Testing, Hemoccult Test) (Stool)

Normal-Negative: Apply small amount of stool on Hemoccult card and close and then send to test site. Open test panel on other side of card and apply 2–3 drops of developer to the test and the positive control panels; read in 30 s. Blue color is positive. Detects >5 mg hemoglobin per gram of feces. Repeat 3 times for maximum yield. (A positive test more informative than a negative test.)

Positive: Any GI tract ulcerated lesion (ulcer, carcinoma, polyp, diverticulosis, inflammatory bowel disease), hemorrhoids, telangiectasias, drugs that cause GI irritation (eg, NSAIDs) swallowed blood, ingestion of rare red meat, certain foods (horseradish, turnips, vitamin C [>500 mg/d], antacids may result in false-negative test)

T_3 RU (Resin Uptake; Thyroxine-Binding Globulin Ratio) (Serum)
- 30–40%

Used in conjunction with a T_4 to yield the Free T_4 Index [FTI], an estimate of the free T_4.

Increased: Hyperthyroidism, medications (phenytoin, steroids, heparin, aspirin, others), nephrotic syndrome

Decreased: Hypothyroidism, medications (iodine, propylthiouracil, others), any cause of increased thyroxine binding globulin (TBG), such as oral estrogen or pregnancy

Testosterone (Serum)
- Male free: 9–30 ng/dL, total 300–1200 ng/dL
- Female, see following data:

Sample Collection	Normal Values (female)
Follicular phase	20–80 ng/dL
Midcycle peak	20–80 ng/dL
Luteal phase	20–80 ng/dL
Postmenopause	10–40 ng/dL

Increased: Adrenogenital syndrome, ovarian stromal hypertheco-sis, polycystic ovaries, menopause, ovarian tumors

Decreased: Hypogonadism, hypopituitarism, Klinefelter's syn-drome, male andropause

Thrombin Time (Blood)

- 10–14 s
- Collection: blue top tube

Measures conversion of fibrinogen to fibrin and fibrin polymeriza-tion. Detects the presence of heparin and hypofibrinogenemia; an aid in the evaluation of prolonged PTT.

Increased: Systemic heparin, DIC, fibrinogen deficiency, congeni-tally abnormal fibrinogen molecules

Thyroglobulin (Serum)

- 1–20 ng/mL (mg/L)
- Collection: tiger top tube

Useful for following patients with non-medullary thyroid carcino-mas

Increased: Differentiated thyroid carcinomas (papillary, follicular), Graves' disease, nontoxic goiter

Decreased: Hypothyroidism, testosterone, steroids, phenytoin

Thyroid-Stimulating Hormone (TSH) (Serum)

- 0.7–5.3 mU/mL
- Collection: tiger top tube

Excellent screening test for hyperthyroidism and hypothyroidism. Differentiates between a low normal and a decreased TSH.

Increased: Hypothyroidism

Decreased: Hyperthyroidism. Less than 1% of hypothyroidism is from pituitary or hypothalamic disease resulting in a decreased TSH.

Thyroxine (T₄ Total) (Serum)

- 5–12 mg/dL (SI 65–155 nmol/L)
- Males >60 years, 5–10 mg/dL (SI: 65–129 nmol)
- Females: 5.5–10.5 µg/dL (SI 71–135 nmol/L)
- Collection: tiger top tube

Good screening test for hyperthyroidism. Measures bound and free T_4 and, hence, can be affected by TBG levels.

Increased: Hyperthyroidism, exogenous thyroid hormone, estrogens, pregnancy, severe illness, euthyroid sick syndrome

Decreased: Hypothyroidism, euthyroid sick syndrome, any cause of decreased TBG

Thyroxine-Binding Globulin (TBG) (Serum)

- 21–52 mg/dL (270–669 nmol/L)
- Collection: tiger top tube

Increased: Hypothyroidism, pregnancy, oral contraceptives, estrogens, hepatic disease, acute porphyria

Decreased: Hyperthyroidism, androgens, anabolic steroids, prednisone, nephrotic syndrome, severe illness, surgical stress, phenytoin, hepatic disease

Thyroxine Index, Free (FTI) (Serum)

- 6.5–1.25

Practically speaking, the FTI is equivalent to the free thyroxine. Useful in patients with clinically suspected hyper- or hypothyroidism. Determined as follows:

Thyroxine (total T_4) × T_3 resin uptake

Increased: Hyperthyroidism, large-dose β blockers, psychiatric illnesses

Decreased: Hypothyroidism, phenytoin (Dilantin)

Toxin Screen (Urine)

- Normal = negative

Tests for common drugs of abuse, often used for employment screening for critical jobs. Assay will vary by facility and may include tests for amphetamines, barbiturates, benzodiazepines, marijuana (cannabinoid metabolites), cocaine metabolites, opiates, and phencyclidine.

Transferrin (Serum)

- 220–400 mg/dL (SI 2.20–4.0 g/L)
- Collection: tiger top tube, avoid hemolysis

Used in the workup of anemias; transferrin levels can also be assessed by TIBC.

Increased: Acute and chronic blood loss, iron deficiency, hemolysis, oral contraceptives, pregnancy, viral hepatitis

Decreased: Anemia of chronic disease, cirrhosis, nephrosis, hemochromatosis, malignancy

Triglycerides (Serum)

- Males: recommended 40–160 mg/dL (SI 0.45–1.81 mmol/L)
- Females: recommended 35–135 mg/dL (SI 0.40–1.53 mmol/L)
- Can change with age
- Collection: tiger top tube
- Fasting preferred

Increased: Nonfasting specimen, hyperlipoproteinemias (types I, IIb, III, IV, and V), hypothyroidism, liver diseases, poorly controlled diabetes mellitus, alcoholism, pancreatitis, AMI, nephrotic syndrome, familial, medications (oral contraceptives, estrogens, betablockers, cholestyramine)

Decreased: Malnutrition, malabsorption, hyperthyroidism, Tangier disease, medications (nicotinic acid, clofibrate, gemfibrozil) congenital abetalipoproteinemia

Triiodothyronine (T$_3$ Radioimmunoassay) (Serum)

- 120–195 ng/dL (SI 1.85–3.00 nmol/L)
- Collection: tiger top tube

Useful when hyperthyroidism is suspected, but T$_4$ is normal (T3 thyrotoxicosis); not useful in the diagnosis of hypothyroidism

Increased: Hyperthyroidism, T$_3$ thyrotoxicosis, pregnancy, exogenous T$_4$, any cause of increased TBG, such as oral estrogen or pregnancy

Decreased: Hypothyroidism and euthyroid sick state, any cause of decreased TBG

Troponin, Cardiac-Specific (Serum)

- Troponin I <0.35 ng/mL
- Troponin T (TT) <0.2 µg/L

Used to diagnose AMI; increases rapidly at 3–12 h, peaks at 24 h, and may stay high for several days (troponin I 5–7 days, troponin T up to 14 days). More cardiac specific than creatine kinase-MB

Positive: Myocardial damage, including MI, myocarditis (false-positive result: renal failure)

24-h Urine Studies

A wide variety of diseases, most of them endocrine, can be diagnosed by assays of 24-h urine samples.

Calcium, Urine

Normal: On a calcium-free diet <150 mg/24 h (3.7 mmol/d), average calcium diet (600–800 mg/24 h) 100–250 mg/24 h (2.5–6.2 mmol/d)

Increased: Hyperparathyroidism, hyperthyroidism, hypervitaminosis D, distal renal tubular acidosis (type I), sarcoidosis, immobilization, osteolytic lesions (bony metastasis, multiple myeloma), Paget's disease, glucocorticoid excess, immobilization, furosemide

Decreased: Medications (thiazide diuretics, estrogens, oral contraceptives), hypothyroidism, renal failure, steatorrhea, rickets, osteomalacia

Catecholamines, Fractionated
Used to evaluate neuroendocrine tumors, including pheochromocytoma and neuroblastoma.
   Avoid caffeine and methyldopa (Aldomet) before test

Normal: Values are variable and depend on the assay method used. Norepinephrine 15–80 mg/24 h (SI 89–473 nmol/24 h), epinephrine 0–20 mg/24 h (SI 0–118 nmol/24 h), dopamine 65–400 mg/24 h (SI 384–2364 nmol/24 h).

Increased: Pheochromocytoma, neuroblastoma, epinephrine administration, presence of drugs (methyldopa, tetracyclines cause false increases)

Cortisol, Free
Used to evaluate adrenal cortical hyperfunction, screening test of choice for Cushing's syndrome

Normal: 10–110 mg/24 h (SI 30–300 nmol)

Increased: Cushing's syndrome (adrenal hyperfunction), stress during collection, oral contraceptives, pregnancy

Creatinine
- See page 292

Uric Acid (Urate) (Serum)

- Males 3.4–7 mg/dL (SI 202–416 mmol/L)
- Females 2.4–6 mg/dL (SI 143–357 mmol/L)
- To convert mg/dL to mmol/L, multiply by 59.48
- Collection: tiger top tube

Increased uric acid is associated with increased catabolism, nucleoprotein synthesis, or decreased renal clearing of uric acid (ie, thiazide diuretics or renal failure).

Increased: Gout, renal failure, destruction of massive amounts of nucleoproteins (leukemia, anemia, chemotherapy, toxemia of pregnancy), drugs (especially diuretics), lactic acidosis, hypothyroidism, PCKD, parathyroid diseases

Decreased: Uricosuric drugs (salicylates, probenecid, allopurinol), Wilson's disease, Fanconi's syndrome

Urinalysis, Normal Values

1. **Appearance:** "Yellow, clear," or "straw-colored, clear"
2. **Specific gravity**
   a. Neonate: 1.012
   b. Infant: 1.002–1.006
   c. Child and adult: 1.001–1.035 (typical with normal fluid intake 1.016–1.022)
3. **pH**
   a. Newborn/neonate: 5–7
   b. Child and adult: 4.6–8.0
4. **Negative for:** bilirubin, blood, acetone, glucose, protein, nitrite, leukocyte esterase, decreasing substances
5. **Trace:** Urobilinogen
6. **RBC count:** Male 0–3/HPF, female 0–5/HPF
7. **WBC count:** 0–4/HPF
8. **Epithelial cells:** Occasional
9. **Hyaline casts:** Occasional
10. **Bacteria:** None
11. **Crystals:** Some limited crystals based on urine pH (see below)

Differential Diagnosis for Routine Urinalysis

Appearance

Colorless: Diabetes insipidus, diuretics, excess fluid intake

Dark: Acute intermittent porphyria, advanced malignant melanoma

Cloudy: Urinary tract infection (UTI; pyuria), amorphous phosphate salts (normal in alkaline urine), blood, mucus, bilirubin

Pink/Red:
Heme(+): Blood, hemoglobin, sepsis, dialysis, myoglobin
Heme(–): Food coloring, beets, sulfa drugs, nitrofurantoin, salicylates

Orange/Yellow: Dehydration, phenazopyridine (Pyridium), rifampin, bile pigments

Brown/Black: Myoglobin, bile pigments, melanin, cascara, iron, nitrofurantoin, alkaptonuria

Green/Blue: Urinary bile pigments, indigo carmine, methylene blue

Foamy: Proteinuria, bile salts

pH
Acidic: High-protein (meat) diet, ammonium chloride, mandelic acid and other medications, acidosis, (due to ketoacidosis [starvation, diabetic], COPD)

Basic: UTI, renal tubular acidosis, diet (high in vegetables, milk, immediately after meals), sodium bicarbonate therapy, vomiting, metabolic alkalosis

Specific Gravity
Usually corresponds with osmolarity except with osmotic diuresis. Value >1.023 indicates normal renal concentrating ability. Random value 1.003–1.030.

Increased: Volume depletion; CHF; adrenal insufficiency; diabetes mellitus; SIADH; increased proteins (nephrosis); if markedly increased (1.040–1.050), suspect artifact or excretion of radiographic contrast medium

Decreased: Diabetes insipidus, pyelonephritis, glomerulonephritis, water load with normal renal function

Bilirubin
Positive: Obstructive jaundice (intrahepatic and extrahepatic), hepatitis. (*Note:* False-positive results occur with stool contamination.)

Blood
Note: If the dipstick is positive for blood, but no RBCs are seen, free hemoglobin may be present; a transfusion reaction may have occurred from lysis of RBCs (RBCs will lyse if the pH is <5 or >8);

or myoglobin may be present because of a crush injury, burn, or tissue ischemia.

Positive: Stones, trauma, tumors (benign and malignant, anywhere in the urinary tract), urethral strictures, coagulopathy, infection, menses (contamination), polycystic kidneys, interstitial nephritis, hemolytic anemia, transfusion reaction, instrumentation (Foley catheter, etc)

Glucose
Positive: Diabetes mellitus, pancreatitis, pancreatic carcinoma, pheochromocytoma, Cushing's disease, shock, burns, pain, steroids, hyperthyroidism, renal tubular disease, iatrogenic causes. (*Note:* Glucose oxidase technique in many kits is specific for glucose and will not react with lactose, fructose, or galactose.)

Ketones
Detects primarily acetone and acetoacetic acid and not β-hydroxybutyric acid.

Positive: Starvation, high-fat diet, DKA, vomiting, diarrhea, hyperthyroidism, pregnancy, febrile states (especially in children)

Nitrite
Many bacteria will convert nitrates to nitrite. (See also section on leukocyte esterase, below.)

Positive: Infection (negative test does not rule out infection because some organisms, such as *Streptococcus faecalis* and other gram-positive cocci, do not produce nitrite, and the urine must also be retained in the bladder for several hours to allow the nitrite reaction to take place)

Protein
Indication by dipstick of persistent proteinuria should be quantified by 24-h urine studies.

Positive: Pyelonephritis, glomerulonephritis, glomerular sclerosis (diabetes), nephrotic syndrome, myeloma, postural causes, preeclampsia, inflammation and malignancies of the lower tract, functional causes (fever, stress, heavy exercise), malignant hypertension, CHF

Leukocyte Esterase
Test detects 5 WBCs/HPF or lysed WBCs. When combined with the nitrite test, it has a positive predictive value of 74% for UTI if both tests are positive and a negative predictive value >97% if both tests are negative.

Positive: UTI (false-positive result: vaginal/fecal contamination)

Reducing Substances
Positive: Glucose, fructose, galactose, false-positives (vitamin C, salicylates, antibiotics, etc)

Urobilinogen
Positive: Cirrhosis, CHF with hepatic congestion, hepatitis, hyperthyroidism, suppression of gut flora with antibiotics

Urinary Indices in Renal Failure (Urine)

Use Table II–8 to help differentiate the causes (renal or prerenal) of oliguria. (See also Oliguria and Anuria, page 205.)

Urine Sediment

Many laboratories no longer do microscopic examinations unless specifically requested or if evidence exists for an abnormal finding on dipstick test (such as positive leukocyte esterase).

Red Blood Cells (RBCs): Trauma, pyelonephritis, genitourinary TB, cystitis, prostatitis, stones, tumors (malignant and benign), coagulopathy, and any cause of blood on dipstick test. (See previous section on blood pH, page 274.)

White Blood Cells (WBCs): Infection anywhere in the urinary tract, TB, renal tumors, acute glomerulonephritis, radiation, interstitial nephritis (analgesic abuse)

TABLE II–8. URINARY INDICES

Index	Prerenal	Renal (ATN)[a]
Urine osmolality (mOsm/kg)	> 500	< 350
Urinary sodium (mEq/L)	< 20	> 40
Urine/serum creatinine	> 40	> 20
Urine/serum osmolarity	> 1.2	< 1.2
Fractional excreted sodium (%)[b]	< 1	< 1.2
Renal failure index (RFI)(%)[c]	> 1	> 1

[a]Acute tubular necrosis (intrinsic renal failure)
[b]Fractional excreted sodium (%)

$$= \frac{Urine\ Sodium\ /\ Serum\ Sodium}{Urine\ Creatinine\ /\ Serum\ Creatinine} \times 100$$

[c] Renal Failure Index (%)

$$= \frac{Urine\ Sodium}{Urine\ Creatinine\ /\ Serum\ Creatinine} \times 100$$

Epithelial Cells: ATN, necrotizing papillitis. (Most epithelial cells are from an otherwise unremarkable urethra.)

Parasites: Trichomonas vaginalis, *Schistosoma haematobium* infection

Yeast: *Candida albicans* infection (especially in diabetics, immunosuppressed patients, or if a vaginal yeast infection is present)

Spermatozoa: Normal in males immediately after intercourse or nocturnal emission

Crystals
Abnormal. Cystine, sulfonamide, leucine, tyrosine, cholesterol
Normal. Acid urine: Oxalate (small square crystals with a central cross), uric acid. *Alkaline urine:* Calcium carbonate, triple phosphate (resemble coffin lids)

Contaminants: Cotton threads, hair, wood fibers, amorphous substances (all usually unimportant)

Mucus: Large amounts suggest urethral disease (normal from ileal conduit or other forms of urinary diversion)

Glitter Cells: WBCs lysed in hypotonic solution

Casts: Localizes some or all of the disease process to the kidney itself.

Hyaline Casts: (Acceptable unless they are "numerous"), benign hypertension, nephrotic syndrome, after exercise

RBC Casts: Acute glomerulonephritis, lupus nephritis, SBE, Goodpasture's disease, after a streptococcal infection (post–streptococcal glomerulonephritis), vasculitis, malignant hypertension

WBC Casts: Pyelonephritis, acute interstitial nephritis, glomerulonephritis

Epithelial (Tubular) Casts: Tubular damage, nephrotoxin, virus

Granular Casts: Breakdown of cellular casts, leads to waxy casts; "dirty brown granular casts" typical for ATN

Waxy Casts: (End stage of granular cast.) Severe chronic renal disease, amyloidosis.

Fatty Casts: Nephrotic syndrome, diabetes mellitus, damaged renal tubular epithelial cells

Broad Casts: Chronic renal disease

Vanillylmandelic Acid (VMA) (Urine)

VMA is the urinary product of epinephrine and norepinephrine; good screening test for pheochromocytoma, also used to diagnose and follow up neuroblastoma and ganglioneuroma

Normal: <7–9 mg/24 h (35–45 mmol/L)

Increased: Pheochromocytoma, other neural crest tumors (ganglioneuroma, neuroblastoma), factitious (chocolate, coffee, tea, methyldopa)

VDRL Test (Venereal Disease Research Laboratory) or Rapid Plasma Reagin (RPR) (Serum)

- Normal = nonreactive
- Collection: tiger top tube

Good screening for syphilis. Almost always positive in secondary syphilis, but frequently becomes negative in late syphilis. Also, in some patients with HIV infection, the VDRL can be negative in primary and secondary syphilis.

Positive (Reactive): Syphilis, SLE, pregnancy and drug addiction. If reactive, confirm with FTA-ABS (false-positive results with bacterial or viral illnesses).

Vitamin B$_{12}$ (Extrinsic Factor, Cyanocobalamin) (Serum)

- >100–700 pg/mL (SI 74–516 pmol/L)
- Collection: tiger top tube

Increased: Excessive intake, myeloproliferative disorders

Decreased: Inadequate intake (especially strict vegetarians), malabsorption, hyperthyroidism, pregnancy

WBC Morphology: Differential Diagnosis (Blood)

The following gives conditions associated with certain changes in the normal morphology of WBCs.

- *Auer Rods:* AML

- **Döhle's Inclusion Bodies:** Severe infection, burns, malignancy, pregnancy
- **Toxic Granulation:** Severe illness (sepsis, burn, high temperature)
- **Hypersegmentation:** Megaloblastic anemias

Xylose Tolerance Test (D-Xylose Absorption Test) (Urine)

- Xylose 5 g in 5-h urine specimen after PO dose of xylose 25 g or 1.2 g after 5-g oral dose
- Collection: Patient is NPO after midnight except for water
- After 8 AM void, 25 g of D-xylose (or 5 g if GI irritation is a concern) is dissolved in water 250 mL
- Additional water 750 mL is drunk and the urine collected for the next 5 h.

Used to assess proximal bowel function; differentiates between malabsorption due to pancreatic insufficiency or intestinal problems.

Decreased: Celiac disease (nontropical sprue, gluten-sensitive enteropathy), false decrease with renal disease

Zinc (Serum)

- 60–130 mg/dL (SI 9–20 mmol/L)
- Collection: check with laboratory; special collection to limit contamination

Increased: Atherosclerosis, CAD

Decreased: Inadequate dietary intake (parenteral nutrition, alcoholism); malabsorption; increased needs, such as pregnancy or wound healing; acrodermatitis enteropathica; dwarfism

III. Bedside Procedures

Procedure Basics

Universal Precautions Universal precautions should be used whenever an invasive procedure exposes the operator to potentially infectious body fluids. Not all patients infected with transmissible pathogens can be reliably identified. Because pathogens transmitted by bloody and body fluids pose a hazard to personnel caring for such patients, particularly during invasive procedures, certain precautions are now *required* for *routine* care of **all** patients whether or not they have been placed on isolation precautions of any type. The Centers for Disease Control and Prevention calls these *universal precautions*.

1. Wash hands before and after **all** patient contact.
2. Wash hands before and after **all** invasive procedures.
3. Wear gloves in **every** instance in which contact with blood or body fluid is certain or likely. For example, wear gloves for all venipunctures, for all intravenous (IV) starts, for IV manipulation, and for wound care.
4. Wear gloves in **every** instance in which contact with any body fluid is likely, including urine, feces, wound secretions, respiratory tract secretions, thoracentesis fluid, paracentesis fluid, etc.

5. Wear gloves once and discard. Do not wear the same pair to perform tasks on 2 different patients or 2 different tasks at different sites on the same patient.
6. Use barrier precautions, including a gown, mask, and protective eyewear for invasive procedures whenever significant splatter or aerosol generation is likely. Always wear a mask when eye protection is worn and vice versa.

Accidental Needle Sticks The US Food and Drug Administration has recommended the use of safer needle devices and has specifically recommended that a device provide a barrier between the hands and the needle after use. Needlestick injury is a cause of occupational injury among health care workers in the United States. The Occupational Safety and Health Administration has estimated that 600,000 to 800,000 needle stick injuries occur on the job each year. Health care workers are at risk of transmission of >20 different bloodborne pathogens (eg, human immunodeficiency virus, hepatitis B and C viruses). Although it is not possible to completely eliminate the risk of needlestick injury, research estimates that 62–88% of sharp injuries could be decreased through the use of devices and procedures designed to protect health care workers from exposed needles. Different self-shielding needle devices are now on the market (see section on IV techniques for examples).

Informed Consent Patients should be counseled before any procedure concerning the reasons for the procedure, possible alternatives, and the potential risks and benefits. Explaining the various steps will make the patient more cooperative and the procedure easier on both parties. In general, procedures such as bladder catheterization, nasogastric (NG) intubation, or venipuncture do not require a written informed consent beyond normal hospital sign-in protocols. More invasive procedures, such as thoracentesis or lumbar puncture, require written consent and must be obtained by a licensed physician. Check with your hospital for specific informed consent guidelines.

Latex Allergy Individuals with certain medical conditions or occupations that are heavily exposed to products containing natural rubber latex may became sensitized to natural rubber latex and develop allergic reactions. It is estimated that 7% of health care workers have allergic reactions; patients with spina bifida have an incidence of 18–40%. Any group of patients frequently and intensely exposed to latex, repeated surgical procedures and treatments, eg, intermittent catheterization, are at increased risk. Local and systemic allergic reactions can often be dramatic and occasionally life threatening. The treatment is as for any allergic reaction (remove exposure, epinephrine, and steroids).

If a patient has latex allergy, it should be noted on prominently displayed signs and the patient should wear an alert bracelet. Latex is found in significant quantity in common items beyond just gloves (ie, anesthesia masks, catheters, condoms, diaphragms, douche bulbs, endotracheal tubes, hemodialysis components, NG tubes, drains, syringes, others) and consumer products (eg, balloons, rubber bands, scuba diving equipment, underwear). Most hospitals currently have an inventory of "latex-free" products and operating rooms have "latex allergy" procedures in place. Nitrile gloves are becoming commonplace in hospital settings due to this growing problem.

Arterial Line Placement

Indications
- Continuous blood pressure readings (eg, critically ill patient, titration of pressors)
- Facilitate frequent arterial blood gas measurements or other blood draws

Contraindications
- Arterial insufficiency with poor collateral circulation
- Thrombolytic therapy or coagulopathy (relative)

Materials
- Minor procedure and instrument tray
- Heparin flush solution (1:1000 dilution)
- Arterial line setup per local intensive care unit routine (transducer, tubing, and pressure bag with pre-heparinized saline, monitor)
- Arterial line catheter kit **or** 20-gauge catheter over needle, 1½–2 inch with 0.025-inch guidewire (optional)

Procedure (Figure III–1)
1. The radial artery is most frequently used and is described here. Other sites, in decreasing preference, are ulnar, dorsalis pedis, femoral, brachial, and axillary arteries. Never puncture the radial and ulnar arteries in the same hand because this may compromise blood supply to the hand and fingers.
2. Prepare the flush bag, tubing, and transducer, paying particular attention to removing the air bubbles.
3. Place the extremity on an armboard with a roll of gauze behind the wrist to hyperextend the joint. Prep with povidone–iodine or chlorhexidine gluconate and drape with sterile towels.
4. Wear sterile gloves, a mask, and eye protection.
5. Palpate the artery, and choose the puncture site where it appears most superficial. Raise a small skin wheal at the puncture site with 1% lidocaine using a 25-gauge needle.

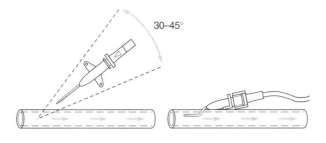

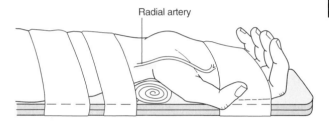

Radial artery

Figure III–1. Technique of radial artery catheterization. *(Reproduced, with permission, from Gomella TL, ed. Neonatology: Basic Management, On-Call Problems, Diseases, Drugs, 5th ed. Copyright (c) 2004 by The McGraw-Hill Companies, Inc.)*

6. See Figure III–1. While palpating the path of the artery with the nondominant hand, advance a 20-gauge (preferably 1½-inch long) catheter-over-needle assembly into the artery at a low (<30 degree) angle. Once a "flash" of blood is seen in the hub, advance the entire unit 1–2 mm so that the needle and catheter are in the artery. If blood flow in the hub stops, carefully pull the entire unit back until flow is re-established. Once the catheter is in the artery, hold the needle steady, and advance the catheter over the needle into the artery. The catheter should slide smoothly into the artery. Activate the safety button on the catheter to automatically shield the needle. Check for arterial blood flow from the catheter. A catheter that does not spurt blood is not in position. Briefly occlude the artery with manual pressure while the pressure tubing is connected. *Note:* The pressure tubing system must be pre-flushed to clear all air bubbles before connection.

7. If placement is not successful, apply pressure to the site for 5 minutes and reattempt 1 or 2 more times. If still not successful, move to another site.

8. Suture in place with 3-0 silk and apply a sterile dressing. Splint the dorsum of the wrist to limit mobility and provide catheter stability.

9. If larger vessels such as the femoral artery are used, one can employ the **Seldinger technique** for cannulation. Locate the vessel lumen with a small-gauge, thin-walled needle. Pass a 0.035-inch floppy-tipped J-wire ("J" describes the configuration of the end of the floppy wire) guidewire into the lumen. While maintaining control of the wire, remove the needle and pass a larger catheter over the wire into the vessel. Use a 16-gauge catheter assembly at least 6 inches long for the femoral artery.

10. Some institutions suggest that you replace arterial lines at a different site every 3–4 days (or per local protocol) to decrease risk of infection. The literature is somewhat controversial regarding this practice.

11. Always compare the arterial line pressure with a standard cuff pressure. An occasional difference is normal (10–20 mm Hg) and should be considered when monitoring the blood pressure.

Complications Thrombosis, hematoma, arterial embolism, arterial spasm, arterial insufficiency with tissue loss, infection, hemorrhage, pseudoaneurysm formation

Arterial Puncture

Indications
- Blood gas determinations (arterial blood gas) and when arterial blood is needed for chemistry determinations (eg, ammonia levels).

Materials
- Cup of ice
- Blood gas-sampling kit **or** 3- to 5-mL syringe
- 23- to 25-gauge needle for radial artery, 20- to 22-gauge needle for femoral artery
- Heparin (1000 U/mL) 1 mL
- Alcohol or povidone–iodine swabs

Procedure
1. Use "heparinized" syringe for blood gas and a "nonheparinized" syringe for chemistry determinations. If a blood gas kit is not available, a 3- to 5-mL syringe can be heparinized by drawing up 1 mL of 1:1000 solution of heparin through a small-gauge needle (23–25 gauge) into the syringe and pulling the plunger all the way back. The heparin is then expelled, leaving only a small coating.

2. In order of preference, use radial, femoral, and brachial arteries. For the radial artery, perform an **Allen test** to verify patency of the ulnar artery. You should not risk damage to the radial artery if there is poor flow in the ulnar artery. To perform the Allen test, the patient makes a tight fist. Occlude the radial and ulnar arteries at the wrist and have the patient open the hand. While maintaining pressure on the radial artery, release the ulnar artery. If the ulnar artery is patent, the hand flushes red within 6 seconds. A radial puncture can be safely performed. If the flushing is delayed or part of the hand or remains pale, do **not** perform the radial puncture. Choose an alternative site. Doppler ultrasound can also be used to determine whether the ulnar artery is patent.

3. For the femoral artery, use the mnemonic **NAVEL** to locate groin structures. Palpate the femoral artery just below the inguinal ligament. From lateral to medial the structures are **N**erve, **A**rtery, **V**ein, **E**mpty space, **L**igament (NAVEL).

4. While wearing gloves, a mask, and eye protection, palpate the chosen artery carefully; lidocaine subcutaneously can be used, but this turns a "1-stick procedure" into a "2-stick procedure." Palpate the artery proximally and distally with 2 fingers or trap the artery between 2 fingers placed on either side of the vessel. Hyperextension of the joint brings the radial and brachial arteries closer to the surface.

5. Prep the area with a povidone–iodine solution or chlorhexidine gluconate.

6. Hold the syringe like a pencil, with the needle bevel up, and enter the skin at a 60- to 90-degree angle. Often you can feel the arterial pulsations as you approach the artery.

7. While maintaining a slightly negative pressure on the syringe, obtain blood on the downstroke or on slow withdrawal (after both sides of the artery have been punctured). Aspirate very slowly. A good arterial sample requires only minimal back pressure. If a glass syringe or special blood-gas syringe is used, the barrel usually fills spontaneously and it is not necessary to pull on the plunger.

8. If the vessel is not encountered, withdraw the needle without coming out of the skin and redirect.

9. After obtaining the sample, withdraw the needle quickly and apply **firm** pressure at the site for ≥**5 minutes** (longer if the patient has anticoagulation). Apply pressure even if a sample was not obtained to prevent a hematoma or pseudoaneurysm. Activate the needle reshielding mechanism, if there is one.

10. If the sample is for a blood-gas determination, expel any air from the syringe, mix the contents thoroughly by twirling the syringe between your fingers, remove and dispose of the needle assembly, and make the syringe airtight with a cap. Place

the syringe in an ice bath if more than a few minutes will elapse before the sample is processed. Note the inspired oxygen concentration and time of day on the laboratory slip.

Bladder Catheterization

Indications
- Relieving urinary retention
- Collect an uncontaminated urine specimen for diagnostic purposes
- Monitoring urinary output in critically ill patients
- Performing bladder tests (cystogram, cystometrogram)

Contraindications
- Urethral disruption, often associated with pelvic fracture
- Acute prostatitis (relative contraindication)

Materials
- Prepackaged bladder catheter tray (may or may not include a catheter)
- Catheters of choice (Figure III–2):

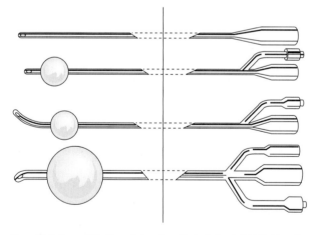

Figure III–2. Types of bladder catheters (from the top): the straight "Robinson" or red rubber catheter, Foley catheter with standard 5-mL balloon, the Coudé catheter, and "3-way" irrigating catheter with 30-mL balloon. Catheters have been shortened for illustrative purposes. *(Reproduced, with permission, from Gomella LG, ed.* Clinician's Pocket Reference, *10th ed. Copyright (c) 2004 by The McGraw-Hill Companies, Inc.)*

Foley: Balloon at the tip to keep it in the bladder. Use a 16F–18F for adults (the higher the number, the larger the diameter). Irrigation catheters ("3-way Foley") should be larger (20F–22F).

Coudé: An elbow-tipped catheter useful in males with prostatic hypertrophy (the catheter is passed with the tip pointing to 12 o'-clock).

Red rubber catheter (Robinson): Plain rubber or latex catheter without a balloon, usually used for "in-and-out catheterization" in which urine is removed but the catheter is not left indwelling.

Procedure
1. Use strict aseptic technique.
2. Have the patient lie supine in a well-lighted area; females should place knees flexed wide and heels together to provide adequate exposure of the meatus.
3. Get all the materials ready before you attempt to insert the catheter. Open the kit and put on the gloves. Open the prep solution and soak the cotton balls. Apply the sterile drapes.
4. Inflate and deflate the balloon of the Foley catheter to ensure its proper function. Coat the end of the catheter with lubricant jelly.
5. For females, use 1 gloved hand to prep the urethral meatus in a pubis-toward-anus direction; hold the labia apart with the other gloved hand. With uncircumcised males, retract the foreskin to prep the glans; use a gloved hand to hold the penis.
6. Do not touch or insert the catheter with the hand used to hold the penis or labia (the "dirty" hand). Use the disposable forceps in the kit to prep and then use the free gloved hand (the "clean" hand) to insert the catheter.
7. In the male, **stretch** the penis upward perpendicular to the body to eliminate any internal folds in the urethra that might lead to a false passage. Use **steady, gentle** pressure to advance the catheter. A slight resistance may be felt as the catheter passes the external sphincter and prostate gland. Encourage the patient to take slow deep breaths and not "bear down." Any significant resistance encountered may represent a stricture or false passage of the catheter and requires urologic consultation. In males with benign prostatic hypertrophy, a Coudé tip catheter may facilitate passage. Keep the catheter tip directed anteriorly. Other helpful tricks used to get a catheter to pass in a male are to make sure that the penis is well stretched and to instill sterile water-based surgical lubricant (K-Y jelly) 30–50 mL into the urethra with a catheter-tipped syringe before passage of the catheter. Viscous lidocaine jelly for urologic use can also be used to help

lubricate and relieve the discomfort of difficult catheter placement. Allow ≥5 minutes after instillation of the lidocaine jelly for the anesthetic effect to take place.

8. In males and females, insert the catheter to the hilt of the drainage end. Compress the penis toward the pubis. These maneuvers ensure that the balloon inflates in the bladder and not in the urethra. Inflate the balloon with sterile water 5–10 mL (do not use saline). After inflation, pull the catheter back so that the balloon comes to rest on the bladder neck. There should be good urine return when the catheter is in place. If a large amount of lubricant jelly was placed into the urethra, the catheter may need to be flushed with sterile saline to clear the excess lubricant. A catheter that will not irrigate is in the urethra, not the bladder.

9. Any male who is uncircumcised should have the foreskin repositioned to prevent edema of the glans after the catheter is inserted.

10. Catheters in females can be taped to the leg. In males, the catheter can be taped to the abdominal wall to decrease stress on the posterior urethra and help prevent stricture formation. The catheter is usually attached to a gravity drainage bag or some device for measuring the amount of urine. Many new kits come with the catheter already secured to the drainage bag. These systems are considered "closed" and should not be opened if at all possible.

11. If blood or clots are present, the bladder should be gently irrigated with a catheter-tipped syringe and normal saline. The urology service should be consulted because there may have been insertion trauma (false passage) or the patient may need a 3-way catheter placed to allow continuous bladder irrigation.

12. For sample collection or determination of residual urine, a straight red rubber catheter without a balloon (Robinson catheter) can be used according to the previously noted technique.

Central Venous Catheterization

Indications

- Administration of fluids and medications (peripheral access preferred)
- Administration of hyperalimentation solutions or other hypertonic fluids (eg, amphotericin B) that damage peripheral veins
- Measurement of central venous pressure
- Acute dialysis or plasmapheresis (Shiley catheter)
- Insertion of a pulmonary artery catheter or transvenous pacemaker

Contraindications
- Coagulopathy dictates the use of the femoral or median basilic vein approach to minimize complications.

Background A central venous catheter (or **"central line"**) is a catheter introduced into the superior or inferior vena cava or 1 of their main branches. One technique (**Seldinger technique**) involves puncturing the vein with a small needle through which a thin guidewire is placed. The needle is withdrawn, and an intravascular appliance or a sheath through which a smaller catheter will be placed is introduced into the vein over the guidewire. Another technique involves puncturing the vein with a larger-bore needle through which the intravascular catheter will fit. This section focuses on the more common **Seldinger technique** and placement of a triple-lumen catheter or a sheath through which a smaller catheter (eg, a pulmonary artery catheter) can be placed. The internal subclavian and jugular approaches are commonly used; the femoral approach, although infrequently utilized, offers some advantages in particular situations (see below). The peripherally inserted central catheter (PICC) line is designed for more long-term outpatient administration of medications and is described on page 371.

Materials Commercially available trays provide all the necessary needles, wires, sheaths, dilators, suture materials, and anesthetics. If needles, guidewires, and sheaths are collected from different places, it is very important to make sure that the needle will accept the guidewire, that the sheath and dilator will pass over the guidewire, and that the appliance to be passed through the sheath will indeed fit the inside lumen of the sheath. Supplies should include the following items:

- Minor procedure and instrument tray; 1% lidocaine (may be mixed 1:1 with sodium bicarbonate 1 mEq/L to neutralize the solution and decrease the pain of injection)
- Guidewire (usually 0.035-inch floppy-tipped J wire)
- Vessel dilator
- Intravascular appliance (triple-lumen catheter or a sheath through which a pulmonary artery catheter could be placed)
- Heparinized flush solution of 1:100 U heparin 1 mL in normal saline 10 mL (to fill lumens before placement to prevent clotting during placement)
- Mask, sterile gown, mask, and eye protection

Subclavian Approach (Left or Right) The left subclavian approach affords a gentle, sweeping curve to the apex of the right ventricle (preferred site for temporary transvenous pacemaker without fluoroscopy). *Caution:* The thoracic duct is on the left side, and the dome of the pleura rises higher on the left.

1. Place the patient flat or head down (Trendelenburg position) with the head in the center or turned to the opposite side (*note:* the "ideal" position is controversial and is based on operator preference and experience). Placing a towel roll along the patient's spine may allow the patient's shoulder to fall posteriorly, thus providing better access to the vein.

2. Use sterile technique (povidone–iodine or chlorhexidine gluconate prep, sterile gown, sterile gloves, mask, eye protection, and a sterile field).

3. Use a 25-gauge needle to make a small skin wheal 2 cm below the midclavicle with 1% lidocaine. Next, a larger needle (eg, 22-gauge) is used to anesthetize the deeper tissues and locate the vein.

4. Attach the large-bore, venipuncture needle supplied with the kit to a 10-mL syringe and introduce it into the site of the skin wheal.

5. Advance the needle under the clavicle, aiming for a location halfway between the suprasternal notch and the base of the thyroid cartilage. The vein is encountered under the clavicle, just medial to the lateral border of the clavicular head of the sternocleidomastoid muscle. In most patients this is roughly 2 fingerbreadths lateral to the sternal notch. Apply gentle pressure on the needle at the skin entrance site to assist in lowering the needle under the clavicle (Figure III–3).

6. Apply back pressure as the needle is advanced deep to the clavicle, but above the first rib, and watch for a "flash" of blood.

7. Free return of blood indicates entry into the subclavian vein. Remember that occasionally the vein is punctured through *both* walls, and a flash of blood may not appear as the needle is advanced. Therefore, if a free return of blood does not occur on needle advancement, withdraw the needle slowly with intermittent pressure. A free return of blood heralds the entry of the end of the needle into the lumen. Bright red blood that forcibly enters the syringe indicates that the subclavian artery has been entered. If the arterial entry occurs, remove the needle. In most patients, the surrounding tissue will tamponade any bleeding from the arterial puncture. *Note:* The artery is under the clavicle, so holding pressure has little effect on bleeding.

8. Using the Seldinger technique, gently advance the J-tipped guidewire through the needle and withdraw the needle. The pulse or electrocardiogram should be monitored during wire passage because the wire can induce ventricular arrhythmias. Arrhythmias usually resolve by pulling the wire out several

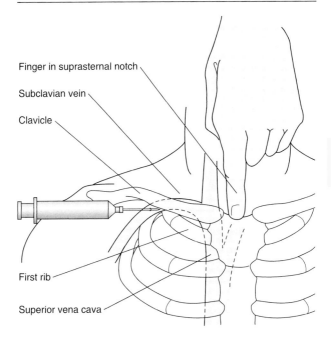

Figure III–3. Technique for subclavian vein catheterization. *(Reproduced, with permission, from Gomella LG, ed.* Clinician's Pocket Reference, *10th ed. Copyright (c) 2004 by the McGraw-Hill Companies, Inc.)*

centimeters. Nick the skin with a no. 11 blade and advance the dilator approximately 5 cm; remove the dilator and advance the catheter in over the guidewire (use the brown port on the triple-lumen catheter). While advancing the dilator or the catheter over the wire, periodically ensure that the wire moves freely in and out. When placing a Cordis (multiport catheter sheath system), advance the catheter and dilator over the guidewire as 1 unit. If the wire does not move freely, it usually is kinked, and the catheter or dilator should be removed and repositioned. Maintain a grip on the guidewire at all times. Remove the wire and attach the IV tubing. Note that the wire used to insert a single-lumen catheter is shorter than the wire supplied with the triple-lumen catheter. This is most critical when exchanging a triple-lumen for a single-lumen catheter; use the longer triple-lumen wire and insert the wire into the brown port. Shiley (hemodialysis) catheters also are placed using the Seldinger technique.

9. Aspirate and flush each port with a heparinized saline solution. Alternatively, attach the catheter directly to an IV solution and place the IV bag below the level of the insertion site to ensure a good backflow of blood into the tubing. If no backflow occurs, the catheter may be kinked or not in the proper position.

10. Securely suture the assembly in place with 2-0 or 3-0 silk. Apply an occlusive dressing with an antimicrobial ointment.

11. Obtain an upright chest radiograph immediately to verify the location of the catheter tip and to rule out pneumothorax. Ideally, the catheter tip lies in the superior vena cava at its junction with the right atrium (about the fifth thoracic vertebra). Malpositioned catheters, which lie in the neck veins, may only be used only for saline infusion and not for monitoring or total parenteral nutrition infusion.

12. Catheters that cannot be manipulated at the bedside into the chest can usually be positioned properly in the interventional radiology suite by using fluoroscopy.

Right Internal Jugular Vein Approach There are 3 different sites for access to the right internal jugular vein: anterior (medial to the sternocleidomastoid muscle belly), middle (between the two heads of the sternocleidomastoid muscle belly), and posterior (lateral to the sternocleidomastoid muscle belly). The middle approach is most common and uses well-defined landmarks: percutaneous entry should be made at the apex of the triangle formed by the 2 heads of the sternocleidomastoid muscle and the clavicle (Figure III–4). The major disadvantage of the internal jugular site is patient discomfort (difficult to dress, uncomfortable when turning the head). Ultrasound guidance (see below) should be used for this procedure.

Procedure

1. Place the patient in the **Trendelenburg** (head down) position with the head turned to the left.

2. Use sterile technique (povidone–iodine or chlorhexidine gluconate prep, sterile gown, sterile gloves, mask, eye protection, and a sterile field).

3. Use a 25-gauge needle to make a small skin wheal with 1% lidocaine in the area to be explored, as indicated above. Next, a larger needle (eg, 22-gauge) is used to anesthetize the deeper tissues and locate the vein.

4. Use a small-bore needle (21-gauge) with syringe to locate the internal jugular vein. It may help to have a small amount of anesthetic in the syringe to inject during exploration if the patient has discomfort. Some prefer to leave this needle and sy-

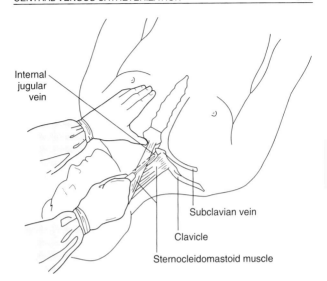

Figure III–4. Technique for internal jugular vein catheterization, central approach. *(Reproduced, with permission, from Gomella LG, ed.* Clinician's Pocket Reference, *10th ed. Copyright (c) 2004 by The McGraw-Hill Companies, Inc.)*

ringe in the vein and then place the large-bore needle directly adjacent to and parallel to the smaller needle and into the vein. This is commonly called the "finder needle" technique.

5. Direct the needle through the skin wheal caudally, directed toward the ipsilateral nipple and at a 30-degree angle to the frontal plane. If the vein is not entered, withdraw the needle slightly and redirect it 5–10 degrees more laterally. Apply intermittent back pressure.

6. If a portable ultrasound device (Site-Rite) is available, it should be used to positively identify the vein, thus helping to avoid injury to the artery or other structures in the neck. The transducer is placed in a sterile sleeve, with a generous amount of ultrasound gel surrounding the face of the transducer. The transducer and sleeve are then used on the sterile field to localize the jugular vein. The vein, unlike the artery, is easily compressed by the probe. Respiratory variation may also be noted. By passing the needle alongside the guide notches on the transducer (be careful not to puncture the sterile sleeve and keep the bevel of the needle "up" to provide a brighter reflection), the needle can be passed into the vein

under direct vision. Note that it is still possible to overshoot and pass the needle through the posterior wall of the vein. Apply back pressure and watch for a "flash" of blood, as you would with any venipuncture.

7. If bright red blood forcibly fills the syringe, the carotid artery has been punctured. Remove the needle and apply firm pressure for 10 minutes.
8. Follow steps 8 through 12 as described for the subclavian technique.

Left Internal Jugular Vein Approach The procedure is similar to the right internal jugular vein approach. In addition to the usual complications, this approach has unique complications, including inadvertent left brachiocephalic vein and superior vena cava puncture with intravascular wires, catheters, and sheaths and laceration of the thoracic duct with chylothorax.

Femoral Vein Approach This approach is relatively safe (arterial and venous sites are easily compressible) and it is impossible to cause pneumothorax from this site. Placement can be accomplished without interrupting cardiopulmonary resuscitation. This site can be used to place different intravascular appliances, including triple-lumen catheters, temporary pacemakers, and pulmonary artery catheters. However, there are several major disadvantages with this approach including a high risk of sepsis, the immobilization it causes, an increased risk of deep vein thrombosis, and a frequent need for fluoroscopy to ensure proper placement of pulmonary artery catheters or transvenous pacemakers. Femoral lines should be used **only** when other sites are not practical and should be removed **within 24 hours**.

Procedure
1. Place the patient in the supine position.
2. Use sterile technique (povidone–iodine or chlorhexidine gluconate prep, sterile gown, sterile gloves, mask, eye protection, and a sterile field). Administer local anesthesia with lidocaine. The site of percutaneous entry should be 1–2 cm below the inguinal crease to minimize irritation and infection.
3. Palpate the femoral artery. Use the mnemonic NAVEL to locate the vein.
4. Guard the artery with the fingers of 1 hand.
5. Explore for the vein just medial to the operator's fingers with a needle and syringe as described above.
6. It may be helpful to have a small amount of anesthetic in the syringe to inject with exploration.
7. Direct the needle cephalad at an angle at about 30 degrees angle and insert below the femoral crease.

8. Puncture is heralded by the return of venous, nonpulsatile blood on application of negative pressure to the syringe.
9. Follow steps 8 through 12 as described for the subclavian technique.

Complications Complications are pneumothorax, hemothorax, hydrothorax, arterial puncture with hematoma, catheter tip embolus, and air embolus. When you suspect an air embolus, place the patient with head down and turned on the left side to keep the air in the right atrium; attempt to aspirate the air through the catheter. Obtain an immediate portable chest radiograph to see if air is present in the heart. Other risks include sepsis, deep vein thrombosis, or puncture of the iliac vessels with retroperitoneal hemorrhage when using the femoral approach.

Chest Tube Placement
(Closed Thoracostomy, Tube Thoracostomy)
(See also Section I, Problem 13, page 63)

Indications
- Pneumothorax (simple or tension)
- Hemothorax, hydrothorax, chylothorax, or empyema evacuation
- Pleurodesis for chronic recurring pneumothorax or effusion that is refractory to standard management (eg, malignant effusion)

Materials
- Chest tube (adult: 22F–24F for pneumothorax, 32F–38F for hemothorax or pleural effusion; newborn: 12F–18F, 1–2 years 14F–24F, 5 years 20F–32F, >5 years as for adult)
- Water-seal drainage system (Pleur-Evac, etc) with connecting tubing to wall suction
- Minor procedure tray and instrument tray
- Silk or nylon suture (0 to 2-0)
- Petrolatum gauze (Vaseline) (optional)
- 4 × 4 gauze dressing and cloth tape
- Pulse oximeter monitoring (recommended)

Background A chest tube is usually placed to control an ongoing intrathoracic process that cannot be managed by simple thoracentesis (page 381). The traditional methods of chest tube placement are described. Percutaneous tube thoracostomy kits are also available based on the Seldinger technique (used for small pneumothoraces when there is no risk of ongoing air leak, but is contraindicated in significant conditions, eg, empyema, major pneumothorax >20%, tension pneumothorax, chronic effusions).

Procedure

> If a patient manifests signs of a tension pneumothorax (acute
> shortness of breath, hypotension, distended neck veins,
> tachypnea, tracheal deviation) before a chest tube is placed,
> urgent treatment is needed. Insert a 14-gauge needle into the
> chest in the second intercostal space in the midclavicular line
> to rapidly decompress the tension pneumothorax and proceed
> with chest tube insertion.

1. Before placing the tube, review the chest radiograph unless an
   emergency does not allow enough time. For a pneumothorax,
   choose a high anterior site (second or third intercostal space,
   midclavicular line, or subaxillary position). Subaxillary is most
   cosmetic. Place a low lateral chest tube in the fifth or sixth intercostal space in the midaxillary line and direct posteriorly for fluid
   removal (usually corresponds to the inframammary crease). In
   traumatic pneumothorax, use a low lateral site because it usually is associated with bleeding. Rarely, a loculated apical
   pneumothorax or effusion may require placement of an anterior
   tube in the second intercostal space at the midclavicular line.
2. Choose the appropriate chest tube. Use a 24F–28F tube for
   pneumothorax and 36F for fluid removal. A "**thoracic catheter**"
   has multiple holes and works best for nearly all purposes.
3. Prep the area with povidone–iodine solution or chlorhexidine
   gluconate and drape it with sterile towels. Use lidocaine (with
   or without epinephrine) to anesthetize the skin, intercostal
   muscle, and periosteum of the rib; start at the center of the rib
   and gently work over the top. Remember, the neurovascular
   bundle runs under the rib (Figure III–5). The needle then can
   be gently "popped" through the pleura and the aspiration of air
   or fluid confirms the correct location for the chest tube. Sedation may be helpful in elective situations.
4. Make a 2- to 3-cm transverse incision over the center of the rib
   with a no. 15 or 11 scalpel blade. Use a blunt-tipped clamp to dis-
   sect over the top of the rib and create a subcutaneous tunnel.
5. Puncture the parietal pleura with the hemostat and spread the
   opening. **Be careful not to injure the lung parenchyma
   with the hemostat tips.** Insert a gloved finger into the pleural
   cavity to gently clear any clots or adhesions and to make certain the lung is not accidentally punctured by the tube. Palpation of lung with the tip of the finger will also confirm that one
   is in the pleural space and not in the peritoneal space.
6. Carefully insert the tube into the desired position with a hemostat or gloved finger as a guide. Attach the end of the tube to
   a water-seal or Pleur-Evac suction system. Trocars are not

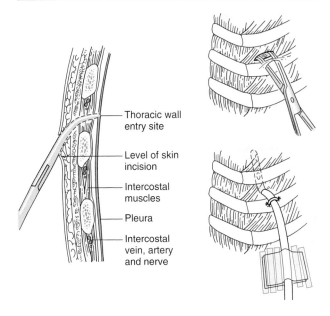

Thoracic wall entry site

Level of skin incision

Intercostal muscles

Pleura

Intercostal vein, artery and nerve

Figure III–5. Chest tube technique, demonstrating the location of the neurovascular bundle and the creation of the subcutaneous tunnel. *(Reproduced, with permission, from Gomella TL, ed.* Neonatology: Basic Management, On-Call Problems, Diseases, Drugs, *5th ed. Copyright (c) 2004 by The McGraw-Hill Companies, Inc.)*

recommended for chest tube placement without considerable prior experience.

7. Suture the tube in place. Place a heavy silk (0 or 2-0) suture through the incision next to the tube. Tie the incision together and then tie the ends around the chest tube. Make sure to wrap the suture around the tube several times. Alternatively, a purse string suture (or "U stitch") can be placed around the insertion site. Make sure all of the suction holes are in the chest cavity before the tube is secured.

8. Cover the insertion site with plain gauze. Make the dressing as airtight as possible with tape and secure all connections in the tubing to prevent accidental loss of the water seal. Some physicians prefer to wrap the insertion site with petroleum jelly (Vaseline or Xeroform) gauze; however, these materials can be problematic (not water soluble and act as foreign bodies), inhibit wound healing, and may not actually seal the site.

9. Start suction (usually −20 cm in adults, −16 cm in children) and take a portable chest radiograph immediately to check the placement of the tube and to evaluate for residual pneumothorax or fluid. Check the position of the "last hole."
10. When placing a chest tube to drain an effusion, be sure not to drain more than 800–1000 mL every few hours. The tube should be clamped if that amount has already drained to avoid the development of "flash" pulmonary edema.

Chest Tube Removal

1. Verify the pneumothorax or hemothorax is cleared. Check for an air leak by having the patient cough; observe the water-seal system for bubbling that indicates a system (tubing) leak or a persistent pleural air leak.
2. Take the tube off suction **but not off water seal** and cut the retention suture. Have the patient inspire deeply and perform the Valsalva maneuver while you apply pressure with petrolatum gauze or with a sufficient amount of antibiotic ointment on 4 × 4 gauze with additional 4 × 4 gauze squares. Pull the tube rapidly while the patient performs the Valsalva maneuver and make an airtight seal with tape. Check an "upright" exhalation chest x-ray film for pneumothorax.

Cricothyrotomy (Needle and Surgical)

Background Cricothyrotomy is an emergency procedure that should be performed when obtaining an airway and using endotracheal or orotracheal intubation is impossible.

Indications
- When immediate mechanical ventilation is indicated, but an endotracheal or orotracheal tube cannot be placed (eg, severe maxillofacial trauma, excessive oropharyngeal hemorrhage).

Contraindications
- Surgical cricothyrotomy is contraindicated in children <12 years; use needle approach.

Basic Materials
- Oxygen connecting tubing, high-flow oxygen source (tank or wall)
- Bag ventilator

Needle Cricothyrotomy
- 12- to 14-gauge catheter over needle (Angiocath or other)
- 6- to 12-mL syringe
- 3-mm pediatric endotracheal tube adapter

Surgical Cricothyrotomy (Minimum Requirements)
- Minor procedure and instrument tray plus tracheal spreader if available
- No. 5–7 tracheostomy tube (6F–8F endotracheal tube can be substituted)
- Tracheostomy tube adapter to connect to bag-mask ventilator

Procedures
Needle Cricothyrotomy
1. With the patient supine, place a roll behind the shoulders to gently hyperextend the neck.
2. Palpate the cricothyroid membrane, which resembles a notch located between the caudal end of the thyroid cartilage and the cricoid cartilage. Prep the area with povidone–iodine solution. Local anesthesia can be used if the patient is awake.
3. Mount the syringe on the 12- or 14-gauge catheter-over-needle assembly, and advance through the cricothyroid membrane at a 45-degree angle, and apply back pressure on the syringe until air is aspirated.
4. Advance the catheter and remove the needle. Attach the hub to a 3-mm endotracheal tube adapter that is connected to the oxygen tubing. Allow the oxygen to flow at 15 L/min for 1–2 seconds on and then 4 seconds off by the use of a Y-connector or a hole in the side of the tubing to turn the flow on and off.
5. The needle technique is only useful for about 45 minutes because the exhalation of CO_2 is suboptimal.

Surgical Cricothyrotomy
1. Follow steps 1 and 2 as for needle cricothyrotomy.
2. Make a 3- to 4-cm vertical skin incision through the cervical fascia and strap muscles in the midline over the cricothyroid membrane. Expose the cricothyroid membrane and make a horizontal incision. Insert the knife handle and rotate it 90 degrees to open the hole in the membrane. Alternatively, a hemostat or tracheal spreader can be used to dilate the opening.
3. Insert a small (5–7 mm) tracheostomy tube, inflate the balloon (if present), and secure in position with the attached cotton tapes.
4. Attach to oxygen source and ventilate. Listen to the chest for symmetrical breath sounds.
5. A surgical cricothyrotomy should be replaced with a formal tracheostomy after the patient has been stabilized and generally within 24–36 hours.

Complications
- Bleeding, esophageal perforation, subcutaneous emphysema, pneumomediastinum, and pneumothorax, CO_2 retention (especially with the needle procedure)

Endotracheal Intubation

Indications
- Airway management during cardiopulmonary resuscitation
- Any indication for using mechanical ventilation (respiratory failure, coma, general anesthesia, etc)

Contraindications
- Massive maxillofacial trauma (relative)
- Fractured larynx
- Suspected cervical spinal cord injury (relative)

Materials
- Endotracheal tube of appropriate size (Table III–1)
- Laryngoscope handle and blade (straight [Miller] or curved [MAC]; no. 3 for adults, no. 1–1.5 for small children)
- 10-mL syringe, adhesive tape, benzoin
- Suction equipment (Yankauer suction)
- Malleable stylet (optional)
- Oropharyngeal airway

Technique (Figure III–6)
1. Orotracheal intubation is most commonly used and is described here. In suspected cervical spine injury, nasotracheal intubation is preferred.
2. Any patient who is hypoxic or apneic must be ventilated before attempting endotracheal intubation (bag mask or mouth to mask). Avoid prolonged periods of no ventilation if the intubation is difficult. A rule of thumb is to hold your breath while attempting intubation. When you need to take a breath, so must the patient. Resume ventilation and reattempt intubation in a minute or so.
3. Extend the laryngoscope blade to 90 degrees to verify the light is working and check the balloon on the tube (if present) for leaks.

TABLE III–1. RECOMMENDED ENDOTRACHEAL TUBE SIZES

Patient	Internal Diameter (mm)
Premature infant	2.5–3.0 (uncuffed)
Newborn infant	3.5 (uncuffed)
3–12 months	4.0 (uncuffed)
1–8 years	4.0–6.0 (uncuffed)[a]
8–16 years	6.0–7.0 (cuffed)
Adult	7.0–9.0 (cuffed)

[a]Rough estimate is to measure the patient's little finger.

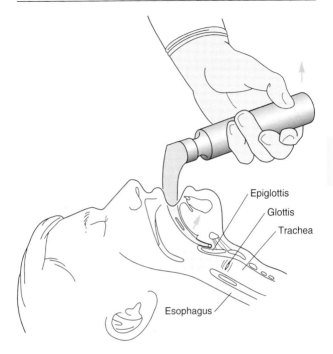

Figure III–6. Endotracheal intubation using a curved laryngoscope blade. *(Reproduced, with permission, from Gomella LG, ed.* Clinician's Pocket Reference, *10th ed. Copyright (c) 2004 by The McGraw-Hill Companies, Inc.)*

4. Place the patient's head in the "sniffing position" (neck extended anteriorly and the head extended posteriorly). Use suction to clear the upper airway if needed.
5. Hold the laryngoscope in the left hand, hold the mouth open with the right hand, and use the blade to push the tongue to patient's left while keeping it anterior to the blade. Advance the blade carefully toward the midline until the epiglottis is visualized. Use suction if needed.
6. If the **straight laryngoscope blade** is used, pass it under the epiglottis and **lift** upward to visualize the vocal cords. If the **curved blade** is used, place it anterior to the epiglottis (into the vallecula) and gently lift anteriorly. In either case, do **not** use the handle to pry the epiglottis open, but rather gently lift to expose the vocal cords.

7. While maintaining visualization of the cords, grasp the tube in your dominant hand and pass it through the cords. With more difficult intubations, the malleable stylet can be used to direct the tube.

8. In patients who may have eaten recently, gentle pressure placed over the cricoid cartilage by an assistant helps to occlude the esophagus and prevent aspiration during intubation. "Cricoid pressure" can also help visualize the vocal cords in patients whose larynx is situated more anteriorly than usual.

9. When using a cuffed tube (adult and older children), gently inflate air with a 10-mL syringe until the seal is adequate (about 5 mL). Ventilate the patient while auscultating and visualizing both sides of the chest to verify positioning. If the left side does not seem to be ventilating, it may signify that the tube has been advanced down the right mainstem bronchus. Withdraw the tube 1–2 cm and recheck the breath sounds. Also auscultate over the stomach to ensure the tube is not mistakenly placed in the esophagus. Confirm positioning with a chest radiograph. The tip of the endotracheal tube should be a few centimeters above the carina.

10. Tape the tube in position and insert an oropharyngeal airway to prevent the patient from biting the tube. Consider an orogastric tube to prevent regurgitation.

Complications Bleeding, oral or pharyngeal trauma, improper tube positioning (esophageal intubation, right mainstem bronchus), aspiration, tube obstruction or kinking

Gastrointestinal Intubation

Indications
- Gastrointestinal decompression: ileus, obstruction, pancreatitis, postoperatively
- Lavage of the stomach with gastrointestinal bleeding or drug overdose
- Prevention of aspiration in an obtunded patient
- Feeding a patient who is unable to swallow

Materials
- Gastrointestinal tube of choice (see following list)
- Lubricant jelly
- Catheter tip syringe
- Glass of water with a straw, stethoscope

Types of Gastrointestinal Tubes

1. **Nasogastric tubes**
   Salem-sump tube: A double-lumen tube; the smaller tube is an air intake vent so that continuous suction can be applied.

This is the best tube for irrigation and lavage because it will not collapse on itself. If a Salem-sump tube stops working even after it is repositioned, often a "shot" of air from a catheter-tipped syringe in the air vent will clear the tube. The Salem-sump tube has radiopaque markings.

2. **Feeding tubes**

   Although any NG tube can be used as a feeding tube, it is preferable to place a specially designed nasoduodenal feeding tube. These are of smaller diameter (usually 8F) and are more pliable and comfortable for the patient. Weighted tips tend to travel into the duodenum, which may help prevent regurgitation and aspiration. Most are supplied with stylets that facilitate positioning, especially if fluoroscopic guidance is needed. Always verify the position of the feeding tube with a radiograph before starting tube feeding. Commonly used tubes include the mercury-weighted varieties (**Keogh tube, Duo-Tube, Dobbhoff, Entriflex**), the tungsten-weighted (**Vivonex tube**), and the unweighted pediatric feeding tubes.

3. **Miscellaneous gastrointestinal tubes**

   a. **Sengstaken–Blakemore tube:** A triple-lumen tube used exclusively for the control of bleeding esophageal varices by tamponade. One lumen is for gastric aspiration, the second is for the gastric balloon, and the third is for the esophageal balloon. Other types include the **Linton** and **Minnesota** tubes. Before placing this device, it is critically important to read the instructions.

   b. **Ewald tube:** An orogastric tube used almost exclusively for gastric evacuation of blood or drug overdose. The tube is usually double lumen and large diameter (18F–36F).

Procedure (for NG and Feeding Tubes)

1. Inform the patient of the nature of the procedure and encourage cooperation if the patient is able. Choose the nasal passage that appears most open. Have the patient sitting up if able.

2. Lubricate the distal 3–4 inches of the tube with a water-soluble jelly (K-Y Jelly or viscous lidocaine) and insert the tube gently along the floor of the nasal passageway. Maintain gentle pressure that will allow the tube to pass into the nasopharynx. Have the patient flex the neck slightly from neutral.

3. When the patient can feel the tube in the back of the throat, ask the patient to swallow small amounts of water through a straw as you advance the tube 2–3 inches at a time.

4. To be sure that the tube is in the stomach, aspirate gastric contents or blow air into the tube with a catheter-tipped syringe and listen over the stomach with your stethoscope for a "pop" or "gurgle." The position of feeding tubes **must** be veri-

fied by a chest radiograph before institution of feedings to prevent accidental bronchial instillation of tube feedings.

5. NG tubes are attached to low wall suction (Salem-sump type tubes with a vent) or to intermittent suction (Levin type tubes); the latter allows the tube to fall away from the gastric wall between suction cycles.

6. Feeding and pediatric feeding tubes in adults are more difficult to insert because they are more flexible. Many are provided with stylets that make their passage easier. These stylets must be used with caution (see step 7). Feeding tubes are best placed into the duodenum or jejunum to decrease the risk of aspiration. Administering metoclopramide (Reglan) 10 mg IV 10 min before insertion of the tube may assist in placing the tube into the duodenum.

7. Do not "freeze" a tube or place it in ice water to make it stiff before insertion. Overly stiff tubes or tubes with very rigid stylets can cause a great deal of trauma, particularly in obtunded or intubated patients. Never force a tube if it meets significant resistance. Always try passing a tube without a stylet first, and use a tube with a stylet only if your initial attempts are unsuccessful. In an intubated patient, it may be useful to pass the tube to about 30 cm and obtain a chest radiograph. If the tube is inadvertently passed into the bronchus, this will be apparent on the film, and a complication such as a tension pneumothorax can be avoided. Fluoroscopic or endoscopic guidance may also be used in situations when a tube does not pass easily.

8. Once the feeding tube is in the stomach, the bell of the stethoscope is placed on the right side of the patient's midabdomen. As the tube is advanced, air is injected to confirm progression of the tube to the right, toward the duodenum. If the sound of the air becomes fainter, the tube is probably curling in the stomach. Pass the tube until a slight resistance is felt, heralding the presence of the tip of the tube at the pylorus. Holding constant pressure and slowly injecting water through the tube are often rewarded with a "give," which signifies passage through the pylorus. The tube often can be advanced far into the duodenum with this method. The duodenum usually provides constant resistance that will give with slow injection of water. Placing the patient in the right lateral decubitus position may help the tube enter the duodenum.

9. Tape the tube securely in place but do not allow it to apply pressure to the ala of the nose. Patients have been disfigured because of ischemic necrosis of the nose caused by a poorly positioned NG tube.

10. **A chest radiograph must be obtained before starting any feeding through a tube to verify its placement in the gastrointestinal tract.**

Complications
- Inadvertent passage into the trachea may provoke coughing or gagging in the patient.
- Aspiration.
- If the patient is unable to cooperate, the tube often becomes coiled in the oral cavity.
- The tube is irritating and may cause a small amount of bleeding in the mucosa of the nose, pharynx, or stomach. The drying and irritation can be lessened by throat lozenges or antiseptic spray.
- Intracranial passage in patient with a basilar skull fracture.
- Esophageal perforation.
- Esophageal reflux caused by the tube-induced incompetence of the distal esophageal sphincter.
- Sinusitis from edema of the nasal passages that blocks drainage from the nasal sinuses.

IV Techniques

Indication
- IV access for the administration of fluids, blood, or medications (other techniques include central venous catheters, page 340, and PICC lines, page 371)

Materials
- IV fluid
- Connecting tubing
- Tourniquet
- Alcohol swab
- Intravenous cannulas
- Antiseptic ointment, dressing, and tape

Technique
1. It helps to rip the tape into strips, attach the IV tubing to the solution, and flush the air out of the tubing before you begin.
2. The upper, nondominant extremity is the site of choice for an IV line, unless the patient is being considered for placement of permanent hemodialysis access. In this instance, the upper nondominant extremity should be "saved" as the access site for hemodialysis. If the patient has previously undergone an axillary lymph node dissection (eg, some breast cancer surgeries), the IV line should be started on the other side. Choose a distal vein (dorsum of the hand) so that, if the vein is lost, you can reposition the IV more proximally. Also avoid the leg because of the increased risk of thrombophlebitis.
3. Apply a tourniquet above the proposed IV site. Use the techniques described in the section on venipuncture to help expose the vein. Carefully clean the site with an alcohol or

povidone–iodine swab. If a large-bore IV is to be used (16 or 14 gauge), local anesthesia (lidocaine injected with a 25-gauge needle) is helpful.

4. Stabilize the vein distally with the thumb of your free hand. Using the catheter-over needle assembly, enter the vein directly or enter the skin alongside the vein first and then stick the vein along the side at about a 20-degree angle. Once the vein is punctured, blood should appear in the "flash chamber." For lower needle assembly, the next steps will vary if you are using a standard catheter over needle device or a self-shielding device.

   a. **Standard catheter over needle.** Advance a few more millimeters to be sure that **both** the needle **and** the tip of the catheter have entered the vein. Thread the catheter into the vein while maintaining traction on the skin. Remove the tourniquet, compress the vein, and stabilize the catheter hub. Connect the IV fluid.

   b. After the flashback is seen, lower the catheter assembly to almost parallel to the skin. Advance the entire unit before attempting to thread catheter. Thread catheter into vein while maintaining traction. Next, release the tourniquet and apply pressure beyond catheter tip, making sure that digital pressure is maintained beyond catheter tip. Press the white button and the needle retracts into a shield. Connect the IV line to the catheter.

5. With the IV fluid running, observe the site for signs of induration or swelling that indicate improper placement or damage to the vein.

6. Tape the IV securely in place; apply a drop of povidone–iodine or antibiotic ointment and apply a sterile dressing. Ideally, the dressing should be changed every 24–48 hours to help decrease infections. Armboards are also useful to help maintain an IV site.

7. *Important point:* Never reinsert the needle into the catheter because this can result in shearing the catheter.

8. **"Butterfly"** or **"scalp vein"** needle can sometimes be used. This is a small metal needle with plastic "wings" on the side. It is very useful in infants who often have poor peripheral veins but prominent scalp veins, children, and adults who have small, fragile veins.

9. Troubleshooting difficult IV placement
   • If the veins are deep and difficult to locate, a small 3- to 5-mL syringe can be mounted on the catheter assembly. Proper positioning inside the vein is determined by aspiration of blood. If blood specimens are needed on a patient who also needs an IV, this technique can be used to start the IV and to collect samples at the same time.

- If no extremity vein can be found, try the external jugular. Placing the patient in the head down position can help distend the vein. This IV site is difficult to maintain and is uncomfortable for the patient, so it should be changed to another line as soon as feasible.
- If all these fail, the next alternative may be a central venous line insertion (page 340).

Joint Aspiration (Arthrocentesis): Diagnostic and Therapeutic

Indications
- **Diagnostic.** Evaluate new-onset arthritis; to rule out infection in an acute or chronic, unremitting joint effusion.
- **Therapeutic.** Instill steroids, maintain drainage of septic arthritis; relief of tense hemarthrosis or effusion.

Contraindications Cellulitis at injection site. Relative contraindication: bleeding disorder; caution if coagulopathy or thrombocytopenia is present or if the patient is receiving anticoagulants.

Materials
- Minor procedure tray (18- or 20-gauge needle; smaller for finger or toe).
- Ethyl chloride spray can be substituted for lidocaine.
- Two heparinized tubes for cell count and crystal examination.
- Note microbiology laboratory preference for transporting fluid for bacterial, fungal, acid-fast bacillus (AFB) culture, and Gram's stain; Thayer–Martin plate used for *Neisseria gonorrhoeae*.
- A syringe containing a long-acting corticosteroid such as methylprednisolone (Depo-Medrol) or triamcinolone is optional for therapeutic arthrocentesis.

Procedures, General
1. Obtain informed consent after describing the procedure and complications.
2. Determine the optimal site for aspiration (see next section), identify landmarks, and mark site with indentation or sterile marking pen. Avoid injection of tendons.
3. If aspiration is followed by corticosteroid injection, maintaining a sterile field with sterile implements minimizes infection.
4. Clean the area with povidone–iodine, dry, and wipe over the aspiration site with alcohol. Povidone–iodine can render cultures negative. Let the alcohol dry before beginning procedure.
5. Anesthetize the puncture site with lidocaine by using a 25-gauge needle; do **not** inject into the joint space; lidocaine is

bactericidal. Avoid Lidocaine preparations with epinephrine, especially in a digit. Alternatively, spray the area with ethyl chloride ("freeze spray") just before needle aspiration.

6. Insert the aspirating needle after applying a small amount of vacuum to the syringe. When the capsule is entered, fluid usually flows easily. Remove as much fluid as possible and reposition the syringe if necessary.

7. If corticosteroid is to be injected, remove the aspirating syringe from the needle, which is still in the joint space. (*Note:* Ensure that the syringe can easily be removed from the needle before step 6.) Attach the syringe containing corticosteroid, pull back on the plunger to ensure you are not in a vein, and inject contents. Never inject steroids when there is any possibility of an infected joint. Remove the needle and apply pressure to the area (leakage of subcutaneous steroids can lead to localized atrophy of the skin). In general, the equivalent of methylprednisolone 40 mg is injected into large joints such as the knee and 20 mg into medium-size joints such as the ankle or wrist. Warn the patient that a postinjection "flare" (pain several hours later) is managed with ice and nonsteroidal anti-inflammatory drugs.

8. Note volume aspirated from joint. The knee typically contains 3.5 mL of synovial fluid; in inflammatory, septic, or hemorrhagic arthritis, volumes can be larger. A bedside test for viscosity is to allow a drop of fluid to fall from the tip of the needle. Normal synovial fluid is highly viscous and forms a several-inch long string; decreased viscosity is seen in infection. A **mucin clot test** (normally forms in <1 minute; delayed result suggests inflammation), once a standard test for rheumatoid arthritis, is not currently routinely performed.

9. Joint fluid is usually sent for:
   - Cell count and differential (purple or green top tube).
   - Microscopic crystal examination using polarized light microscopy (purple or green top tube); **normally** no debris, crystals, or bacteria are seen; urate crystals are present with gout; calcium pyrophosphate in pseudogout.
   - Glucose (red top tube).
   - Gram's stain, and cultures for bacteria, fungi, and AFB as indicated (check with your laboratory or deliver immediately in a sterile tube with no additives).
   - Cytology if a malignant effusion is suspected clinically.

Arthrocentesis of the Knee (Figure III–7A)

1. Fully extended the knee with the patient supine. Wait until the patient has a relaxed quadriceps muscle because its contraction approximates the patella against the femur, making aspiration painful.

2. Insert the needle posterior to the *lateral* portion of the patella into the patellar-femoral groove. Direct the advancing needle slightly posteriorly and inferiorly

Arthrocentesis of the Wrist (Figure III–7B)

- The easiest site for aspiration is between the navicular bone and radius on the dorsal wrist. Locate the distal radius between the tendons of the extensor pollicis longus and the extensor carpi radialis longus to the second finger. This site is just ulnar to the anatomic snuff box. Direct the needle perpendicular to the mark.

Arthrocentesis of the Ankle (Figure III–7C)

1. The most accessible site is between the tibia and the talus. Position the angle of the foot to leg at 90 degrees. Make a mark lateral and anterior to the medial malleolus and medial

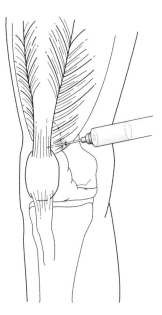

Figure III–7. A: Arthrocentesis of the knee. **B:** Arthrocentesis of the wrist. **C:** Arthrocentesis of the ankle. *(Reproduced, with permission, from Haist SA, Robbins JB, eds. Internal Medicine On Call, 4th ed. Copyright (c) 2005 by The McGraw-Hill Companies, Inc.)*

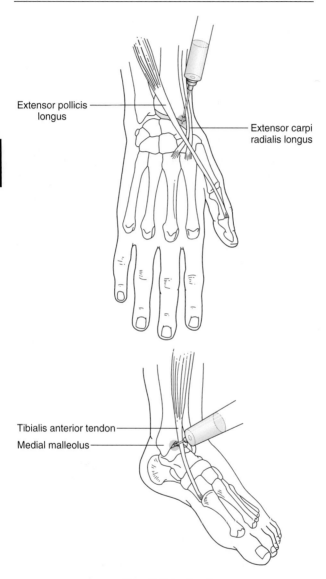

Extensor pollicis longus

Extensor carpi radialis longus

Tibialis anterior tendon

Medial malleolus

Figure III–7. *(continued)*

and posterior to the tibialis anterior tendon. Direct the advancing needle posteriorly toward the heel.

2. The **subtalar ankle joint** does not communicate with the ankle joint and is difficult to aspirate even by an expert. Be aware that "ankle pain" may originate in the subtalar joint rather than in the ankle.

Synovial Fluid Interpretation

Noninflammatory arthritis: Osteoarthritis, traumatic, aseptic necrosis, osteochondritis desiccans

Inflammatory arthritis: Gout (usually associated with increased serum uric acid), pseudogout, rheumatoid arthritis, rheumatic fever, collagen–vascular disease

Septic arthritis: Pyogenic bacterial (*Staphylococcus aureus*, *N gonorrhoeae*, and *Staphylococcus epidermidis* are most common), tuberculosis.

Hemorrhagic: Hemophilia or other bleeding diathesis, trauma, with or without fracture.

Complications Complications are infection, bleeding, and pain. Postinjection flare of joint pain and swelling can occur after steroid injection and may persist for up to 24 hours. This complication is felt to be a crystal-induced synovitis due to the crystalline suspension used in long-acting steroids.

Lumbar Puncture (LP)

Indications
- **Diagnostic purposes:** Analysis of cerebrospinal fluid (CSF) for conditions such as meningitis, encephalitis, Guillain-Barré syndrome, staging work-up for lymphoma, and others.
- Measurement of CSF pressure or its changes with various maneuvers (Valsalva, etc).
- **Injection of various agents:** Contrast medium for myelography, antitumor drugs, analgesics, and antibiotics.

Contraindications
- Increased intracranial pressure (papilledema, mass lesion)
- Infection near the puncture site
- Planned myelography or pneumoencephalography
- Coagulation disorders

Materials
- A sterile, disposable LP kit
  or
- Minor procedure tray
- Spinal needles (21-gauge for adults, 22-gauge for children)

Background The objective of an LP is to obtain a sample of CSF from the subarachnoid space. Specifically, during an LP the fluid is obtained from the **lumbar cistern,** the CSF located between the termination of the spinal cord (conus medullaris) and the termination of the dura mater at the coccygeal ligament. The cistern is surrounded by the subarachnoid membrane and the overlying dura. Located within the cistern are the filum terminale and the nerve roots of the cauda equina. When an LP is done, the main body of the spinal cord is avoided and the nerve roots of the cauda are simply pushed out of the way by the needle. The termination of the spinal cord in the adult is usually between L_1 and L_2, and in the pediatric patient between L_2 and L_3. The safest site for an LP is the interspace between L_4 and L_5. An imaginary line drawn between the iliac crests (the supracristal plane) intersects the spine at the L_4 spinous process or the L_4–L_5 interspace. A spinal needle introduced between the spinous processes of L_4 and L_5 penetrates the layers in the following order: skin, supraspinous ligament, interspinous ligament, ligamentum flava, epidural space (contains loose areolar tissue, fat, and blood vessels), dura, "potential space," subarachnoid membrane, and subarachnoid space (lumbar cistern).

Technique
1. Examine the fundus for evidence of papilledema and review the computed tomogram or magnetic resonance image of the head, if available. Discuss the relative safety and lack of discomfort to the patient to dispel any myths. Some clinicians prefer to call the procedure a "subarachnoid analysis" rather than a spinal tap. As long as the procedure and the risks are outlined, most patients will agree to the procedure. Have the patient sign an informed consent form.
2. Place the patient in the lateral decubitus position close to the edge of the bed or table. The patient (held by an assistant, if possible) should be positioned with knees pulled up toward stomach and head flexed onto chest. This position enhances flexion of the vertebral spine and widens the interspaces between the spinous processes. Place a pillow beneath the patient's side to prevent sagging and ensure alignment of the spinal column. In an obese patient or a patient with arthritis or scoliosis, the sitting position, ie, leaning forward, may be preferred.
3. Palpate the supracristal plane (see under Background) and carefully determine the location of the L_4–L_5 interspace.
4. Open the kit, put on sterile gloves, and prep the area with povidone–iodine solution in a circular fashion to cover several interspaces. Next, drape the patient.
5. With a 25-gauge needle and lidocaine, raise a skin wheal over the L_4–L_5 interspace. Anesthetize the deeper structures with a 22-gauge needle.

6. Examine the spinal needle with a stylet for defects and then insert it into the skin wheal and into the spinous ligament. Hold the needle between your index and middle fingers, with your thumb holding the stylet in place. Direct the needle cephalad at a 30- to 45-degree angle in the midline and parallel to the bed.

7. Advance through the major structures and pop into the subarachnoid space through the dura. An experienced operator can feel these layers, but an inexperienced one may need to periodically remove the stylet to look for return of fluid. It is important to always replace the stylet before advancing the spinal needle. The needle may be withdrawn, however, with the stylet removed. This technique may be useful if the needle has passed through the back wall of the canal. Direct the bevel of the needle parallel to the long axis of the body so that the dural fibers are separated rather than sheared. This method helps cut down on "spinal headaches."

8. If no fluid returns, it is sometimes helpful to rotate the needle slightly. If still no fluid appears, and you think that you are within the subarachnoid space, inject air 1 mL because it is not uncommon for a piece of tissue to clog the needle. **Never** inject saline or distilled water. If no air returns and if spinal fluid cannot be aspirated, the bevel of the needle probably lies in the epidural space; advance it with the stylet in place.

9. When fluid returns, attach a manometer and stopcock and measure the pressure. Normal opening pressure is 70–180 mm of water in the lateral position. Increased pressure may be due to a tense patient, congestive heart failure, ascites, subarachnoid hemorrhage, infection, or a space-occupying lesion. Decreased pressure may be due to needle position or obstructed flow (you may need to leave the needle in for a myelogram because if it is moved, the subarachnoid space may be lost).

10. Collect 0.5- to 2.0-mL samples in serial, labeled containers. Send them to the laboratory in this order:
    - **First tube for bacteriology:** Gram's stain, routine culture and sensitivity (C&S), AFB, and fungal cultures and stains
    - **Second tube for glucose and protein:** In addition, if multiple sclerosis is suspected, order electrophoresis to detect oligoclonal banding and assay for myelin basic protein
    - **Third tube for cell count:** Complete blood cell count with differential
    - **Fourth tube for special studies as clinically indicated:** Venereal Disease Research Laboratory (neurosyphilis), counterimmunoelectrophoresis for bacterial antigens such as *Haemophilus influenzae*, *Streptococcus pneumoniae*, and *Neisseria meningitidis*, polymerase chain reaction assay for tuberculous meningitis or herpes simplex en-

cephalitis (allows rapid diagnosis). If *Cryptococcus neoformans* is suspected (most common cause of meningitis in patients who have acquired immunodeficiency syndrome), India ink preparation and cryptococcal antigen (latex agglutination test) should be used.

Note: Some clinicians prefer to send the first and last tubes for a complete blood cell count because this procedure permits a better differentiation between a **subarachnoid hemorrhage** and a **traumatic tap.** In a traumatic tap, the number of red blood cells in the first tube should be much larger than that in the last tube. In a subarachnoid hemorrhage, the cell counts should be equal, and **xanthochromia** of the fluid should be present, indicating the presence of old blood.

11. Withdraw the needle and place a dry, sterile dressing over the site.
12. Instruct the patient to remain recumbent for 6–12 hours and encourage an increased fluid intake to help prevent "spinal headaches."
13. Interpret the results (Table III–2).

TABLE III–2. DIFFERENTIAL DIAGNOSIS OF CEREBROSPINAL FLUID

Condition	Color	Opening Pressure (mmH$_2$O)	Protein (mg/100 mL)	Glucose (mg/100 mL)	Cells (#/mL)
Adult (normal)	Clear	70–180	15–45	45–80	0–5 lymphs
Newborn (normal)	Clear	70–180	20–120	2/3 serum glucose	40–60 lymphs
Viral infection	Clear or opalescent	Normal or slightly increased	Normal or slightly increased	Normal	10–500 lymphs (polys early)
Bacterial infection	Opalescent or yellow, may clot	Increased	50–1500	Lower, usually <20	25–10,000 polys
Granulomatous (TB, fungal)	Clear or opalescent	Often lower	Higher, but usually <500	Lower, usually 20–40	10–500 lymphs
Subarachnoid hemorrhage	Bloody or xanthochromic after 2–8 h	Usually lower	Higher	Normal	WBC/RBC ratio same as blood

RBC = red blood cell; TB = tuberculosis; WBC = white blood cell.

Complications
- **Spinal headache:** This is the most common complication (about 20%) and appears within the first 24 h after. It is relieved when the patient is lying down and is aggravated when the patient sits up. It is characterized by a severe throbbing pain in the occipital region and can last a week. It is thought to be caused by intracranial traction caused by the acute volume depletion of CSF and by persistent leakage from the puncture site. To help prevent spinal headaches, keep the patient recumbent for 6–12 hours, encourage the intake of fluids, use the smallest needle possible, and keep the bevel of the needle parallel to the long axis of the body to help prevent a persistent CSF leak. If the headache persists, a blood patch (peripheral blood injected into the epidural space, usually performed by anesthesia service) may be needed to seal the leak.
- **Trauma to nerve roots or to the conus medullaris:** Much less frequent (some anatomic variation does exist, but it is very rare for the cord to end below L_3). If the patient suddenly complains of paresthesia (numbness or shooting pains in the legs), stop the procedure.
- **Herniation of either the cerebellum or the medulla:** Occurs rarely, during or after a spinal tap, usually in a patient with increased intracranial pressure. This complication can often be reversed medically if it is recognized early.
- **Meningitis.**
- Bleeding in the subarachnoid/subdural space can occur with resulting paralysis especially if the patient is receiving anticoagulants or has severe liver disease with a coagulopathy.

Paracentesis

Indications
- To determine the cause of ascites
- To determine if intra-abdominal bleeding is present or if a viscus has ruptured (diagnostic peritoneal lavage is considered a more accurate test; see preceding procedure)
- Therapeutic removal of fluid when distention is pronounced or respiratory distress is associated with it (acute treatment only)

Contraindications
- Abnormal coagulation factors
- Bowel obstruction, pregnancy
- Uncertainty if distention is due to peritoneal fluid or to a cystic structure (ultrasound can usually differentiate)

Materials
- Minor procedure tray
- Catheter-over-needle assembly (Angiocath Autoguard, Insyte Autoguard, 18–20 gauge with a 1½-inch needle)

- 20- to 60-mL syringe
- Sterile specimen containers

Procedure Peritoneal paracentesis is surgical puncture of the peritoneal cavity for the aspiration of fluid. Ascites is indicated by abdominal distention, shifting dullness, and a palpable fluid wave.

1. Explain the procedure and have the patient sign an informed consent form. Have the patient empty the bladder, or place a Foley catheter if voiding is impossible or if significant mental status changes are present.
2. The entry site is usually the midline 3–4 cm below the umbilicus. Avoid old surgical scars because the bowel may be adhering to the abdominal wall. Alternatively, the entry site can be in the left or right lower quadrant midway between the umbilicus and the anterior superior iliac spine or in the patient's flank, depending on the percussion of the fluid wave. Avoid the rectus abdominus due to bleeding potential. Ultrasound may be used to mark out a site where free fluid appears under the abdominal wall and where no bowel loops are present. If the patient moves, ultrasound must be repeated because the abdominal contents will shift.
3. Prep and drape the area and raise a skin wheal with lidocaine over the entry site.
4. A "Z" track technique will help limit persistent leakage of peritoneal fluid after the tap. Manually retract the skin caudally and release traction on the skin when the peritoneum is entered. With the catheter mounted on the syringe, go through the anesthetized area while aspirating. There is resistance as the fascia is entered. When you get free return of fluid, leave the catheter in place, remove the needle or activate the self-shielding mechanism. Begin to aspirate; reposition the catheter because of abutting bowel as needed.
5. Aspirate the amount of fluid needed for tests (20–30 mL). If the tap is therapeutic, 10–15 L can be safely removed. The removal of a large volume can be facilitated by the use of vacuum container bottles (500 mL–1 L) supplied at most hospitals. Tubing is first connected to the catheter and then to the vacuum container bottles.
6. Apply a sterile, 4 × 4 gauze square and apply pressure with tape.
7. Depending on the clinical picture of the patient, send samples for cell count including differential, total protein, albumin, amylase, lactate dehydrogenase, glucose, cytology, culture, and stains.

Complications Peritonitis, perforated viscus (bowel, bladder), hemorrhage, precipitation of hepatic coma if patient has severe liver disease, oliguria, hypotension.

Diagnosis of Ascitic Fluid The older classification of ascitic fluid as transudative or exudative is no longer used. The etiology of ascites is found more likely to be found by determining the serum to ascites albumin gradient. See Table III–3 to interpret the results of ascitic fluid analysis.

Pericardiocentesis

Indications
- Emergency treatment of cardiac tamponade
- Diagnose cause of pericardial effusion

Contraindications
- Minimal pericardial effusion (<200 mL)
- After coronary artery bypass grafting due to risk of injury to grafts
- Uncorrected coagulopathy

Materials
- Electrocardiographic machine
- Prepackaged pericardiocentesis kit **or** procedure and instrument tray with pericardiocentesis needle or 16- to 18-gauge needle 10 cm long

Background Cardiac tamponade results in decreased cardiac output, increased right atrial filling pressures, and a pronounced pulsus paradoxus.

TABLE III–3. DIFFERENTIAL DIAGNOSIS OF ASCITIC FLUID.
TRANSUDATIVE ASCITES: CIRRHOSIS, NEPHROSIS, CONGESTIVE HEART FAILURE. **EXUDATIVE ASCITES:** MALIGNANCY, PERITONITIS (TB, PERFORATED VISCUS), HYPOALBUMINEMIA.

Lab Value	Transudate	Exudate
Specific gravity	<1.016	>1.016
Protein (ascitic fluid)	<3 g/100 mL	> 3 g/100 mL
Protein (ascitic to serum ratio)	<0.5	>0.5
LDH (ascitic to serum ratio)	<0.6	>0.6
Ascitic fluid LDH	<200 IU	>200 IU
Glucose (serum to ascitic ratio)	<1	>1
Fibrinogen (clot)	No	Yes
White blood cells	<500/μL	>1000/μL
Red blood cells		>100/μL

[a]Food fibers: Found in most causes of a perforated viscus. Cytology: Bizarre cells with large nuclei may represent reactive mesothelial cells and not a malignancy; malignant cells suggest a tumor. LDH = lactate dehydrogenase; TB = tuberculosis.

Procedure

1. If time permits, use sterile prep and draping with gown, mask, and gloves.
2. Draining the pericardium can be approached through the left paraxiphoid or the left parasternal fourth intercostal space. The paraxiphoid is safer, more commonly used, and described here (Figure III–8).
3. Anesthetize the insertion site with lidocaine. Connect the needle with an alligator clip to a chest lead (brown) on the electrocardiographic machine. Attach the limb leads and monitor the machine.
4. Insert the pericardiocentesis needle just to the left of the xiphoid and directed upward 45 degrees toward the left shoulder.

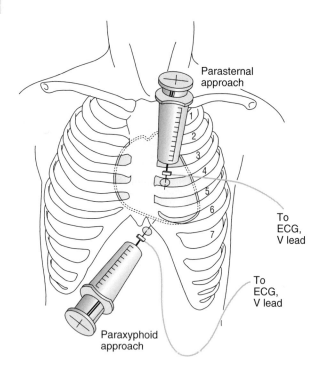

Figure III–8. Techniques for pericardiocentesis. The paraxiphoid approach is the most popular. *(Reproduced, with permission, from Stillman RM, ed.* Surgery, Diagnosis, and Therapy. *Originally published by Appleton & Lange. Copyright (c) 1989 by The McGraw-Hill Companies, Inc.)*

5. Aspirate while advancing the needle until the pericardium is punctured and the effusion is tapped. If the ventricular wall is felt, withdraw the needle slightly. In addition, if the needle contacts the myocardium, pronounced ST-segment elevation will be noted on the electrocardiogram.

6. If performed for cardiac tamponade, removal of as little as 50 mL of fluid dramatically decreases blood pressure and right atrial pressure.

7. Blood from a bloody pericardial effusion is usually defibrinated and will not clot, whereas blood from the ventricle will clot.

8. Send fluid for hematocrit, cell count, or cytology if indicated.
   - **Serous fluid:** Consistent with congestive heart failure, bacterial infection, tuberculosis, hypoalbuminemia, or viral pericarditis.
   - **Bloody fluid (hematocrit >10%):** May result from trauma; be iatrogenic; or due to myocardial infarction, uremia, coagulopathy, or malignancy (lymphoma, leukemia, breast, lung most common).

9. If continuous drainage is necessary, use a guidewire to place a 16-gauge IV catheter and connect to a closed drainage system.

Complications Arrhythmia, ventricular puncture, lung injury.

Peripherally Inserted Central Catheter (PICC Line)

Indications
- Home infusion of hypertonic or irritating solutions and drugs
- Long-term infusion of medications (antibiotics, chemotherapeutics)
- Total parenteral nutrition
- Repetitive venous blood sampling

Contraindications
- Infection over placement site
- Failure to identify veins in an arm with a tourniquet in place

Materials
- PICC catheter kit (contains most items necessary including the silastic long-arm line, eg, Introsyte Autoguard system)
- Tourniquet, sterile gloves, mask, sterile gown, heparin flush, 10-mL syringes

Background Installation of a PICC allows for central venous access through a peripheral vein. Typically, a long-arm catheter is placed into the basilic or cephalic vein and is threaded into the subclavian vein/superior vena cava. PICCs are useful for long-term home infusion therapies. The design of PICC catheters can vary, and the operator should be familiar with the features of the device (attached hub or detachable hub designs).

Procedure

1. Explain the procedure to the patient and then obtain informed consent. Position the patient in a sitting or reclining position with the elbow extended and the arm in a dependent position. The arm should be externally rotated.

2. Using a measuring tape, determine the length of the catheter required. Measure from the extremity vein insertion site to the subclavian vein.

3. Wear mask, gown, protective eyewear, and sterile gloves. Prep and drape the skin in the standard fashion. Set up an adjacent sterile working area.

4. Anesthetize the skin at the proposed area of insertion. Apply a tourniquet above the proposed IV site.

5. Trim the catheter to the appropriate length. Most PICC lines have an attached hub, and the distal end of the catheter is cut to the proper length. Flush with heparinized saline.

6. Insert the catheter and introducer needle (usually 14-gauge) into the chosen arm vein as detailed in the section on IV techniques (page 357). Once the catheter is in the vein, push the white button on the Introsyte device to shield the needle. Discard the needle assembly.

7. Place the PICC line in the catheter and advance (use a forceps if provided by the manufacturer of the kit to advance the PICC line). Remove the tourniquet and gradually advance the catheter the requisite length. Remove the inner stiffening wire slowly once the catheter has been adequately advanced.

8. Peel away the introducer catheter. Attach the Luer-lock and flush the catheter again with heparin solution. Attempt to also aspirate blood to verify patency.

9. Attach the provided securing wings and suture in place. Apply a sterile dressing over the insertion site.

10. Confirm placement in the central circulation with a chest radiograph. Always document the type of PICC, the length inserted, and the site of its radiologically confirmed placement.

11. If vein cannulation is difficult, a surgical cutdown may be necessary to cannulate the vein. If the catheter will not advance, fluoroscopy may be helpful.

12. Instruct the patient on the maintenance of the PICC, The PICC should be flushed with heparinized saline after each use. Dressing changes should be performed at least every 7 days under sterile conditions. Patient must be instructed to evaluate the PICC site for signs and symptoms of infection. Patient must also be instructed to come to the emergency room for evaluation of any fevers.

13. For venous samples, a specimen of at least the catheter volume (1–3 mL) must first be withdrawn and then discarded. The PICC must always be flushed with heparinized saline after each blood draw.

PICC Removal
1. Position the patient's arm at a 90-degree angle to his body. Remove the dressing and gently pull the PICC out.
2. Apply pressure to site for 2–3 minutes. Always measure the length of the catheter and check prior documentation to ensure that the PICC line has been removed in its entirety. If a piece of a catheter is left behind, an emergency interventional radiology consult is in order.

Complications Site bleeding, clotted catheter, subclavian thrombosis, infection, broken catheter (leakage or embolization), and arrhythmia (the catheter is inserted too far).

Peritoneal Lavage

Indications
- **Diagnostic peritoneal lavage** is used in the evaluation of intra-abdominal trauma (bleeding, perforation). (*Note:* Spiral computed tomography of the abdomen has largely replaced this as an initial screening for intra-abdominal trauma in the emergency setting.)
- Acute peritoneal dialysis and management of severe pancreatitis.

Contraindications
- None are absolute. Relative contraindications include multiple abdominal procedures, pregnancy, known retroperitoneal injury (high false-positive rates) cirrhosis, morbid obesity, and any coagulopathy.

Materials
- Prepackaged diagnostic peritoneal lavage or peritoneal dialysis tray

Procedure
1. A Foley catheter and an NG or orogastric tube **must** be in place. Prep the abdomen from above the umbilicus to the pubis.
2. The site of choice is in the midline 1–2 cm below the umbilicus. Avoid the site of old surgical scars (danger of adherent bowel). If an infraumbilical scar or pelvic fracture is present, then a supraumbilical approach is recommended.

3. Infiltrate the skin with lidocaine with epinephrine. Incise the skin in the midline vertically and expose the fascia.
4. Pick up the fascia and incise it or puncture it with the trocar and peritoneal catheter. Caution is needed to avoid puncturing any organs. Use 1 hand to hold the catheter near the skin and to control the insertion while using the other hand to apply pressure to the end of the catheter. After entering the peritoneal cavity, remove the trocar and direct the catheter inferiorly into the pelvis.
5. During a diagnostic lavage, gross blood indicates a positive tap. If no blood is encountered, instill lactated Ringer's solution or normal saline 10 mL/kg (about 1 L in adults) into the abdominal cavity.
6. Gently agitate the abdomen to distribute the fluid and after 5 minutes drain off as much fluid as possible into a bag on the floor. (Minimum fluid for a valid analysis is 200 mL in an adult.) If the drainage is slow, try instilling additional fluid while carefully repositioning the catheter.
7. Send the fluid for analysis (amylase, bile, bacteria, hematocrit, and cell count). See Table III–4 for interpretation.
8. Remove the catheter and suture the skin. If the catheter is inserted for pancreatitis or peritoneal dialysis, suture the catheter in place.
9. A negative diagnostic peritoneal lavage does not rule out retroperitoneal trauma. A false-positive diagnostic peritoneal

TABLE III–4. DIAGNOSTIC PERITONEAL LAVAGE FINDINGS THAT SUGGEST INTRA-ABDOMINAL TRAUMA.

Positive	>20 mL gross blood on free aspiration (10 mL in children)
	≥100,000 RBC/mL
	≥500 WBC/mL (if obtained >3 h after injury)
	≥175 U amylase/dL
	Bacteria on Gram's stain
	Bile (by inspection or chemical determination of bilirubin contents)
	Food particles (microscopic analysis of strained or spun specimen)
Intermediate	Pink fluid on free aspiration
	50,000–100,000 RBC/mL in blunt trauma
	100–500 WBC/mL
	75–175 U amylase/dL
Negative	Clear aspirate
	≤100 WBC/μL
	≤75 U amylase/dL

RBC = red blood cells; WBC = white blood cells.
Source: (Reprinted, with permission, from: Way, L., Doherty GM, eds. Current Surgical Diagnosis and Treatment, 11th ed. McGraw-Hill, 2003.

lavage can be caused by a pelvic fracture or bleeding induced by the procedure (eg, laceration of an omental vessel).

Complications Infection/peritonitis or superficial wound infection, bleeding, perforated viscus (bladder, bowel).

Pulmonary Artery Catheterization (See also Section I, Problem 62, page 217)

Indications
1. Acute heart failure.
2. Complex circulatory and fluid conditions (burn patients, patients in shock).
3. Diagnosis of cardiac tamponade.
4. Perioperative management (elderly or debilitated patients, patients with severe cardiac or pulmonary diseases).

Materials Central venous catheter equipment; a flow-directed balloon-tipped catheter (aka Swan-Ganz catheter); a 7F catheter with thermistor or pulse oximetry port is most frequently used in adults (Figure III–9A); a sheath, a dilator, a no. 11 blade, and guidewires for catheter insertion (usually supplied as a kit, such as Cordis or Arrow Introducer Kit); connecting tubing; a transducer and monitor; heparin flush solution (1 U heparin/mL normal saline); pressure bags; an electrocardiographic monitor; a crash cart; and rapid access to lidocaine 100-mg bolus for IV use.

Procedure
1. Informed consent is needed. The patient must be on an electrocardiographic monitor, have a working IV in place, and the crash cart should be nearby, because arrhythmias are a frequent complication. Coagulation profile should ideally be normal. Placement may be contraindicated for patients with second-degree heart block.
2. Gown, gloves, mask, cap, and a wide sterile field are needed.
3. Remove the pulmonary artery catheter from the package, place it on a sterile field, and flush all the lumens with heparinized saline. Balance the transducer at the reference point of the midaxillary line with the patient supine. Connect all ports to the monitoring lines. Check the function of the transducer by gently flicking the tip and observing oscillation on the monitor.
4. Check the flow balloon at the end of the catheter by gently inflating with air 1.5 mL (for a 7F catheter). Some operators check the balloon in a cup of sterile water for leaks. If there is the possibility of a left-to-right shunt, carbon dioxide is suggested for inflation. Liquid should not be used to inflate the balloon.

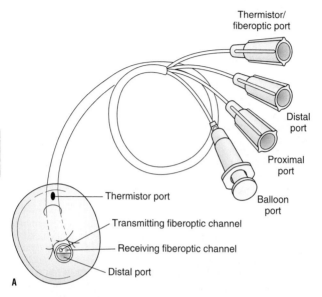

Thermistor/
fiberoptic port

Distal
port

Proximal
port

Thermistor port

Transmitting fiberoptic channel

Receiving fiberoptic channel

Balloon
port

Distal port

A

Figure III–9. A: Example of a pulmonary artery catheter with an oximetric measuring feature. *(Reproduced, with permission, from Gomella LG, ed.* Clinician's Pocket Reference, *10th ed. Copyright (c) 2004 by The McGraw-Hill Companies, Inc.)* **B:** Positioning and pressure waveforms seen as the pulmonary artery catheter is advanced. *(Reproduced, with permission, from Stillman RM, ed.* Surgery, Diagnosis, and Therapy. *Originally published by Appleton & Lange. Copyright (c) 1989 by The McGraw–Hill Companies, Inc.)*

5. Obtain access to a central vein as described in "Central Venous Catheter Placement" by using a guidewire technique. The subclavian access is usually preferred because of the ease of securing the catheter to the relatively flat upper chest wall. The internal jugular and antecubital routes are also acceptable. Avoid the femoral vein, if possible, because of the increased risk of infection and an embolism.

6. Place the guidewire in the introducer set at least halfway into the vein. The patient must be monitored continuously during the procedure because arrhythmia, most frequently ventricular, may occur.

7. Mount the dilator inside the introducer, nick the skin with a no. 11 blade, and advance the assembly slowly over the guidewire.

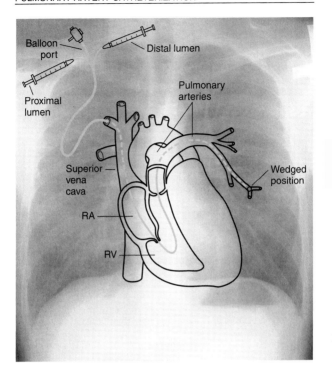

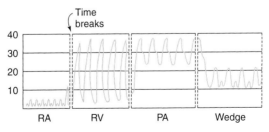

Figure III–9. (continued)

8. Flush the pulmonary artery catheter ports with heparinized saline one more time to remove air bubbles. Remove the guidewire and dilator and leave the introducer in position. Place a finger over the end of the introducer to prevent excessive bleeding or an air embolus. Mount a telescoping clear plastic contamination guard, if necessary, to the hub of the introducer. A rubber gasket assembly usually prevents excessive bleeding before the time the catheter is threaded into the introducer. This guard allows the catheter to be adjusted over a range of approximately 20 cm under sterile conditions after the catheter has been positioned.

9. Slowly advance the catheter to approximately the right atrium. Follow the characteristic patterns as the catheter is advanced (Figure III–9B). Most catheters have markings every 10 cm. The reference lengths to the right atrium are as follows: right internal jugular or subclavian, 10–20 cm; left internal jugular or subclavian, 20–30 cm; left or right antecubital vein, 40–50 cm; left or right femoral vein, 30 cm.

10. While at the approximate level of the right atrium, slowly inflate the balloon of the 7F catheter with air 1.5 mL (0.8 mL for the 5F catheter). Advance the catheter and observe the pressure tracing (Figure III–9B) on the oscilloscope from the distal port to follow the catheter tip as it flows through the right ventricle and out the pulmonary artery. Do not hesitate if ventricular ectopy is seen. Rapidly pass the catheter through the ventricle and use IV lidocaine (50- to 100-mg IV bolus) if the ectopy persists. Once at the pulmonary artery, advance the catheter 10–20 cm farther to obtain the wedge pressure. If multiple attempts fail to successfully pass the catheter out of the pulmonary artery, fluoroscopy may be needed.

TABLE III–5. NORMAL PULMONARY ARTERY CATHETER MEASUREMENTS.

Parameter	Range
Right atrial pressure	1–7 mm Hg
Right ventricular systolic pressure	15–25 mm Hg
Right ventricular diastolic pressure	0–8 mm Hg
Pulmonary artery systolic pressure	15–25 mm Hg
Pulmonary artery diastolic pressure	8–15 mm Hg
Pulmonary artery mean pressure	10–20 mm Hg
Pulmonary capillary wedge pressure	6–12 mm Hg
Systemic vascular resistance[a]	900–1200 dynes/s/cm^5
Cardiac output	3.5–5.5 L/min
Cardiac index	2.8–3.2 L/min

[a][(mean arterial pressure − central venous pressure) × 80]/cardiac output.

11. Deflate the balloon, and the pulmonary artery tracing should reappear. Adjust the catheter as needed so that this pattern is reproduced. **Never** leave the balloon inflated continuously, as pulmonary infarction or an arterial rupture may occur. **Never** leave the balloon inflated while pulling the catheter back. The pulmonary artery tracing should be observed at all times unless the balloon is inflated.

12. Suture the introducer and pulmonary artery catheter in position with 2-0 silk. If there is a contamination shield, extend it about halfway to allow the catheter to be moved, should repositioning be needed.

13. Dress the site with povidone-iodine and gauze or transparent shield dressing (eg, Op-Site).

14. Obtain an immediate portable chest radiograph to verify the proper catheter position and to rule out a pneumothorax. A properly positioned pulmonary artery catheter should follow a smooth curve, and the tip of the catheter should not be farther than 5 cm from the midline and most often in the right pulmonary artery.

15. Normal pulmonary artery parameters are listed in Table III–5, and diagnosis of conditions associated with certain readings are listed in Table III–6.

Complications All complications are associated with central venous catheter placement (see page 340), arrhythmia, pulmonary artery rupture or pulmonary infarction, knotting of catheter or rupture of the balloon, sepsis, and complete heart block.

TABLE III–6. DIFFERENTIAL DIAGNOSIS OF COMMON PULMONARY ARTERY CATHETER READINGS.

Low right atrial pressure: Volume depletion
High right atrial pressure: Volume overload, congestive heart failure, cardiogenic shock, increased pulmonary vascular resistance (hypoxia, ventilator effects of PEEP, pulmonary disease, primary pulmonary hypertension)
Low right ventricular pressures: Volume depletion
High right ventricular pressures: Volume overload, congestive heart failure, cardiogenic shock, increased pulmonary vascular resistance (see above)
High pulmonary artery pressure: Congestive heart failure, increased pulmonary vascular resistance (hypoxia, ventilator effect of PEEP, pulmonary disease), cardiac tamponade
Low wedge pressure: Volume depletion
High wedge pressure: Cardiogenic shock, left ventricular failure, ventricular septal defect, mitral regurgitation and stenosis, severe hypertension, volume overload, cardiac tamponade

PEEP = positive end-expiratory pressure.

Sigmoidoscopy

Indications
1. Workup of gastrointestinal tract bleeding or lower gastrointestinal tract symptoms.
2. Evaluation of trauma.

Materials Gloves, lubricant, Hemoccult paper and developer, sigmoidoscope and light source, an insufflation bag, tissues, long (rectal) swabs and a suction catheter, a proctologic examination table (not essential).

Procedure
1. Enemas and cathartics are not given routinely before sigmoidoscopy, although some clinicians prefer to give a mild prep, such as a Fleet's Enema, just before the examination. Explain the procedure and have the patient sign an informed consent form.
2. Sigmoidoscopy can be performed with the patient in bed lying on his side in the knee-to-chest position, but the best results are obtained with the patient in the "jackknife" position on the proctologic table. Do not position the patient until all materials are at hand and you are ready to start.
3. Converse with the patient to create distraction and to relieve apprehension. Announce each maneuver in advance. Put on gloves before proceeding.
4. Observe the anal region for skin tags, hemorrhoids, fissures, etc. Do a careful rectal examination and a Hemoccult test with a gloved finger using plenty of lubricant.
5. Lubricate the sigmoidoscope well and insert it with the obturator in place. Aim toward the patient's umbilicus initially. Advance 2–3 cm past the internal sphincter and remove the obturator.
6. Always advance under direct vision and make sure that the lumen is always visible (Figure III–10). Insufflation (introducing air) may be used to help visualize the lumen, but remember this may be painful to the patient. It is necessary to follow the curve of the sigmoid toward the sacrum by directing the scope more posteriorly toward the back. A change from a smooth mucosa to concentric rings indicates entry into the sigmoid colon. The scope should reach 15 cm with ease. Use suction and the rectal swabs as needed to clear the way.
7. At this point, the sigmoid curves to the patient's left. Warn the patient that a cramping sensation may be felt. If you ever have difficulty negotiating a curve, **do not force the scope.**
8. After advancing as far as possible, slowly remove the scope; use a small rotary motion to view all surfaces. Observation here is critical. Remember to release the air from the colon before withdrawing the scope.

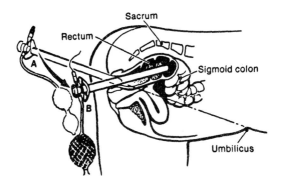

Figure III–10. The sigmoidoscope is advanced under direct vision as shown. *(Reproduced, with permission, from Gomella LG, ed.* Clinician's Pocket Reference, *8th ed. Copyright (c) 1997 by Appleton & Lange.)*

9. Inform the patient that mild cramping may be experienced after the procedure.

Complications Bleeding, perforation, abdominal cramping.

Thoracentesis

Indications
- Determining the cause of a pleural effusion
- Therapeutically removing pleural fluid in the event of respiratory distress
- Aspirating small pneumothoraces where the risk of recurrence is small (ie, postoperative without lung injury)
- Instilling sclerosing compounds (eg, tetracycline) to obliterate the pleural space

Contraindications
- None is absolute (pneumothorax, hemothorax, or any major respiratory impairment on the contralateral side, or coagulopathy).

Materials
- Prepackaged thoracentesis kit with needle or catheter (preferred)
  or
- Minor procedure tray
- 20- to 60-mL syringe, 20- or 22-gauge needle 1½-inch needle, 3-way stopcock
- Specimen containers

Procedure Thoracentesis is the surgical puncture of the chest wall to aspirate fluid or air from the pleural cavity. The area of pleural effusion is dull to percussion with decreased breath sounds. Pleural fluid causes blunting of the costophrenic angles on chest radiograph. Blunting usually indicates that ≥300 mL of fluid is present. If you suspect that <300 mL of fluid is present or you suspect that the fluid is loculated (trapped and not free flowing), a lateral decubitus film is helpful. Loculated effusions do not layer out. Thoracentesis can be done safely on fluid visualized on lateral decubitus film if ≥10 mm of fluid is measurable on the decubitus film. Ultrasound may also be used to localize a small or loculated effusion.

1. Explain the procedure and have the patient sign an informed consent form. Have the patient sit up comfortably, preferably leaning forward slightly on a bedside tray table. Ask the patient to practice increasing intrathoracic pressure by using the Valsalva maneuver or by humming.

2. The usual site for thoracentesis is the posterior lateral aspect of the back superior to the diaphragm but inferior to the top of the fluid level. Confirm the site by counting the ribs based on the radiograph and percussing out the fluid level. Avoid going below the eighth intercostal space because of the risk of peritoneal perforation.

3. Use sterile technique, including gloves, povidone–iodine prep, and drapes. Thoracentesis kits come with an adherent drape with a hole in it.

4. Make a skin wheal over the proposed site with a 25-gauge needle and lidocaine. Change to a 22-gauge, 1½-inch needle and infiltrate up and over the rib; try to anesthetize the deeper structures and the pleura. During this time, you should be aspirating back for pleural fluid. Once fluid returns, note the depth of the needle and mark it with a hemostat. This gives you an approximate depth. Remove the needle.

5. Use a hemostat to measure the 14- to 18-gauge thoracentesis needle to the same depth as the first needle. Penetrate through the anesthetized area with the thoracentesis needle. **Make sure that you "march" over the top of the rib** to avoid the neurovascular bundle that runs below the rib. With the 3-way stopcock attached, advance the thoracentesis catheter through the needle, withdraw the needle from the chest, and place the protective needle cover over the end of the needle to prevent injury to the catheter. Next, aspirate the amount of pleural fluid needed. Turn the stopcock and evacuate the fluid through the tubing. **Never remove >1000–1500 mL per tap!** This may result in hypotension or the development of pulmonary edema due to re-expansion of compressed alveoli.

6. Have the patient hum or do the Valsalva maneuver as you withdraw the catheter. This maneuver increases intrathoracic pressure and decreases the chances of a pneumothorax. Place a sterile dressing over the site.

7. Obtain a chest radiograph to evaluate fluid level and rule out a pneumothorax. An expiratory film is preferred because it is superior in identifying a small pneumothorax.

8. Distribute specimens in containers, label slips, and send them to the laboratory. Always order measurements for pH, specific gravity, protein, lactate dehydrogenase, cell count and differential count, glucose, Gram's stain and cultures, acid-fast cultures and smears, and fungal cultures and smears. Optional laboratory studies are cytology if you suspect a malignancy, amylase if you suspect an effusion secondary to pancreatitis (usually on the left) or esophageal perforation, and a Sudan stain and triglycerides (>110 mg/dL) if a chylothorax is suspected.

TABLE III–7. DIFFERENTIAL DIAGNOSIS OF PLEURAL FLUID.
TRANSUDATE: NEPHROSIS, CONGESTIVE HEART FAILURE (CHF), CIRRHOSIS.
EXUDATE: INFECTION (PNEUMONIA, TB), MALIGNANCY, EMPYEMA, PERITONEAL DIALYSIS, PANCREATITIS, CHYLOTHORAX.

Lab Value	Transudate	Exudate
Specific gravity	<1.016	>1.016
Protein (pleural fluid)	<2.5 g/100 mL	> 3 g/100 mL
Protein ration (pleural fluid to serum ratio)	<0.5	>0.5
LDH ratio (pleural fluid to serum ratio)	<0.5	>0.6
Pleural fluid LDH	<200 IU	>200 IU
Fibrinogen (clot)	No	Yes
Cell count and differential	Very low WBC	Suspect an inflammatory exudate (early polys, later monos)

Grossly bloddy tap: Trauma, pulmonary infarction, tumor, and iatrogenic causes.

pH: The pH of pleural fluid is usually > 7.3. If between 7.2 and 7.3, suspect TB or malignancy or both. If < 7.2, suspect an empyema.

Glucose: Normal pleural fluid glucose is 2/3 serum glucose pleural fluid glucose is much lower than serum glucose in effusions due to rheumatoid arthritis (0–16 mg/100 mL).

Triglycerides and positive sudan stain: Chylothorax.

Complications
- Pneumothorax, hemothorax, infection, pulmonary laceration, hypotension, hypoxia due to ventilation–perfusion mismatch in the newly aerated lung segment.

Differential Diagnosis of Pleural Fluid A **transudate** suggests nephrosis, congestive heart failure, or cirrhosis; an **exudate** infection (pneumonia, tuberculosis) suggests malignancy, empyema, peritoneal dialysis, pancreatitis, or chylothorax. See Table III–7, page 383, for the differential diagnosis.

$\text{IV}.$ Fluids & Electrolytes

FLUID ADMINISTRATION

Basic principles govern internal and external exchanges of water and salt. The following requirements that are explained below are all in reference to a 70-kg male. Daily water losses include approximately 250 mL as stool, 800–1500 mL as urine, and approximately 600–900 mL as insensible losses per day. Urine output must exceed 500–800 mL/day to excrete the products of catabolism (>20–30 mL/h). Daily sodium requirements are 50–90 mEq/day, and potassium requirements are approximately 50 mEq/day. There is much variability from the 70-kg male; therefore, clinical judgment is prudent in assessing any patient.

A. **Calculation of Maintenance Fluid Administration**
  1. **Normal Adult Patients**. Maintenance fluid replacement is aimed at replacing fluids lost during the course of the day as stated above. Calculations do not reflect any pre-existing deficits or ongoing losses. The simplest way to determine the 24-hour fluid requirement is the "kg method":

     • For the first 10 kg of body weight: 100 mL/kg per day plus
     • For the second 10 kg of body weight: 50 mL/kg per day plus
     • For weight >20 kg: 20 mL/kg per day

     Divide the sum of the above by 24 hours to determine the hourly rate.

     For example, a 70-kg person would receive 1000 mL/day (for the first 10 kg), 500 mL/day (for the second 10 kg), and 1000 mL/day (20 mL/kg for the final 50 kg), or a total of 2500 mL/day.

     To provide adequate glucose and electrolyte balance, a mixture of 5% dextrose (D5) and 0.5 normal saline (NS) with KCl 20 mEq/L should be used. This is applicable for the patient with normal renal function, a patient not receiving other fluids (such as enteral or parenteral nutrition support), and a patient with normal electrolytes. In these special situations, fluid administration guidelines must be appropriately modified.
  2. **Pediatric patients.** In general, children require less sodium than adults, so 0.25 NS is used instead of 0.5 NS. There are 2 methods used to calculate maintenance fluid requirements in the pediatric patient:
     a. **Body weight method:** As outlined in A-1.

b. **Body surface area method:** Maintenance fluids are 2000 mL/m² per day. Divide by 24 to get the flow rate per hour (not accurate for infants <10 kg in body weight). To calculate the surface area, use the body surface area nomogram in Appendix A.

B. **Specific Replacement Fluids.** Table IV–1 lists general guidelines for the daily production and composition of various body fluids. It is important to replace high-output losses with fluids of similar composition. You can use the data listed in Table IV–1 with these guidelines, and the information in Table IV–2 to write orders for fluid replacement.

1. **Gastric (nasogastric tube, emesis).** D5 and 0.5 NS with KCl 20 mEq/L.
2. **Diarrhea.** D5 and 0.5 NS with KCl 15 mEq/L. Use body weight as a replacement guide (about 1 L for each 1-kg or 2.2-lb lost).
3. **Small bowel.** Five percent dextrose in lactated Ringer solution (D5LR) with HCO_3 25 mEq/L (half ampule).
4. **Bile.** D5LR with HCO_3 25 mEq/L (half ampule).
5. **Pancreatic fluid.** D5LR with HCO_3 50 mEq/L (1 ampule).
6. **Burn patients** (Figure IV–1). The "Parkland formula" follows.

Total fluid required during the first 24 hours = (percentage of second- and third-degree burns) × (body weight in kg) × 4 mL

Replace with lactated Ringer's solution over 24 hours:

TABLE IV–1. COMPOSITION AND DAILY PRODUCTION OF BODY FLUIDS

Fluid	Electrolytes (mEq/L)				Average Daily Production[a] (mL)
	Na	Cl	K	HCO	
Sweet	50	40	5	0	Varies
Saliva	10	15	26	50	1500
Gastric juice	60–100	100	10	0	1500–2000
Duodenum	130	90	5	0–10	300–2000
Bile	145	100	5	15–35	100–000
Pancreatic juice	140	75	5	70–115	100–800
Ileum	140	100	5	15–30	2000–3000
Diarrhea	50	40	35	45	—

[a]In adults.

TABLE IV–2. COMPOSITION OF COMMONLY USED CRYSTALLOIDS.

Fluid	Glucose (gm/L)	Na	Cl (mEq/L)	K	Ca	HCO₃ᵃ	Mg	HPO4	KCal/L
D5W	50	—	—	—	—	—	—	—	170
D10W	100	—	—	—	—	—	—	—	340
D20W	200	—	—	—	—	—	—	—	680
D50W	500	—	—	—	—	—	—	—	1700
1/2 NS (0.45% NaCl)	—	77	77	—	—	—	—	—	0
3% NS	513	513	—	—	—	—	—	—	0
NS (0.9% NaCl)	—	154	154	—	—	—	—	—	0
D5 1/4 NS	50	38	38	—	—	—	—	—	17
D5 1/2 NS (0.45% NaCl)	50	77	77	—	—	—	—	—	17
D5 NS (0.9% NaCl)	50	154	154	—	—	—	—	—	17
D5LR	50	130	110	4	3	27	—	—	18
Lactated Ringer solution	—	130	110	4	3	27	—	—	<1
Ionosol MB	50	25	22	20	—	23	3	3	17
Normosol M	50	40	40	13	—	16	3	—	17

ᵃHCO³ is administered in these solutions as lactate that is converted to bicarbonate.
D5 = 5% dextrose; D5W = 5% dextrose in water; D10W = 10% dextrose in water; D20W = 20% dextrose in water; D50W = 50% dextrose in water; D5LR = 5% dextrose in lactated Ringer solution; NS = normal saline.

- Half total during first 8 hours (from time of burn)
- One-fourth total during second 8 hours
- One-fourth total during third 8 hours

   C. Composition of Commonly Used Parenteral Fluids.
   See Table IV–2 for the composition of commonly used parenteral fluids.

   D. Fluid Administration in the Surgical Patient. In addition to administration of maintenance fluids, surgery patients often need administration of fluids to replenish deficits, most commonly referred to as "third-space losses." It is important to use urine output and vital signs as a guide for administration of this additional fluid.

ELECTROLYTES

Specific electrolyte abnormalities are discussed in Section I as individual problems.

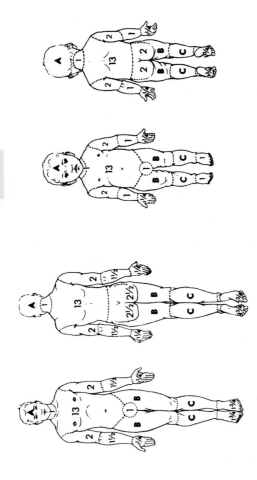

FIGURE IV-1. Tables for estimating the extent of burns in adults and children. In adults, a reasonable system for calculating the percentage of body burned is the "rule of nines": Each arm equals 9%; the head equals 9%; the anterior and posterior trunks each equal 18%; each leg equals 18%; and the perineum equals 1%. (*Reproduced, with permission, from Demling RH. Burns & other thermal injuries. In: Way LW, Doherty GM, eds.* Current Surgical Treatment & Diagnosis, *11th ed. Copyright (c) 2003 by The McGraw-Hill Companies, Inc.*)

A. **Hyponatremia: see Problem 47, page 174**
B. **Hypernatremia: see Problem 42, page 158**
C. **Hypokalemia: see Problem 46, page 170**
D. **Hyperkalemia: see Problem 41, page 155**
E. **Hypocalcemia: see Problem 44, page 165**
F. **Hypercalcemia: see Problem 39, page 147**

REFERENCES

Berry SM. *The Mont Reid Hand Book,* 5th ed. St. Louis: Mosby; 1997.
Marino PL. *The ICU Book,* 2nd ed. Baltimore: Williams & Wilikins; 1998.
Scwartz SI, et al. *Principles of Surgery,* 7th ed. New York: McGraw-Hill; 1999.

V. Nutritional Management of the Surgical Patient

Adequate nutritional support is of paramount importance in the care of the surgical patient. A suboptimal response to therapy is more common in the malnourished patient, and complications such as poor wound healing, impaired organ function, and compromised immunity may be more commonly observed. Nutritional support, whether enteral or parenteral, when used appropriately, can help prevent nutrition-related morbidities in the surgical patient. There are no data supporting the use of routine nutritional support in the preoperative period except in the severely malnourished patient.

Assessment

Differentiation of acute from chronic malnutrition is helpful in deciding when to initiate nutritional support. Acute malnutrition, also called **kwashiorkor** or **acute hypoalbuminemia**, is defined as starvation that occurs during catabolic stress such as surgery, infection, burn, or trauma and is a more aggressive nutritional insult than simple starvation for a brief period. Chronic malnutrition, also called **marasmus,** is characterized by growth retardation, wasting of muscle and subcutaneous fat, and maintenance of an appetite. Frequently in the surgical patient, these 2 nutritional insults may be superimposed, causing combined protein-calorie malnutrition. The most recent guidelines from the American Society for Parenteral and Enteral Nutrition state that: "patients should be considered malnourished or at risk of developing malnutrition if they have inadequate nutrient intake for 7 d or more, or if they have a weight loss of 10% or more of their pre-illness body weight." The formula for determination of percentage weight loss is:

$$\% \text{ Weight loss} = \frac{(\text{usual weight} - \text{present weight})}{\text{usual weight}} \times 100$$

Formal evaluation is important to identify patients at nutritional risk and to provide a baseline to assess the achievement of therapeutic goals with specialized nutritional support. The patient's history is useful to evaluate weight loss and dietary intolerance (eg, glucose or lactose and disease states that may influence nutritional tolerance). Anthropometric evaluations such as midarm muscle circumference and triceps skinfold thickness have much interobserver variability and are generally not useful unless performed by an experienced evaluator. Absolute lymphocyte count and response to skin test antigens provide insight to the patient's immune function. Visceral protein markers, such as prealbumin, fibronectin, and transferrin, may be helpful in evaluating nutritional insult and catabolic stress. Although the most commonly quoted laboratory parameter of nutritional status is serum albumin, its concentration often reflects hydration status and metabolic response to injury (ie, acute-phase response) more than the nutritional state of the patient. This is true particularly in the patient who has intravascular volume deficits. Because of its long half-life, serum albumin level may be normal in the malnourished patient. Prealbumin and fibronectin are superior as indicators of malnutrition only because of their shorter half-life (2 and 1 days, respectively). However, these serum proteins as indicators of malnutrition are subject to the same limitations because they are affected by catabolic stress.

Urinary urea nitrogen (UUN) collected during a 24-hour period is an important tool to evaluate nitrogen balance and the adequacy of a patient's nutritional regimen.

- Nitrogen balance = nitrogen input − nitrogen output
- Nitrogen input = protein (g)/6.25 (6.25 g protein contains 1 g nitrogen)
- Nitrogen output = 24-hour UUN + 4 g/day (nonurinary loss).

Certain disease states, eg, high-output fistulas or massive diarrhea, will increase the amount of nonurinary losses for nitrogen.

Example of Nitrogen Balance Calculation

A patient receives 2 L of total parenteral nutrition (TPN) per 24 hours with 27.5 g synthetic amino acid (protein) solution per liter.

1. 27.5 g protein/L × 2 L = 55 g protein/24 hours.
2. Recall that 1 g nitrogen = 6.25 g protein.
3. Nitrogen input = 55 g protein at 6.25 g protein/g nitrogen = 8.8 g nitrogen.
4. Patient voided 22.5 dL urine/24 hours with UUN 66 mg/dL.
5. Nitrogen lost in urine = 22.5 dL × 66 mg/dL = 1485 mg or about 1.5 g.
6. Add 4.0 g for nonurine nitrogen loss.
7. Nitrogen output = 1.5 g + 4.0 = 5.5 g
8. Nitrogen balance = input − output = 8.8 − 5.5 = positive 3.3 g nitrogen.

A positive nitrogen balance ensures that the amount of protein being administered is sufficient to cover the losses of endogenous protein, which occur secondary to catabolism. Once positive balance has been achieved, protein replacement has been optimized. This may not be possible in the acute phase of injury in severe trauma or burn patients. Thus a minimization of loss (2–4 g/day) may be the goal during this period. A negative nitrogen balance indicates insufficient protein replacement for the degree of skeletal muscle loss. Under most circumstances, an attempt to achieve positive balance should be made.

Several considerations including pre-existing illnesses and coexisting metabolic abnormalities are commonly present in the critically ill patient. Pre-existing conditions such as hepatic insufficiency, congestive heart failure, and renal impairment must be taken into consideration when instituting nutritional support. For example, a high carbohydrate load for patients with respiratory failure can lead to a significant increase in CO_2 production. It is important to correct coexisting metabolic abnormalities, such as hypophosphatemia or hyperglycemia, before instituting nutritional support, in particular parenteral nutrition. It is not usually critically important to correct other metabolic abnormalities before instituting TPN.

The decision to begin nutritional support is not an "on-call problem" in the literal sense. It is never a decision that must be made late at night by the house officer. Rather, it should be a considered decision made by the team responsible for the care of the patient. Clear indications for nutritional support include:

- Weight loss ≥12% of body weight (or weight <85% of ideal body weight).
- Expected >5 days of no oral intake.
- Inadequate nutrient intake for ≥7 days.
- Albumin <3.5 g/dL, transferrin <200 mg/dL.

Hospital Diets

There different standard dietary formulations available in the hospital. Most hospitals have a reference that provides details of the available diets. In addition, registered dieticians are available for consultation. This service should be used when questions arise about the use of specialized diets and dietary supplements in the care of individual patients.

Regular. Used for adult patients without dietary restrictions. The composition is based on recommended dietary allowances.

Soft. Calorically and nutritionally similar to a regular diet, but tender foods are used (this is not a ground/pureed diet). Useful in patients with oral problems that prevent chewing of food.

Mechanical Soft. Uses ground foods, also useful for those with chewing difficulties (eg, edentulous patients).

Pureed. Foods are ground finely, also useful in patients with difficulty chewing or swallowing.

Clear Liquids. Usually used in the immediate preoperative or postoperative period, particularly in the transition from nonoral to starting oral feedings. This diet leaves little residue and requires minimal digestive activity for absorption. In general, this diet should not be used for >3 days without supplementation.

Full Liquids. Includes foods that are liquid at room temperature, such as milk or milk products (puddings, ice cream, etc). This diet previously was used widely as a transitional diet from clear liquids to regular, but it is currently used less often. This diet can be difficult for many patients because it contains high-fat, lactose-containing ingredients.

Low Fiber (Residue). Indicated for patients with colitis, ileitis, or diarrhea. Decreases fecal volume.

High Fiber. Useful for atonic constipation, diverticular disease, irritable bowel syndrome, and diabetes.

Diabetic (ADA). Used for patients with insulin-dependent or non–insulin-dependent diabetes mellitus. These diets are prescribed at a specified number of calories per day (eg, 2000 calories ADA, 2400 calories ADA, etc). Assessment by a clinical dietician helps to determine the appropriate calorie level and to help the patient maintain the correct diet after leaving the hospital.

Reduction. Used to assist in weight loss to achieve ideal body weight. Assessment by a clinical dietician is helpful in determining the appropriate caloric level.

Pediatric. Usually ordered as "diet for age."

Hyperlipidemia. Used for patients with lipid abnormalities. Diet is written as type I, IIa, IIb, III, IV, or V depending on the patient's diagnosis.

Low Fat. Designed to limit fat intake to approximately 50 g/day. Indicated for some diseases of the gallbladder, liver, or pancreas.

Protein Restricted. Useful in patients with renal failure or hepatic disorders. Specify number of grams of protein to be given.

Sodium Restricted. Used for management of patients with congestive heart failure, hypertension, or other diseases that result in fluid retention. Specify amount of sodium in milligrams or grams. Sodium restriction at levels <1000 mg/day is not recommended because of the poor palatability of such diets. The average person in the United States consumes 12.5–15 g salt per day.

Potassium Restricted. Used mostly for patients with renal failure. Specify in grams or milliequivalents. A typical renal diet is limited to 40 mEq potassium daily.

Nutritional Requirements

Overall, nutritional requirements are the same whether feeding the patient enterally or parenterally. Appropriate calculations of calories and protein are important to achieve optimal anabolism and avoid the metabolic complications associated with overfeeding.

Caloric Requirements. Caloric requirements are dictated by the patient's needs for energy to support metabolic processes and activity. Catabolic patients with stresses from infections, burns, surgery, or trauma require additional energy to allow for the increased basal metabolic rate and increased metabolic demands associated with these conditions. Using the appropriate weight to predict energy needs is important for the patient who is not at ideal body weight. For an underweight patient, it is important to use the actual weight to avoid the complications associated with overfeeding. Similarly, for the overweight patient, it is important to estimate the amount of mass that is metabolically active to avoid unnecessary metabolic stress. This weight is 25% of the difference between ideal weight and actual weight added to ideal weight.

Ideal body weight:

Males: 50 kg + 2.3 kg/inch >5 feet.
Females: 45.5 kg + 2.3 kg/inch >5 feet.

Metabolically active weight for obese patients = actual weight − ideal body weight × 0.25 + ideal body weight.

The amount of energy to support the metabolic process can be estimated from a number of equations or a nomogram. The Harris-Benedict equation is frequently used to provide an estimation of basal energy expenditure (see below). Predicted basal energy expenditure should be approximately 22 kcal/kg when calculated correctly. To estimate a patient's caloric requirement, basal energy expenditure is multiplied by a factor for activity and injury.

Factors used to adjust basal energy expenditure are fewer than originally published as the risks of overfeeding became apparent. Modified factors are presented in Table V–1. Overall, total caloric provisions (protein + nonprotein calories) should not exceed 25–30 kcal/kg for the nonstressed patient and 30–35 kcal/kg for the catabolically stressed patient. The burn victim will have higher requirements based on the amount of body surface area involved. In general, target nutritional support can be estimated to be:

Nonstressed: 25–30 kcal/kg daily.
Stressed: 30–35 kcal/kg daily.

TABLE V–1. CALCULATION OF CALORIC REQUIREMENTS. THE CALCULATION RELIES ON THE HARRIS-BENEDICT EQUATION FOR MEN AND WOMEN AND IS ADJUSTED FOR ACTIVITY LEVEL OR INJURY FACTORS.

Caloric requirement (men) = 66.47 + (13.75 × wgt [kg]) + (5.0 × hgt (cm))
− (6.76 × age [yrs]) × (activity factor) × (injury factor)

Caloric requirement (women) = 655.10 + (9.56 × wgt[kg]) + (1.65 × hgt [cm])
− (4.68 × age [yrs]) × (activity factor) × (injury factor)

Activity	Factor
Paralyzed	1.1
Confined to bed	1.2
Out of bed	1.3
Normal activity	1.5
Injury (choose highest factors)	
Surgery	
Minor	1.1
Major	1.1–1.3
Infection	
Minor	1.1
Severe	1.1–1.3
Trauma	
Skeletal	1.2–1.3
Head injury with steroids	1.6
Burns	
Up to 20% BSA	1–1.5
20–40% BSA	1.5–1.85
>40% BSA	1.85–1.95

BSA = body surface area.

Protein Requirements. Protein is required to minimize endogenous net catabolism by supporting anabolic processes. Daily maintenance protein requirements are 0.8–1 g/kg. Patients with mild to moderate physiologic stress require 1.2–1.5 g/kg per day. Those with severe injuries may require as much as 2.5 g/kg per day. Protein administration may be limited by relative hepatic or renal insufficiency. For patients with a history of hepatic encephalopathy, protein doses >0.8 g/kg are rarely tolerated. Such patients may benefit from amino acid formulations with higher concentrations of branched-chain amino acids.

Carbohydrates & Fat. In general, the caloric goal is achieved with carbohydrate and fat when feeding a patient parenterally. The protein is not counted as calories in the acutely stressed patient. Conceptually, this is to provide adequate calories for nitrogen incorporation and to allow adequate protein for tissue anabolism, although this practice differs in various medical centers. Optimal ratios of calorie to nitrogen to achieve nutritional anabolism are estimated to be 150:1 for the nonstressed patient and 100:1 for the catabolic patient. On average, protein consists of 16% nitrogen.

Most calories are provided as carbohydrate. This is consistent with the typical diet. Carbohydrate administration, enterally or parenterally, may be limited owing to hyperglycemia, increased CO_2 production, or fatty liver infiltration. In general, the maximal glucose administration tolerated is 4–5 mg/kg per minute or 20–25 kcal/kg per day.

A minimum amount of fat must be given to the parenterally fed patient to prevent the development of essential fatty acid deficiency. This minimum is 4% of total calories in the form of linoleic acid. However, additional fat calories are used to provide energy and to decrease the metabolic stress of glucose in the intolerant patient. Maximal intravenous (IV) fat administration is 1–2.5 g/kg per day. Fat emulsions should not be infused in patients with triglyceride values >300–400 mg/dL. Although at one time practitioners considered IV fat emulsion contraindicated in pancreatitis, IV fat may be a better tolerated fuel source for patients with pancreatitis without hypertriglyceridemia. IV fat emulsion has been associated with impaired immune function in animal studies. For this reason, IV fat emulsion should not be administered to acutely septic patients or to patients during the immediate perioperative period.

Determining the Route of Nutritional Support

Having determined that nutritional support is indicated, select the route to be used. Clinical and laboratory studies demonstrate that the intestinal tract plays a critical role in the progress of numerous disease states. Enteral nutrition helps to preserve gut morphology, is better tolerated metabolically, and is less expensive. In addition, in animal studies, enteral nutrition has been shown to prevent translocation of bacteria across the gut mucosa; therefore, enteral nutrition may have a role in preventing septicemia. Further, there is no advantage to parenteral nutrition in the patient with a functioning gastrointestinal tract. Parenteral nutrition does not achieve greater anabolism or provide greater control over a patient's nutritional regimen. Thus, parenteral nutrition is indicated **only** when the enteral route is not usable. In other words: **"If the gut works, use it."**

The factors involved in choosing the route for enteral nutrition include duration, gastrointestinal tract pathophysiology, and risk for aspiration. Nasally placed tubes are the most frequently used. Patient comfort is maximized when a small-bore flexible tube is used. However, such tubes do not allow monitoring of residual volumes that may be significant when gastric emptying is questionable. Patients at risk for aspiration require longer tubes into the jejunum or duodenum. When long-term feeding is anticipated, a tube enterostomy is required. Percutaneous endoscopic gastrostomy tubes are usually placed without general anesthesia. However, patients with tumors, gastrointestinal obstruction, adhesions from prior upper-abdominal surgery, or abnormal anatomy may require open surgical placement. A jejunal feeding tube may be threaded through a percutaneous endoscopic gastrostomy tube for small bowel feeding. Placement of a needle catheter or Witzel jejunostomy during surgery generally allows earlier postoperative feeding with an elemental formulation than if one had to wait for the return of gastric emptying and colonic function (see page 354 for enteral tube placement procedures).

Some patients, because of their disease states, cannot be fed enterally and require parenteral feedings. Enteral nutrition is avoided for patients with active, massive gastrointestinal bleeding, obstruction, high-output fistulas, or short-gut syndrome. Other contraindications for enteral feeding include severe diarrhea of small bowel origin, peritonitis, severe acute pancreatitis, shock, or intestinal hypomotility.

1. Enteral Nutrition. Enteral nutrition is best tolerated when instilled into the stomach because there are fewer problems with osmolarity or feeding volumes. Remember that the stomach serves as a barrier to hyperosmolarity, thus the use of isotonic feedings is mandated only when instilling nutrients directly into the small intestine. The use of gastric feedings is thus preferable and should be used whenever appropriate. Patients at risk for aspiration or with impaired gastric emptying may need to be fed past the pylorus into the jejunum or the duodenum. Feedings through a jejunostomy placed at the time of surgery can often be initiated on the first postoperative day, thus obviating parenteral nutrition.

Although enteral nutrition is generally safer than parenteral nutrition, aspiration can be a significant morbid event in the care of a patient. Appropriate monitoring for residual volumes in addition to keeping the head of the bed elevated can help prevent this complication. A significant residual may be defined as 2 times the instillation rate. This can be managed by a number of methods. There may be a transient postoperative ileus best managed by waiting. Metoclopramide or erythromycin may be useful pharmacologic therapy. Patients who have been tolerating feedings and who develop a new high residual should be carefully assessed for the cause, concentrating on intra-abdominal infections.

The question of when to start enteral feedings in the postoperative patient must be clarified. Often the presence of bowel sounds is used as the single criterion. It is important to realize that the presence of bowel sounds may not be a reliable indicator of gastrointestinal motility. The passage of flatus indicates colonic motility and, because the colon is the last part of the gastrointestinal tract to regain motility after laparotomy in most cases, this may be a more useful indicator.

However, a more global approach to assessment of the gastrointestinal tract is warranted. If feeding into the stomach, gastric emptying should be evaluated. In general, when an adult patient drains 600 mL/24-hour shift on nasogastric suction, the pylorus is functioning appropriately. Clamping of the nasogastric tube to evaluate gastric emptying is contraindicated because it exposes the patient to the risk of aspiration unnecessarily. Tolerance to enteral feeding can be assessed with the instillation of an isotonic diet given for 24 hours at 30 mL/h as a trial. Feeding intolerance is characterized by vomiting, abdominal distention, diarrhea, or large gastric residual volumes.

Nutritional components and osmolality of the enteral product help classify the formulations to simplify selection. The protein component can be supplied as intact proteins, partially digested hydrolyzed proteins, or crystalline amino acids. Each gram of protein provides 4 cal when oxidized. The carbohydrate source may be intact complex starches, glucose polymers, or simpler disaccharides such as sucrose. Carbohydrates provide 4 cal/g. Fat in enteral products usually is supplied as long-chain fatty acids. However, some enteral products contain medium-chain triglycerides, which are transported directly into the portal circulation rather than by chyle production. Because medium-chain triglyceride oil does not contain essential fatty acids, it cannot be used as the sole fat source. Long-chain fatty acids provide 9 cal/g and medium-chain triglyceride oil provides 8 cal/g.

The osmolality of an enteral product is determined primarily by the concentration of carbohydrates, electrolytes, amino acids, or small peptides. The clinical importance of osmolality is often debated. Hyperosmolal formulations with osmolalities >450 mosm/L may contribute to diarrhea by acting in a manner similar to osmotic cathartics. Hyperosmolal feedings are well tolerated when delivered into the stomach (as opposed to the small bowel) because gastric secretions dilute the feeding before it leaves the pylorus to traverse the small bowel. Thus, feedings administered directly to the small bowel (eg, through feeding jejunostomy) should not exceed 450 mOsm/L.

On the basis of osmolality and macronutrient content, the clinician can classify enteral products into several categories. Low osmolality formulas are isotonic and contain intact macronutrients. They usually provide 1 cal/mL and require approximately 2 L to provide the recommended daily allowance for vitamins. These products are appropriate for the general patient population. Two examples are Ensure and Isocal.

High-density formulas may provide up to 2 cal/mL. These concentrated solutions are hyperosmolar and also contain intact nutrients. The recommended daily allowance for vitamins can be met with volumes ≤1500 mL. These products are used for volume-restricted patients. Examples are Nutren 2.0 and Ensure Plus HN Liquid.

Chemically defined or elemental formulas provide the macronutrients in the predigested state. These formulations are usually hyperosmolar and have poor palatability. Patients with compromised nutrient absorptive abilities or gastrointestinal function may benefit from elemental type feedings. Vivonex TEN and Peptamen are 2 such products.

Several enteral formulas have been developed that have been altered for various disease states. Products for pulmonary patients, such as Pulmocare, contain a larger percentage of calories from fat to decrease the carbon dioxide load from the metabolism of excess glucose. A low-carbohydrate, high-fat product for persons with diabetes is available that also contains fiber that may help regulate glucose control. Other fiber-containing enteral feedings are available to help regulate bowel function, eg, Enrich. Patients with hepatic insufficiency may benefit from formulations that contain a higher concentration of the branched-chain amino acids and fewer aromatic amino acids in an attempt to correct their altered serum amino acid profile, eg, Hepatic-Aid II. Formulas that contain only essential amino acids have been marketed for the patient with renal failure. The clinical usefulness of many specialty products remains controversial.

Oral supplements differ from other enteral feedings by design so that they are more palatable to improve compliance. Further, oral supplements contain lactose, which is inappropriate for patients with lactase deficiency, whereas most enteral products do not contain lactose.

Guidelines for ordering enteral feedings are outlined in Table V–2. In summary, when using enteral feedings:

- Determine nutritional needs.
- Assess gastrointestinal tract function and appropriateness of enteral feedings.
- Determine fluid requirements and volume tolerance on the basis of overall status and concurrent disease states.
- Select an appropriate enteral feeding product.

TABLE V–2. ROUTINE ORDERS FOR ENTERAL NUTRITION.

1. Confirm tube placement.
2. Elevate head of bed to 45 degrees.
3. Check gastric residuals in patients receiving gastric feedings. Hold feeding is >1.5–2 × infusion rate. Significant residuals should be reinstilled and rechecked in 1 hour. If continues to be elevated, hold tubefeeding and begin nasogastric suction.
4. Check patient's weight 3 times week.
5. Record strict input and output.
6. Routine laboratory studies.

- Verify that the regimen selected satisfies micronutrient requirements.
- Monitor and assess nutritional status to evaluate the need for changes in the selected regimen.

Complications of Enteral Nutrition

A. Diarrhea. A common complication of enteral feeding is diarrhea. It occurs in about 10–60% of patients who receive enteral feedings. The clinician must be certain to evaluate the patient for other causes of diarrhea (see Section I, Problem 22, page 93). Formula-related causes include contamination, excessive cold temperature, lactose intolerance, osmolality, and the method and/or route of delivery. Eliminate potential causes before using antidiarrheal medications:

- Check medication profile for possible drug-induced cause.
- Rule out *Clostridium difficile* colitis for patients receiving antibiotics.
- Attempt to decrease rate.
- Change formulation: limit lactose, decrease osmolality.
- Use pharmacologic therapy only after eliminating controllable causes.

B. Constipation. Although less common than diarrhea, constipation can occur in the enterally fed patient. Check to be sure that adequate fluid volume is being given. Patients with additional requirements may benefit from water boluses or dilution of the enteral formulation. Fiber can be added to help regulate bowel function.

C. Aspiration. Aspiration is a serious complication of enteral feedings and is more likely to occur in the patient with diminished mental status. The best approach here is prevention, accomplished by elevating the patient's head and carefully monitoring residual fluid volume. Before instituting enteral feedings, one should further evaluate any patient who has suspected aspiration or is assessed to be at increased risk of aspiration. Such a patient may not be a candidate for gastric feedings and may require small bowel feedings (see Section I, Problem 8, page 31).

D. Drug Interactions. Vitamin K content of various enteral products varies from 22 mg to 156 mg/1000 cal. This can significantly affect the anticoagulation profile of a patient who receives warfarin. Tetracycline products should not be administered 1 hour before or 2 hours after enteral feedings to avoid the inhibition of absorption. Similarly, enteral feedings should be stopped 2 hours before and after the administration of phenytoin.

2. Parenteral Nutrition. *Peripheral Versus Central Parenteral Nutrition.* The use of **total parenteral nutrition** necessitates a central venous catheter with its concomitant risks. Although some patients require TPN, others have nutritional needs that can be met better with the use of **peripherally administered parenteral nutrition (PPN).**

The limiting factor in the use of PPN is the osmolality of the solution. Because centrally administered fluids are rapidly diluted at the catheter tip, osmolality is not a concern; conversely, peripherally administered fluids of high osmolality rapidly result in venous sclerosis owing to the relatively low flow and slow dilution of these fluids. Thus, only patients with modest nutritional requirements will be able to meet these criteria for the necessarily low-calorie–containing solutions that can be administered peripherally.

PPN can have up to 900 mOsm/kg and can be prepared from amino acid mixtures (5%), dextrose solutions (10%), and fat emulsions (20%). They have a low caloric density (0.3–0.6 kcal/mL) compared with TPN solutions and thus can only provide 1200–2300 kcal/day in 2000–3500 mL solution. Thus, with PPN, the ability to provide caloric needs in relatively small volumes is lost; this may be clinically significant for patients who require fluid restriction.

In general, the largest-bore IV catheter should be used. The site should be changed frequently, usually every 72 hours. Fat emulsion can be given through a Y-connector or by using a 3-in-1 bag as is commonly used for centrally administered parenteral nutrition. Septic complications are uncommon, but thrombophlebitis can occur at the infusion site.

Although peripherally administered parenteral nutrition alleviates some of the complications associated with central TPN, its use is limited by the inability to provide the level of nutritional support frequently needed in the surgical patient. Patients with large nutrition requirements owing to stress or chronic malnutrition, high electrolyte needs, fluid restrictions, or prolonged IV feeding are inappropriate candidates for PPN.

Prescribing TPN (Central TPN). Central vein infusions allow greater concentrations of macronutrients and electrolytes. Therefore, central TPN is much more flexible in meeting a patient's nutritional requirements. With the use of permanent types of catheters (eg, tunneled subclavian catheter, implantable port, or a peripherally inserted central line), TPN can be administered in the hospital or home setting, depending on the patient's overall clinical condition.

When calculating caloric provision of parenteral nutrition, IV fat emulsion 10% provides 1.1 kcal/mL, and 20% provides 2 kcal/mL. IV dextrose provides 3.4 kcal/g rather than 4 kcal/g because it is a monohydrate and therefore less calorically dense.

Centrally administered TPN is given through a central venous catheter (placed percutaneously or an operatively placed tunneled catheter; see Section III, page 340). The solutions are usually >1900 mOsm/kg and contain ≥1 kcal/mL. Thus the usual infusion of 2000–2500 L/day provides ≥2000–2500 kcal/day. This is sufficient to meet the nutritional needs of most surgical patients.

The solutions are formulated in the hospital pharmacy and are typically ordered by using a standard "checklist" that is available in most hospitals. A commonly used method uses a single infusion bag that contains all components to be infused over a 24-hour period. A typical 24-hour single bag will contain

Amino acids (10%) 1000 mL
Dextrose (50%) 500 mL
Fat emulsion (20%) 500 mL
Total 2000 mL
Electrolytes and vitamins to create a solution containing all nutrient requirements:
Sodium 30 mEq/L
Potassium 30 mEq/L
Phosphate 15 mmol/L
Magnesium 8 mEq/L
Calcium gluconate 4.7 mEq/L
Chloride 50 mEq/L
Acetate 70 mEq/L

These values represent commonly used amounts but must be adapted to the nutritional and electrolyte needs of individual patients, and must consider concurrent disease states, such as renal or hepatic failure.

Electrolyte administration must also be changed to reflect losses. Salts are usually administered as chloride or acetate, usually in similar amounts. However, patients losing fluid by nasogastric suction require increased amounts of chloride. Similarly, patients with high-output pancreatic or small bowel fistulae will require more acetate.

Trace elements are added daily. Commercially available mixtures are usually adequate to provide needed amounts. Similarly, vitamins are usually added as premade mixtures. In addition to these mixtures, the clinician must administer vitamin K 5–10 mg intramuscularly weekly. Increased amounts of zinc are necessary with small bowel losses.

Starting TPN (Table V–3). TPN is usually begun at 25–50 mL/h, with increases of 25 mL/h until the precalculated final rate is achieved. Glucose is carefully monitored, especially in the early phase of TPN administration because glucose intolerance is very

TABLE V–3. SAMPLE ORDERS FOR PATIENTS ON CENTRAL TPN

Routine orders on starting TPN
    Specify infusion (typically start 25–50 mL/hr for 24 h: if tolerating well, especially
        sugars, can increase up to 2 L/d)
    Daily electrolytes
    Liver funtions test twice weekly
    CBC daily
    Vital signs qshift
    Fingerstick blood sugar shift
    Strict intake and output
    Prealbumin

Routine orders once stabilized on TPN
    Electrolytes and liver function tests twice weekly
    Weight weekly
    Prealbumin (weekly)
    Urinary nitrogen (weekly)

CBC = complete blood cell count; TPN = total parenteral nutrition.

common. Be sure to check serum electrolytes (especially PO_4) and glucose before starting TPN. Remember that glucose intolerance in a patient who had normal glucose levels while on TPN may be an early sign of sepsis. If a patient is undergoing surgery, TPN usually is tapered to help prevent stress-related hyperglycemia and assist in fluid administration.

Stopping TPN. Although commonly practiced, weaning is generally not necessary. Most patients tolerate cessation of TPN, especially if they are taking oral nutrition at the time TPN is stopped. If there are concerns about hypoglycemia, the TPN rate can be halved for 1 hour and then stopped completely. When TPN solution is stopped in a patient who is not on another form of feeding, then peripherally infused 10% dextrose solution is used to avoid hypoglycemia.

Complications. Complications associated with parenteral nutrition are generally divided into mechanical, infectious, and metabolic problems.

A. Mechanical Complications. After placement of the central venous catheter, a chest radiograph is obtained to evaluate the catheter tip position and the presence of a pneumothorax. The tip should be at the atriocaval junction. A catheter tip well into the right ventricle can cause arrhythmias and may damage the tricuspid valve. Pneumo- and hydrothorax should be controlled with appropriate chest tube drainage.

B. Infectious Complications. The use of central lines always has the potential for infectious problems. Always consider infection in a patient with new glucose intolerance on TPN. The line is usually the source of infection. Once suspected, the line should be removed. If TPN is still necessary, then a new site should be used. The catheter tip should be carefully removed and cultured. Secondary infection of the catheter, ie, seeding from another septic site, is also possible and may necessitate catheter removal.

C. Hyperglycemia. The most frequently occurring metabolic complication is hyperglycemia. Hyperglycemia for the patient receiving TPN is defined as a glucose level >200 mg/dL. The approach to hyperglycemia should be dictated by first determining its cause. The initial step in this process is to assess the appropriateness of overall caloric provisions and to clarify the fuel sources. Carbohydrate calories in excess of 30–35 kcal/kg should be decreased. For patients who are diabetic, are on steroids, or are otherwise glucose intolerant, glucose in excess of 150–200 g/day may be tolerated poorly. Fat calories should be increased to approximately 30% of the nonprotein calories in the nonseptic patient. If, after adjustments, hyperglycemia persists, a review of the patient's clinical condition and medications would be warranted.

Patients with new-onset hyperglycemia should always be evaluated for an infection. Corticosteroids are the leading culprit in hyperglycemia. For patients with infections or changing steroid doses, management of hyperglycemia can be achieved with sliding scale insulin or insulin infusions when the patient is in the intensive care unit. Insulin should not be incorporated in the TPN of patients with new-onset hyperglycemia because their hyperglycemia is due to increased hepatic gluconeogenesis and a relative insulin resistance and not to a lack of endogenously released insulin. Hyperglycemia associated with parenteral nutrition generally requires aggressive sliding scale coverage (Table V–4). Only regular insulin should be used to manage hyperglycemia in pa-

TABLE V–4. SLIDING SCALE DOSAGE FOR SUBCUTANEOUS INSULIN ADMINISTRATION.

| Blood Sugar (mg/dL) | Dose of Regular Insulin (in units) | |
	Adequate Renal Function	Renal Failure
200–250	5	2
251–300	10	4
301–350	15	6
351–400	20	8

tients on TPN. Patients who are stable on a given amount of insulin may have the insulin placed in the TPN bag.

Insulin infusions are typically compounded by adding regular insulin 150 U to 0.9% sodium chloride solution 150 mL. The infusion is started at 1–2 U/h and titrated upward to maintain the serum glucose at 80–120 mg/dL. Recent evidence shows that the careful control of serum glucose in this range can decrease morbidity and length of stay. When insulin infusions exceed 8–10 U/h, insulin resistance is probably occurring. At this point, it is often best to discontinue the TPN and correct the hyperglycemia.

D. Refeeding Syndrome. Often when malnutrition is recognized, the inclination is to rapidly and aggressively initiate specialized nutritional support. Unfortunately, this approach is associated with more hazards than the underlying malnutrition. The refeeding syndrome and morbidity associated with overfeeding are real clinical hazards associated with parenteral and enteral nutrition. The refeeding syndrome is a constellation of severe fluid and electrolyte shifts that are associated with initiating nutrition in the chronically malnourished individual.

Typically, hypophosphatemia, hypomagnesemia, and hypokalemia are the electrolyte abnormalities that can result in cardiac and respiratory dysfunction and failure. Thiamine deficiency, hyperglycemia, and volume overload have also occurred. The best approach to the refeeding syndrome is prevention. TPN should be started at ≤1000 kcal or 20 kcal/kg on the first day and titrated according to a patient's tolerance, as defined by glucose monitoring and electrolyte values. Empiric replacement of vitamins, phosphorus, magnesium, and potassium is appropriate in the patient at risk.

E. Electrolyte Abnormalities. In general, when electrolyte deficiencies are present in the patient before initiating TPN, it is best to correct the problems and delay IV feeding. Electrolyte deficiencies that occur once the patient is receiving parenteral nutrition should be corrected with runs outside parenteral nutrition. If the patient has increased maintenance requirements because of chronic gastrointestinal losses or other reasons, the maintenance requirements should be incorporated into the parenteral nutrition mixture. The use of inadequate or excessive amounts of any additive results in the corresponding electrolyte abnormality. The amount of the corresponding electrolyte must be adjusted to correct the abnormality.

F. Acid-Base Disturbances. Hyperchloremic metabolic acidosis is fairly common in patients receiving TPN and may result from bicarbonate loss, which can be caused by severe diarrhea, pancreatic fistulae, or small bowel losses. Therapy is to administer more Na and K as acetate salts (instead of Cl salt).

G. Impaired Liver Function Tests. Hepatic and biliary complications associated with parenteral nutrition are generally characterized by the duration of parenteral nutrition. Abnormal liver function tests are common in short-term and long-term patient populations. The most common hepatic complication associated with short-term TPN administration is hepatic steatosis. This fatty liver infiltration is thought to be a result of overfeeding, especially of carbohydrate calories. The incidence of hepatic steatosis has decreased with the introduction of IV fat emulsion and the growing consideration of conservative caloric feeding. Biliary sludge formation and cholelithiasis with its associated complications have been noted in patients who received TPN for ≥3 weeks. Biliary stasis caused by lack of stimulation resulting from bowel rest or short gut is thought to be the primary mechanism. Long-term TPN administration is associated with hepatic steatonecrosis. Its pathogenesis is unclear at this time.

The diagnosis of TPN-associated hepatotoxicity is a diagnosis of exclusion. Once other causes have been ruled out, management of hepatotoxicity includes reformulation of the caloric regimen, cyclic administration of TPN, and metronidazole.

H. Prerenal Azotemia. Excessive amino acid infusion with inadequate calorie administration can result in prerenal azotemia. Increasing serum urea nitrogen levels should be monitored but often are not controlled until levels reach >100 mg/dL. Increased levels are controlled by decreasing amino acid intake and increasing calories administered as glucose. Prerenal azotemia resulting from intravascular volume depletion should be ruled out.

I. Bleeding Abnormalities. These can be caused by inadequate amounts of vitamin K, iron deficiency, folate deficiency, or vitamin B_{12} deficiency. Adjust the nutrient administration to the required amount.

J. Overfeeding. It is imperative to nutritionally support a patient on a rational and quantitative basis. To do this, the clinician must know the requirements for each nutritional component. Energy requirements are dependent on gender, weight, height, age, energy expenditure, and severity of injury. Overfeeding places patients at risk for hepatic complications, increased carbon dioxide production, and hyperglycemia.

3. TPN in Specific Disease States. Administration of TPN must be changed for patients with certain diseases.

Cardiac Failure. Fluid administration is limited in these patients. Instead of the usual 1 mL water per calorie (as in tube feedings), water is given at 0.5 mL/cal. Alternatively, water can be given at a rate equal to 500 mL (insensible losses) plus measured losses. Protein can be limited to 0.8–1 g/kg, and sodium limited to 0.5–1.5 g/day.

Diabetes. Use increased calories from fat in these patients to limit the carbohydrate calories and provide sufficient calories for protein anabolism. Insulin can be added to the bag in a patient who has stable insulin requirements. In general, fat should provide ≤50% of total caloric intake and ≤2.5 g/kg per day.

Hepatic Dysfunction. Patients with hepatic dysfunction usually benefit from increased amounts of branched-chain amino acids (leucine, valine, and isoleucine) and decreased amounts of aromatic amino acids, which are precursors to centrally active amines and thus contribute to hepatic encephalopathy. Specialized mixtures of amino acids are available and should be used only for patients with hepatic encephalopathy. Lipid emulsions should be limited in those patients with severe hepatic dysfunction.

Renal Disease. These patients have a number of specific restrictions that must be carefully accounted for in the administration of TPN including fluid, protein, potassium, magnesium, and sodium. Protein must be restricted to 0.6–0.8 g/kg per day for patients not undergoing dialysis. Patients receiving hemodialysis generally require 1.2 g/kg protein per day, and patients undergoing peritoneal dialysis need 1.5 g/kg. The latter patient also absorbs approximately 500 kcal/day dextrose from the dialysate, which must be considered when designing their nutritional regimen. Patients on hemodialysis may receive the usual protein load of 1–1.5 g/kg per day. For these patients, specially formulated amino acid mixtures are used that contain larger amounts of essential amino acids. In general, TPN for patients who have renal failure should not contain potassium or magnesium. Decreased sodium may also be necessary.

Pulmonary Dysfunction. Carbohydrate metabolism (including overfeeding) results in production of CO_2. Thus, patients who have impaired ventilation and already may retain CO_2 are further stressed when high carbohydrate loads are administered. This problem may be managed by increasing the percentage of calories provided by fat (up to 50%). Overall, calories should not exceed 30–35 kcal/kg. These patients also may be sensitive to phosphate depletion and should be monitored carefully for the development of hypophosphatemia. Once identified, this is managed with phosphate supplementation.

REFERENCES

ASPEN Board of Directors. Guidelines for the use of parenteral and enteral nutrition in adult and pediatric patients. *JPEN* 17:6SA, 1993.

Finney SJ, et al. Glucose control and mortality in critically ill patients. *JAMA* 290:2041–7, 2003.

Gomella LG. Total parenteral nutrition. In: Gomella LG, ed. *Clinician's Pocket Reference,* 10th ed. New York: McGraw-Hill; 2004.

VI. Blood Component Therapy

APPROACH TO THE BLEEDING PATIENT

When called to evaluate a patient for a low hemoglobin/hematocrit level (Hb/Hct) or for active bleeding, as in all such situations, start with the ABCs (airway, breathing, and circulation). Once the airway and breathing are controlled, heart rate, blood pressure, and the need for blood components/transfusions or just intravenous fluid must be assessed. First, obtain good intravenous access with 2 large-bore intravenous lines, ≥16 gauge, and order a complete blood cell count and coagulation studies (prothrombin time, partial thromboplastin time, and platelet count). A type and screen or type and cross should also be ordered, depending on the clinical situation.

Questions to ask include:

- What is the current Hb/Hct level?
- What is the previous Hb/Hct level?
- Is the patient on any anticoagulants?

An attempt should be made to assess the location and amount of the patient's bleeding, and the patient's vital signs should be monitored very closely. "Transfusion triggers" have changed during the past several years, and it is no longer mandatory to maintain a particular Hb level (eg, 10 g/dL) in all patients. Considerations include a patient's age, the presence of comorbid conditions, including risk factors for coronary artery disease (hypertension, diabetes mellitus, smoking, age >50 years in men, and hypercholesterolemia) and rapidity of the bleeding and decrease in Hb/Hct level. Perhaps the most important consideration regarding transfusion for a low Hct level is the patient's own physiologic response to that loss of blood volume. In young healthy patients, Hb, in certain clinical situations, has been allowed to decrease as low as 6 g/dL (note females have a lower baseline Hct level than do males of the same age). Oxygen delivery is partly dependent on the Hb/Hct levels. Several studies suggest that, for noncritically ill patients, the threshold for transfusion is Hb of 7–8 g/dL. However, this level does not appear to be acceptable for patients with significant risk factors for coronary artery disease or for patients with symptomatic anemia, tachycardia, etc. Having a Hb level of 8 g/dL or even 10 g/dL in light of ongoing active bleeding (eg, lower/upper gastrointestinal tract) may also be an indication for transfusion because Hb takes time to equilibrate. Continued blood loss may cause the next Hb measurement to be only 6 g/dL when one does not consider ongoing blood loss. It should be remembered that a decrease in Hb level may be a **late** sign of active bleeding.

BLOOD BANKING PROCEDURES

Type & Screen. The blood bank will type the patient's blood and screen it for antibodies. If a rare antibody is found, the physician usually will be notified. When there is a reasonable chance that the patient may need blood in the immediate future, it is advisable to **type and crossmatch** a bleeding patient. If one waits until the laboratory test indicates a low Hct and a transfusion is immediately required, it takes another hour for a unit of crossmatched blood to be ready. Many intensive care units have blood analyzers to rapidly and accurately determine Hct (among other tests). Once a type and screen has been sent, crossmatched blood is usually available in <1 hour.

Type & Cross. The blood bank will type and screen the patient's blood and match the patient with specific donor units. The number of units to be crossed and held must be specified. If the request is made "stat," the bank will set up blood immediately and usually hold it for 12 hours. For routine requests, the blood is set up at a date and time that the physician specifies, and the blood is usually held for 36–48 hours.

BLOOD BANK PRODUCTS & BLOOD COMPONENT THERAPY

Tables VI–1 and VI–2 list products used in blood component therapy and some common indications for their use.

TRANSFUSION PROCEDURE

1. Draw a clot tube ("red top") and sign the laboratory slips to verify it is the sample from the correct patient.
2. Make sure that the patient has good venous access for the transfusion ($\geq$18 gauge is preferred in an adult).
3. Verify the information with another person. *Note:* Nearly all hospitals have defined protocols for this procedure; check guidelines for your specific institution.
4. Blood products to be transfused may be mixed with only isotonic normal saline. Using hypotonic products, such as 5% dextrose in water, may result in hemolysis of the blood in the tubing. Lactated Ringer solution should not be used because the calcium could chelate the anticoagulant citrate.
5. When transfusing large volumes of packed red cells (6–8 U), it is necessary to also transfuse platelets and fresh frozen plasma periodically (dilutional thrombocytopenia is the most

TABLE VI–1. BLOOD BANK PRODUCTS THAT USUALLY REQUIRE A "CLOT TUBE" TO BE SENT FOR TYPING

Product	Description	Common Indications
Whole blood	No elements removed; 1 U = 450 mL ; contains red cells, white cells, plasma and platelets (platelets may be nonfunctional)	Not for routine use; acute massive bleeding: open heart surgery; neonatal total exchange
PRBC (also see page 367)	Most plasma removed; unit = 250–300 mL: 1 U should raise Hct 3%	Replacement in chronic and acute (PRBC) blood loss, GI bleeding, trauma
Universal pedi-packs	250–300 mL divided into 3 bags; contains red cells, some white cells, some plasma and platelets	Transfusion for infants
Platelets (also see page 367)	1 "pack" should raise count by 5–8000; "6–pack" means a pool of platelets from 6 U of blood; 1 pack = about 50 mL	Decreased production or destruction (ie, aplastic anemia, acute leukemia, postchemo, etc); counts <5000 (risk of spontaneous hemorrhage); counts 5–30,000 if risk of bleeding (headache, GI losses, contiguous petechiae) or active bleeding; counts <50,000 if life-threatening bleed or preop; counts <100,000 in some cases of post-CABG bleeding or with neuro- or ophthalmic. surgery; usually not indicated in idiopathic thrombocytopenic purpura or thrombotic thrombocytopenic purpura unless life-threatening bleed or preoperatively
Leukocyte poor red cells	Most WBCs removed less antigenic; 1 U = 200–250 mL	Previous fabrile transfusion reactions; patients requiring multiple transfusions (eg, leukemia)
Washed RBCs	Like leukocyte poor red cells but WBC almost completely removed; 1 U = 300 mL	As for leukocyte poor red cells, but very expensive and much more purified

(continued)

TABLE VI–1. BLOOD BANK PRODUCTS THAT USUALLY REQUIRE A "CLOT TUBE" TO BE SENT FOR TYPING. (*continued*)

Product	Description	Common Indications
Cryoprecipitated antihemophilic factor ("cryo")	Contains factor VIII, factor XIII, von Willebrand's factor, and fibrinogen; 1 U = 10 mL	Hemophilia A (factor VIII deficiency), when safer factor VIII concentrate not available; von Willebrand disease; fibrinogen deficiency, fibrin surgical glue
Fresh frozen plasma (FFP)	Contains factors II, VII, IX, X, XI, XII, XIII and heat labile V and VII; about 1 h to thaw; 150–250 mL (400–600 mL if single donor pheresis)	Emergency reversal of Coumadin; massive transfusion (>5 L in adults); Hypoglobinemia (IV immune globulin preferred); suspected or documented coagulopathy (congenital or acquired) with active bleeding or before surgery; clotting factor replacement when concentrate unavailable; no longer recommended for volume replacement
Single donor plasma	Like FFP, but lacks factors V and VIII; about 1 h to thaw; 150–200 mL	No longer routinely used for plasma replacement; stable clotting factor replacement; Coumadin reversal, Hemophilia B (Christmas disease)
RhoGam (RhoD immune globulin)	Antibody against Rh factor	Rh⁻ mother with Rh⁺ baby within 72 hr of delivery

CABG = coronary bypass grafting; FFP = fresh frozen plasma; GI = gastrointestinal; PRBC = packed red blood cells; RBC = red blood cell; WBC = white blood cell.

common complication of multiple transfusions). Studies demonstrate higher mortality rates for patients not given platelets and factors early during a massive resuscitation. Also, a calcium replacement is sometimes needed because the preservative used in blood (citrate) is a calcium binder, and hypocalcemia can result after large amounts of blood are transfused. Also, the blood should be warmed, if at all possible, in all transfusions. In cases in which massive resuscitation efforts are necessary, warming is essential to prevent hypothermia, coagulopathy, and cardiac arrhythmias. Massive blood transfusions are associated with transfusion-related acute lung injury and possibly disseminated intravascular coagulation.

TABLE VI–2. BLOOD BANK PRODUCTS THAT ARE DISPENSED BY MOST HOSPITAL PHARMACIES AND ARE ORDERED AS MEDICATION

Product	Description	Common Indications
Factor VIII (purified antihemophilic factor)	From pooled plasma, pure factor VIII	Routine for hemophilia A (factor VII deficiency); increased hepatitis risk
Factor IX concentrate (prothrombin complex)	Increased hepatitis risk; factors II, VII, IX, and X equivalent to 2 U of plasma	Active bleeding in Christmas disease (hemophilia B or factor IX deficiency)
Immune serum globulin	Precipitate from plasma; gamma globulin	Immune globulin deficiency: disease prophylaxis (eg,. hepatitis A, measles)
5% albumin or 5% plasma protein fraction	Precipitate from plasma (see Section IX)	Plasma volume expanders in acute blood loss
25% albumin	Precipitate from plasma	Hypoalbuminemia, volume expander, burns; draws extravascular fluid into circulation

BLOOD GROUPS

Table VI–3 presents information on the major blood groups and their relative occurrences. O– is the universal donor and AB+ is the universal recipient.

TRANSFUSION FORMULAS

Red Blood Cells

As a rule of thumb, 1 U packed red cells increases Hct by 3% (Hb by 1 g/dL) in the average adult. To roughly determine the volume of whole blood or packed red cells needed to increase Hct to a specific amount, use the following formula:

$$\text{Volume of cells} = \frac{\text{Total blood volume of patient x (desired Hct} - \text{actual Hct)}}{\text{Hct of transfusion product}}$$

Platelets

Some clinicians seek platelet counts >100,000 before major surgery and >50,000 for minor surgery. The occurrence of spontaneous hemorrhage is thought to occur with platelet counts

TABLE VI–3. BLOOD GROUPS

Type (ABO/Rh)	Occurrences	Can Usually Receive Blood From
O^+	1 in 3	O $(^{+/-})$
O^-	1 in 15	O $(^-)$
A^+	1 in 3	A $(^{+/-})$ or O $(^{+/-})$
A^-	1 in 16	A $(^-)$ or O $(^-)$
B^+	1 in 12	B $(^{+/-})$ or O $(^{+/-})$
B^-	1 in 67	B $(^-)$ or O $(^-)$
AB^+	1 in 29	AB, A, B or O (all $^+$ or $^-$)
AB^-	1 in 167	AB, A, B or O (all $^-$)

<20,000. However, in the experience of many surgeons disorders that cause thrombocytopenia such as splenic abnormalities, hematologic cancers, or other disorders often do not cause bleeding even with platelet counts as low as 5000. The exact platelet count needed to avoid the morbidity of bleeding in a thrombocytopenic patient is undefined because bleeding may be the result of poorly functioning platelets (eg, with a normal platelet count) and a decreased number of platelets. After administration of 1 U multiple donor platelets, the count should increase 5–8000/mL within 1 hour of transfusion and to 4500/mL within 24 hours. Normally, stored platelets that are transfused should survive in vivo 6–8 days after infusion. Clinical factors (disseminated intravascular coagulation, alloimmunization) can significantly shorten these intervals.

COAGULATION FACTORS

Blood products are often used to replenish coagulation factors that are diminished from a variety of causes, most commonly secondary to massive transfusions in the surgical population. It is important to use the correct blood product to ensure that the desired factor is replaced and to avoid use of blood products that carry some risk to patients. The composition of commonly used blood products and the factors contained therein are listed in Table VI–4. This information in addition to that listed in Table VI–2 should be used to guide administration of commonly used blood products.

EMERGENCY TRANSFUSIONS

The transfusion of non-crossmatched blood is occasionally necessary in cases of trauma and/or massive hemorrhage. Type-specific blood (ABO and Rh-matched only) is usually available in 10

TABLE VI–4. COMPOSITION OF COMMONLY USED BLOOD PRODUCTS

Product	Description	Typical Volume
Whole blood	Erythrocytes, white cells, plasma, and platelets	400–500 mL
PRBC	Erythrocytes, with most plasma removed	250–300 mL
Platelets	Thrombocytes	1–50 packs
FFP	Factors II, V, VII, IX, X, XI, XII, XIII	150–200 mL
Cryoprecipitate	Factors VII and VIII, fibrinogen	1–10 U

FFP = fresh frozen plasma; PRBC = packed red blood cells.
Source: (Adapted from Lefor AT, ed. Critical Care On Call. New York: McGraw-Hill; 2002, p 364.)

minutes and can be used. If even this time is too long, type O, Rh-negative, packed red cell blood can be used. Most blood banks can do a complete crossmatch within 1 hour. As per advanced trauma life support protocol, a 2-L challenge of crystalloid is used to support blood pressure; however, when hypotension persists or there are massive ongoing blood losses, transfusion of non-cross-matched (universal donor) blood may be warranted.

TRANSFUSION REACTIONS

See Section I, Problem 69 ("Transfusion Reaction"), page 238. More than 85% of adverse hemolytic transfusion reactions relate to clerical error.

AUTOLOGOUS BLOOD TRANSFUSIONS

Because of concerns over the transmission of disease by blood transfusion therapy, prehospital autologous blood banking (predeposit phlebotomy) has become popular in the elective surgery patient. General guidelines for autologous banking include good overall health status, Hct >34%, and arm veins that can accommodate a 16-gauge needle. Patients can usually donate up to 1 U every 3–7 days until 3–7 days before surgery (individual blood banks have their own specifications), depending on the needs of the planned surgery. Iron supplements (eg, ferrous gluconate 325 mg orally 3 times daily) are usually given before and several months after the donation. Units of whole blood can be held for up to 35 days.

DIRECTED DONOR BLOOD PRODUCTS

Because of concerns over disease transmission, this form of donation is becoming more widely used, although this varies by region. This involves a person, often a relative, donating blood for a specific patient. This cannot be used in the emergency setting because it takes up to 48 hours to process the blood for transfusion. These units are usually stored as packed red blood cells and released into the general transfusion pool 8 hours after surgery unless otherwise requested.

APHERESIS

Apheresis procedures are used to collect single-donor platelets (platelet pheresis) or white blood cells (leukophoresis); the remaining components are returned to the donor. Therapeutic apheresis is the separation and removal of a particular component to achieve a therapeutic effect (eg, erythrocytophoresis to control polycythemia).

TRANSFUSION-TRANSMITTED DISEASE

Before administering a transfusion, the risks of the procedure should be explained to the patient and/or the patient's family, and an informed consent should be obtained. An exception to this practice is in emergency/trauma cases where this is not practical. The current risk of contracting human immunodeficiency virus (HIV) from a blood transfusion based on data from 2001 is 0.005%. The risk of hepatitis B is estimated to be 0.047%, that of human T-lymphotropic virus is 0.013%, and that of hepatitis C is 0.234%. As can be seen, hepatitis C is the most common form of hepatitis transmitted by transfusions. The most common infectious agent transmitted is cytomegalovirus, which is a concern in immunocompromised patients.

The greatest risk is with pooled factor products, such as concentrates of factor VIII. Use of albumin, globulins, and the new genetically engineered factor VIII concentrates involves no risk of hepatitis or HIV.

OTHER OPTIONS

Blood Product Substitutes

Red blood cell substitutes currently in development include hemoglobin-based oxygen carriers, perfluorocarbon emulsions, and liposome-encapsulated Hb. The 2 major types of blood substitutes, hemoglobin-based oxygen carriers and perfluorocarbon emulsions, are in phase II and III clinical trials. Potential advantages would include eliminating the risk of passing on HIV and hepatitis and using these products for patients who refuse blood transfusions.

Erythropoietin. Erythropoietin stimulates erythrocyte production in patients with anemia of chronic renal failure and other conditions. It can also stimulate erythropoiesis in the autologous donor to enable additional donation.

REFERENCES

Goodnough LT, et al. Transfusion medicine. *N Engl J Med* 340:438–525, 1999.

Hebert PC, et al. A multicenter, randomized, controlled clinical trial of transfusion requirements in critical care. *N Engl J Med* 340:409–17, 1999.

Winslow RM. New transfusion strategies: red cell substitutes. *Annu Rev Med* 50:337–53, 1999.

Zou S, et al. Probability of viremia with HBV, HCV, HIV and HTLV among tissue donors in the United States. *N Engl J Med* 351:751–9, 2004.

VII. Ventilator Management

INDICATIONS & VENTILATOR SETUP

I. Indications for Ventilator Support

A. Hypoxemic Respiratory Failure. The inability to oxygenate is an important indication for ventilator support. An arterial partial pressure of oxygen (Pa_{O_2}) <60 mm Hg on >50% inspired fraction of oxygen (FI_{O_2}) constitutes hypoxemic respiratory failure. Although these patients can sometimes be managed with higher FI_{O_2} delivery systems (eg, noninvasive positive pressure ventilation, delivered by mask), they are at high risk for respiratory arrest and should be closely monitored in an intensive care unit. These delivery systems are at a significant disadvantage compared with mechanical ventilation because it is difficult to continuously maintain a high FI_{O_2} delivery. Further, these methods require a patient who is awake and cooperative and has no gastric distention or nausea/vomiting. Worsening of the respiratory status necessitates prompt intubation and initiation of ventilator support. One of the most common causes for pure hypoxemic respiratory failure in surgical patients is acute respiratory distress syndrome (ARDS) in which the high shunt fraction leads to refractory hypoxemia.

B. Ventilatory Failure. Some criteria for defining ventilatory failure are presented in Table VII–1. In general, ventilatory failure is based on the degree of hypercarbia. An arterial partial pressure of carbon dioxide (Pa_{CO_2}) >50 mm Hg indicates ventilatory failure; however, many patients with chronic pulmonary conditions, such as chronic obstructive pulmonary disease (COPD), will have chronic ventilatory failure with renal compensation (retaining HCO_3^-) to adjust the pH toward normal. Thus, absolute pH is often a better guide than Pa_{CO_2} in determining the need for ventilator assistance. A respiratory acidosis with a rapidly decreasing pH or an absolute pH ≤7.24 is an indication for ventilator support. Examples of ventilatory failure include the patient with drug overdose in whom there is a sudden loss of central respiratory drive with uncontrolled hypercarbia, neuromuscular disease, and COPD.

C. Mixed Respiratory Failure. Most patients who require ventilator support have failure of ventilation and oxygenation (eg, COPD with acute bronchitis). The indications for

TABLE VII–1. CRITERIA FOR DIAGNOSIS OF ACUTE RESPIRATORY FAILURE.

Parameter	Normal	Respiratory Failure
Respiratory rate	12–20	>35
Vital capacity (mL/kg body wt)[a]	65–75	<15
FEV_1 (mL/Kg body wt)[a]	50–60	≤10
Inspiratory force (cm H_2O)	75–100	≥25
Compliance (mL/cm H_2O)	100	<20
Pao_2 (mm/cm H_2O)	80–95 Room air	<70
A-aDo_2 (mm Hg) (Fio_2 = 1.0)	25–65	>450
Os/Ot (%)	5–8	>20
$Paco_2$	35–45	>55[b]
VD/VT	0.2–0.3	>0.60

[a]Ideal body weight should be used.
[b]Chronic lung disease constitutes the exception.
A-aDo_2 = alveolar-arterial oxygen gradient; FEV_1 = forced expiratory volume in 1 second; Fio_2 = fraction of inspired oxygen; Os/Ot = shunt fraction; $Paco_2$ = partial pressure of carbon dioxide in arterial blood; Pao_2 = partial pressure of oxygen in arterial blood; VD/VT = ratio of dead space to tidal volume.
Source: (Reproduced, with permission, from Demling RH, Goodwin CW. Pulmonary dysfunction. In: Willmore DW, ed. Care of the Surgical Patient. Scientific American, 1989.)

ventilator support remain the same as those listed above. The threshold for initiating ventilator support will be even lower for patients with ventilation and oxygenation failure, because oxygen management may further compound hypercarbia. Bronchospasm alters the ventilation-perfusion ratio relations, leading to worsening hypoxemia. Perhaps the most important element in decision making for the initiation of ventilator support is clinical judgment. It is far easier to initiate ventilator support and withdraw it later than to avoid this therapy and end up with a critically ill or dead patient.

D. Neuromuscular Failure. This is a category of ventilatory failure but deserves special mention because the management is different. Hypercarbia occurs just before respiratory arrest; thus, criteria other than arterial blood gases (ABGs) are needed.

1. In progressive tachypnea, breathing rates >24/min are an early sign of respiratory failure. A progressive increase in the respiratory rate or sustained breathing rates >30/min is an indication for ventilatory support.

2. Abdominal paradox indicates dyssynergy of chest wall muscles and diaphragm contraction with impending

respiratory failure. It is manifested by inward movement of the abdominal wall during inspiration rather than the normal outward motion.

3. A vital capacity <15 mL/kg (1000 mL for a person with normal body size) is associated with acute respiratory failure and an inability to clear secretions. Similarly, a negative inspiratory force –25 cm H_2O implies impending respiratory arrest. A rapidly decreasing vital capacity or a vital capacity <1000 mL requires initiation of respirator support.

II. **Endotracheal Intubation** (see Section III, page 352). Endotracheal intubation can be a difficult and potentially hazardous part of ventilator initiation. Skill and experience are required for correct placement of the endotracheal tube. Aspiration, esophageal intubation, and right main stem bronchus intubation are the most common complications. Five-point auscultation is used to confirm proper placement (anterior and lateral chest wall on the right and left sides, plus the stomach). The most accurate method of confirming proper placement is by measuring expired CO_2. The current standard of care is the use of a monitoring device that can demonstrate the presence of CO_2 by color change.

Key factors in successful intubation are complete preparation of all supplies before attempting intubation, proper hand placement, and proper use of the laryngoscope. Intubation can be accomplished by 3 routes: nasotracheal intubation, orotracheal intubation, or tracheostomy. When one encounters an unexpectedly difficult intubation, an immediate call for additional, more experienced personnel is a necessity and an indication of good clinical judgment. An immediate postintubation portable chest radiograph should always be obtained.

A. **Nasotracheal Intubation.** This can be accomplished blindly and in an awake patient. It requires experience and adequate local anesthesia. Complications include esophageal intubation, nosebleeds, kinking of the endotracheal tube (ETT), and postobstructive sinusitis. A smaller ETT is usually required for nasotracheal versus orotracheal intubation; this leads to greater work of breathing because of increased resistance, difficulties with adequate suctioning, and higher ventilation pressures. Nasotracheal ETTs may be more comfortable than orotracheal ETTs. Nasotracheal intubation should not be attempted by those without experience in an emergency setting. Newer ventilators are able to compensate for the greater work of breathing by using tubing compensation, but older machines that do not have this technique can lead to difficulties during weaning.

B. **Orotracheal Intubation.** Placement of orotracheal tubes requires some neck mobility to allow hyperextension of the neck for direct visualization of the vocal cords. Adequate sedation is necessary for safe placement without aspiration.

C. **Tracheostomy.** Cricothyroidotomy is the surgical procedure most often done in the acute setting for upper airway obstruction; however, in patients who require >14–21 days of ventilator support, conversion to formal surgical tracheostomy is recommended to prevent tracheal stenosis and vocal cord damage. Tracheostomy tubes facilitate the weaning process by decreasing tube resistance because the tube is shorter and has a larger radius. Patients are able to eat and they find the tubes more comfortable.

III. Ventilator Setup

A. **The Ventilator.** Almost all modern adult ventilators are cycled by time and flow (volume) and can be used in adults and in children >2 years. Children <2 years and infants are usually managed on pressure-limited continuous flow. Pressure-controlled ventilation is an alternate mode of support most frequently used for patients with ARDS. High frequency or "jet" ventilators are not commonly used and are indicated only in patients with tracheobronchial fistulas and in preterm infants with severe respiratory distress. Elaborate alarm systems are present to alert personnel to inadequate ventilation, high pressure, disconnection of the ETT, and so forth.

   Minute ventilation is defined as tidal volume × respiratory rate. Thus, ventilation may be adjusted by changing the respiratory rate, the tidal volume, or both. Tidal volumes >12 mL/kg may cause overdistention of alveoli and increase the risk of pneumothorax. Based on recent studies, the initial tidal volume is set at 6–8 mL/kg. Oxygenation is adjusted by changing FIO_2 and positive end-expiratory pressure (PEEP; Figure VII–1). Prolonged FIO_2 >60% may cause pulmonary fibrosis due to oxygen toxicity. Thus, down-adjustment to "safe levels" sufficient to maintain O_2 saturation >90% should be attempted and verified by ABGs. If an O_2 saturation >90% cannot be maintained when decreasing the FIO_2 <60%, other means, eg, increasing PEEP, can be used.

B. **Modes of Ventilation**
   1. **Control mode** delivers a set rate and tidal volume irrespective of patient efforts and is used for patients who are paralyzed or unable to initiate a breath. (Rarely, if ever, used.)

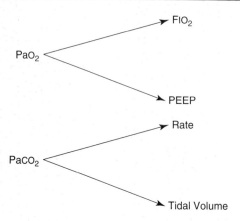

Figure VII–1. A simple way to remember the ventilator parameters that affect PaO_2 and $PaCO_2$.

2. **Assist control** (AC) mode allows patient triggering of machine breaths once a threshold of inspiratory flow or effort is made. It also supplies a backup rate in case of apnea or paralysis, so that the patient receives at least the set rate number of breaths. This mode provides the full specified tidal volume each time the threshold effort is achieved.

3. **Intermittent mandatory ventilation** (IMV) provides a set number of machine-initiated breaths per minute and allows the patient to take spontaneous breaths between machine-initiated breaths. Synchronized IMV (SIMV) allows synchronization of the IMV breaths with patient efforts and is the generally preferred method because it avoids breath-stacking. As the ventilator's rate is decreased, the patient assumes more and more of the work of breathing. All efforts by the patient between synchronized breaths must overcome the resistance of the tubing unless pressure support is added. This mode is well tolerated by patients who continue to require mechanical ventilation but are awake and otherwise stable.

4. **Pressure support ventilation** (PSV) is used to help decrease the inspiratory work of breathing by the patient. Pressure support supplies a positive pressure when the patient initiates a breath. PEEP and pressure

support must be specified, and the patient sets the flow, respiratory rate, and tidal volume. **Continuous positive airway pressure** (CPAP) is the same as PSV and is basically an older term for the same function. The key differentiating point for this ventilator mode is that there is *no set respiratory rate*. The patient must have respiratory drive. A set amount of continuous pressure is applied during inspiration and expiration (0–30 cm H_2O). There are no ventilator-delivered breaths. The amount of support provided by the machine during patient inspirations can be specified by increasing the pressure support. Patients are started with a high-pressure support that is gradually decreased over time. PSV can be used as a "weaning mode" (see below).

5. **High frequency (jet) ventilation** is only used in specific situations. The process relies on low airway pressure, low tidal volumes (4 mL/kg), and very high rates (typically 100–400 cycles/min). Use of this mode results in permissive hypercapnia.

6. **Pressure-controlled ventilation (PCV)**

   a. **Pressure versus volume.** This mode of ventilation relies on pressure settings instead of volume settings to control gas flow to the patient. This mode is currently most commonly used for patients with ARDS or other diseases that require markedly increased FIO_2 for prolonged periods. The major differences in this mode of ventilation are (1) the ability to deliver inverse ratio ventilation without erratic pressure changes and (2) a lack of ability to maintain constant minute ventilation. Pressure control ventilation should be implemented only when the patient is chemically paralyzed or deeply sedated. Inverse ratio ventilation is most effective when patients cannot initiate spontaneous respirations. Bilevel is a breath mode in which the patient has the ability to breathe spontaneously at 2 levels of PEEP. Its pressure waveform resembles PCV but differs in its ability to allow unrestricted spontaneous breathing at the upper and lower pressure levels. Therefore, only a minimally necessary degree of ventilatory augmentation needs to be applied. Spontaneous breaths in bilevel can be augmented with pressure support.

   b. **Settings.**

      i. **Oxygenation** is controlled by manipulation of the FIO_2 and the PEEP. Oxygenation can further be increased by extending the time spent in inspiration. The I:E ratio refers to the ratio of time spent in inspiration to time spent in expiration. The I:E ratio (or I time) can directly be regulated in PCV.

ii. **Ventilation** is controlled by regulating the respiratory rate and manipulation of the pressure delivered. Pressure delivered is referred to as *delta P. *Delta P is the difference between the peak inspiratory pressure (PIP) and the PEEP. This pressure differential affects the volume delivered in the inspiratory time specified.

iii. **Initial settings** for PCV should be performed at the patient's bedside with the respiratory therapist present. The PIP should be determined while still on volume control. Baseline oxygen saturation and hemodynamics should also be obtained. Respiratory rate, PEEP, and Fio_2 should be left unchanged. Initial *delta P should be the PIP minus the PEEP multiplied by a factor of 0.66, ie, $0.66 \times (PIP - PEEP)$. The I:E ratio can generally be started at 1:1.5 or 1:2. This signifies that, for each second spent in inspiration, the ventilator allows 1.5 or 2 seconds for exhalation.

After conversion to pressure control, several parameters must be observed, including tidal volume, oxygen saturation, and blood pressure. The pressure/volume graphs must be inspected. This graph is generated by many modern ventilators and graphically depicts the pressure and volume changes during inspiration and expiration. The graph is important to ensure that the settings allow enough time in expiration to prevent auto-PEEP. Auto-PEEP occurs when inspirations are initiated by the ventilator before complete expiration from the previous cycle. Auto-PEEP can cause an increase in the work of breathing to result in cardiovascular sequelae, such as hypotension.

iv. **Example of conversion**
AC Mode
Fio_2: 100%
Rate: 20 breaths/min
PEEP: 10 cm H_2O
Observed PIP: 70 cm H_2O
PIP – PEEP: 60 cm H_2O
Pressure Control Mode (new settings)
Fio_2: 100%
Rate: 20 breaths/min
*Delta P: 40
I:E ratio: 1:1.5

c. **Special considerations for PCV.** Several factors should be considered for patients who require PCV. All changes to rate or I:E ratios should be followed by monitoring the pressure volume cycle graphs. Changes to PCV generally require additional time to be reflected in measurements of blood gases. Inspiratory time can be maximized by using the pressure/volume cycle graphs to minimize the portion of time spent in expiration. This can be accomplished by manipulating the I:E ratio such that inspiration occurs immediately after complete exhalation.

In addition, inspiratory time can be increased if the respiratory rate can be decreased and then the inspiration/expiration cycle time can be increased. I:E ratios can be manipulated to reverse the natural tendency of expiration time to exceed inspiration time. Most clinicians limit the inverse ratio ventilation to 3:1.

d. **Common errors with PCV.** There are 2 common problems that can arise after conversion to PCV. The first occurs after ventilator setting changes. In particular, rate changes can be associated with subsequent inappropriate I:E ratios if they have not been specified. Second, inverse ratio ventilation becomes ineffective when paralytic agents are allowed to become subtherapeutic, and the patient struggles to breathe against the settings of the ventilator.

7. **Airway pressure release ventilation** mode is used in patients who can breathe spontaneously, and it applies a high level of CPAP that is terminated for a brief period. This release period allows clearance of CO_2. It has been shown in some studies to improve oxygen delivery in patients with ARDS.

C. Initial Ventilator Settings

1. Initial ventilator settings are dictated by the underlying condition and previous ABG results. There are 5 parameters to order when writing initial ventilator orders: **FIO_2, PEEP, rate, tidal volume, and mode**. The patient's partial pressure of oxygen is affected by the FIO_2 and the PEEP level. The patient's partial pressure of carbon dioxide (PCO_2) is affected by the rate and the tidal volume (see Figure VII–1).

a. **Fraction of inspired oxygen.** Most commonly, the ventilator is started at 100% oxygen. The problem with high oxygen concentrations is toxicity, and this phenomenon is related to time. Many clinicians recommend 100% until the first blood gas result is available. This should not exceed 1 hour to minimize any toxic effect. In general, try to keep FIO_2 <50% to maintain acceptable oxygenation (generally >90% saturation on ABG). Patients who have been in the operating room and monitored by the anesthesiologist may often be started on lower O_2 concentrations as recommended by the anesthesiologist in the PACU.

b. **Positive-end expiratory pressure.** PEEP is usually begun at a level of 5 cm H_2O pressure. Higher levels of PEEP are added when trying to wean a patient from high levels of oxygen (FIO_2 >60%). PEEP is associated with an increased risk of alveolar rupture (which can result in a tension pneumothorax) and decreased cardiac output, depending on the mean intrathoracic pressure. Hemodynamic monitoring is usually needed for high levels of PEEP.

c. **Rate.** Normal respiratory rate is 12–20 breaths/min. Initially the ventilator should be set at 12 breaths/min.

d. **Tidal volume.** Normal tidal volume is 6–8 mL/kg body weight.

e. **Mode.** There are several modes of operation of most volume-cycled ventilators, including AC, IMV, SIMV, etc, as discussed in detail above. A basic understanding of these modes is important to order the optimum support for a given patient.

   An attempt should be made to supply the patient with at least as much minute ventilation as was required before intubation. Thus, patients with pulmonary edema, ARDS, or neuromuscular disease may require minute ventilation of 14–22 L/min. The patient with COPD should not be overventilated initially. Such patients may have chronically high bicarbonate because of renal compensation, and overventilation could cause severe alkalosis and prolong the weaning phase significantly.

2. **Secondary ventilator controls.** Most major ventilator controls (inspired oxygen, tidal volume, PEEP, rate, and mode) are ordered by the physician and accomplish the major control of the ventilator's functions. However, there are a series of secondary ventilator controls that can be used to "optimize" or fine-tune the ventilator. Often, secondary controls are determined by local protocol. However, secondary ventilator control settings can be specified, including:

a. **Peak inspiratory pressure.** This represents the maximum pressure generated and is typically set at

20–30 cm H_2O. Pressures >45 cm are associated with significant barotrauma. If the PIP is >35–40 cm, then a change of ventilator mode to PCV may be indicated.

   b. Inspiratory/expiratory ratio. Normal is approximately 1:3. Higher ratios favor oxygenation, and lower ratios enhance CO_2 removal. Most ventilator alarms sound if the parameters chosen result in an I:E ratio <1:1. Inverse I:E ratio ventilation in patients with severe hypoxemia is usually performed in PCV or airway pressure release ventilation modes with a deeply sedated or paralyzed patient.

D. Additional Orders

  1. Restraint of the patient's hands and feet should be considered because the natural reaction to the ETT after awakening is to pull it out. Orders should be as per hospital protocols.

  2. Place a nasogastric tube to decompress the stomach and/or to continue administration of essential oral medications and monitor gastric pH.

  3. Consider placement of an arterial catheter. An arterial line provides a continuous monitor for blood pressure and the ability to easily obtain ABGs.

  4. Obtain an immediate portable chest radiograph to confirm ETT placement and to reassess the patient if respiratory status changes. In addition, daily chest radiographs should be obtained to confirm the position of the ETT.

  5. Manage any additional conditions that might influence respiratory status (eg, maximize bronchodilators, frequent chest physiotherapy and suctioning, or diuretics when indicated).

  6. Implement a "bundle" of 3 prophylactic measures. (1) Administer low-molecular-weight heparin and the use of sequential compression devices on the lower extremities (as indicated) for deep venous thrombotic prophylaxis. These may decrease the incidence of pulmonary embolism while the patient is immobilized. (2) Stress ulceration bleeding can be prevented by judicious use of agents such as antacids, ranitidine (Zantac), or sucralfate (Carafate). (3) The head of the bed should be elevated. These 3 interventions, when used together, have been shown to decrease the incidence of ventilator-associated complications.

  7. Ventilated patients should be sedated as per hospital protocols. Pain medication is administered according to the patients' needs.

ROUTINE MODIFICATION OF VENTILATOR SETTINGS

ABGs should be monitored and the ventilator adjusted to yield a normal pH (7.37–7.44) and a PaO_2 >60 mm Hg on <60% O_2. Once correlation of the oxygen saturation by pulse oximeter and the blood gas has been established, the ABGs for oxygenation can be minimized. Continuous pulse oximetry is the standard of care.

I. Ventilator Changes to Affect Pao_2

A. To Decrease. FIO_2 should be decreased in increments of 10–20%, with ABGs or oximetry checked between increments. The "rule of 7s" states that there will be a 7 mm Hg decrease in Pao_2 for each 1% decrease in FIO_2.

B. To Increase

1. Ventilation has some effect on PaO_2 (as shown by the alveolar gas equation); therefore, correction of hypercarbia will improve oxygenation.

2. PEEP can be added in increments of 2–4 cm H_2O. PEEP recruits previously collapsed alveoli, holds them open, and restores functional residual capacity to a more physiologic level. It counteracts pulmonary shunts and increases PaO_2. PEEP increases intrathoracic pressure and thus may impede venous return and decrease cardiac output. This is particularly true in the presence of volume depletion and shock. The effects of PEEP have a slower onset than changes in FIO_2 and may require several hours to become apparent.

3. Increase I:E ratio, which can be affected even in AC mode by changing the waveforms in which the specified tidal volume is delivered.

II. Ventilator Changes to Affect $Paco_2$

A. To Decrease

1. Increase the rate.
2. Increase the tidal volume.
3. Check for leaks in the system.

B. To Increase

1. Decrease the rate.
2. Decrease the tidal volume.
3. If necessary, the ventilator mode should be changed. It often is necessary to determine the optimum mode for that particular patient. More sedation may be required to optimize ventilator support.

    The cause of hyperventilation should be determined (eg, anxiety or sepsis) and managed appropriately. Always inspect the ventilator for artificial causes of increased respiratory rate, eg, condensation within the tubing can cause water movement that can be mistaken for patient efforts at inspiration. In addition, adjusting the sensitivity of the ventilator to trigger ventilator breaths may be helpful.

TROUBLESHOOTING

Common problems with intubated patients are discussed in Section I. Typical ventilator management problems discussed include

- Agitation, Problem 72, page 246.
- High FIO_2, Problem 73, page 249.
- High peak pressure, Problem 74, page 253.
- Low $PaCO_2$/high $PaCO_2$, Problem 75, page 255.

WEANING

I. **Requirements.** Once the underlying cause of respiratory failure has been corrected, the patient is weaned from the ventilator. Optimally, the weaning process begins at the time of intubation.

   A. **Stabilization.** The underlying disease is under optimum control.

   B. **Initiation of Weaning.** The process is typically begun in the early morning. The following list of parameters is reasonable to begin the formal weaning process, which ends with extubation.
- $PaO_2 = 60$ mm Hg on 5-cm PEEP and $FIO_2 < 0.5$.
- Minute ventilation <10 L/min.
- Negative inspiratory force more negative than −20 cm water.
- Vital capacity >800 mL.
- Tidal volume >300 mL.
- Resolution of underlying process.

II. **Techniques.** The formal weaning process may take hours or days, depending on the patient's baseline respiratory status, debility caused by the underlying disease process, etc. There are many techniques used to wean a patient from the ventilator, and there is no one best technique. In general, a mode of ventilation is selected, and fewer machine breaths are given as the patient begins taking spontaneous breaths between machine breaths. SIMV is commonly used for this purpose. For example, a patient breathing at a rate of 14 breaths/min in AC mode is switched to SIMV mode with a rate of 14 breaths/min. The rate is then decreased to 10, 6, 4, and then to 0 breaths/min. Once the machine rate is decreased to 2 or 0 and the patient is tolerating it well (as indicated by ABG results, patient respiratory rate, etc), then 1 of 2 techniques is commonly used just before extubation.

A. CPAP and Pressure Support. In this method, the patient is switched to the spontaneous breathing mode, which, in modern ventilators, is the CPAP mode. Anywhere from 0 to 30 cm pressure may be used, but generally the lowest level possible (usually 0–5 cm) is preferred. Pressure support may be used concomitantly to augment spontaneous breaths by the patient. It can then be progressively decreased as the patient increases tidal volumes. For example, pressure support levels of 25, then 20, then 15, and finally 10 can be used while monitoring the patient's breathing rate, tidal volumes, and ABGs. This method requires an alert, cooperative patient who is spontaneously breathing. Machine backup functions remain in place in case of apnea or other inadequate parameters. Placing the patient on CPAP with pressure support and physiologic levels of PEEP is referred to as "tubing compensation," where the ventilator calculates (in newer ventilator models) the resistance of the ETT and ventilator tubing and provides just enough pressure support to eliminate the additional work of breathing needed to overcome this resistance. This method of weaning is preferred by many clinicians.

B. T-Piece (or T-tube bypass). The ETT is connected to a constant flow of O_2 (usually 40–50%). If the patient tolerates breathing independently, the length of time off the respirator is progressively increased. It is particularly easy to use for patients with no underlying lung disease (eg, in a patient recovering from a drug overdose). There are 3 significant drawbacks to this technique: (1) no alarms are available because the patient is totally disconnected from the ventilator; (2) it is time consuming for the respiratory therapists and nurses; and (3) it is much more work than breathing spontaneously without an ETT. This is due to the relatively small diameter of the tube. Therefore, patients are usually placed on a T-piece for intervals <2 hours at a time. The use of the T-piece is generally considered inferior and should not be used, especially with tubing compensation supplied by modern ventilators.

III. Timing. Deciding when to extubate the patient is part of the art of medicine. Nevertheless, fulfilling certain criteria will help achieve success. The following extubation parameters (as discussed earlier) are acceptable.

- Respiratory rate <30 breaths/min.
- ABGs show a pH >7.35 and adequate oxygenation.
- The patient is awake and alert.
- A normal gag reflex is present.
- The stomach is not distended.
- Control of the underlying disease process.
- Minimize secretions.

IV. Postextubation. After extubation, it is important that the patient be encouraged to cough frequently. Respiratory therapies should be continued. Incentive spirometry should be used several times an hour while the patient is awake to encourage deep breathing. The patient must be carefully observed for stridor, respiratory muscle fatigue, or other signs of failure. Oxygen should be given at the same level or at a level slightly higher than was given through the respirator before intubation, usually by face mask. The ABGs should be checked 2–4 hours after extubation to confirm adequate ventilation and oxygenation.

REFERENCES

Acute respiratory distress syndrome network. Ventilation with lower tidal volumes as compared with traditional tidal volumes for acute lung injury and the acute respiratory distress syndrome. *N Engl J Med* 342:1301–8, 2000.

Brower RG, et al. Higher versus lower positive end expiratory pressures in patients with the acute respiratory distress syndrome. *N Engl J Med* 351:327–36, 2004.

Derdak S. High frequency oscillatory ventilation for acute respiratory distress syndrome in adult patients. *Crit Care Med* 31(suppl):S317–23, 2003.

Kaplan LJ, et al. Airway pressure release ventilation increases cardiac performance in patients with acute lung injury/adult respiratory distress syndrome. *Crit Care* 5:221–6, 2001.

VIII. Management of Perioperative Complications

This section details specific surgical complications that can occur in the postoperative period and sometimes require action by the house officer while "on call." They are listed by complication, rather than by operation, because they can result from many different operations.

Certain complications occur acutely and initial diagnosis and management may be life saving (eg, neck hematoma, bronchial stump leak). Each management section includes a discussion on **Immediate Action** that details plans for life-threatening problems. (The **Immediate Action** appears in a shaded box, whereas other management suggestions appear in regular typeface.)

Other complications discussed here are more subacute, but early recognition and management with an understanding of the differential diagnosis and pathophysiology of the problem lead to optimal outcomes. This section does not provide a comprehensive listing of the various specific complications that can occur after general surgical procedures because most of these problems are fixed or chronic (eg, recurrent laryngeal nerve injury, short gut syndrome) and have no acute management issues.

Acute Gastric Dilatation

A. Operations. Major thoracic procedures and some abdominal operations (eg, open splenectomy) if a nasogastric tube is not functioning or was not placed intraoperatively.

B. Pathophysiology. Acute gastric dilatation is the thoracic equivalent of an ileus limited to the foregut.

C. Diagnosis. Tachypnea, tachycardia, diaphoresis, or hiccups. Often the patients do not highlight abdominal distress. Pay attention to the gastric shadow on a chest radiograph in this post-thoracotomy patient population (see Problem 38, page 145).

D. Management.

> **Immediate Action: Place a nasogastric tube, or make the tube that is in place functional.** The problem is rapidly resolved by decompression with a nasogastric tube.

E. Comments. In general, the patients with this problem look clinically ill and more serious diagnoses should be considered and ruled out. An awareness of this condition results in appropriate diagnosis and treatment. Acute gastric dilatation can cause further complications (eg, bleeding) after certain procedures, such as a splenectomy. However, this is rare after laparoscopic splenectomy.

REFERENCE

Todd SR, et al. Acute gastric dilatation revisited. *Am Surg* 66:709–10, 2000.

Anastomotic Leak

A. Operations. This complication occurs after abdominal operations in which 1 hollow viscus (bowel or pancreaticobiliary) is connected to another hollow viscus.

B. Pathophysiology. This complication may be caused by a technical problem with leakage of intestinal contents, bile, pancreatic juice, or urine through an anastomotic suture or staple line. It can be a result of late tissue necrosis or local infection at the site of anastomosis. When it is an esophageal anastomosis, the leak may occur in the neck or the pleural cavity, whereas other sites of leakage will be in the peritoneal cavity.

C. Diagnosis. Fever, leukocytosis, and pain are the hallmarks of this complication. There may be increased or change in drain output or even possible leakage of intestinal contents from the wound. The timing of this complication is typically 5–10 days after the procedure (see also Section I, Problem 78, page 264).

D. Management.

> **Immediate Action: Usually not necessary except in the patient who is septic because of the leak.**

The management must be individualized according to the patient's condition. A small disruption of a suture or staple line may be salvageable without reoperation and should be treated by decreasing passage of material through the lumen by making the patient nonoral (NPO) for bowel anastomoses and possibly inserting a nasogastric tube. Treatment with H_2-receptor blockers and possibly the somatostatin analogue octreotide will decrease bowel and pancreatic secretions and aid in healing. A significant fluid collection of leaked contents adjacent to the anastomosis will need to be drained to facilitate healing. Percutaneous drainage of the leaking anastomosis immediately converts the situation to a bowel, pancreatic, or biliary fistula, allowing assessment of ongoing leak and controlling internal infection. For major disruptions of anastomoses, operative reconstruction will almost always be indicated. Depending on the situation and the clinical condition of the patient, operative reconstruction may be attempted initially or as a temporizing measure (eg, a diverting colostomy for a rectal anastomosis or defunctionalizing the esophagus for a leak in the chest) may be indicated.

E. Comments. Among bowel anastomoses usually performed in general surgical procedures, leaks are a more frequent complication from esophageal and rectal procedures. These areas of the gastrointestinal tract do not have a serosal covering and have somewhat impaired healing compared with small bowel or gastric anastomoses. Another problematic area involves anastomoses of the pancreas to the small intestine such as that performed in the Whipple procedure (pancreaticoduodenectomy).

REFERENCES

Makela JT, et al. Risk factors for anastomotic leakage after left-sided colorectal resection with rectal anastomosis. *Dis Colon Rectum* 46:653–60, 2003.

Sutton CD, et al. Colorectal anastomotic leakage often masquerades as a cardiac complication. *Colorectal Dis* 6:21–2, 2004.

Bronchial Stump Leak

A. Operations. Pneumonectomy.

B. Pathophysiology. Disruption of staple or suture line on the mainstem bronchus after lung resection is the usual problem.

C. Diagnosis. This condition is usually heralded by sudden onset of severe shortness of breath or expectoration of large amounts of serosanguineous fluid. It may present more insidiously with cough, fever, sepsis, or contralateral pneumonia. On chest radiograph there are often new air-fluid levels in the affected hemithorax.

D. Management.

> **Immediate Action: Position patients on their side with the resected side down and the intact lung up. Intubation of the bronchus with a cuffed tube can prevent ongoing aspiration of pleural space fluid.**

After undertaking the immediate action, the chest usually is drained with a chest tube. Intravenous fluids and antibiotics are usually indicated. Although small leaks may seal with tube thoracostomy alone, repeat thoracotomy usually is required, often with flap coverage of the defect. In some cases, this can be accomplished with the videoscopic-assisted thoracic surgery (VATS) techniques.

E. Comments. The incidence of bronchial stump disruption is much lower in the era of mechanical staplers to close the bronchus as opposed to handsewn closures. Nevertheless, the initial management of this complication, in which a patient with 1 lung essentially drowns due to aspiration of fluid, can be life saving.

REFERENCE

Ferguson MK. Thoracoscopy for empyema, bronchopleural fistula and chylothorax. *Ann Thorac Surg* 56: 644–5, 1993.

Early Postoperative Bowel Obstruction

A. Operations. Any major intraperitoneal procedure.

B. Pathophysiology. Mechanical obstruction of the small intestine generally results from twists or kinks (the precursors for later adhesions). The possibility of an internal hernia must be considered on the basis of the initial abdominal procedure the patient underwent.

C. Diagnosis. Abdominal distention, crampy pain, obstipation. Abdominal radiographs will show distended loops of small bowel with air-fluid levels. The main differential diagnosis is between a prolonged postoperative ileus, which is a functional problem, and a true mechanical bowel obstruction, which occurs early in the postoperative course. Radiographic features of an adynamic ileus include a dilated colon primarily indicating no physical obstruction at the level of the small bowel (see Section I, Problem 1, page 1).

D. Management.

> **Immediate Action: Usually not necessary.**

Mechanical bowel obstruction in the early postoperative period (5–20 days) is usually managed in a nonoperative manner in contrast to late postoperative mechanical obstruction, which more commonly requires operative intervention. Decompression with a nasogastric tube and observation usually are indicated. The early adhesions at this time are filmy and unlikely to cause strangulation of the bowel. Also, operative repair at this point is difficult because the bowel is friable and susceptible to intraoperative injury. Although some surgeons advocate the use of a long suction tube that is often identified by the trade name (Cantor tube, Dennis tube, Baker tube, etc) in this situation, there is no evidence that this use is beneficial.

E. Comments. The primary differential diagnosis for early postoperative bowel obstruction is whether it is a true mechanical problem or a prolonged adynamic ileus, which is a functional problem. If a postoperative ileus resolves and the patient tolerates a diet and then develops signs and symptoms of obstruction, it is more obvious but often the problems blend together. Gas patterns on abdominal radiographs help with this diagnosis because in functional ileus the colon is typically most affected, whereas in mechanical obstruction it is the small bowel. Another consideration in a postoperative patient who develops abdominal distention and difficulty tolerating a diet is a focal infectious problem.

REFERENCE

Cheng SP, Liu CL. Early postoperative small bowel obstruction. *Br J Surg* 91:683–91, 2004.

Major Lymphatic Leak

A. Operations. Cervical procedures in the left neck, left subclavian line placement, esophagectomy, or retroperitoneal dissection can lead to thoracic duct or major lymphatic duct injury with subsequent chylothorax or chylous ascites.

B. Pathophysiology. Operative injury to a major lymphatic vessel with a large amount of lymph leaking out of neck incision or accumulating in the pleural or peritoneal space.

C. Diagnosis. High output drainage (500 mL/day) from cervical drain or chest tube with high concentrations of lymphocytes and high triglyceride content. The fluid is usually grossly chylous after fatty meal ingestion. For chylous ascites, postoperative ascites has the fluid characteristics as described above.

D. Management.

> **Immediate Action: Usually not necessary.**

Restrict fatty foods or make the patient NPO with total parenteral nutrition (TPN) to decrease lymph flow and seal the leak. Maintain closed suction drainage system while measuring the volume of output daily. Follow serum albumin and serum total lymphocyte counts, which may be depleted in patients with high output leaks.

If there is persistent drainage, then surgical exploration with suture ligature of leaking lymphatic may be indicated. Preoperative ingestion of a fatty meal may help identify the source of leak intraoperatively.

E. Comments. These major lymphatic leaks are ideally detected as fluid in the surgical field during the initial procedure. Knowledge of the anatomy of the thoracic duct is important to avoid this complication.

REFERENCE

Noel AA, et al. Treatment of symptomatic primary chylous disorders. *J Vasc Surg* 34:785–91, 2001.

Neck Hematoma

A. Operations. Thyroidectomy, parathyroidectomy, carotid artery endarterectomy, cervical esophageal procedures (eg, repair of a Zenker diverticulum).

B. Pathophysiology. Postoperative bleeding into the closed space under the deep cervical fascia where the trachea lies.

C. Diagnosis. Postoperative swelling in the neck with difficulty breathing and stridor. Distortion or deviation of tracheal air column may be seen on radiograph.

D. Management.

> **Immediate Action: Open the skin and deep cervical fascial closure to release the hematoma.** Patients who are stable should be brought to the operating room for this procedure. For patients in whom the airway is compromised, it may be necessary to perform this procedure at the bedside.

Cover the open wound with a sterile dressing before reclosing the incision in the operating room. Avoid attempts at endotracheal intubation because placement of the tube will be difficult as a result of tracheal compression. However, endotracheal intubation may be required.

E. Comments. Any cervical procedure that closes the deep cervical fascia can lead to a trapped hematoma, which can cause tracheal compression and stridor. Opening the wound quickly solves the problem and can be life saving.

Pancreatic Fistula or Fluid Collection

A. Operations. Pancreatic resections or splenectomy where the tail of the pancreas may be injured.

B. Pathophysiology. Any violation of the pancreatic parenchyma transects small pancreatic ducts. The digestive enzymes in exocrine pancreatic juice may prevent normal healing or sealing of minor duct injuries with accumulation of a pancreatic fluid collection high in enzyme content. For this reason it is appropriate to drain any pancreatic resection procedure and high output of fluid from these drains rich in pancreatic juice defines the presence of a pancreatic fistula. Percutaneous drainage of a pancreatic fluid collection postoperatively often leads to continued drainage defining a pancreatic fistula.

C. Diagnosis. High amylase content in fluid from peripancreatic drains placed at the time of pancreatic resection. Pancreatic fluid in a drain has a characteristic "dirty dishwater" brown/gray color. Drain output may increase or change in character with initiation of oral intake.

D. Management.

> **Immediate Actions: Usually not necessary.**

Continued and complete drainage of a pancreatic fistula is an imperative component of treatment, and daily monitoring of drain output in terms of volume with intermittent amylase content checks help assess progress in treatment. Additional measures aimed at decreasing exocrine pancreas stimulation are used to help heal the fistula. Making the patient NPO and using TPN (see Section V, page 397) may be necessary for patients with high-output fistulas. Patients continuing oral intake should be given a non-fat diet to decrease pancreatic stimulation. The somatostatin analogue, octreotide, can be given to decrease exocrine pancreas secretions. For patients undergoing pancreatic procedures, there is evidence that beginning this agent preoperatively decreases postoperative pancreatic leak. When the drain (or fistula) output decreases to acceptable levels (<50 mL/day) with a low amylase content (<3 times the serum level), then octreotide should be stopped. If output remains low, then the drain can be removed.

E. Comments. Dependent on the caliber and location of the pancreatic duct injury, the fistula can be low, mid, or high output. Injuries of the main duct or immediate branches of the main duct and injuries in the pancreatic head, as opposed to the distal pancreas, result in greater problems that are more difficult to heal.

REFERENCES

Munoz-Bongrand N, et al. Conservative management of pancreatic fistula after pancreaticoduodenectomy with pancreaticogastrostomy. *J Am Coll Surg* 199:198–203, 2004.

Popiela T, et al. Risk factors of pancreatic fistula following pancreaticoduodenectomy for periampullary cancer. *Hepatogastroenterology* 51:1484–8, 2004.

Peripheral Lymphatic Leak

A. Operations. Lymph node dissection, vascular procedure with groin or axillary incision.

B. Pathophysiology. Operative injury to lymphatic vessels with leakage of fluid (usually clear) from the incision.

C. Diagnosis. Patients with this complication have a persistently high drain output from postoperative closed drains placed in the operative field. They often have a fluid leak from the wound onto dressings.

D. Management.

> **Immediate Actions: Usually not necessary.**

If the drainage is controlled by a closed system, alternative management options include:

1. Observation with continued drainage including limiting activity, elevation of extremity, and wrapping extremity to decrease drain output.
2. Surgical exploration with suture ligation of leak sites. Preoperative injection of vital dye (methylene blue, etc) subcutaneously in a distal extremity may help identify leak sites. Closed drain placed at this operation and components of treatment option 1 (above) are instituted.
3. Pull drain and observe wound. Sometimes suction drains may induce leakage and removing the drain solves the problem. This plan works best for low-output (75–150 mL/day) lymphatic leaks.

Avoid injecting sclerosing agents (eg, bleomycin, tetracycline) into drains because this management causes discomfort, increases risk of infection, and is not effective in a controlled trial.

When lymph leak occurs as open drainage through the wound, surgical exploration as in treatment option 2 (above) is usually indicated. Open drainage tends to macerate skin and increase the chance of wound infection.

E. Comments. Postoperative lymph leaks are often difficult to resolve quickly even by surgical re-exploration. Attention to detail by clipping or ligating lymphatics at the initial procedure to prevent this complication should be emphasized. Lymph leaks in vascular procedures can lead to more serious secondary complications of graft infection when artificial graft material is present.

Postoperative Adrenal Insufficiency

A. Operations. Any major surgical procedure, but especially after adrenalectomy or radical nephrectomy.

B. Pathophysiology. Acute postoperative adrenal insufficiency may occur for 1 of 2 general reasons. First, the adrenal glands may not respond appropriately to the stress of the surgical procedure because of unrecognized underlying adrenal pathology or because of iatrogenic adrenal suppression owing to steroid medication. A second cause of acute adrenal insufficiency is bilateral adrenal hemorrhage. Patients who are anticoagulated are more susceptible to this complication, but most patients who have this life-threatening problem are not anticoagulated.

C. Diagnosis. This condition is often very difficult to diagnose other than the fact that patients do very poorly for no obvious reason. This must be remembered as a possible explanation for poor progress in the postoperative period. Symptoms include hypotension, confusion, vomiting with inability to eat; however, the electrolyte manifestations of Addison's disease may not occur. Computed tomographic scans of the adrenals may show large bilateral hematomas. The diagnosis can be confirmed by failure to have a cortisol response to corticotropin injection. (See Section II, ACTH Stimulation Test, page 269)

D. Management.

> **Immediate Action: Intravenous steroid administration. Hydrocortisone 100 mg intravenously STAT.**

Once the diagnosis is made (and it often is not realized until a postmortem examination), therapy with stress doses of steroids can be life saving.

E. Comments. Awareness of this very rare, but very serious problem is the most important factor. For patients who are failing rapidly but have no obvious source of infection, are not bleeding, and have no other explanations for a "downward clinical spiral," acute adrenal insufficiency should be considered.

Postoperative Bleeding

A. Operations. Any surgical procedure.

B. Pathophysiology. Surgical bleeding is usually a technical error with a bleeding vessel that was not controlled satisfactorily intraoperatively. Occasionally, because of the primary disease, patients may have a coagulopathy with medical bleeding from dissection planes, which normally would be hemostatic, oozing blood as a result of the inability to form clot.

C. Diagnosis. Minor wound bleeding typically appears as bloody drainage from the wound or a subcutaneous hematoma. Major postoperative bleeding is evident as signs and symptoms of hemorrhagic shock with hypotension, tachycardia, low urine output, and falling hematocrit. (See On Call Problems 23 and 24 relating to drain output, and Problem 47 "Hypotension")

D. Management.

> **Immediate Action: Volume resuscitation, obtain cross-matched blood products, identify source of bleeding.**

For major postoperative surgical bleeding, the principles of care of hemorrhagic shock of any etiology apply. Volume resuscitation that make certain adequate venous access lines available and ordering blood products to control the bleeding are the cornerstones of therapy. Assessment of ongoing bleeding and response to volume resuscitation in terms of blood pressure, urine output, and serial hematocrit measurements guides the decision as to whether the bleeding mandates reoperation. Some situations are clinically obvious, with dramatic acute bleeding and large transfusion requirements for which reoperation is needed as soon as possible. Other clinical situations are more subacute and may not require reoperation. In all cases, measurement of coagulation parameters (including ProTime, prothrombin time, and platelet count) is indicated because some cases of bleeding are primarily a result of coagulopathy, which must be controlled with the appropriate blood products.

Minor bleeding that results in a wound hematoma in a subcutaneous location almost never results in hemodynamically significant blood loss. In most locations, this can be managed with observation, possibly with direct pressure to halt the blood loss. In certain locations, even small hematomas can be symptomatic (see previous section, "Neck Hematoma"). When the subcutaneous bleeding is saturating the wound dressings instead of causing a hematoma, direct pressure often will control the bleeding site. Sometimes the offending vessel is a skin vessel that can be identified by inspecting the wound, and a simple nylon stitch under local anesthesia at the bedside can solve the problem.

E. Comments. An understanding of the volume of blood that can hide in the peritoneal or pleural cavities is needed to appreciate the potential problem that can happen with acute postoperative hemorrhage. Serial measurements of abdominal girth (as is often done) are an insensitive assessment of this potentially life-threatening complication.

Postoperative Intra-abdominal Fluid Collection/Abscess

A. Operations. Any abdominal operation can result in this problem, particularly infected, contaminated, or clean/contaminated procedures.

B. Pathophysiology. Postoperative intra-abdominal fluid serves as a site for infection to develop from organisms that typically originate from the bowel, biliary, or genitourinary tract during the surgical procedure. As patients recover in a supine position, the fluid settles in the most dependent areas of the greater peritoneal cavity in the subphrenic spaces, infrahepatic space (Morrison pouch), paracolic gutters, and pelvis.

C. Diagnosis. This complication may be evident as leukocytosis, fever, increased abdominal pain, referred pain to shoulders or back, or abdominal distention. Often patients who are recovering from an abdominal procedure after making normal progress begin to feel worse or lose their ability to eat.

D. Management.

> **Immediate Action: Usually not necessary.**

Current management involves imaging fluid collections by computed tomography or ultrasound with a radiologically guided aspiration and drainage, if possible. Aspirated fluid should be sent to the laboratory for Gram stain and culture. If the operative procedure involved the pancreas, assay of the fluid for amylase content will indicate a pancreatic source. Checking the creatinine level in the fluid may demonstrate that it is urine. Broad-spectrum antibiotics to control enteric organisms should be initiated as soon as cultures are obtained. For clinically significant fluid collections that cannot be safely approached percutaneously (eg, interloop fluid collections between loops of small bowel), operative drainage may be indicated.

E. Comments. Advancements in radiographic imaging techniques and interventions have revolutionized the management of this postoperative complication.

Postoperative Intestinal Fistula

A. Operations. Abdominal operations where an intestinal anastomosis was created. Reoperative procedures where significant adhesions exist and there is the possibility of an unintentional enterotomy or a leak from a repaired inadvertent enterotomy. Rarely, sutures used for fascial closure may include a bowel segment with subsequent fistula formation.

B. Pathophysiology. Postoperative fistulas require violation of the bowel wall with leakage of intestinal contents, which eventually find a path out of the body to the skin. The most common cause for bowel wall disruption is an anastomotic leak as previously discussed. However, if the bowel wall was injured or made ischemic during the initial procedure, then it may develop into an intestinal leak that is not related to an anastomosis and that can progress to a fistula.

C. Diagnosis. This complication is diagnosed by leakage of intestinal contents to the wound or drain sites.

D. Management.

> **Immediate Action: Usually not necessary.**

Similar to the situations with anatomic leak and intra-abdominal abscess discussed above, the principles of management of an intestinal fistula are bowel rest (use TPN, see Section V, page 397), antibiotics, and control of the leak with drainage of intra-abdominal fluid collections to limit infection. Obtaining radiologic studies, such as computed tomographic scan, to look for undrained fluid collections and possibly a fistulogram by injecting contrast retrograde into the site of the fistula to define the anatomy of the leak are helpful to define the anatomy of the fistula.

Fistulas are usually categorized as low output (<500 mL/day) or high output (>500 mL/day). It is critically important to protect the skin at the site of the fistula. A stoma appliance is usually helpful in this matter as is collecting the effluent. High-output fistulas should be managed as above, but persistent high-output fistulas usually require operative repair; low-output fistulas usually close gradually with nonoperative management as previously outlined (see also Section I, Problem 78, page 264).

E. Comments. The postoperative complications of intra-abdominal fluid collection, anastomotic leak, and intestinal fistula are interrelated problems that can occur together in patients who undergo major abdominal procedures.

REFERENCE

Foster CE, Lefor AT. Gastrocutaneous fistulas: Initial Management. *Surg Clin North Am* 76:1019–33, 1996.

Seroma

A. Operations. Lymph node dissection, mastectomy, any soft tissue resection.

B. Pathophysiology. Accumulation of lymph or serous fluid in deep wound space with normal healing of skin.

C. Diagnosis. This problem is evident as a nontender swelling in the wound that is usually fluctuant. A needle aspirate (performed using sterile technique) reveals serous fluid.

D. Management.

> **Immediate Actions: Usually not necessary.**

Observe for signs of infection or enlargement. Repeated complete aspiration of fluid should be done with a sterile technique. Avoid placing an indwelling drain.

E. Comments. Seromas are more of a nuisance than a symptomatic complication. Secondary problems, such as infection or open lymphatic leak, are more worrisome.

Skin Flap Necrosis

A. Operations. Mastectomy, lymph node dissection, soft tissue tumor resection, neck dissection.

B. Pathophysiology. Ischemic necrosis of skin and subcutaneous tissue resulting from inappropriate construction of a flap or closure of incision under tension that stretches tissues and restricts blood flow.

C. Diagnosis. This is a clinical diagnosis with a variable area of skin along an incision that demarcates and appears with various shades of gray or purple, has little or no capillary refill, and eventually becomes black and necrotic.

D. Management.

> **Immediate Actions: Usually not necessary.**

When flap necrosis is initially suspected, several maneuvers can be done to minimize skin and soft tissue loss. The patient should be well hydrated to ensure adequate tissue perfusion and be placed on oxygen to maximize oxygen tension in the area at risk. Nitropaste may be applied to the endangered area to cause vasodilatation and increase blood flow. When the flap becomes a black eschar, the damage is irreversible, and debridement of the dead tissue with subsequent skin graft or flap coverage should be done as quickly as possible.

E. Comments. Flap necrosis is a vascular, not an infectious, problem at the outset. However, early recognition of this complication and prompt action to increase oxygen delivery to the tissue may salvage some of the ischemic skin flap.

Wound Infection

A. Operations. Any surgical procedure. More common in dirty, contaminated, or clean-contaminated cases.

B. Pathophysiology. The subcutaneous tissue between the skin and fascia is the most susceptible to infection because it is the least vascularized.

C. Diagnosis. Erythema, pain, and warmth at the wound characterize superficial infections. Purulent drainage from a wound in which there is a thick layer of subcutaneous tissue may be the only symptom. Systemic signs, such as fever or leukocytosis, may be present. Inspection of the wound, including palpation to identify and express trapped purulent fluid, confirms the diagnosis.

D. Management.

> **Immediate Actions: Usually not necessary.**

After diagnosing a wound infection, management of superficial cellulitis involves antibiotics. Parenteral antibiotics are indicated for patients with acute surgical wound infections. Antibiotic coverage for enteric organisms is recommended for dirty cases, ie, when the subcutaneous tissue comes into contact with intestinal contents. For most wound infections, the causative organism is a gram-positive bacteria from the skin (*Staphylococcus* species or *Streptococcus* species), and therapy should be directed toward these organisms. If there is suspicion of an abscess or known drainage of pus from the wound, then the wound needs to be opened widely to achieve drainage. The wound is then managed with dressing changes 2–3 times a day and allowed to heal by secondary intention (see also Section I, Problem 78, page 264).

E. Comments. Assessment of postoperative fever includes evaluation and inspection of the surgical incision. Even early postoperative fever mandates inspection of the wound because the source may be an early streptococcal or clostridial infection that can progress rapidly and cause a high morbidity rate.

IX. Commonly Used Medications

This section is a quick reference to commonly used medications. You should be familiar with all of the dosages, indications, contraindications, side effects, and drug interactions of the medications that you prescribe. Such detailed information is beyond the scope of this manual and can be found in the package insert, Physicians' Desk Reference (PDR), or the American Hospital Formulary Service.

Drugs in this section are listed in alphabetic order by generic names. Common uses are listed that include labeled indications and common off-label uses on the basis of recommendations of our editorial board. Some of the more common trade names are listed for each medication. Where no pediatric dose is provided, the implication is that the use of the agent is not well established in this age group or is infrequently used. Drugs under the control of the Drug Enforcement Agency (Schedule 2–5 controlled substances) are indicated by the symbol [C].

CLASSIFICATION

Allergic Disorders

Antihistamines

Cetirizine
Chlorpheniramine
Clemastine fumarate

Diphenhydramine
Fexofenadine

Hydroxyzine
Loratadine

Miscellaneous Agents

Budesonide

Cromolyn

Antidotes

Acetylcysteine
Charcoal
Digoxin immune FAB

Flumazenil
Glucagon
Ipecac syrup

Mesna
Naloxone
Physostigmine

Antimicrobial Agents

Antibiotics

AMINOGLYCOSIDES
Amikacin
Gentamicin

Neomycin
Streptomycin

Tobramycin

CEPHALOSPORINS

Cefaclor
Cefadroxil
Cefazolin
Cefepime
Cefixime
Cefoperazone

Cefotaxime
Cefotetan
Cefoxitin
Cefpodoxime
Ceftazidime
Ceftizoxime

Ceftriaxone
Cefuroxime
Cephalexin
Cephradine
Loracarbef

FLUOROQUINOLONES

Ciprofloxacin
Ciprofloxacin and
 hydrocortisone otic

Gatifloxacin
Levofloxacin
Lomefloxacin

Moxifloxacin
Norfloxacin
Ofloxacin

MACROLIDES

Azithromycin
Clarithromycin

Dirithromycin

Erythromycin

PENICILLINS

Amoxicillin
Amoxicillin-clavulanate
Ampicillin
Ampicillin-sulbactam
Cloxacillin
Dicloxacillin

Mezlocillin
Nafcillin
Oxacillin
Penicillin G aqueous
Penicillin G benzathine
Penicillin G procaine

Penicillin V
Piperacillin
Piperacillin-tazobactam
Ticarcillin
Ticarcillin-clavulanate

TETRACYCLINES

Doxycycline

Tetracycline

MISCELLANEOUS AGENTS

Aztreonam
Clindamycin
Cortisporin, otic
Daptomycin
Drotrecogin alpha
Ertapenem

Fosfomycin
Imipenem-cilastatin
Linezolid
Meropenem
Metronidazole
Mupirocin

Quinupristin/dalfopristin
Silver nitrate
Trimethoprim-sul-
 famethoxazole
Vancomycin
Zidovudine

Antifungals

Amphotericin B cholesteryl
Amphotericin B lipid
 complex
Amphotericin B liposomal
Caspofungin
Ciclopirox

Clotrimazole
Econazole
Fluconazole
Itraconazole

Ketoconazole
Miconazole
Nystatin
Voriconazole

Antimycobacterials

Ethambutol
Isoniazid

Pyrazinamide
Rifampin

Rifapentine

Antivirals

Acyclovir
Amantadine
Famciclovir
Foscarnet
Ganciclovir

Interferon alfacon-1
Interferon alpha-2B and
 ribavirin
Oseltamivir
Ribavirin

Rimantadine
Valacyclovir
Zanamivir

Miscellaneous Agents

Pentamidine

Silver sulfadiazine

Cardiovascular Agents

Alpha-1 Adrenergic Blockers

Doxazosin

Prazosin

Terazosin

Angiotensin-Converting Enzyme Inhibitors

Benazepril
Captopril
Enalapril and enalaprilat
Fosinopril

Lisinopril
Moexipril
Perindopril

Quinapril
Ramipril
Trandolapril

Angiotensin II Receptor Antagonist

Candesartan
Eprosartan

Irbesartan
Losartan

Telmisartan
Valsartan

Antiarrhythmic Agents

Adenosine
Amiodarone
Atropine
Digoxin
Disopyramide
Esmolol

Flecainide
Ibutilide
Lidocaine
Mexiletine
Moricizine

Procainamide
Propafenone
Quinidine
Sotalol
Tocainide

Beta-Blockers

Acebutolol
Atenolol
Atenolol and chlorothiazide
Betaxolol
Bisoprolol

Carteolol
Carvedilol
Labetalol
Metoprolol
Nadolol

Penbutolol
Pindolol
Propranolol
Timolol

Calcium Channel Antagonists

Amlodipine
Bepridil
Diltiazem
Felodipine

Isradipine
Nicardipine
Nifedipine

Nimodipine
Nisoldipine
Verapamil

Centrally Acting Antihypertensive Agents

Clonidine

Methyldopa

Diuretics

Acetazolamide
Amiloride
Bumetanide
Chlorothiazide
Chlorthalidone
Ethacrynic acid
Furosemide

Hydrochlorothiazide
Hydrochlorothiazide and
  amiloride
Hydrochlorothiazide and
  spironolactone
Hydrochlorothiazide and
  triamterene

Indapamide
Mannitol
Metolazone
Spironolactone
Torsemide
Triamterene

Inotropic Agents

Amrinone
Digoxin
Dobutamine

Dopamine
Epinephrine
Isoproterenol

Milrinone
Norepinephrine
Phenylephrine

Lipid-Lowering Agents

Atorvastatin
Cholestyramine
Colesevelam
Colestipol

Fenofibrate
Fluvastatin
Gemfibrozil
Lovastatin

Niacin
Pravastatin
Rosuvastatin
Simvastatin

Vasodilators

Epoprostenol
Fenoldopam
Hydralazine
Isosorbide dinitrate

Isosorbide mononitrate
Minoxidil
Nesiritide

Nitroglycerin
Nitroprusside
Tolazoline

Central Nervous System

Antianxiety

Alprazolam
Buspirone
Chlordiazepoxide
Clorazepate

Diazepam
Doxepin
Hydroxyzine

Lorazepam
Oxazepam
Prazepam

Anticonvulsants

Carbamazepine
Clonazepam
Diazepam
Ethosuximide
Fosphenytoin
Gabapentin

Lamotrigine
Levetiracetam
Lorazepam
Oxcarbazepine
Pentobarbital
Phenobarbital

Phenytoin
Tiagabine
Topiramate
Valproic acid
Zonisamide

Antidepressants

Amitriptyline
Amoxapine
Bupropion
Citalopram
Desipramine
Doxepin
Escitalopram

Fluoxetine
Fluvoxamine
Imipramine
Maprotiline
Mirtazapine
Nefazodone
Nortriptyline

Paroxetine
Phenelzine
Sertraline
Trazodone
Trimipramine
Venlafaxine

Antiparkinson Agents

Amantadine
Benztropine
Bromocriptine
Carbidopa/levodopa

Entacapone
Pergolide
Pramipexole
Procyclidine

Ropinirole
Selegiline
Trihexyphenidyl

Antipsychotics

Chlorpromazine
Clozapine
Fluphenazine
Haloperidol
Lithium carbonate

Olanzapine
Perphenazine
Prochlorperazine
Quetiapine

Risperidone
Thioridazine
Thiothixene
Trifluoperazine

Sedative Hypnotics

Chloral hydrate
Diphenhydramine
Estazolam
Flurazepam
Hydroxyzine

Midazolam
Pentobarbital
Phenobarbital
Propofol

Secobarbital
Temazepam
Triazolam
Zolpidem

Miscellaneous Agents

Nimodipine

Endocrine System

Antidiabetic Agents

Acarbose
Acetohexamide
Chlorpropamide
Glimepiride
Glipizide

Glyburide
Insulin
Metformin
Miglitol
Pioglitazone

Repaglinide
Rosiglitazone
Tolazamide
Tolbutamide

Hormone & Synthetic Substitutes

Cortisone
Desmopressin
Dexamethasone
Fludrocortisone acetate

Glucagon
Hydrocortisone
Methylprednisolone
Metyrapone

Prednisolone
Prednisone
Vasopressin

Hypercalcemia Agents

Calcitonin
Etidronate

Gallium nitrate
Pamidronate

Plicamycin
Zoledronic acid

Osteoporosis Agents

Alendronate
Calcitonin

Raloxifene

Risedronate

Thyroid/Antithyroid

Levothyroxine
Liothyronine

Methimazole
Potassium iodide

Propylthiouracil
Thyroid

Miscellaneous Agents

Demeclocycline

Gastrointestinal Tract

Antacids

Alginic acid
Aluminum hydroxide
Aluminum hydroxide
  with magnesium
  carbonate

Aluminum hydroxide
  with magnesium
  hydroxide
Aluminum hydroxide with
  magnesium hydroxide
  and simethicone

Calcium carbonate
Magaldrate
Simethicone

Antidiarrheal

Bismuth subsalicylate
Diphenoxylate with atropine

Kaolin/pectin
Lactobacillus

Loperamide
Octreotide

Antiemetic

Buclizine
Chlorpromazine
Dimenhydrinate
Dolasetron
Dronabinol

Droperidol
Granisetron
Meclizine
Metoclopramide
Ondansetron

Prochlorperazine
Promethazine
Scopolamine
Thiethylperazine
Trimethobenzamide

Antiulcer

Cimetidine
Famotidine
Lansoprazole

Nizatidine
Omeprazole
Pantoprazole

Rabeprazole
Ranitidine
Sucralfate

Cathartics/Laxatives

Bisacodyl
Docusate calcium

Glycerin suppositories
Lactulose

Mineral oil
Polyethylene glycol-
  electrolyte solution
Docusate potassium
Docusate sodium

Magnesium citrate
Magnesium hydroxide

Psyllium
Sorbitol

Enzymes

Pancreatin

Pancrelipase

Miscellaneous Agents

Alosetron
Dexpanthenol
Dicyclomine
Hyoscyamine
Hyoscyamine, atropine,
  scopolamine, and
  phenobarbital

Infliximab
Mesalamine
Metoclopramide
Misoprostol
Olsalazine

Propantheline
Sulfasalazine
Tegaserod
Vasopressin

Hematologic Modifiers

Anticoagulants

Ardeparin
Argatroban
Dalteparin

Enoxaparin
Fondaparinux sodium
Heparin

Lepirudin
Warfarin

Antiplatelet

Abciximab
Aspirin
Clopidogrel

Eptifibatide
Reteplase

Ticlopidine
Tirofiban

Antithrombin Agents

Alteplase, recombinant
  (TPA)
Aminocaproic acid

Aprotinin
Dextran 40
Reteplase

Streptokinase
Tenecteplase
Urokinase

Hemopoietic Stimulants

Epoetin alfa (Erythropoietin) Filgrastim (G-CSF)

Sargramostim (GM-
  CSF)

Volume Expanders

Albumin

Dextran 40

Hetastarch

Miscellaneous Agents

Antihemophilic factor VIII

Desmopressin

Pentoxifylline

Protamine factor IX
  complex

Immune System

Immunomodulators

Interferon alfa

Interferon alfacon

Immunosuppressive Agents

Antithymocyte globulin
  (ATG)
Azathioprine

Cyclosporine
Daclizumab
Mycophenolate mofetil

Sirolimus
Steroids
Tacrolimus

Vaccine/Serums/Toxoids

CMV immune globulin
Haemophilus B conjugate
Hepatitis A vaccine
Hepatitis B immune
Hepatitis B vaccine

Immune globulin
   intravenous
Pneumococcal 7-valent
Pneumococcal vaccine,
   polyvalent

Tetanus immune
   globulin
Tetanus toxoid globulin

Musculoskeletal Disorders

Antigout Agents

Allopurinol
Colchicine

Probenecid

Sulfinpyrazone

Muscle Relaxants

Aspirin and meprobamate
Baclofen
Carisoprodol
Chlorzoxazone

Cyclobenzaprine
Dantrolene
Diazepam

Metaxalone
Methocarbamol
Orphenadrine

Neuromuscular Blockers

Atracurium
Cisatracurium

Pancuronium
Succinylcholine

Vecuronium

Miscellaneous Agents

Edrophonium

Methotrexate

OB/GYN

Contraceptives

Levonorgestrel Implants

Norgestrel

Estrogen Supplementation

Esterified estrogen
Esterified estrogen with
   methyltestosterone
Estradiol
Estradiol topical

Estradiol transdermal
Estrogen, conjugated
Estrogen, conjugated
   with methyl
   progesterone

Estrogen, conjugated
   with methyl-
   testosterone

Vaginal Preparations

Amino-Cerv pH 5.5 cream
Miconazole

Nystatin
Terconazole

Tioconazole

Miscellaneous Agents

Gonadorelin
Leuprolide
Magnesium sulfate

Medroxyprogesterone
Methylergonovine

Oxytocin
Terbutaline

Ophthalmic Agents

Acetazolamide
Apraclonidine
Artificial tears
Atropine
Bacitracin and polymyxin-
   B (Polysporin)
Betaxolol
Brimonidine
Brinzolamide

Carteolol
Ciprofloxacin
Cromolyn
Cyclopentolate
Diclofenac
Dipivefrin
Dorzolamide
Dorzolamide and timolol
Echothiophate iodine

Erythromycin
Fomivirsen and
   prednisolone
Gentamicin
Ketorolac
Latanoprost
Levobunolol
Levocabastine
Lodoxamide

Naphazoline
   and antazoline
Naphazoline and
   pheniramine
Neomycin, polymyxin-B
   and prednisolone
Norfloxacin
Ofloxacin
Phenylephrine

Pilocarpine
Prednisolone
Neomycin, bacitracin, and
   polymyxin-B
Neomycin, polymyxin-B,
   and dexamethasone
Neomycin, polymyxin-B,
   and hydrocortisone
Rimexolone

Sulfacetamide
Timolol
Tobramycin
Tobramycin and
   dexamethasone
Trifluridine
Tropicamide
Vidarabine

Otic Agents

Antipyrine and
   benzocaine
Hydrocortisone otic

Neomycin, polymyxin-B,
   and hydrocortisone
Ofloxacin otic

Pro Floxin
Triethanolamine
   polypeptide oleate

Pain

Local Anesthetics

Antipyrine and benzocaine
Anusol
Bupivacaine

Capsaicin
Cocaine
Dibucaine

Lidocaine
Lidocaine/prilocaine

Narcotics

Alfentanil
Buprenorphine
Butalbital and
   acetaminophen
Butalbital and aspirin
Butalbital, aspirin,
   and codeine
Butorphanol
Codeine
Codeine with
   acetaminophen
Dezocine

Fentanyl
Fentanyl transdermal
Fentanyl transmucosal
Hydrocodone
Hydrocodone and
   acetaminophen
Hydrocodone and aspirin
Levorphanol
Meperidine
Methadone
Morphine
Nalbuphine

Oxycodone and
   acetaminophen
Oxycodone and aspirin
Oxymorphone
Pentazocine
Propoxyphene
Propoxyphene and
   acetaminophen
Propoxyphene and
   aspirin
Sufentanil

Non-narcotic Agents

Acetaminophen

Tramadol

Nonsteroidal Anti-inflammatory Agents

Aspirin
Aspirin with codeine
Celecoxib
Diclofenac
Diflunisal
Etodolac
Fenoprofen

Flurbiprofen
Ibuprofen
Indomethacin
Ketoprofen
Ketorolac
Meloxicam
Nabumetone

Naproxen
Naproxen sodium
Oxaprozin
Piroxicam
Rofecoxib
Sulindac
Tolmetin

Respiratory Tract

Antitussives & Decongestants

Acetylcysteine
Benzonatate
Codeine
Dextromethorphan
Guaifenesin
Guaifenesin and codeine

Guaifenesin and
   dextromethorphan
Guaifenesin and
   pseudoephedrine
Hydrocodone and
   homatropine

Hydrocodone and
   pseudoephedrine
Hydromorphone and
   guaifenesin
Pseudoephedrine

Bronchodilators

Albuterol
Albuterol and ipratropium
Aminophylline
Bitolterol
Ephedrine

Epinephrine
Isoetharine
Isoproterenol
Levalbuterol
Metaproterenol

Pirbuterol
Salmeterol
Terbutaline
Theophylline

Respiratory Inhalants

Acetylcysteine
Beclomethasone
Cromolyn sodium

Flunisolide
Fluticasone

Ipratropium
Nedocromil

Miscellaneous Agents

Beractant
Montelukast

Zafirlukast

Zileuton

Steroids

Systemic

Betamethasone
Cortisone
Dexamethasone
Hydrocortisone

Methylprednisolone acetate
Methylprednisolone
    succinate

Prednisolone
Prednisone

Topical

Alclometasone
    dipropionate
Amcinonide
Augmented
    betamethasone
Betamethasone
    dipropionate
Betamethasone valerate
Clobetasol propionate

Clocortolone pivalate
Desonide
Desoximetasone
Dexamethasone
Diflorasone diacetate
Fluocinolone acetonide
Fluocinonide
Flurandrenolide
Fluticasone propionate

Halcinonide
Halobetasol
Hydrocortisone
Hydrocortisone acetate
Hydrocortisone butyrate
Hydrocortisone valerate
Mometasone furoate
Prednicarbate
Triamcinolone

Supplements

Calcitriol
Calcium acetate
Calcium chloride
Cholecalciferol
Cyanocobalamin
    (vitamin B_{12})
Ferric sodium gluconate

Ferrous sulfate
Folic acid
Iron dextran
Iron sucrose
Leucovorin
Magnesium oxide
Magnesium sulfate

Phytonadione
    (vitamin K)
Potassium supplements
Pyridoxine (vitamin B_6)
Sodium bicarbonate
Thiamine (vitamin B_1)

Urinary Tract Agents

Ammonium aluminum
Belladonna and opium
    suppositories
Bethanechol
DMSO
Hyoscyamine sulfate

Neomycin-polymyxin
    bladder irrigant
Nitrofurantoin
Oxybutynin
Phenazopyridine

Potassium citrate
Potassium citrate and
    citric acid
Sodium citrate
Trimethoprim

Benign Prostatic Hyperplasia

Doxazosin
Finasteride

Tamsulosin

Terazosin

Miscellaneous Agents

Isotretinoin
Lindane
Megestrol acetate
Metyrosine

Naltrexone
Nicotine transdermal
Sildenafil

Sodium polystyrene
  sulfonate
Witch hazel

GENERIC DRUGS

Abciximab (ReoPro)

COMMON USES: Prevention of acute ischemic complications in patients undergoing percutaneous transluminal coronary angioplasty (PTCA).
DOSAGE: 0.25 mg/kg administered 10–60 min before PTCA, then 0.125 mg/kg/min (10 mg/min) continuous infusion for 12 h.
NOTES: Used concomitantly with heparin; may cause allergic reactions.

Acebutolol (Sectral)

COMMON USES: Hypertension (HTN); ventricular arrhythmias, angina.
DOSAGE: 200–400 mg, PO bid.

Acetaminophen (Tylenol, others)

COMMON USES: Mild pain, headache, fever.
DOSAGE: *Adults:* 650–1000 mg PO or PR q4–6h. *Peds:* 10 mg/kg/dose PO or PR q4–6h.
NOTES: Overdose causes hepatotoxicity and is managed with N-acetylcysteine; charcoal is not usually recommended; it has no anti-inflammatory or platelet-inhibiting action.

Acetaminophen With Codeine
(Tylenol No. 1, No. 2, No. 3, No. 4; Others) [C]

COMMON USES: No. 1, No. 2, No. 3 for mild to moderate pain; No. 4 for moderate to severe pain; antitussive.
DOSAGE: *Adults:* 1–2 tablets q3–4h prn. *Peds:* Acetaminophen 10–15 mg/kg/dose; codeine 0.5–1.0 mg/kg/dose q4–6h (useful elixir dosing guide: 3–6 y, 5 mL/dose; 7–12 y, 10 mL/dose).
NOTES: Capsules contain acetaminophen 325 mg, tablets, 300 mg; codeine 7.5 mg in No. 1, 15 mg in No. 2, 30 mg in No. 3, 60 mg in No. 4; 5-mL elixir contains acetaminophen 120 mg, codeine 12 mg plus alcohol.

Acetazolamide (Diamox)

COMMON USES: Diuresis, glaucoma, alkalinization of urine, refractory epilepsy.
DOSAGE: *Adults:* Diuretic: 250–375 mg IV or PO q24h in divided doses. Glaucoma: 250–1000 mg PO qd in divided doses. *Peds:* Epilepsy: 8–30 mg/kg/24h PO in 4 divided doses. Diuretic: 5 mg/kg/24h PO or IV. Alkalinization of urine: 5 mg/kg/dose PO bid–tid. Glaucoma: 20–40 mg/kg/24h PO in 4 divided doses.
NOTES: Contraindicated in renal failure, sulfa hypersensitivity; follow Na^+ and K^+; watch for metabolic acidosis.

Acetylcysteine (Mucomyst)

COMMON USES: Mucolytic agent as adjuvant therapy of chronic bronchopulmonary diseases and cystic fibrosis; as antidote to acetaminophen hepatotoxicity within 24 h of ingestion.
DOSAGE: *Adults* and *Peds:* Nebulizer: 20% solution 3–5 mL diluted with equal volume of water or normal saline administered tid–qid. Antidote: PO or nasogastric; 140 mg/kg diluted 1:4 in carbonated beverage as loading dose, then 70 mg/kg q4h for 17 doses.
NOTES: Watch for bronchospasm when used by inhalation in asthmatics; activated charcoal adsorbs acetylcysteine when given PO for acute acetaminophen ingestion.

Acyclovir (Zovirax)

COMMON USES: Herpes simplex and herpes zoster viral infections.
DOSAGE: *Adults:* Topical: apply 0.5-inch ribbon q3h. Oral: Initial genital herpes: 200 mg PO q4h while awake; 5 capsules/d for 10 d. Chronic suppression: 400 mg PO bid–tid. Intermittent therapy: as for initial treatment, except treat for 5 d at the earliest prodrome. Herpes zoster: 800 mg PO 5 times/d. Intravenous: 5–10 mg/kg/dose IV q8h. *Peds:* 5–10 mg/kg/dose IV or PO q8h or 750 mg/m^2/24h divided q8h.
NOTES: Adjust dose in renal insufficiency.

Adenosine (Adenocard)

COMMON USES: Paroxysmal supraventricular tachycardia, including that associated with Wolff-Parkinson-White syndrome.
DOSAGE: *Adults:* 6 mg rapid IV, repeated in 1–2 min at 12 mg IV if no response. *Peds:* 0.03–0.25 mg/kg IV bolus; repeat larger dose in 1–2 min if no response.
NOTES: Doses >12 mg are not recommended; caffeine and theophylline antagonize the effects of adenosine.

Albumin (Albuminar, Buminate, Albutein, Others)

COMMON USES: Plasma volume expansion for shock resulting from burns, surgery, hemorrhage, or other trauma.
DOSAGE: *Adults:* 25 g IV initially; subsequent infusions should depend on clinical situation and response. *Peds:* 0.5–1.0 g/kg/dose; infuse at 0.05–0.1 g/min.
NOTES: Contains 130–160 mEq Na$^+$/L. Not typically used for acute resuscitation.

Albuterol (Proventil, Ventolin)

COMMON USES: Management of bronchospasm in reversible obstructive airway disease; prevention of exercise-induced bronchospasm.
DOSAGE: *Adults:* 2–4 inhalations q4–6h; 1 Rotocap inhaled q4–6h; 2–4 mg PO tid–qid. *Peds:* 2 inhalations q4–6h; 0.1–0.2 mg/kg/dose PO, to maximum dose of 2–4 mg PO tid.

Albuterol & Ipratropium (Combivent)

COMMON USES: Management of COPD.
DOSAGE: 2 inhalations qid.

Alfentanil (Alfenta) [C]

COMMON USES: Adjunct in the maintenance of general anesthesia.
DOSAGE: *Adults* and *Peds >12 y:* 8–75 mg/kg IV infusion; total dose depends on duration of operative procedure.

Alginic Acid With Aluminum Hydroxide & Magnesium Trisilicate (Gaviscon)

COMMON USES: Symptomatic relief of heartburn; hiatal hernia.
DOSAGE: 2–4 tablets or 15–30 mL PO qid followed by water.

Allopurinol (Zyloprim, Lopurin)

COMMON USES: Gout, management of hyperuricemia of malignancy, uric acid urolithiasis.
DOSAGE: *Adults:* Initial 100 mg PO qd; usual 300 mg PO qd. *Peds:* Use only for controlling hyperuricemia of malignancy in children; 10 mg/kg/24h divided q6–8h (max 600 mg/24h).
NOTES: Aggravates acute gout episode, do not begin until acute episode resolves. Adjust dose for renal insufficiency.

Alprazolam (Xanax) [C]

COMMON USES: Anxiety and panic disorders; anxiety associated with depression.

DOSAGE: 0.25–2 mg PO tid.
NOTES: Decrease dose in elderly and debilitated patients.

Alteplase, Recombinant [TPA] (Activase)

COMMON USES: Acute MI and pulmonary embolism.
DOSAGE: 100 mg IV over 3 h.
NOTES: May cause bleeding. Also used in acute nonhemorrhagic stroke (see package insert for criteria and dosing)

Aluminum Carbonate (Basaljel)

COMMON USES: Hyperacidity (peptic ulcer, hiatal hernia, etc); supplement to management of hyperphosphatemia in renal disease.
DOSAGE: *Adults:* 2 capsules or tablets or 10 mL (in water) q2h prn. *Peds:* 50–150 mg/kg/24h PO divided q4–6h.

Aluminum Hydroxide (Amphojel, ALternaGEL, Alu-Cap, Alu-Tab)

COMMON USES: See aluminum carbonate.
DOSAGE: *Adults:* 10–30 mL or 2 tablets/capsules PO q4–6h. *Peds:* 5–15 mL PO q4–6h.
NOTES: Can be used in renal failure; may cause constipation.

Aluminum Hydroxide With Magnesium Carbonate (Gaviscon)

COMMON USES: Hyperacidity (peptic ulcer, hiatal hernia, etc).
DOSAGE: *Adults:* 15–30 PO pc and hs. *Peds:* 5–15 mL PO qid or prn.
NOTES: Doses qid are best given after meals and at bedtime; may cause hypermagnesemia.

Aluminum Hydroxide With Magnesium Hydroxide (Maalox)

COMMON USES: Hyperacidity (peptic ulcer, hiatal hernia, etc).
DOSAGE: *Adults:* 10–60 mL or 2–4 tablets PO qid or prn. *Peds:* 5–15 mL PO qid or prn.
NOTES: Doses qid are best given after meals and at bedtime; may cause hypermagnesemia in renal insufficiency.

Aluminum Hydroxide With Magnesium Hydroxide & Simethicone (Mylanta, Mylanta II, Maalox Plus)

COMMON USES: Hyperacidity with bloating.
DOSAGE: *Adults:* 10–60 mL or 2–4 tablets PO qid or prn. *Peds:* 5–15 mL PO qid or prn.
NOTES: May cause hypermagnesemia in renal insufficiency; Mylanta II contains twice the amount of aluminum and magnesium hydroxide as Mylanta.

Amantadine (Symmetrel)

COMMON USES: Management or prophylaxis of influenza A viral infections; Parkinsonism.
DOSAGE: *Adults:* Influenza A: 200 mg PO qd or 100 mg PO bid. Parkinsonism: 100 mg PO qd–bid. *Peds:* 1–9 y: 4.4–8.8 mg/kg/24h to maximum of 150 mg/24h divided qd–bid; >9 y: same as adults.
NOTES: Decrease dose in renal insufficiency.

Amikacin (Amikin)

COMMON USES: Management of serious infections caused by gram-negative bacteria.
DOSAGE: *Adults* and *Peds:* 15 mg/kg/24h divided q8–12h or based on renal function; refer to Aminoglycoside dosing (Table IX–1).
NOTES: May be effective against gram-negative bacteria resistant to gentamicin and tobramycin; monitor renal function carefully for dose adjustments; monitor serum levels (Table IX–2, page 460).

TABLE IX–1. AMINOGLYCOSIDE DOSING.

See Table IX–2, page 460, "Common Drug Levels" for the trough and peak levels of the aminoglycosides gentamicin, tobramycin, and amikacin. Peak levels should be drawn 30 min after the dose is completely infused; trough levels should be drawn 30 min before the dose. As a general rule, draw the peak and trough around the fourth maintenance dose.

Therapy can be initiated with the recommended guidelines that follow. The following calculations are not valid for netilmicin.

Procedure (Adult)

1. Calculate the estimated creatinine clearance (CrCl) based on serum creatinine (SCr), age, and body weight, or you can order a formal creatinine clearance, if time permits.

$$\text{CrCl: Male} = \frac{(140 - \text{age [y]}) \times (\text{body wt. [kg]})}{(\text{SCr [mg / dL]}) \times 72}$$

CrCl: Female $= 0.85 \times$ CrCl

2. Select the loading dose:

Gentamicin: 1.5–2.0 mg/kg   Tobramycin: 1.5–2.0 mg/kg

Amikacin: 5.0–7.5 mg/kg

3. By using Table IX–3, page 461 you can now select the maintenance dose (as a percentage of the chosen loading dose) most appropriate for the renal function of the patient based on CrCl and dosing interval. Bold numbers are the suggested percentages and intervals for any given creatinine clearance.

Amiloride (Midamor)

COMMON USES: HTN and CHF.
DOSAGE: 5–10 mg PO qd.
NOTES: Hyperkalemia may occur; monitor serum potassium levels.

Aminocaproic Acid (Amicar)

COMMON USES: Excessive bleeding resulting from systemic hyperfibrinolysis and urinary fibrinolysis.
DOSAGE: *Adults* and *Peds:* 100 mg/kg IV, then 1 g/m^2/h to maximum of 18 g/m^2/d or 100 mg/kg/dose q8h.
NOTES: Administer for 8 h or until bleeding is controlled; contraindicated in disseminated intravascular coagulation; not for upper urinary tract bleeding; oral form rarely used.

Aminoglutethimide (Cytadren, Elipten, Orimeten)

COMMON USES: Adrenal cortex carcinoma, Cushing's syndrome, and prostate cancer.
DOSAGE: 750–1500 mg/d in divided doses plus dexamethasone 2–5 mg/d or hydrocortisone 20–40 mg/d.
NOTES: Toxicity includes adrenal insufficiency ("medical adrenalectomy"), hypothyroidism, masculinization, hypotension, vomiting, rare hepatotoxicity, rash, myalgia, and fever.

Aminophylline

COMMON USES: Asthma and bronchospasm; apnea of prematurity.
DOSAGE: *Adults:* Acute asthma: load 6 mg/kg IV, then 0.4–0.9 mg/kg/h IV continuous infusion. Chronic asthma: 24 mg/kg/24h PO or PR divided q6h. *Peds:* Load 6 mg/kg IV, then 1.0 mg/kg/h IV continuous infusion.

TABLE IX–2. COMMON DRUG LEVELS.[a]

Drug	Therapeutic Level	Toxic Level
Carbamazepine	8.0–12.0 mg/mL	>15.0 mg/mL
Cyclosporine	150–300 ng/mL (variable)	
Digoxin	0.8–2.0 ng/mL	>2.4 ng/mL
Ethanol		100–200 mg/100 mL (legally drunk most states, labile behavior)
		150–300 mg/100 mL (confusion)
		250–400 mg/100 mL (stupor)
		350–500 mg/100 mL (coma)
		>450 mg/100 mL (death)
Ethosuximide	40.0–100.0 mg/mL	>150.0 mg/mL
Lidocaine	1.5–6.5 mg/mL	>6.0–8.0 mg/mL
Lithium	0.6–1.2 mmol/L	>2.0 mmol/L
Phenobarbital	15.0–40.0 mg/mL	>45.0 mg/mL
Phenytoin	10.0–20.0 mg/mL	>25.0 mg/mL
Procainamide	4.0–10.0 mg/mL	>16.0 mg/mL
Quinidine	3.0–7.0 mg/mL	>7.0 mg/mL
Theophylline	10.0–20.0 mg/mL	>20.0 mg/mL
Valproic acid	50–100 mg/mL	>150 mg/mL

Antibiotic (maintain below upper limit)

	Trough (mg/mL)	Peak (mg/mL)
Amikacin	5.0–7.5	25–35
Gentamicin	1.5–2.0	5–8
Tobramycin	1.5–2.0	5–8
Netilmicin	0.5–2.0	6–10
Vancomycin	5.0–10.0	20–40

[a]Each lab may have values that differ slightly from those provided. Therapeutic levels are usually determined as a trough just before next dose.

NOTES: Individualize dose; signs of toxicity include nausea, vomiting, irritability, tachycardia, ventricular arrhythmias, and seizures; follow serum levels carefully; aminophylline is about 85% theophylline (see Table IX–2); erratic absorption with rectal doses.

Amiodarone (Cordarone)

COMMON USES: Recurrent ventricular fibrillation or hemodynamically unstable ventricular tachycardia.
DOSAGE: *Adults:* Load: 800–1600 mg/d PO for 1–3 wk. Maintenance: 600–800 mg/d PO for 1 mo, then 200–400 mg/d. IV: 15 mg/min for 10 min, then 1 mg/min for 6 h; maintenance dose 0.5 mg/min continuous infusion. *Peds:* 10–15 mg/kg/24h divided q12h PO for 7–10 d, then 5 mg/kg/24h divided q12h or qd (infants and neonates may require larger loading dose).

TABLE IX–3. PERCENTAGE OF LOADING DOSE REQUIRED FOR DOSAGE INTERVAL SELECTED

CrCl (mL/min)	Dosing Interval		
	8 h	12 h	24 h
90	90[a]	—	—
90	86[a]	—	—
70	84[a]	—	—
60	79[a]	91	—
50	74[a]	87	—
40	66	80[a]	—
30	57	72[a]	92
25	51	66[a]	88
20	45	59[a]	83
15	37	50[a]	75
10	29	40	64[a]
7	24	33	55[a]
5	20	28	48[a]
2	14	20	35[a]
0	9	13	25[a]

[a]Suggested dosage intervals. This is only an empirical dose to begin therapy. Serum levels should be monitored routinely for optimal therapy. Use Table IX–2, "Common Drug Levels."
Source (From Hull JH, Sarubbi FA: Gentamicin serum concentrations: Pharmacokinetic predictions. Ann Intern Med 1976;85:183.)

NOTES: Average half-life is 53 d; potentially toxic effects leading to pulmonary fibrosis, liver failure, ocular opacities, and exacerbation of arrhythmias; IV concentrations >0.2 mg/mL should be administered via a central catheter.

Amitriptyline (Elavil)
COMMON USES: Depression, peripheral neuropathy, chronic pain, cluster, and migraine headaches.
DOSAGE: *Adults:* Initially, 50–100 mg PO qhs; may increase to 300 mg qhs. *Peds:* Not recommended if <12 y unless for chronic pain: 0.1 mg/kg qhs initially, then advance over 2–3 wk to 0.5–2 mg/kg qhs.
NOTES: Strong anticholinergic side effects; may cause urinary retention and sedation.

Amlodipine (Norvasc)
COMMON USES: HTN, chronic stable angina, and vasospastic angina.
DOSAGE: 2.5–10 mg PO qd.

Amoxapine (Asendin)
COMMON USES: Depression and anxiety.
DOSAGE: Initially, 150 mg PO qhs or 50 mg PO tid; increase to 300 mg/d.
NOTES: Decrease dose in elderly patients; taper slowly when discontinuing therapy.

Amoxicillin (Amoxil, Larotid, Polymox, Others)

COMMON USES: Management of susceptible gram-positive bacteria (streptococci) and gram-negative bacteria (*H influenzae*, *E coli*, *P mirabilis*; ie, SBE prophylaxis, otitis media, respiratory, skin, and urinary tract infections).
DOSAGE: *Adults:* 250–500 mg PO tid. *Peds:* 25–100 mg/kg/24h PO divided q8h; 200 mg–400 mg PO bid (equivalent to 125 mg–250 mg tid).
NOTES: Cross-hypersensitivity with penicillin; may cause diarrhea; skin rash is common; many hospital strains of *E coli* are resistant.

Amoxicillin/Potassium Clavulanate (Augmentin)

COMMON USES: Management of infections caused by β-lactamase–producing strains of *H influenzae*, *S aureus*, and *E coli*.
DOSAGE: *Adults:* 250–500 mg as amoxicillin PO q8h or 875 mg q12h. *Peds:* 20–40 mg/kg/d as amoxicillin PO divided q8h.
NOTES: Do not substitute 2 250–mg tablets for 1 500-mg tablet or an overdose of clavulanic acid will occur; may cause diarrhea and gastrointestinal (GI) intolerance. This is a combination of a β-lactamase antibiotic and a β-lactamase inhibitor.

Amphotericin B (Fungizone)

COMMON USES: Severe, systemic fungal infections (eg, *Candida* spp, histoplasmosis, etc); bladder irrigation for fungal infections.
DOSAGE: *Adults* and *Peds:* Test dose of 1 mg, then 0.25–1.5 mg/kg/24h IV over 4–6 h. Doses often range from 25 to 50 mg qd or every other day. Total dose varies with indication. Bladder irrigation: 50 mg in 1 L sterile water irrigated over 24 h; used for 2–7 d or until culture is negative.
NOTES: Severe side effects with IV infusion; monitor renal function; hypokalemia and hypomagnesemia may be seen from renal wasting; pretreat with acetaminophen and antihistamines (Benadryl) to help minimize adverse effects such as fever; topical and oral forms are available.

Amphotericin B Lipid Complex (Abelcet)

COMMON USES: Invasive fungal infection in persons refractory or intolerant to conventional amphotericin B.
DOSAGE: 5 mg/kg/d IV administered as single daily dose; infuse at rate of 2.5 mg/kg/h.
NOTES: Filter solution with a 5-mm filter needle; do not mix in electrolyte-containing solutions. If infusion exceeds 2 h, gently mix contents of the bag.

Amphotericin B Liposomal (AmBisome)

COMMON USES: Invasive fungal infection in persons refractory or intolerant to conventional amphotericin B.
DOSAGE: *Adults* and *Peds:* 3 to 5 mg/kg/d, infused over 60–120 min.

Ampicillin (Amcill, Omnipen)

COMMON USES: Management of susceptible gram-negative (*Shigella*, *Salmonella*, *E coli*, *H influenzae*, *P mirabilis*) and gram-positive (streptococci) bacteria.
DOSAGE: *Adults:* 500 mg to 2 g PO, IM, or IV q6h. *Peds:* Neonates <7 d: 50–100 mg/kg/24h IV divided q8h. Term infants: 75–150 mg/kg/24h divided q6–8h IV or PO. Infants >1 mo and children: 100–200 mg/kg/24h divided q4–6h IM or IV; 50–100 mg/kg/24h divided q6h PO up to 250 mg/dose. Meningitis: 200–400 mg/kg/24h divided q4–6h IV.
NOTES: Cross-hypersensitivity with penicillin; can cause diarrhea and skin rash; many hospital strains of *E coli* are now resistant.

Ampicillin/Sulbactam (Unasyn)

COMMON USES: Control of infections caused by β-lactamase–producing organisms of *S aureus*, *Enterococcus* spp, *H influenzae*, *P mirabilis*, and *Bacteroides* species.

DOSAGE: *Adults:* 1.5–3.0 g IM or IV q6h. *Peds:* Dosed by ampicillin content 100–200 mg /kg/d (Unasyn 150–300 mg) divided q6h; max daily dose ampicillin 8 g/d (Unasyn 12 g).
NOTES: 2:1 ratio of ampicillin/sulbactam; adjust dose in renal failure; observe for hypersensitivity reactions.

Amrinone (Inocor)

COMMON USES: Short-term management of CHF.
DOSAGE: *Adults* and *Peds:* Initially give IV bolus of 0.75 mg/kg over 2–3 min followed by maintenance dose of 5–10 mg/kg/min.
NOTES: Not to exceed 10 mg/kg/d; incompatible with dextrose-containing solutions; monitor for fluid and electrolyte changes and renal function during therapy.

Antihemophilic (AHF) Factor [Factor VIII] (Monoclate, Others)

COMMON USES: Management of classic hemophilia A with factor VIII deficiency.
DOSAGE: *Adults* and *Peds:* AHF 1 U/kg increases factor VIII concentration in the body by approximately 2%. Units required = body weight (kg) × (desired factor VIII increase as percentage of normal) × (0.5). Prophylaxis of spontaneous hemorrhage: 5% normal. Hemostasis after trauma or surgery: 30% normal. Head injuries, major surgery, or bleeding: 80–100% normal. Patient's percentage of normal level of factor VIII concentration must be ascertained before dosing for these calculations. Typical dosing is 20–50 U/kg/dose given q12–24h.
NOTES: Not effective in controlling bleeding of patients with von Willebrand's disease; derived from pooled human plasma.

Antithymocyte Globulin [ATG] (Atgam)

COMMON USES: Management of allograft rejection in renal transplant patients.
DOSAGE: *Adults:* 10–30 mg/kg/d. *Peds:* 5–25 mg/kg/d.
NOTES: Do not administer to a patient with a history of severe systemic reaction to any other equine gamma-globulin preparation; discontinue therapy if severe unremitting thrombocytopenia or leukopenia occurs.

Aprotinin (Trasylol)

COMMON USES: Decrease or prevention of blood loss in patients undergoing CABG.
DOSAGE: Large dose: 2 million KIU load, 2 million KIU for pump prime dose, followed by 500,000 KIU/h until surgery ends. Small dose: 1 million KIU load, 1 million KIU for pump prime dose, followed by 250,000 KIU/h until surgery ends. Maximum total dose is 7 million KIU.
NOTES: 1000 KIU = 0.14 mg aprotinin.

Ardeparin (Normiflo)

COMMON USES: Prevention of DVT and pulmonary embolism after knee replacement.
DOSAGE: 35–50 U/kg SC q12h. Begin day of surgery and continue <14 d.
NOTES: Laboratory monitoring is not necessary.

Artificial Tears [OTC] (Tears Naturale, others)

COMMON USES: Dry eyes.
DOSAGE: 1–2 drops tid–qid.

Aspirin (Bayer, Ecotrin, St. Joseph, ASA, Others)

COMMON USES: Mild pain, headache, fever, inflammation, prevention of emboli, MI, and transient ischemic attack (TIA).
DOSAGE: *Adults:* Pain, fever: 325–650 mg q4–6h PO or PR. Rheumatoid arthritis: 3–6 g/d PO in divided doses. Platelet inhibitory action: 325 mg PO qd. Prevention of MI: 160–325 mg PO qd. TIA: 1.3 g/d PO divided bid–qid. *Peds:* Caution: use linked to Reye's syndrome; avoid use with viral illness in children. Antipyretic: 10–15 mg/kg/dose PO or PR q4h up to 80 mg/kg/24h. Rheumatoid

arthritis: 60–100 mg/kg/24h PO divided q4–6h (monitor serum levels to maintain level at 15–30 mg/dL).

NOTES: GI upset and erosion are common adverse reactions; discontinue use 1 wk before surgery to avoid postop bleeding complications.

Aspirin With Codeine (Empirin No. 1, No. 2, No. 3, No. 4) [C]

COMMON USES: Relief of mild to moderate pain.

DOSAGE: *Adults:* 1–2 tablets PO q3–4h prn. *Peds:* Aspirin 10 mg/kg/dose; codeine 0.5–1.0 mg/kg/dose q4h.

NOTES: Codeine 7.5 mg in No. 1, 15 mg in No. 2, 30 mg in No. 3, 60 mg in No. 4.

Atenolol (Tenormin)

COMMON USES: HTN, angina, after MI, antiarrhythmic, acute alcoholic withdrawal.

DOSAGE: *Adults:* HTN and angina: 50–100 mg PO qd. AMI: 5 mg IV × 2 doses, then 50 mg PO bid.

Atenolol & Chlorthalidone (Tenoretic)

COMMON USES: HTN.

DOSAGE: 50–100 mg PO qd.

Atorvastatin (Lipitor)

COMMON USES: Control high levels of cholesterol and triglycerides plus dietary modifications.

DOSAGE: Initial dose 10 mg/d, may be increased to 80 mg/d.

NOTES: May cause myopathy, monitor liver function tests (LFTs) regularly.

Atracurium (Tracrium)

COMMON USES: Adjunct to anesthesia to facilitate endotracheal intubation.

DOSAGE: *Adults* and *Peds:* 0.4–0.5 mg/kg IV bolus, then 0.08–0.1 mg/kg every 20–45 min prn.

NOTES: Patient must be intubated and on controlled ventilation. Use adequate amounts of sedation and analgesia.

Atropine

COMMON USES: Preanesthetic, symptomatic bradycardia, asystole; organophosphate poisoning, bronchodilator, mydriatic and cycloplegic for eye examination, uveitis, reversal of neuromuscular blockade with neostigmine or edrophonium.

DOSAGE: *Adults:* Emergency cardiac care, bradycardia: 0.5 mg IV q5min up to 2.0 mg total. Asystole 1.0 mg IV, repeat in 5 min. Preanesthetic: 0.3–0.6 mg IM/IV/SC. Ophthalmic: 1–2 drops qid or 1/4 inch of 1% ointment; refraction, administer 1 h before examination. *Peds:* Emergency cardiac care: 0.01–0.03 mg/kg IV q2–5 min up to 1.0 mg total dose; minimum dose 0.1 mg. Preanesthetic: 0.01 mg/kg/dose SC/IM/IV (max 0.4 mg).

NOTES: Can cause blurred vision, urinary retention, dry mucous membranes.

Azathioprine (Imuran)

COMMON USES: Adjunct for the prevention of rejection after organ transplantation; rheumatoid arthritis; systemic lupus erythematosus.

DOSAGE: *Adults* and *Peds:* 1–3 mg/kg/d IV or PO.

NOTES: May cause GI intolerance; injection should be handled with appropriate precautions.

Azithromycin (Zithromax)

COMMON USES: Management of acute bacterial exacerbations of COPD, mild community-acquired pneumonia, pharyngitis, otitis media, skin and skin structure infections, nongonococcal urethritis, and PID. Management and prevention of *Mycobacterium avium* complex (MAC) infections in HIV-infected persons.

DOSAGE: *Adults:* PO: Respiratory tract: 500 mg on first day, followed by 250 mg PO qd for 4 more days. Nongonococcal urethritis: 1 g as a single dose. Pre-

vention of MAC: 1200 mg PO once a week. IV: 500 mg for ≥2 d, followed by 500 mg PO for total of 7–10 d. *Peds:* Otitis media: 10 mg/kg PO on day 1, then 5 mg/kg/d on days 2–5. Pharyngitis: 12 mg/kg/d PO for 5 d.
NOTES: Should be taken before meals.

Aztreonam (Azactam)

COMMON USES: Infections caused by aerobic gram-negative bacteria where beta-lactam may not be useful, including *Enterobacter*, *H influenzae*, *Pseudomonas* sepsis, UTI, skin infections, intra-abdominal and gynecologic infections
DOSAGE: *Adults:* 1–2 g IV/IM q6–12h. *Peds:* Premature infants: 30 mg/kg/dose IV q12h. Term infants, children: 30–50 mg/kg/dose q6–8h.
NOTES: Not effective against gram-positive or anaerobic bacteria; may be given to penicillin-allergic patients.

Bacitracin & Polymyxin B (Polysporin)

COMMON USES: Blepharitis, conjunctivitis, and prophylactic management of corneal abrasions.
DOSAGE: Apply q3–4h.

Baclofen (Lioresal)

COMMON USES: Spasticity secondary to severe chronic disorders such as multiple sclerosis or spinal cord lesions.
DOSAGE: 5 mg PO tid initially, increase every 3 d to maximum effect; max 80 mg/d.
NOTES: Caution in patients with seizure disorder and neuropsychiatric disturbances.

Beclomethasone (Beconase, Vancenase Nasal Inhalers)

COMMON USES: Allergic rhinitis refractory to conventional therapy with antihistamines and decongestants.
DOSAGE: *Adults:* 1 spray intranasally bid–qid. *Peds:* 6–11 y: 1 spray intranasally tid.
NOTES: Nasal spray delivers 42 mg/dose.

Beclomethasone (Beclovent Inhaler, Vanceril Inhaler)

COMMON USES: Chronic asthma.
DOSAGE: *Adults:* 2–4 inhalations tid–qid (max 20/d). *Peds:* 1–2 inhalations tid–qid (max 10/d).
NOTES: Not effective for acute asthmatic attacks; may cause oral candidiasis.

Belladonna & Opium Suppositories (B & O Supprettes) [C]

COMMON USES: Control of bladder or rectal spasms; moderate to severe pain.
DOSAGE: Insert 1 suppository rectally q4–6h prn. (15A = powdered opium 30 mg; belladonna extract 16.2 mg. 16A = powdered opium 60 mg; belladonna extract 16.2 mg.)
NOTES: Anticholinergic side effects; caution subjects about sedation, urinary retention, constipation.

Benazepril (Lotensin)

COMMON USES: Hypertension.
DOSAGE: 10–40 mg PO qd.
NOTES: May cause symptomatic hypotension in patients taking diuretics; may cause a nonproductive cough.

Benzonatate (Tessalon Perles)

COMMON USES: Symptomatic relief of nonproductive cough.
DOSAGE: 100 mg PO tid.
NOTES: May cause sedation.

Benztropine (Cogentin)

COMMON USES: Management of Parkinson's disease and drug-induced extrapyramidal disorders.
DOSAGE: 1–6 mg PO, IM, or IV in divided doses.
NOTES: Anticholinergic side effects.

Bepridil (Vascor)

COMMON USES: Management of chronic stable angina, HTN, and CHF.
DOSAGE: 200–400 mg PO daily (adjust dose after 10 d).
NOTES: May cause serious ventricular arrhythmias, including torsade de pointes and agranulocytosis.

Beractant (Survanta)

COMMON USES: Prevention/management of respiratory distress syndrome (RDS) in premature infants.
DOSAGE: 4 mL/kg intratracheally; up to 4 doses in the first 48 h of life ≥6 h apart; additional therapy based on clinical response.

Betamethasone, Systemic (Celestone, Others) (also see Table IX–4 below, and Table IX–7, page 524.)

COMMON USES: Steroid replacement, anti-inflammatory, immunosuppressive.
DOSAGE: 0.6–7.2 mg/d PO divided bid–tid; up to 9 mg/d IM; intra-articular 0.5–2.0 mL.

Betaxolol (Kerlone)

COMMON USES: HTN, ocular for glaucoma.
DOSAGE: 10–20 mg PO, qd; ophthalmic: 1–2 drops of solution or suspension bid.

TABLE IX–4. COMPARISON OF SYSTEMIC GLUCOCORTICOIDS (see page 522)

Drug	Relative Equivalent Dose (mg)	Activity	Mineralocorticoid Duration	Route
Betamethasone	0–0.75	0	36–72 h	PO, IM
Cortisone (Cortone)	25.00	2	8–12 h	PO, IM
Dexamethasone (Decadron)	0.75	0	36–72 h	PO, IV
Hydrocortisone (Solu-Cortef, Hydrocortone)	20.00	2	8–12 h	PO, IM, IV
Methylprednisolone acetate (Depo-Medrol)	4.00	0	36–72 h	PO, IM, IV
Methylprednisolone Succinate (Solu-Medrol)	4.00			PO, IM, IV
Prednisone (Deltasone)	5.00	1	12–36 h	PO
Prednisolone (Delt-Cortef)	5.00	1	12–36 h	PO, IM, IV

Bethanechol (Urecholine, Duvoid, Others)

COMMON USES: Neurogenic atony of the bladder with urinary retention, acute postoperative and postpartum functional (nonobstructive) urinary retention.
DOSAGE: **Adults:** 10–50 mg PO tid–qid or 5 mg SC tid–qid and prn. **Peds:** 0.3–0.6 mg/kg/24h PO divided tid–qid or Z\c the oral dose SC.
NOTES: Contraindicated in bladder outlet obstruction, asthma, coronary artery disease; do not administer IM or IV.

Bicarbonate, see Sodium Bicarbonate

Bisacodyl (Dulcolax, others)

COMMON USES: Constipation, bowel prep.
DOSAGE: **Adults:** 5–10 mg PO or 10 mg rectally prn. **Peds:** <2 y: 5 mg rectally prn; >2 y: 5 mg PO or 10 mg rectally prn.
NOTES: Do not use with an acute abdomen or bowel obstruction; do not chew tablets; do not give within 1 h of antacids or milk.

Bismuth Subsalicylate (Pepto-Bismol, Others)

COMMON USES: Indigestion, nausea, and diarrhea.
DOSAGE: **Adults:** 2 tablets or 30 mL PO prn. **Peds:** 3–6 y: 1/3 tablet or 5 mL PO prn; 6–9 y: 2/3 tablet or 10 mL PO prn; 9–12 y: 1 tablet or 15 mL PO prn.

Bisoprolol (Zebeta)

COMMON USES: HTN.
DOSAGE: 5–10 mg qd.

Bitolterol (Tornalate)

COMMON USES: Prophylaxis and management of asthma and reversible bronchospasm.
DOSAGE: **Adults:** and children >12 y: 2 inhalations q8h.

Bromocriptine (Parlodel)

COMMON USES: Parkinsonian syndrome.
DOSAGE: Parkinson's: 1.25 mg PO bid initially, titrated to effect.
NOTES: Nausea and vertigo are common side effects.

Budesonide (Rhinocort, Pulmicort)

COMMON USES: Management of allergic and nonallergic rhinitis, management of asthma.
DOSAGE: **Intranasal:** 2 sprays in each nostril bid. **Oral inhaled:** 1–4 inhalations twice daily. **Peds:** 1–2 inhalations twice daily.

Bumetanide (Bumex)

COMMON USES: Edema from CHF, hepatic cirrhosis, and renal disease.
DOSAGE: **Adults:** 0.5–2.0 mg PO daily; 0.5–1.0 mg IV q8–24h. **Peds:** 0.015–0.1 mg/kg/dose PO, IV, IM q6–24h.
NOTES: Monitor fluid and electrolyte status during treatment.

Bupivacaine (Marcaine, Sensorcaine)

COMMON USES: Local infiltration anesthesia, lumbar epidural.
DOSAGE: Dependent on the procedure, vascularity of the tissues, depth of anesthesia, and degree of muscle relaxation required. Maximum infiltration dose in 70–kg adult is 0.25% 70 mL.

Buprenorphine (Buprenex) [C]

COMMON USES: Relief of moderate to severe pain.
DOSAGE: 0.3 mg IM or slow IV push every 6 h prn.
NOTES: May induce withdrawal syndrome in opioid-dependent subjects.

Bupropion (Wellbutrin, Zyban)

COMMON USES: Management of depression, adjunct to smoking cessation.
DOSAGE: Depression: 100–450 mg/d divided bid–tid. Smoking: 150 mg daily for 3 d, then 150 mg twice daily.
NOTES: Has been associated with seizures; avoid use of alcohol and other CNS depressants.

Buspirone (BuSpar)

COMMON USES: Short-term relief of anxiety.
DOSAGE: 5–10 mg PO tid.
NOTES: No abuse potential. No physical or psychological dependence.

Butalbital & Acetaminophen (Fioricet, Medigesic, Phrenilin, Phrenilin Forte, Sedapap-10, Others) [C]

COMMON USES: Tension headache, pain.
DOSAGE: 1–2 PO q4h prn, max 6 tabs/d.
NOTES: Butalbital habit forming; Medigesic caps: butalbital 50 mg, caffeine 40 mg, and acetaminophen 325 mg; Phrenilin Forte caps: butalbital 50 mg and acetaminophen 650 mg; Fioricet Tabs: butalbital 50 mg, caffeine 40 mg, and acetaminophen 325 mg; Phrenilin Tabs: butalbital 50 mg and acetaminophen 325 mg; Sedapap-10: butalbital 50 mg and acetaminophen 650 mg.

Butalbital & Aspirin (Fiorinal, Lanorinal, Marnal, Others) [C]

COMMON USES: Tension headache, pain
DOSAGE: 1–2 PO q4h prn, max 6 tabs/d.
NOTES: Butalbital habit forming; Fiorinal, Lanorinal, Marnal Caps and Tabs: Butalbital 50 mg, caffeine 40 mg, and aspirin 325 mg.

Butalbital, Aspirin, & Codeine (Fiorinal With Codeine) [C]

COMMON USES: Moderate pain.
DOSAGE: 1–2 PO q4h prn, max 6/d.
NOTES: Butalbital may be habit forming; may cause sedation; contains butalbital 50 mg, caffeine 40 mg, aspirin 325 mg, and codeine 30 mg.

Butorphanol (Stadol) [C]

COMMON USES: Analgesic for moderate to severe pain; migraine headache.
DOSAGE: 1–4 mg IM or 0.5–2 mg IV every 3–4 h prn; 1 spray in 1 nostril (1 mg) re-evaluate in 60–90 min and repeat if needed; repeat 2-dose sequence prn in 3–4 h.
NOTES: May induce withdrawal syndrome in opioid-dependent patients.

Calcitrol (Rocaltrol)

COMMON USES: Decrease high parathyroid hormone levels, hypocalcemia associated with dialysis.
DOSAGE: *Adults:* renal failure 0.25 mg PO, qd increase 0.25 mg/d every 4–6 wk prn; 0.5 mg 3 times/wk IV, increase as needed. *Hyperparathyroidism:* 0.5–2.0 mg/d. *Peds:* renal failure 15 ng/kg/d, increase prn typical maintenance 30–60 ng/kg/d. *Hyperparathyroidism:* <5 y, 0.25–0.75 mg/d; >6 y, 0.5–2.0 mg/d.
NOTES: 1,25 Dihydroxycholecalciferol, a vitamin D analogue; monitor dosing to keep calcium levels within normal range.

Calcitonin (Cibacalcin, Miacalcin)

COMMON USES: Paget's disease of bone; hypercalcemia; osteogenesis imperfecta, postmenopausal osteoporosis.
DOSAGE: Paget's salmon form: 100 U/d IM/SC initially, 50 U/d or 50–100 U q1–3d maintenance. Paget's human form: 0.5 mg/d initially; maintenance: 0.5 mg 2–3 times/wk or 0.25 mg/d, max 0.5 mg bid. Hypercalcemia salmon calcitonin: 4 U/kg IM/SC q12h; increase to 8 U/kg q12h, max q6h. Osteoporosis salmon calcitonin: 100 U/d IM/SC; Intranasal: 200 U = 1 nasal spray/d.

NOTES: Human (Cibacalcin) and salmon forms; human only approved for Paget's bone disease.

Calcium Acetate

COMMON USES: End-stage renal disease associated with hyperphosphatemia.
DOSAGE: 2–4 tabs PO with meals.
NOTES: Can cause hypercalcemia, monitor levels.

Calcium Carbonate (Alka-Mints, Caltrate, Tums, Os-Cal, Others)

COMMON USES: Hyperacidity associated with peptic ulcer disease, hiatal hernia, etc; calcium supplementation.
DOSAGE: 500 mg to 2.0 g PO prn.

Calcium Salts (Chloride Gluconate)

COMMON USES: Calcium replacement, ventricular fibrillation, electromechanical dissociation, management of hyperphosphatemia in end-stage renal disease.
DOSAGE: *Adults:* Replacement: 1–2 g PO qd. Cardiac emergencies: calcium chloride 0.5–1.0 g IV every 10 min or calcium gluconate 1–2 g IV every 10 min. *Peds:* Replacement: 200–500 mg/kg/24h PO or IV divided qid. Cardiac emergency: gluconate salt 100 mg/kg/dose IV every 10 min.
NOTES: Calcium chloride contains 270 mg (13.6 mEq) elemental calcium per gram, and calcium gluconate contains 90 mg (4.5 mEq) elemental calcium per gram.

Candesartan (Atacand)

COMMON USES: Management of HTN.
DOSAGE: 2–32 mg/d, usual dose 16 mg once daily.
NOTES: Monitor blood pressure (BP) and titrate to effect; maximum BP response within 2 wk.

Capsaicin (Zostrix, others)

COMMON USES: Topical analgesic (after herpetic neuralgia, arthritis, postop pain).
DOSAGE: Over-the-counter (OTC) form, apply tid–qid.

Captopril (Capoten)

COMMON USES: Management of HTN, CHF, and diabetic nephropathy.
DOSAGE: *Adults:* Hypertension: Initially, 25 mg PO bid–tid; titrate to a maintenance dose every 1–2 wk by 25-mg increments per dose (max 450 mg/d) to desired effect. CHF: Initially, 6.25–12.5 mg PO tid; titrate to desired effect. *Peds:* Infants <2 mo, 0.05–0.1 mg/kg/dose PO tid–qid. *Children:* Initially, 0.15 mg/kg/dose PO; double q2h until BP is controlled, to max 6 mg/kg/d; maintenance: 0.5–0.6 mg/kg/d PO divided bid–qid.
NOTES: Use with caution in renal failure. Give 1 h before meals; can cause rash, proteinuria, and cough.

Carbamazepine (Tegretol)

COMMON USES: Epilepsy; trigeminal neuralgia.
DOSAGE: *Adults:* 200 mg PO bid initially; increase by 200 mg/d; usual 800–1200 mg/d. *Peds:* 6–12 y: 100 mg/dose PO bid or 10 mg/kg/24h PO divided qd–bid initially; increase to a maintenance dose of 20–30 mg/kg/24h divided tid–qid.
NOTES: Can cause severe hematologic side effects; monitor CBC count; monitor serum levels (see Table IX–2, page 460); generic products are not interchangeable.

Carbidopa/Levodopa (Sinemet)

COMMON USES: Parkinson's disease.
DOSAGE: Start at 10/100 PO bid–tid; titrate as needed.

NOTES: May cause psychiatric disturbances, orthostatic hypotension, dyskinesias, and cardiac arrhythmias.

Caspofungin (Cancidas)

COMMON USES: Aspergillosis, invasive, refractory and esophageal candidiasis.
DOSAGE: 70 mg IV load, then 50 mg IV daily.
NOTES: Dose adjustments for hepatic and renal impairment.

Carisoprodol (Soma)

COMMON USES: Adjunct to sleep and physical therapy for the relief of painful musculoskeletal conditions.
DOSAGE: 350 mg PO qid.
NOTES: Avoid alcohol and other CNS depressants; also available with codeine 16 mg per tablet [C].

Carteolol (Cartrol, Ocupress Ophthalmic)

COMMON USES: Management of HTN; ophthalmic solution for increased intraocular pressure.
DOSAGE: 2.5–5 mg PO qd; ophthalmic 1 drop eye/eyes bid.

Carvedilol (Coreg)

COMMON USES: Management of HTN and CHF.
DOSAGE: HTN: 6.25–12.5 mg twice daily. CHF: 3.125–25 mg twice daily.
NOTES: Take with food to slow absorption and decrease incidence of orthostatic hypotension.

Cefaclor (Ceclor)

COMMON USES: Management of infections caused by susceptible bacteria involving the upper and lower respiratory tract, skin, bone, urinary tract, abdomen, and gynecologic system (*S aureus*, *S pneumoniae*, *H influenzae*).
DOSAGE: *Adults:* 250–500 mg PO tid. *Peds:* 20–40 mg/kg/d PO divided tid.
NOTES: Second-generation cephalosporin; more gram-negative activity than first-generation cephalosporins.

Cefazolin (Ancef, Kefzol)

COMMON USES: Management of infections caused by susceptible strains of *Streptococcus*, *Staphylococcus*, *E coli, Proteus,* and *Klebsiella* involving the skin, bone, upper and lower respiratory tract, and urinary tract.
DOSAGE: *Adults:* 1–2 g IV q8h. *Peds:* 50–100 mg/kg/d IV divided q8h.
NOTES: Widely used for surgical prophylaxis; first-generation cephalosporin.

Cefepime (Maxipime)

COMMON USES: Control of UTIs and pneumonia caused by susceptible *S pneumoniae*, *S aureus*, *K pneumoniae*, *E coli*, *P aeruginosa*, and *Enterobacter* spp.
DOSAGE: 1–2 g IV q12h for 5–10 d; UTI 500 mg IV q12h.
NOTES: Fourth-generation cephalosporin; improved gram-positive coverage over third generation.

Cefixime (Suprax)

COMMON USES: Control of infections caused by susceptible bacteria involving the respiratory tract, skin, bone, urinary tract, meningitis, and septicemia; single dose to control gonorrhea.
DOSAGE: *Adults:* 200–400 mg PO bid–qd. *Peds:* 8 mg/kg/d PO divided bid–qd, max 400 mg/d.
NOTES: Third-generation cephalosporin; use suspension to manage otitis media.

Cefonicid (Monocid)

COMMON USES: Control of infections caused by susceptible bacteria: respiratory, skin, bone and joint, urinary, gynecologic, and septicemia.

DOSAGE: 1 g IM/IV q24h.
NOTES: Second-generation cephalosporin.

Cefoperazone (Cefobid)

COMMON USES: Control of infections caused by susceptible bacteria: respiratory, skin , urinary tract, sepsis; as a third-generation cephalosporin, cefoperazone has activity against gram-negative bacilli (eg, *E coli*, *Klebsiella*, and *Haemophilus*) but variable activity against *Streptococcus* and *Staphylococcus* spp; it has activity against *P aeruginosa*, but less than ceftazidime.
DOSAGE: *Adults:* 2–4 g/d, divided q12h IM/IV; 12 g/d max. *Peds:* 100–150 mg/kg/d divided q8–12h IM/IV.
NOTES: Third-generation cephalosporin; active against gram-negatives but variable activity against *Staphylococcus* and *Streptococcus*; some activity against *Pseudomonas*.

Cefotaxime (Claforan)

COMMON USES: Control of infections caused by susceptible bacteria involving the respiratory tract, skin, bone, urinary tract, meningitis, and septicemia.
DOSAGE: *Adults:* 1–2 g IV q4–12h. *Peds:* 100–200 mg/kg/d IV divided q6–8h.
NOTES: Third-generation cephalosporin.

Cefotetan (Cefotan)

COMMON USES: Control of infections caused by susceptible bacteria involving the upper and lower respiratory tract, skin, bone, urinary tract, abdomen, and gynecologic system.
DOSAGE: *Adults:* 1–2 g IV q12h. *Peds:* 40–80 mg/kg/d IV divided q12h.
NOTES: Second-generation cephalosporin; more gram-negative activity than first-generation cephalosporins; has anaerobic activity.

Cefoxitin (Mefoxin)

COMMON USES: Control of infections caused by susceptible bacteria involving the upper and lower respiratory tract, skin, bone, urinary tract, abdomen, and gynecologic system.
DOSAGE: *Adults:* 1–2 mg IV q6h. *Peds:* 80–160 mg/kg/d divided q4–6h.
NOTES: Second-generation cephalosporin; more gram-negative activity than first-generation cephalosporins; has anaerobic activity.

Cefpodoxime (Vantin)

COMMON USES: Control of infections caused by susceptible bacteria involving the respiratory tract (community-acquired pneumonia due to *S pneumonia* or non–beta-lactamase *H influenzae*, otitis media, pharyngitis, tonsillitis, skin, bone, urinary tract, gonorrhea, meningitis, and septicemia.
DOSAGE: *Adults:* 200–400 mg PO q12h. *Peds:* >6 mo, 10 mg/kg/d PO divided bid.
NOTES: Second-generation cephalosporin; drug interactions with agents increasing gastric pH.

Ceftazidime (Fortaz, Ceptaz, Tazidime, Tazicef)

COMMON USES: Control of infections caused by susceptible bacteria involving the respiratory tract, skin, bone, urinary tract, meningitis, and septicemia.
DOSAGE: *Adults:* 1–2 g IV q8h. *Peds:* 30–50 mg/kg/d IV divided q8h.
NOTES: Third-generation cephalosporin; useful in patients with pseudomonal infections at risk for nephrotoxicity; empiric therapy in febrile granulocytopenic patients.

Ceftizoxime (Cefizox)

COMMON USES: Control of infections caused by susceptible bacteria involving the respiratory tract, skin, bone, urinary tract, meningitis, and septicemia.
DOSAGE: *Adults:* 1–2 g IV q12–8h. *Peds:* 150–200 mg/kg/d IV divided q6–8h.
NOTES: Third-generation cephalosporin

Ceftriaxone (Rocephin)

COMMON USES: Control of infections caused by susceptible bacteria involving the respiratory tract, skin, bone, urinary tract, meningitis, chancroid, uncomplicated gonorrhea, and septicemia.

DOSAGE: *Adults:* 1–2 g IV q12–24h; gonococcus (GC) and chancroid <45kg, 125 mg IM; >45 kg, 250–mg IM single dose. *Peds:* 50–100 mg/kg/d IV divided q12–24h.

NOTES: Third-generation cephalosporin.

Cefuroxime (Ceftin [Oral], Zinacef [Parenteral])

COMMON USES: Control of infections caused by susceptible bacteria involving the upper and lower respiratory tract, skin, bone, urinary tract, abdomen, and gynecologic system.

DOSAGE: *Adults:* 750 mg–1.5 g IV q8h or 250–500 mg PO bid. *Peds:* 100–150 mg/kg/d IV divided q8h or 20–30 mg/kg/d PO divided bid.

NOTES: Second-generation cephalosporin; more gram-negative activity than first-generation cephalosporins; IV crosses the blood-brain barrier.

Celecoxib (Celebrex)

COMMON USES: Osteoarthritis and rheumatoid arthritis.

DOSAGE: 100–200 mg once or twice daily.

Cephalexin (Keflex, Keftab)

COMMON USES: Control of infections caused by susceptible strains of *Streptococcus, Staphylococcus, E coli, Proteus,* and *Klebsiella* involving the skin, bone, upper and lower respiratory tract, and urinary tract.

DOSAGE: *Adults:* 250–500 mg PO qid. *Peds:* 25–100 mg/kg/d PO divided qid.

NOTES: First-generation cephalosporin.

Cephradine (Velocef)

COMMON USES: Control of susceptible bacterial infections, including group A beta-hemolytic *Streptococcus.*

DOSAGE: *Adults:* 2–4 g/d in 4 divided doses (8 g/d max). *Peds:* >9 mo: 25–100 mg/kg/d divided q6–12h (4 g/d max).

NOTES: First-generation cephalosporin.

Cetirizine (Zyrtec)

COMMON USES: Allergic rhinitis and chronic urticaria.

DOSAGE: *Adults* and *Children >6 y:* 5–10 mg/d.

Charcoal, Activated (SuperChar, Actidose, Liqui-Char)

COMMON USES: Emergency management for poisoning by most drugs and chemicals.

DOSAGE: *Adults:* Acute intoxication: 30–100 g/dose. GI dialysis: 25–50 g q4–6h. *Peds:* Acute intoxication: 1–2 g/kg/dose. GI dialysis: 5–10 g/dose q4–8h.

NOTES: Administer with a cathartic; liquid dosage forms are in sorbitol base; powder mixed with water; protect airway in lethargic or comatose patient.

Chloral Hydrate (Noctec) [C]

COMMON USES: Nocturnal and preoperative sedation.

DOSAGE: *Adults:* Hypnotic: 500 mg to 1 g PO or PR 30 min before sleep or procedure. Sedative: 250 mg PO or PR tid. *Peds:* Hypnotic: 50 mg/kg/24h PO or PR 30 min before sleep or procedure. Sedative: 25 mg/kg/24h PO or PR tid.

NOTES: Mix syrup in a glass of water or fruit juice.

Chlordiazepoxide (Librium) [C]

COMMON USES: Anxiety, tension, alcohol withdrawal.

DOSAGE: *Adults:* Mild anxiety, tension: 5–10 mg PO tid–qid or prn. Severe anxiety, tension: 25–50 mg IM or IV tid–qid or prn. Alcohol withdrawal: 50–100 mg IM

or IV; repeat in 2–4 h if needed, up to 300 mg in 24 h; gradually taper daily. **Peds:** 0.5 mg/kg/24h PO or IM divided q6–8h.
NOTES: Decrease dose in elderly patients; absorption of IM doses can be erratic.

Chlorothiazide (Diuril)

COMMON USES: HTN, edema, CHF.
DOSAGE: **Adults:** 500 mg to 1.0 g PO or IV qd–bid. **Peds:** 20–30 mg/kg/24h PO divided bid.
NOTES: Contraindicated in anuria.

Chlorpheniramine (Chlor-Trimeton, Others)

COMMON USES: Seasonal rhinitis, allergic reactions.
DOSAGE: **Adults:** 4 mg PO or IV q4–6h or 8–12 mg PO bid of sustained release (SR). **Peds:** 0.35 mg/kg/24h PO divided q4–6h or 0.2 mg/kg/24h SR.
NOTES: Anticholinergic side effects and sedation are common. Available in many OTC combinations (eg, acetaminophen, phenylephrine, pseudoephedrine).

Chlorpromazine (Thorazine)

COMMON USES: Psychotic disorders, apprehension, intractable hiccups, control of nausea and vomiting.
DOSAGE: **Adults:** Acute anxiety, agitation: 10–25 mg PO or PR bid–tid. Severe symptoms: 25 mg IM, can repeat in 1 h, then 25–50 mg PO or PR tid. Hiccups: 25–50 mg PO bid–tid. **Peds:** 2.5–6.0 mg/kg/24h PO, PR or IM divided q4–8h.
NOTES: Beware of extrapyramidal side effects, sedation, has alpha-adrenergic blocking properties.

Chlorpropamide (Diabinese)

COMMON USES: Management of non–insulin-dependent diabetes mellitus.
DOSAGE: 100–500 mg qd.
NOTES: Use with caution in renal insufficiency.

Chlorthalidone (Hygroton)

COMMON USES: HTN, edema associated with CHF, steroid and estrogen therapy.
DOSAGE: **Adults:** 50–100 mg PO qd. **Peds:** 2 mg/kg/dose PO 3 times/wk or 1–2 mg/kg PO daily.
NOTES: Contraindicated in anuric patients.

Chlorzoxazone (Paraflex, Parafon Forte DSC)

COMMON USES: Adjunct to rest and physical therapy for the relief of discomfort associated with acute, painful musculoskeletal conditions.
DOSAGE: **Adults:** 250–500 mg PO tid–qid. **Peds:** 20 mg/kg/d or 600 mg/m^2/d divided in 3–4 doses.

Cholecalciferol [Vitamin D$_3$] (Delta D)

COMMON USES: Dietary supplement for management of vitamin D deficiency.
DOSAGE: 400–1000 IU PO daily.
NOTES: cholecalciferol 1 mg = vitamin D activity 40,000 IU.

Cholestyramine (Questran)

COMMON USES: Adjunctive therapy to decrease serum cholesterol in patients with primary hypercholesterolemia; relief of pruritus associated with partial biliary obstruction.
DOSAGE: Individualize dose to 4 g 1–6 times daily.
NOTES: Mix cholestyramine 4 g in noncarbonated beverage 2–6 oz.

Cimetidine (Tagamet)

COMMON USES: Duodenal ulcer; ulcer prophylaxis in hypersecretory states, such as trauma, burns, surgery, Zollinger-Ellison syndrome; and gastroesophageal reflux disease (GERD).

DOSAGE: *Adults:* Active ulcer: 2400 mg/d IV continuous infusion or 300 mg IV q4–6h; 400 mg PO bid or 800 mg qhs. Maintenance therapy: 400 mg PO qhs. GERD: 800 mg PO bid; maintenance 800 mg PO hs. *Peds:* Neonates: 10–20 mg/kg/24h PO or IV divided q4–6h. Children: 20–40 mg/kg/24h PO or IV divided q4–6h.

NOTES: Extend dosing interval with renal insufficiency; decrease dose in elderly patients.

Ciprofloxacin (Cipro, Ciloxan Ophthalmic)

COMMON USES: Broad-spectrum activity against a variety of gram-positive and gram-negative aerobic bacteria (UTI, prostatitis, sinusitis, skin, infectious diarrhea, osteomyelitis, ocular infections).

DOSAGE: *Adults:* 250–750 mg PO q12h or 200–400 mg IV q12h. Ophthalmic: 1–2 drops in eye(s) q2h while awake. *Peds:* Not recommended for use in children <18 y because of cartilage effects.

NOTES: Little activity against streptococci; drug interactions with theophylline, caffeine, sucralfate, and antacids. Nausea, vomiting, and abdominal discomfort are common side effects. Contraindicated in pregnancy.

Cisatrocurium (Nimbex)

COMMON USES: Adjunct to general anesthesia to aid with endotracheal intubation, surgery, and muscle relaxation during mechanical intubation.

DOSAGE: *Adults:* 0.15–2 mg/kg IV bolus followed by maintenance infusion of 1–2 µg/kg/min. *Peds 2–12 y:* 0.1 mg/kg IV bolus followed by maintenance infusion 1–2 µg/kg/min.

NOTES: Hoffman elimination. No dose adjustments for renal or hepatic insufficiency.

Citalopram (Celexa)

COMMON USES: Management of depression.

DOSAGE: Initially, 20 mg/d, may be increased to 40 mg/d.

Clarithromycin (Biaxin)

COMMON USES: Control of upper and lower respiratory tract infections, skin, *H pylori* infections, and infections caused by non-tuberculosis (atypical) *Mycobacterium*; prevention of MAC infections in HIV-infected individuals.

DOSAGE: *Adults:* 250–500 mg PO bid. *Mycobacterium:* 500–1000 mg PO bid. *Peds:* 7.5 mg/kg/dose PO bid.

NOTES: Increases theophylline and carbamazepine levels; avoid concurrent use with cisapride; causes metallic taste.

Clemastine (Tavist [OTC])

COMMON USES: Allergic rhinitis.

DOSAGE: 1.34–2.68 mg (1–2 tabs) tid, max 8.04 mg/d.

Clindamycin (Cleocin)

COMMON USES: Susceptible strains of streptococci, pneumococci, staphylococci, and gram-positive and gram-negative anaerobes, no activity against gram-negative aerobes. Topical agent for severe acne, and vaginal infections.

DOSAGE: *Adults:* 150–450 mg PO qid; 300–600 mg IV q6h or 900 mg IV q8h. Topical: apply bid. Vaginal: 1 full applicator instilled at bedtime for 1 wk. *Peds:* Neonates: 15–20 mg/kg/24h divided q6–8h. Children >1 mo: 15–40 mg/kg/24h divided q6–8h (4 g/d).

NOTES: Beware of diarrhea that may represent pseudomembranous colitis caused by *C difficile*.

Clonazepam (Klonopin) [C]

COMMON USES: Lennox-Gastaut syndrome, akinetic and myoclonic seizures, absence seizures.

DOSAGE: *Adults:* 1.5 mg/d PO in 3 divided doses; increase by 0.5–1.0 mg/d every 3 d prn up to 20 mg/d. *Peds:* 0.01–0.05 mg/kg/24h PO divided tid; increase to 0.1–0.2 mg/kg/24h divided tid.

NOTES: CNS side effects including sedation.

Clonidine (Catapres)

COMMON USES: HTN, opioid, and tobacco withdrawal.

DOSAGE: *Adults:* 0.10 mg PO bid adjusted daily by 0.1–0.2-mg increments (max 2.4 mg/d). *Peds:* 5–25 mg/kg/24h divided q6h.

NOTES: Dry mouth, drowsiness, sedation occur frequently; more effective for HTN when combined with diuretics, rebound HTN can occur with abrupt cessation of doses >0.2 mg bid.

Clonidine Transdermal (Catapres TTS)

COMMON USES: HTN.

DOSAGE: Apply 1 patch every 7 d to a hairless area on the upper arm or torso; titrate according to individual therapeutic requirements.

NOTES: TTS-1, TTS-2, TTS-3 (delivers clonidine 0.1, 0.2, 0.3 mg/d, respectively, for 1 wk). Doses >2 TTS-3 are usually not associated with increased efficacy.

Clopidogrel (Plavix)

COMMON USES: Decrease atherosclerotic events.

DOSAGE: 75 mg once daily.

NOTES: Prolongs bleeding time, use with caution in persons at risk of bleeding from trauma, etc.

Clorazepate (Tranxene) [C]

COMMON USES: Acute anxiety disorders, acute alcohol withdrawal symptoms, and adjunctive therapy in partial seizures.

DOSAGE: *Adults:* 15–60 mg/d PO in single or divided doses. Elderly and debilitated patients: Initiate therapy at 7.5–15 mg/d in divided doses. Alcohol withdrawal: Day 1: Initially, 30 mg; followed by 30–60 mg in divided doses. Day 2: 45–90 mg in divided doses. Day 3: 22.5–45 mg in divided doses. Day 4: 15–30 mg in divided doses. *Peds:* 3.75–7.5 mg/dose bid, to a maximum of 60 mg/d divided bid–tid.

NOTES: Monitor patients with renal and hepatic impairment because drug may accumulate; CNS depressant effects.

Clotrimazole (Lotrimin, Mycelex)

COMMON USES: Control of candidiasis and tinea infections.

DOSAGE: Orally: 1 troche dissolved slowly in mouth 5 times/d for 14 d. Vaginal: Cream: 1 applicator qhs for 7–14 d; Tablets: 100 mg vaginally qhs for 7 d or 200 mg (2 tablets) vaginally qhs for 3 d or 500-mg tablet vaginally hs for 3 d. Topical: Apply 3–4 times daily for 10–14 d.

NOTES: Oral prophylaxis commonly used in immunosuppressed patients.

Cloxacillin (Cloxapen)

COMMON USES: Control of respiratory, skin, bone, joint infections caused by susceptible strains of penicillinase-producing *Staphylococcus*.

DOSAGE: *Adults:* 250–500 mg PO qid. *Peds:* 50–100 mg/kg/d divided qid.

NOTES: Take on an empty stomach.

Clozapine (Clozaril)

COMMON USES: Severe schizophrenia that does not respond to standard therapy.

DOSAGE: Initially 25 mg qd–bid, increase dose to 300–450 mg/d over 2 wk. Maintain patient at smallest dose possible.

NOTES: Has limited distribution. Contact local pharmacy for drug availability. Monitor blood counts frequently because of the risk of agranulocytosis. May cause drowsiness and seizures.

Cocaine [C]

COMMON USES: Topical anesthetic for mucous membranes.
DOSAGE: Apply topically smallest amount of topical solution that provides relief; 1 mg/kg max.

Codeine [C]

COMMON USES: Mild to moderate pain; symptomatic relief of cough.
DOSAGE: *Adults:* Analgesic: 15–60 mg PO, SC/IM qid prn. Antitussive: 5–15 mg PO or SC q4h prn. *Peds:* Analgesic: 0.5–1.0 mg/kg/dose PO or SC q4–6h prn. Antitussive: 1.0–1.5 mg/kg/24h divided q4h, max 30 mg/24h.
NOTES: Most often used in combination with acetaminophen for pain or with agents such as terpin hydrate as an antitussive; 120 mg IM equivalent to 10 mg morphine IM.

Colchicine

COMMON USES: Acute gout.
DOSAGE: Initially, 0.5–1.2 mg PO or IV, then 0.5–1.2 mg every 1–2 h until GI side effects develop (max 8 mg/d).
NOTES: Caution in elderly patients and patients with renal impairment. Colchicine 1–2 mg IV within 24–48 h of an acute attack can be diagnostic and therapeutic in monoarticular arthritis.

Colestipol (Colestid)

COMMON USES: Adjunctive therapy to decrease serum cholesterol in patients with primary hypercholesterolemia.
DOSAGE: 15–30 g/d divided into 2–4 doses.
NOTES: Do not use dry powder; mix with beverages, soups, cereals, etc.

Cortisone

See Table IX–4, page 466, and "Steroids," page 522.

Cromolyn Sodium (Intal, NasalCrom, Opticrom)

COMMON USES: Adjunct to the prophylaxis of asthma; prevention of exercise-induced asthma; allergic rhinitis; ophthalmic allergic manifestations.
DOSAGE: *Adults* and *Peds* >12 years: Inhalation: 20 mg (as powder in capsule) inhaled qid or metered-dose inhaler 2 puffs qid. Oral: 200 mg 4 times/d 15–20 min before meals, up to 400 mg 4 times/d. Nasal instillation: Spray once in each nostril 2–6 times/d. Ophthalmic: 1–2 drops in each eye 4–6 times/d. *Peds:* Inhalation: 2 puffs qid of metered-dose inhaler. Oral: Infants <2 y: 20 mg/kg/d in 4 divided doses. 2–12 y: 100 mg 4 times/d before meals.
NOTES: Has no benefit in acute situations; may require 2–4 wk for maximal effect in perennial allergic disorders.

Cyanocobalamin/Vitamin B$_{12}$

COMMON USES: Pernicious anemia and other vitamin B$_{12}$ deficiency states.
DOSAGE: *Adults:* 100 mg IM or SC qd for 5–10 d, then 100 mg IM twice a week for 1 mo, then 100 mg IM monthly. *Peds:* 100 mg qd IM or SC for 5–10 d, then 30–50 mg IM every 4 wk.
NOTES: Oral absorption highly erratic, altered by many drugs and not recommended; for use with hyperalimentation; see Section V, page 390.

Cyclobenzaprine (Flexeril)

COMMON USES: Adjunct to rest and physical therapy for the relief of muscle spasm associated with acute painful musculoskeletal conditions.
DOSAGE: 10 mg PO tid.
NOTES: Do not use >2–3 wk; has sedative and anticholinergic properties.

Cyclosporine (Sandimmune, Neoral)

COMMON USES: Prophylaxis of organ rejection in kidney, liver, heart, and bone marrow transplants in conjunction with adrenal corticosteroids; other autoimmune diseases.

DOSAGE: *Adults* and *Peds:* Oral: 15 mg/kg/d beginning 12 h before transplantation; after 2 wk, taper the dose by 5 mg/wk to 5–10 mg/kg/d. IV: 5–6 mg/kg/d divided q12–24h. If the patient is unable to take the drug PO, give half the PO dose IV, switch to PO as soon as possible.

NOTES: May increase serum urea nitrogen and creatinine, which may be confused with renal transplant rejection; should be administered in glass containers; has many drug interactions; Neoral and Sandimmune are not interchangeable. See Table IX–2, page 460 for drug levels.

Cytomegalovirus Immune Globulin [CMV-IVIG] (CytoGam)

COMMON USES: Attenuation of primary CMV disease associated with transplantation.

DOSAGE: Administered for 16 wk after transplantation; see product information for dosing schedule.

Daclizumab (Zenapax)

COMMON USES: Prevention of acute organ rejection.

DOSAGE: *Adults* and *Peds:* 1 mg/kg IV per dose; first dose before transplantation followed by 4 doses 14 d apart after transplantation.

Dalteparin (Fragmin)

COMMON USES: Unstable angina, non–Q-wave MI, prevention of ischemic complications because of clot formation in patients on concurrent aspirin, prevention of DVT after surgery.

DOSAGE: Angina/MI: 120 IU/kg (max 10,000 IU) SC q12h with aspirin. DVT prophylaxis: 2500–5000 IU SC 1–2 h before surgery, then once daily for 5–10 d. Systemic anticoagulation: 200 IU/kg SC once daily or 100 IU/kg SC twice daily.

NOTES: Predictable antithrombotic effects eliminate need for laboratory monitoring.

Dantrolene Sodium (Dantrium)

COMMON USES: Management of clinical spasticity resulting from upper motor neuron disorders such as spinal cord injuries, strokes, cerebral palsy, or multiple sclerosis; control of malignant hyperthermic crisis.

DOSAGE: *Adults:* Spasticity: Initially, 25 mg PO qd, titrate to effect by 25 mg up to maximum dose of 100 mg PO qid prn. *Peds:* Initially, 0.5 mg/kg/dose bid, titrate by 0.5 mg/kg to effectiveness up to maximum dose of 3 mg/kg/dose qid prn. *Adults* and *Peds:* Malignant hyperthermia therapy: Continuous rapid IV push beginning at 1 mg/kg until symptoms subside or 10 mg/kg is reached. Postcrisis follow-up: 4–8 mg/kg/d in 3–4 divided doses for 1–3 d to prevent recurrence.

NOTES: Monitor alanine and aspartate aminotransferases closely.

Daptomycin (Cubicin)

COMMON USES: Control of complicated skin infections caused by susceptible gram positive organisms such as *E. faecalis, S. aureus* (including methicillin-resistant *S aureus*), *S agalactiae, S dysgalactiae,* and *S pyogenes.*

DOSAGE: 4 mg/kg every 24 h for 7–14 d.

NOTES: Monitor serum creatinine phosphokinase levels weekly. Adjust dose for renal impairment.

Demeclocycline (Declomycin)

COMMON USES: Management of SIADH.

DOSAGE: SIADH: 300–600 mg PO q12h; antimicrobial: 150–300 mg PO q12h.

NOTES: Decrease dose in renal failure. May cause diabetes insipidus.

Desipramine (Norpramin)

COMMON USES: Endogenous depression.

DOSAGE: 25–200 mg/d in single or divided doses; usually as a single bedtime dose.

NOTES: Many anticholinergic side effects, including blurred vision, urinary retention, and dry mouth.

Desmopressin (DDAVP, Stimate)

COMMON USES: Diabetes insipidus; bleeding due to hemophilia A and type I von Willebrand's disease (parenteral); nocturnal enuresis.

DOSAGE: Diabetes insipidus: *Adults:* Intranasal, 0.1–0.4 mL (10–40 mg) daily in 2–3 divided doses; 0.5–1 mL (2–4 mg) IV/SC daily in 2 divided doses. If converting from intranasal to parenteral dosing, use 1/10 of intranasal dose. *Peds:* 3 mo to 12 y: intranasal 0.05–0.3 mL/d in single or 2 doses. Hemophilia A and von Willebrand's disease (type I): *Adults* and *Peds* >10 kg: 0.3 mg/kg diluted to 50 mL with NS infuse over 15–30 min. *Peds* < 10 kg: Same as above with dilution to 10 mL with normal saline. Nocturnal enuresis: *Peds* >6 y: 20 mg (0.2 mL) qhs, adjust as needed 10–40 mg.

NOTES: In very young and old patients, adjust fluid intake to avoid water intoxication and hyponatremia.

Dexamethasone, Neomycin, Polymyxin-B (Maxitrol)

See page 506.

Dexamethasone, Systemic (Decadron, Dexasone, others)

See "Steroids," page 522, and Table IX–4, page 466.

Dexpanthenol (Lopan-Choline, Ilopan)

COMMON USES: Minimize paralytic ileus, control postoperative distention.

DOSAGE: *Adults:* Relief of gas: 2–3 tablets PO tid. Prevention of postoperative ileus: 250–500 mg IM stat, repeat in 2 h, then q6h as needed. Ileus: 500 mg IM stat, repeat in 2 h, followed by doses every 6 h, if needed.

NOTES: Do not use if obstruction is suspected.

Dextran 40 (Macrodex, Rheomacrodex)

COMMON USES: Plasma expander for adjunctive therapy in shock; prophylaxis of DVT and thromboembolism; adjunct in peripheral vascular surgery.

DOSAGE: Shock: 10 mL/kg infused rapidly with maximum dose of 20 mL/kg in the first 24 h; total daily dose beyond 24 h should not exceed 10 mL/kg and should be discontinued after 5 d. Prophylaxis of DVT and thromboembolism: 10 mL/kg IV on day of surgery followed by 500 mL IV daily for 2–3 d; then 500 mL IV every 2–3 d based on patient's risk factors for up to 2 wk.

NOTES: Observe for hypersensitivity reactions; monitor renal function and electrolytes.

Dextromethorphan (Vicks Formula 44, Many Others)

COMMON USES: To control nonproductive cough.

DOSAGE: *Adults:* 10–20 mg PO q4h prn. *Peds:* 1–2 mg/kg/24h divided tid–qid.

NOTES: May be found in many OTC combination products with guaifenesin, acetaminophen and pseudoephedrine.

Diazepam (Valium) [C]

COMMON USES: Anxiety, alcohol withdrawal, muscle spasm, status epilepticus, and preoperative sedation.

DOSAGE: *Adults:* Status epilepticus: 0.2–0.5 mg/kg/dose IV q15–30 min to 30 mg max. Anxiety, muscle spasm: 2–10 mg PO or IM q3–4h prn. Preoperative: 5–10 mg PO or IM 20–30 min before procedure; can be given IV just before procedure. Alcohol withdrawal: Initially, 2–5 mg IV, may require up to 1000–2000 mg in 24-h period for severe withdrawal symptoms. *Peds:* Status epilepticus: <5 y:

0.2–0.5 mg/kg/dose IV q15–30min up to maximum of 5 mg; >5 y: may administer up to maximum of 10 mg. Sedation, muscle relaxation: 0.04–0.2 mg/kg/dose q2–4h IM or IV up to maximum of 0.6 mg/kg in 8 h, or 0.12–0.8 mg/kg/24h PO divided tid–qid.

NOTES: Do not exceed 5 mg/min IV in adults because respiratory arrest can occur; absorption of IM dose may be erratic.

Dibucaine (Nupercainal, [OTC])

COMMON USES: Hemorrhoids and minor skin conditions.
DOSAGE: Insert into rectum with applicator bid and after each bowel movement.

Diclofenac (Cataflam, Voltaren)

COMMON USES: Management of arthritis (rheumatoid, osteoarthritis) and pain; ophthalmic as an adjunct to cataract surgery.
DOSAGE: 50–75 mg PO bid; ophthalmic 1 drop in eye; qid 24 h postop for up to 2 wk.

Dicloxacillin (Dynapen, Dycill)

COMMON USES: Control of infections caused by susceptible strains of *S aureus* and *Streptococcus.*
DOSAGE: *Adults:* 250–500 mg qid. *Peds:* 12.5–25 mg/kg/d divided qid.
NOTES: Take on an empty stomach.

Dicyclomine (Bentyl)

COMMON USES: Management of functional irritable bowel syndromes.
DOSAGE: *Adults:* 20 mg PO qid titrated to a maximum dose of 160 mg/d or 20 mg IM q6h. *Peds* >6 mo: 5 mg/dose tid–qid; children: 10 mg/dose tid–qid.
NOTES: Anticholinergic side effects may limit dose.

Diflunisal (Dolobid)

DOSAGE: Pain: 500 mg PO bid. Osteoarthritis: 500–1500 mg PO in 2–3 divided doses. Supplied tablets 250, 500 mg.
NOTES: May prolong PT.

Digoxin (Lanoxin, Lanoxicaps)

COMMON USES: CHF, atrial fibrillation and flutter, and paroxysmal atrial tachycardia.
DOSAGE: *Adults:* PO digitalization: 0.50–0.75 mg PO, then 0.25 mg PO q6–8h to a total dose of 1.0–1.5 mg. IV/IM digitalization: 0.25–0.50 mg IM/IV, then 0.25 mg q4–6h, total dose of about 1 mg. Maintenance: 0.125–0.500 mg PO/IM/IV qd (average daily dose 0.125–0.250 mg). *Peds:* Preterm infants: Digitalization: 30 mg/kg PO or 25 mg/kg IV; give 1/2 dose initially, then 1/4 dose at 8- to 12-h intervals for 2 doses. Maintenance: 10 mg/kg/24h PO or 6–8 mg/kg/24h IV divided q12h. Term infants to 2 y: Digitalization: 65–75 mg/kg PO or 50 mg/kg IV; give 1/2 dose initially, then 1/4 dose at 8- to 12-h intervals for 2 doses. Maintenance: 15–20 mg/kg/24h PO or 12–15 mg/kg/24h IV divided q12h. 2–10 y: Digitalization: 30–40 mg/kg PO or 25 mg/kg IV; give 1/2 dose initially, then 1/4 dose at 8- to 12-h intervals for 2 doses. Maintenance: 8–10 mg/kg/24h PO or 6–8 mg/kg/24h IV divided q12h. >10 y: Same as for adults.
NOTES: Can cause heart block; low potassium can potentiate toxicity; decrease dose in renal failure; symptoms of toxicity include nausea and vomiting, headache, fatigue, visual disturbances (yellow-green halos around lights), and cardiac arrhythmias (see Table IX–2, page 460); IM injection can be painful and has erratic absorption.

Digoxin Immune FAB (Digibind)

COMMON USES: Management of life-threatening digoxin intoxication.

DOSAGE: *Adults* and *Peds:* Based on serum level and patient's weight. See dosing charts provided with the drug. Empiric where overdose is not known, 20 vials (760 mg) IV in adults.

NOTES: Each vial will bind approximately digoxin 0.6 mg; in renal failure, may require redosing in several days because of breakdown of the immune complex.

Diltiazem (Cardizem, Dilacor)

COMMON USES: Management of angina pectoris, prevention of reinfarction, hypertension; atrial fibrillation or flutter, and paroxysmal SVT.

DOSAGE: Oral: 30 mg PO qid initially; titrate to 180–360 mg/d in divided doses as needed. SR: 60–120 mg PO bid, titrate to effect, max 360 mg/d. Continuous dose: 180–300 mg PO qd. IV: 0.25 mg/kg IV bolus over 2 min; may repeat dose in 15 min at 0.35 mg/kg. May begin continuous infusion of 5–15 mg/h.

NOTES: Contraindicated in sick-sinus syndrome, AV block, and hypotension. Cardizem CD and Dilacor XR are not interchangeable.

Dimenhydrinate (Dramamine)

COMMON USES: Prevention and management of nausea, vomiting, dizziness, or vertigo of motion sickness.

DOSAGE: *Adults:* 50–100 mg PO q4–6h, max 400 mg/d; 50 mg IM/IV prn. *Peds:* 5 mg/kg/24h PO or IV divided qid.

NOTES: Anticholinergic side effects.

Dimethyl Sulfoxide DMSO (Rimso 50)

COMMON USES: Interstitial cystitis.

DOSAGE: Intravesical, 50 mL, retain for 15 min; repeat q2 wk until relief.

Diphenhydramine (Benadryl, Others)

COMMON USES: Allergic reactions, motion sickness, potentiate narcotics, sedation, cough suppression, control of extrapyramidal reactions.

DOSAGE: *Adults:* 25–50 mg PO, IV or IM bid–tid. *Peds:* 5 mg/kg/24h PO or IM divided q6h (max 300 mg/d).

NOTES: Anticholinergic side effects including dry mouth, urinary retention; causes sedation; increase dosing interval in moderate to severe renal failure.

Diphenoxylate With Atropine (Lomotil) [C]

COMMON USES: Control diarrhea.

DOSAGE: *Adults:* Initially 5 mg PO tid or qid until under control, then 2.5–5.0 mg PO bid. *Peds* >2 y: 0.3–0.4 mg/kg/24h divided bid–qid.

NOTES: Atropine-type side effects.

Dirithromycin (Dynabac)

COMMON USES: Control of bronchitis, community-acquired pneumonia, and skin and skin structure infections.

DOSAGE: 500 mg PO qd for 7–14 d.

NOTES: Absorption is enhanced when taken with food.

Disopyramide (Norpace, NAPAmide)

COMMON USES: Suppression and prevention of premature ventricular contractions.

DOSAGE: *Adults:* 400–800 mg/d divided q6h for regular release products and q12h for SR products. *Peds:* <1 y: 10–30 mg/kg/24h PO; 1–4 y: 10–20 mg/kg/24h PO; 4–12 y: 10–15 mg/kg/24h PO; 12–18 y: 6–15 mg/kg/24h PO.

NOTES: Has anticholinergic side effects (urinary retention); negative inotropic properties may induce CHF; decrease dose in impaired hepatic function.

Dobutamine (Dobutrex)

COMMON USES: Short-term use in patients with cardiac decompensation secondary to depressed contractility.

DOSAGE: ***Adults*** and ***Peds:*** Continuous IV infusion of 2.5–15 mg/kg/min; rarely 40 mg/kg/min may be required; titrate according to response.
NOTES: Monitor electrocardiogram for increased heart rate, BP, and ectopic activity; monitor pulmonary wedge pressure and cardiac output.

Docusate Calcium (Surfak, others)

Docusate Potassium (Dialose)

Docusate Sodium (DOSS, Colace, Others)

COMMON USES: Constipation-prone patient; adjunct to painful anorectal conditions (hemorrhoids).
DOSAGE: ***Adults:*** 50–500 mg PO qd. ***Peds:*** Infants to 3 y: 10–40 mg/24h divided qd–qid; 3–6 y: 20–60 mg/24h divided qd–qid; 6–12 y: 40–120 mg/24h divided qd–qid.
NOTES: No significant side effects, no laxative action.

Dolasetron (Anzemet)

COMMON USES: Prevention of nausea and vomiting associated with chemotherapy.
DOSAGE: ***Adults*** and ***Peds:*** 1.8 mg/kg IV as a single dose. ***Adults:*** 100 mg PO as a single dose. ***Peds:*** 1.8 mg/kg PO up to 100 mg as a single dose.
NOTES: May cause prolongation of the QT interval.

Dopamine (Intropin, Dopastat)

COMMON USES: Short-term use in patients with cardiac decompensation secondary to decreased contractility; increases organ perfusion.
DOSAGE: ***Adults*** and ***Peds:*** 5 µg/kg/min by continuous infusion titrated by increments of 5 µg/kg/min to maximum of 50 mg/kg/min based on effect.
NOTES: Dose >10 µg/kg/min may decrease renal perfusion; monitor urinary output; monitor electrocardiogram for increased heart rate, BP, and ectopic activity; monitor pulmonary capillary wedge pressure (PCWP) and carbon monoxide if possible.

Doxazosin (Cardura)

COMMON USES: Control of HTN and benign prostatic hypertrophy (BPH).
DOSAGE: HTN: Initially 1 mg PO qd; may be increased to 16 mg PO qd. BPH: Initially 1 mg PO qd, may be increased to 8 mg PO qd.
NOTES: Doses >4 mg increase the likelihood of excessive postural hypotension; use qhs dosing to limit.

Doxepin (Sinequan, Adapin)

COMMON USES: Control depression or anxiety.
DOSAGE: 50–150 mg PO qd usually qhs but can be in divided doses.
NOTES: Anticholinergic, central nervous system, and cardiovascular side effects.

Doxycycline (Vibramycin)

COMMON USES: Broad-spectrum antibiotic including activity against *Rickettsia*, *Chlamydia*, and *M pneumoniae*.
DOSAGE: ***Adults:*** 100 mg PO q12h first day, then 100 mg PO qd or bid or 100 mg IV q12h. ***Peds*** >8 y: 5 mg/kg/24h PO up to a maximum of 200 mg/d, divided qd or bid.
NOTES: Useful for chronic bronchitis; tetracycline of choice for patients with renal impairment.

Dronabinol (Marinol) [C]

COMMON USES: Nausea and vomiting associated with cancer chemotherapy; appetite stimulation.
DOSAGE: ***Adults*** and ***Peds:*** Antiemetic: 5–15 mg/m^2/dose q4–6h prn. ***Adults:*** Appetite: 2.5 mg PO before lunch and supper.

NOTES: Principal psychoactive substance present in marijuana; many CNS side effects.

Droperidol (Inapsine)

COMMON USES: Nausea and vomiting, premedication for anesthesia.
DOSAGE: *Adults:* Nausea: 1.25–2.5 mg IV prn; Premedication: 2.5–10 mg IV. *Peds:* 0.1–0.15 mg/kg/dose.
NOTES: May cause drowsiness, moderate hypotension, and occasionally tachycardia.

Edrophonium (Tensilon)

COMMON USES: Diagnosis of myasthenia gravis; acute myasthenic crisis; curare antagonist; paroxysmal atrial tachycardia (PAT).
DOSAGE: *Adults:* Test for myasthenia gravis: 2 mg IV in 1 min; if tolerated, give 8 mg IV; a positive test is a brief increase in strength. PAT: 10 mg IV to a maximum of 40 mg. *Peds:* Test for myasthenia gravis: total dose 0.2 mg/kg. Give 0.04 mg/kg as a test dose. If no reaction occurs, give the remainder of the dose in 1-mg increments to a maximum of 10 mg.
NOTES: Can cause severe cholinergic effects; keep atropine available.

Efavirenz (Sustiva)

COMMON USES: HIV-1 infections in combination with ≥2 other agents.
DOSAGE: *Adults:* 600 mg qd at bedtime. *Peds:* See insert, based on body weight.

Enalapril (Vasotec)

COMMON USES: Management of HTN and CHF.
DOSAGE: *Adults:* 2.5–5 mg/d PO titrated by effect to 10–40 mg/d as 1–2 divided doses, or 1.25 mg IV q6h. *Peds:* 0.05–0.08 mg/kg/dose PO q12–24h.
NOTES: Initial dose can produce symptomatic hypotension, especially with concomitant diuretics; discontinue diuretic for 2–3 d before initiation if possible; monitor closely for increases in serum potassium; may cause a nonproductive cough.

Enoxaparin (Lovenox)

COMMON USES: Prevention of DVT.
DOSAGE: 30 mg SC twice daily.
NOTES: Does not significantly affect bleeding time, platelet function, PT or aPTT.

Entacapone (Comtan)

COMMON USES: Management of Parkinson's disease.
DOSAGE: 200 mg administered concurrently with each levodopa/carbidopa dose to a maximum of 8 times/d.

Ephedrine

COMMON USES: Acute bronchospasm, nasal congestion, hypotension, narcolepsy, enuresis, myasthenia gravis.
DOSAGE: *Adults:* 25–50 mg IM/SC or 5–25 mg/dose slow IV every 10 min to maximum of 150 mg/d or 25–50 mg PO q3–4h prn. *Peds:* 0.2–0.3 mg/kg/dose IM or IV q4–6h prn.

Epinephrine (Adrenalin, Sus-Phrine, Others)

COMMON USES: Cardiac arrest, anaphylactic reactions, acute asthma.
DOSAGE: *Adults:* Emergency cardiac care: 0.5–1.0 mg (5–10 mL of 1:10,000) IV every 5 min to response. Anaphylaxis: 0.3–0.5 mL of 1:1000 dilution SC; may repeat q10–15 min to maximum of 1 mg/dose and 5 mg/d. Asthma: 0.3–0.5 mL of 1:1000 dilution SC repeated at 20-min to 4-h intervals or 1 inhalation (metered dose) repeated in 1–2 min or suspension 0.1–0.3 mL SC for extended effect. *Peds:* Emergency cardiac care: 0.1 mL/kg of 1:10,000 dilution IV q3–5 min to response.

NOTES: Sus-Phrine offers sustained action; in acute cardiac settings can be given via endotracheal tube if a central line is not available.

Epoetin Alfa (Epogen, Procrit)

COMMON USES: Management of anemia associated with chronic renal failure, zidovudine therapy in HIV-infected patients, and patients receiving cancer chemotherapy; decreased transfusions associated with surgery.

DOSAGE: *Adults* and *Peds:* 50–150 U/kg 3 times weekly; adjust the dose every 4–6 wk as needed. Surgery: 300 U/kg/d for 10 d before surgery.

NOTES: May cause HTN, headache, tachycardia, nausea, and vomiting; store in refrigerator.

Epoprostenol (Flolan)

COMMON USES: Management of pulmonary HTN.

DOSAGE: 4 ng/kg/min IV continuous infusion; make adjustments based on clinical status and package insert guidelines.

NOTES: Availability through a pharmacy benefit manager (PBM).

Eprosartan (Teveten)

COMMON USES: Management of HTN.

DOSAGE: 400–800 mg daily as single dose or twice daily.

NOTES: Avoid use during pregnancy.

Eptifibatide (Integrilin)

COMMON USES: Management of acute coronary syndrome.

DOSAGE: 180 mg/kg IV bolus, followed by 2 mg/kg/min continuous infusion.

Ertapenem (Invanz)

COMMON USES: Management of acute pelvic infections, community-acquired pneumonia, intra-abdominal infections, complicated skin and urinary tract infections.

DOSAGE: 1 g IV once a day.

Erythromycin (E-Mycin, Ilosone, Erythrocin, ERYC, Others)

COMMON USES: Infections caused by group A streptococci (*S pyogenes),* alphahemolytic streptococci, and *N gonorrhoeae* infections in penicillin-allergic patients, *S pneumoniae, M pneumoniae,* and *Legionella.*

DOSAGE: *Adults:* 250–500 mg PO qid or 500 mg to 1 g IV qid. *Peds:* 30–50 mg/kg/24h PO or IV divided q6h, to a maximum of 2 g/d.

NOTES: Frequent mild GI disturbances; estolate salt is associated with cholestatic jaundice; erythromycin base not well absorbed from the GI tract; some forms such as ERYC are better tolerated with respect to GI irritation; lactobionate salt contains benzyl alcohol so use with caution in neonates; base formulation not absorbed and used as part of the "Nichols-Condon Bowel Prep."

Escitalopram (Lexapro)

COMMON USES: Management of depression and generalized anxiety disorders.

DOSAGE: 10–20 mg/d.

Esmolol (Brevibloc)

COMMON USES: Supraventricular tachycardia, noncompensatory sinus tachycardia.

DOSAGE: Initial 500 mg/kg load over 1 min, then 50 mg/kg/min for 4 min; if inadequate response, repeat loading dose and follow with maintenance infusion of 100 mg/kg/min for 4 min; continue titration process by repeating loading dose followed by incremental increases in the maintenance dose of 50 mg/kg/min for 4 min until desired heart rate is reached or a decrease in BP occurs; average dose is 100 mg/kg/min.

NOTES: Monitor closely for hypotension; decreasing or discontinuing infusion will reverse hypotension in approximately 30 min.

Estrogen, Conjugated (Premarin)

COMMON USES: Moderate to severe vasomotor symptoms associated with menopause; atrophic vaginitis; palliative therapy of advanced prostatic carcinoma; prevention of estrogen deficiency induced osteoporosis.
DOSAGE: 0.3–1.25 mg/d PO cyclically; prostatic carcinoma requires 1.25–2.5 mg PO tid.
NOTES: Do not use in pregnancy; associated with an increased risk of endometrial carcinoma, gallbladder disease, thromboembolism, and possibly breast cancer; generic products are not equivalent.

Ethacrynic Acid (Edecrin)

COMMON USES: Edema, CHF, ascites, any time rapid diuresis is desired.
DOSAGE: *Adults:* 50–200 mg PO qd or 50 mg IV prn. *Peds:* 1 mg/kg/dose IV. Repeated doses are not recommended.
NOTES: Contraindicated in anuria; many severe side effects. Only loop diuretic without a sulfonamide component.

Ethambutol (Myambutol)

COMMON USES: Pulmonary tuberculosis and other mycobacterial infections.
DOSAGE: *Adults* and *Peds* >12 y: 15–25 mg/kg PO daily as single dose.
NOTES: May cause vision changes and GI upset.

Ethosuximide (Zarontin)

COMMON USES: Absence seizures.
DOSAGE: *Adults:* 500 mg qd PO initially; increase by 250 mg/d every 4–7 d as needed. *Peds:* 20–40 mg/kg/24h PO qd to a maximum of 1500 mg/d.
NOTES: Blood dyscrasias, CNS and GI side effects may occur; use caution in patients with renal or hepatic impairment. See drug levels on page 460.

Etidronate (Didronel)

COMMON USES: Hypercalcemia of malignancy, hypertrophic ossification associated with spinal cord injury, Paget's disease, postmenopausal osteoporosis.
DOSAGE: Hypercalcemia: 7.5 mg/kg IV in NS over 2 h daily for 3 d, then 20 mg/kg/d PO for 1 mo. Ossification: 20 mg/kg/d for 2 wk, then 10 mg/kg/d for 10 wk.

Etodolac (Lodine)

COMMON USES: Control of arthritis and pain.
DOSAGE: 200–400 mg PO bid–qid.

Factor IX Complex (AlphaNine, Mononine)

COMMON USES: Rapid reversal of increased INR with severe bleeding secondary to warfarin use.
DOSAGE: 25–50 U/kg infused over 10 min.
NOTES: Vitamin K should be given concomitantly.

Famciclovir (Famvir)

COMMON USES: Management of acute herpes zoster (shingles) and genital herpes infections.
DOSAGE: Zoster: 500 mg PO q8h. Simplex: 125–250 mg PO bid.

Famotidine (Pepcid)

COMMON USES: Short-term therapy of active duodenal ulcer and benign gastric ulcer; maintenance therapy for duodenal ulcer, hypersecretory conditions, GERD, and heartburn.
DOSAGE: *Adults:* Ulcer: 20–40 mg PO hs or 20 mg IV q12h. Hypersecretory: 20–160 mg PO q6h. GERD: 20 mg PO bid; maintenance 20 mg PO hs. Heartburn: 10 mg PO prn heartburn. *Peds:* 1–2 mg/kg/d.
NOTES: Decrease dose in severe renal insufficiency.

Felodipine (Plendil)

COMMON USES: Management of HTN.
DOSAGE: 5–20 mg PO qd.
NOTES: Closely monitor BP in elderly patients and patients with impaired hepatic function; doses >10 mg should not be used in these patients.

Fenoldopam (Corlopam)

COMMON USES: Management of hypertensive emergency.
DOSAGE: Initial dose 0.03–0.1 mg/kg/min IV continuous infusion, titrate to effect every 15 min with 0.05–0.1 mg/kg/min increments, max 1.6 mg/kg/min.
NOTES: Avoid concurrent use with beta-blockers.

Fenoprofen (Nalfon)

COMMON USES: Management of arthritis and pain.
DOSAGE: 200–600 mg q4–8h, to a maximum of 3200 mg/d.

Fentanyl (Sublimaze) [C]

COMMON USES: Short-acting analgesic used in conjunction with anesthesia.
DOSAGE: *Adults* and *Peds:* 0.025–0.15 mg/kg IV/IM titrated to effect.
NOTES: Causes significant sedation.

Fentanyl Transdermal System (Duragesic) [C]

COMMON USES: Management of chronic pain.
DOSAGE: Apply patch to upper torso every 72 h. Dose is calculated from the narcotic requirements for the previous 24 h. Transdermal patches deliver 25, 50, 75, and 100 mg/h.
NOTES: Fentanyl 0.1 mg is equivalent to morphine 10 mg IM.

Fentanyl Transmucosal System (Actiq, Fentanyl Oralet) [C]

COMMON USES: Induction of anesthesia and breakthrough cancer pain.
DOSAGE: *Adults* and *Peds:* Anesthesia: 5–15 mg/kg. Pain: 200, 300, or 400 mg consumed over 15 min, titrate to appropriate effect.

Ferric Sodium Gluconate (Ferrlecit)

COMMON USES: Iron deficiency anemia; iron supplementation.
DOSAGE: 125 mg in NS 100 mL over 1 h.
NOTES: Initial test dose 2 mL (25 mg) in NS 50 mL over 1 h.

Ferrous Sulfate

COMMON USES: Iron deficiency anemia; iron supplementation.
DOSAGE: *Adults:* 100–200 mg/d of elemental iron divided tid–qid. *Peds:* 1–2 mg/kg/24h divided qd–bid.
NOTES: May turn stools and urine dark; can cause GI upset, constipation; vitamin C taken with ferrous sulfate increases absorption of iron especially in patients with atrophic gastritis.

Fexofenadine (Allegra)

COMMON USES: Relief of allergic rhinitis.
DOSAGE: *Adults* and *Peds >12 y:* 60 mg twice daily.

Filgrastim [G-CSF] (Neupogen)

COMMON USES: To decrease the incidence of infection in febrile neutropenic patients and control of chronic neutropenia.
DOSAGE: *Adults* and *Peds:* 5 mg/kg/d SC or IV as a single daily dose.
NOTES: May cause bone pain. Discontinue therapy when absolute neutrophil count (ANC) >10,000 cells/µl.

Finasteride (Proscar, Propecia)

COMMON USES: Treatment of BPH and androgenetic alopecia.
DOSAGE: BPH (Proscar): 5 mg PO qd. Alopecia (Propecia): 1 mg PO qd.

NOTES: Will decrease prostate-specific antigen levels; may take 3–6 mo to see effect on urinary symptoms.

Flecainide (Tambocor)

COMMON USES: Life-threatening ventricular arrhythmias.

DOSAGE: 100 mg PO q12h; increase in increments of 50 mg q12h every 4 d to maximum of 400 mg/d.

NOTES: May cause new or worsened arrhythmias; therapy should be initiated in the hospital; may dose q8h if patient is intolerant or uncontrolled at q12h interval; drug interactions with propranolol, digoxin, verapamil, and disopyramide; may cause CHF.

Fluconazole (Diflucan)

COMMON USES: Oropharyngeal and esophageal candidiasis; cryptococcal meningitis; *Candida* infections of the lungs, peritoneum, and urinary tract; prevention of candidiasis in bone marrow transplant patients on chemotherapy or radiation; and candidal vaginitis.

DOSAGE: *Adults:* 100–400 mg PO or IV qd. Vaginitis: 150 mg PO as a single dose. *Peds:* 3–6 mg/kg PO or IV qd.

NOTES: Adjust dose in renal insufficiency; PO dosing produces the same blood levels as IV dosing, so the PO route should be used whenever possible.

Fludrocortisone Acetate (Florinef)

COMMON USES: Partial therapy for adrenocortical insufficiency.

DOSAGE: *Adults* and *Peds >1 y:* 0.05–0.1 mg PO qd. Infants: 0.1–0.2 mg PO qd.

NOTES: For adrenal insufficiency, must be used in conjunction with a glucocorticoid supplement; dosing changes based on plasma renin activity.

Flumazenil (Romazicon)

COMMON USES: For complete or partial reversal of the sedative effects of benzodiazepines.

DOSAGE: 0.2 mg IV over 15 s, dose may be repeated if the desired level of consciousness is not obtained to a maximum dose of 1 mg.

Flunisolide (AeroBid)

COMMON USES: Control of bronchial asthma in patients requiring chronic corticosteroid therapy.

DOSAGE: *Adults:* 2–4 inhalations bid. *Peds:* 2 inhalations bid.

NOTES: May cause oral candidiasis; not for acute asthma attack.

Fluoxetine (Prozac, Sarafem)

COMMON USES: Management of depression, obsessive-compulsive disorders, and bulimia, premenstrual dysphoric disorder (PMDD).

DOSAGE: Initially, 20 mg PO qd; titrate to a maximum of 80 mg/24h; doses >20 mg/d should be divided. Bulimia: 60 mg once daily in the morning.

NOTES: May cause nausea, nervousness, and weight loss.

Fluphenazine (Prolixin, Permitil)

COMMON USES: Psychotic disorders.

DOSAGE: 0.5–10 mg/d in divided doses PO q6–8h; average maintenance 5.0 mg/d or 1.25 mg IM initially, then 2.5–10 mg/d in divided doses q6–8h prn.

NOTES: Decrease dose in elderly patients; monitor liver functions; may cause drowsiness; do not administer concentrate with caffeine, tannic acid, or pectin-containing products.

Flurazepam (Dalmane) [C]

COMMON USES: Insomnia.

DOSAGE: *Adults* and *Peds >15 y:* 15–30 mg PO qhs prn.

NOTES: Decrease dose in elderly patients.

Flurbiprofen (Ansaid)

COMMON USES: Management of arthritis.
DOSAGE: 50–100 mg bid–qid to 300 mg/d max.

Fluticasone Oral (Flovent, Flovent Rotadisk)

COMMON USES: Long-term management of asthma.
DOSAGE: *Adults & adolescents:* 2–4 puffs bid. *Peds* 4–11 y: 50 mg twice daily.
NOTES: Counsel patients carefully on use of device multidose inhaler 44, 110, or 220 mg/activation; Rotadisk dry powder 50, 100, and 250 mg/activation; risk of thrush.

Folic Acid

COMMON USES: Macrocytic anemia.
DOSAGE: *Adults:* Supplement: 0.4 mg PO qd; pregnancy: 0.8 mg PO qd; folate deficiency: 1.0 mg PO qd–tid. *Peds:* Supplement: 0.04–0.4 mg/24h PO, IM, IV, or SC; folate deficiency: 0.5–1.0 mg/24h PO, IM, IV, or SC

Fomvirsen (Vitravene)

COMMON USES: CMV retinitis in AIDS patients who do not respond to other therapies.
DOSAGE: 6.6 mg intraocular injection every other week for 2 wk followed by 1 injection once every 4 wk.

Fondaparinux (Arixtra)

COMMON USES: Prevention of DVT after hip or knee replacement surgery.
DOSAGE: 2.5 mg SC once daily.
NOTES: Does not significantly affect bleeding time, platelet function, PT, or aPTT.

Foscarnet (Foscavir)

COMMON USES: Management of CMG; acyclovir-resistant herpes infections.
DOSAGE: Induction: 60 mg/kg IV q8h for 14–21 d. Maintenance: 90–120 mg/kg IV qd (Monday–Friday).
NOTES: Dose must be adjusted for renal function; nephrotoxic; monitor ionized calcium closely (causes electrolyte abnormalities); administer through a central venous catheter.

Fosfomycin (Monurol)

COMMON USES: Uncomplicated UTI in women.
DOSAGE: 3 g in water (1 dose).

Fosinopril (Monopril)

COMMON USES: Control HTN.
DOSAGE: Initially, 10 mg PO qd; may be increased to a maximum of 80 mg/d PO divided qd–bid.
NOTES: Decrease dose in elderly patients, unnecessary to adjust dose for renal insufficiency, may cause a nonproductive cough and dizziness.

Fosphenytoin (Cerebyx)

COMMON USES: Management of status epilepticus.
DOSAGE: Loading 15–20 mg phenytoin equivalents/kg, maintenance 4–6 mg phenytoin equivalents/kg/d.
NOTES: Dosed as phenytoin equivalents; administer at <150 mg phenytoin equivalents/min to prevent hypotension.

Furosemide (Lasix)

COMMON USES: Edema, HTN, CHF.
DOSAGE: *Adults:* 20–80 mg PO or IV qd or bid. *Peds:* 1 mg/kg/dose IV q6–12h; 2 mg/kg/dose PO q12h–24h.

NOTES: Monitor for hypokalemia; use with caution in hepatic disease; large doses of the IV form may cause ototoxicity.

Gabapentin (Neurontin)

COMMON USES: Adjunctive therapy in the management of partial seizures, chronic pain.

DOSAGE: 900–1800 mg/d PO in 3 divided doses.

NOTES: It is not necessary to monitor serum gabapentin levels.

Gallium Nitrate (Ganite)

COMMON USES: Management of hypercalcemia of malignancy.

DOSAGE: 100–200 mg/m^2/d for 5 d.

NOTES: Can cause renal insufficiency; 1% acute optic neuritis.

Ganciclovir (Cytovene, Vitrasert)

COMMON USES: Management and prevention of CMV retinitis and prevention of CMV disease in transplant recipients.

DOSAGE: *Adults* and *Peds:* IV: 5 mg/kg IV q12h for 14–21 d, then maintenance with 5 mg/kg IV qd for 7 d/wk or 6 mg/kg IV qd for 5 d/wk. *Adults:* PO: After induction, 1000 mg PO tid. Prevention: 1000 mg PO tid.

NOTES: Not a cure for CMV; granulocytopenia and thrombocytopenia are the major toxicities; injection should be handled with appropriate precautions; take capsules with food.

Gatifloxacin (Tequin)

COMMON USES: Management of acute exacerbation of chronic bronchitis, sinusitis, community-acquired pneumonia, UTIs.

DOSAGE: 400 mg PO or IV once daily

NOTES: Avoid use with antacids; do NOT use in children <18 y or in pregnant or lactating women; reliable activity against *S pneumoniae*.

Gentamicin (Garamycin)

COMMON USES: Serious infections caused by susceptible *Pseudomonas*, *Proteus*, *E coli*, *Klebsiella*, *Enterobacter*, and *Serratia* and for initial therapy of gram-negative sepsis.

DOSAGE: *Adults:* 3–5 mg/kg/24h IV divided q8–24h. *Peds:* Infants >7 d: 2.5 mg/kg/dose IV q12–24h; children: 2.5 mg/kg/d IV q8h. See Table IX–1, page 459.

NOTES: Nephrotoxic and ototoxic; decrease dose with renal insufficiency; monitor creatinine clearance and serum concentration for dosing adjustments; see Table IX–2, page 460.

Glimepiride (Amaryl)

COMMON USES: Control of non–insulin-dependent diabetes mellitus.

DOSAGE: 1–4 mg once daily.

Glipizide (Glucotrol)

COMMON USES: Control of non–insulin-dependent diabetes mellitus.

DOSAGE: 5–15 mg qd–bid.

Glucagon

COMMON USES: Management of severe hypoglycemia in diabetic patients with sufficient liver glycogen stores.

DOSAGE: *Adults:* 0.5–1.0 mg SC, IM, or IV repeated after 20 min as needed. *Peds:* Neonates: 0.3 mg/kg/dose SC, IM, or IV q4h prn; children: 0.03–0.1 mg/kg/dose SC, IM or IV repeated after 20 min prn.

NOTES: Administration of glucose IV is necessary; ineffective in states of starvation, adrenal insufficiency, or chronic hypoglycemia. Used as antidote for beta-blocker toxicity.

Glyburide (DiaBeta, Micronase)

COMMON USES: Management of non–insulin-dependent diabetes mellitus.
DOSAGE: Non-micronized: 1.25–10 mg qd–bid. Micronized: 1.5–6 mg qd–bid.

Glycerin Suppository

COMMON USES: Constipation.
DOSAGE: *Adults:* 1 adult suppository PR, prn. *Peds:* 1 infant suppository PR, qd–bid prn.

Granisetron (Kytril)

COMMON USES: Prevention of nausea and vomiting associated with emetogenic cancer therapy.
DOSAGE: *Adults* and *Peds:* 10 mg/kg IV 30 min before initiation of chemotherapy. *Adults:* 1 mg PO 1 h before chemotherapy, then q12 h.

Guaifenesin (Robitussin, Others)

COMMON USES: Symptomatic relief of dry nonproductive cough; expectorant.
DOSAGE: *Adults:* 200–400 mg (10–20 mL) PO q4h. *Peds:* 2–5 y: 50–100 mg (2.5–5 mL) PO q4h; 6–11 y: 100–200 mg (5–10 mL) PO q4h.

Guaifenesin & Codeine (Robitussin AC, Brontex, others) [C]

COMMON USES: Antitussive with expectorant.
DOSAGE: *Adults:* 10 mL or 1 tab PO q6–8h. *Peds:* 2–6 y: codein 1–1.5 mg/kg/d divided dose q4–6h. 6–12 y: 5 mL q4h. >12 y: 10 mL q4h, max 60 mL/24h.
NOTES: Brontex tab contains codeine 10 mg; Brontex liquid codeine 2.5 mg per 5 mL; others codeine 10 mg per 5 mL.

Guaifenesin & Dextromethorphan (Many OTC Brands)

COMMON USES: Cough due to upper respiratory irritation.
DOSAGE: *Adults* and *Peds:* >12 y: 10 mL PO q6h. 2–6 y: 2.5 mL q6–8h, 10 mL/d max. 6–12 y: 5 mL q6–8h, 20 mL/d max.

Haloperidol (Haldol)

COMMON USES: Management of psychotic disorders; schizophrenia; agitation; Tourette's disorders; hyperactivity in children.
DOSAGE: *Adults:* Moderate symptoms: 0.5–2.0 mg PO bid–tid. Severe symptoms or agitation: 3–5 mg PO bid–tid or 1–5 mg IM q4h prn (max 100 mg/d). *Peds:* 3–6 y: 0.01–0.03 mg/kg/24h PO qd; 6–12 y: initially, 0.5–1.5 mg/24h PO, increase by 0.5 mg/24h to maintenance of 2–4 mg/24h (0.05–0.1 mg/kg/24h) or 1–3 mg/dose IM q4–8h to 0.1 mg/kg/24h max. For Tourette's, up to 15 mg/24h PO.
NOTES: Can cause extrapyramidal symptoms, hypotension; decrease dose in elderly patients.

Heparin Sodium

COMMON USES: Control and prevention of venous thrombosis and pulmonary emboli, atrial fibrillation with emboli formation, acute arterial occlusion.
DOSAGE: *Adults:* Prophylaxis: 3000–5000 U SC q8–12h. Control of thrombosis: Loading dose 50–75 U/kg IV, then 10–20 U/kg IV qh (adjust based on PTT). *Peds:* Infants: Load 50 U/kg IV bolus, then 20 U/kg/h IV infusion. Children: Load 50 U/kg IV, then 15–25 U/kg/h continuous infusion or 100 U/kg/dose q4h IV intermittent bolus.
NOTES: Follow PTT, thrombin time, or activated clotting time to assess effectiveness; heparin has little effect on the PT; with proper dose PTT is about 1 to 1.5 times the control; can cause thrombocytopenia; follow platelet counts.

Hepatitis A Vaccine (Havrix)

COMMON USES: High-risk exposure to hepatitis A (travelers, health care workers, etc).
DOSAGE: *Adults:* 1 mL IM, booster 6–12 mo. *Peds:* 0.5 mL IM on days 1 and 30, booster 6–12 mo.

Hepatitis B Immune Globulin (HyperHep, H-BIG)

COMMON USES: Exposure to materials positive for hepatitis B immune globulin: blood, plasma, or serum (accidental needle-stick, mucous membrane contact, oral ingestion).
DOSAGE: *Adults* and *Peds:* 0.06 mL/kg IM,5 mL max; within 24 h of needle-stick or percutaneous exposure; within 14 d of sexual contact; repeat at 1 and 6 mo after exposure.
NOTES: Administered in gluteal or deltoid muscle; if exposure continues, should receive hepatitis B vaccine.

Hepatitis B Vaccine (Engerix–B, Recombivax HB)

COMMON USES: Prevention of type B hepatitis in high-risk individuals.
DOSAGE: *Adults:* 3 IM doses of 1 mL each, the first 2 given 1 mo apart, the third 6 mo after the first. *Peds:* 0.5 mL IM dose given on the same schedule as adults.
NOTES: IM injections for adults and older children to be administered in the deltoid; injections in other children to be administered in anterolateral thigh; may cause fever, injection site soreness; derived from recombinant DNA technology.

Hetastarch (Hespan)

COMMON USES: Plasma volume expansion as an adjunct in management of shock due to hemorrhage, surgery, burns, and other trauma.
DOSAGE: 500–1000 mL (do not exceed 1500 mL/d) IV at a rate not to exceed 20 mL/kg/h.
NOTES: Not a substitute for blood or plasma; contraindicated in patients with severe bleeding disorders, severe CHF, or renal failure with oliguria or anuria.

Hydralazine (Apresoline)

COMMON USES: Moderate to severe HTN.
DOSAGE: *Adults:* 10 mg PO qid, increase to 25 mg qid to 300 mg/d max. *Peds:* 0.75–3 mg/kg/24h PO divided q12–6h.
NOTES: Caution with impaired hepatic function, coronary artery disease; compensatory sinus tachycardia can be eliminated with the addition of propranolol; chronically high doses can cause SLE-like syndrome; SVT can occur after IM administration.

Hydrochlorothiazide (HydroDIURIL, Esidrix, Others)

COMMON USES: Edema, HTN, CHF.
DOSAGE: *Adults:* 25–100 mg PO qd in single or divided doses. *Peds:* 2–3 mg/kg/24h PO divided bid.
NOTES: Hypokalemia is frequent; hyperglycemia, hyperuricemia, hyperlipidemia, and hyponatremia are common side effects.

Hydrochlorothiazide & Amiloride (Moduretic)

COMMON USES: HTN, adjunctive therapy for CHF.
DOSAGE: 1–2 tablets PO qd.
NOTES: Should not be given to patients with diabetes or renal failure.

Hydrochlorothiazide & Spironolactone (Aldactazide)

COMMON USES: Edema (CHF, cirrhosis), HTN.
DOSAGE: 1–8 tablets (25–200 mg each component per day) 1–2 divided doses.

Hydrochlorothiazide & Triamterene (Dyazide, Maxzide)

COMMON USES: Edema, HTN.

DOSAGE: Dyazide: 1–2 capsules PO qd–bid. Maxzide: 1 tablet PO qd.
NOTES: Can cause hyperkalemia and hypokalemia; follow serum potassium.

Hydrocortisone

See "Steroids," page 522.

Hydrocodone & Acetaminophen (Lorcet, Vicodin, Others) [C]

COMMON USES: Moderate to severe pain; hydrocodone has antitussive properties.
DOSAGE: 1–2 PO q4–6h prn.
NOTES: Many different combinations; specify hydrocodone/acetaminophen dose: 2.5/500, 5/400, 5/500, 7.5/400, 10/400, 7.5/500, 7.5/650, 7.5/750, 10/325, 10/400, 10/500, 10/650; Elixir and solution: hydrocodone 2,5 mg/acetaminophen 167 mg per 5 mL.

Hydrocodone & Aspirin (Lortab ASA, Others) [C]

COMMON USES: Moderate to severe pain.
DOSAGE: 1–2 PO q4–6h prn.
NOTES: Hydrocodone 5 mg/aspirin 500 mg per tablet.

Hydrocodone & Guaifenesin (Hycotuss expectorant, Others) [C]

COMMON USES: Nonproductive cough associated with respiratory infection.
DOSAGE: *Adults* and *Peds:* >12 y: 5 mL q4h, pc and hs; <2 y: 0.3 mg/kg/d divided qid; 2–12 y: 2.5 mL q4h pc and hs.

Hydrocodone & Homatropine (Hycodan, Others) [C]

COMMON USES: Relief of cough.
DOSAGE: *Adults:* 5–10 mg q4–6h. *Peds:* 0.6 mg/kg/d divided tid–qid.
NOTES: Dose based on hydrocodone; syrup hydrocodone 5 mg/5 mL; tablet hydrocodone 5 mg.

Hydrocodone & Ibuprofen (Vicoprofen) [C]

COMMON USES: Moderate to severe pain (<10 d).
DOSAGE: 1–2 tablets q4–6h prn.
NOTES: Hydrocodone 7.5 mg/ibuprofen 200 mg/tablet.

Hydrocodone & Pseudoephedrine (Entuss-D, Histussin-D, Others) [C]

COMMON USES: Cough and nasal congestion.
DOSAGE: 5 mL qid, prn
NOTES: Hydrocodone 5 mg/5 mL

Hydrocodone, Chlorpheniramine, Phenylephrine, Acetaminophen, & Caffeine (Hycomine) [C]

COMMON USES: Cough and symptoms of upper respiratory infections.
DOSAGE: 1 PO, q4h, prn.
NOTES: Hydrocodone 5 mg/tab.

Hydromorphone (Dilaudid) [C]

COMMON USES: Moderate to severe pain.
DOSAGE: 1–4 mg PO, IM, IV, SC or PR q4–6h prn.
NOTES: 1.5 mg IM equivalent to morphine 10 mg IM.

Hydroxyzine (Atarax, Vistaril)

COMMON USES: Anxiety, tension, sedation, itching.
DOSAGE: *Adults:* Anxiety or sedation: 50–100 mg PO or IM qid or prn (max 600 mg/d); itching: 25–50 mg PO or IM tid–qid. *Peds:* 0.6–1.0 mg/kg/24h PO or IM q6h.

NOTES: Useful in potentiating the effects of narcotics; not for IV use; drowsiness, anticholinergic effects are common.

Hyoscyamine (Anaspaz, Cystospaz, Levsin, Others)

COMMON USES: Spasm associated with GI and bladder disorders.
DOSAGE: *Adults:* 0.125–0.25 mg (1–2 tabs) SL 3–4 times a day, pc and hs; 1 capsule q12h (SR [Cystospaz-M, Levsinex]).

Hyoscyamine, Atropine, Scopolamine, & Phenobarbital (Donnatal, Others)

COMMON USES: Irritable bowel, spastic colitis, peptic ulcer, spastic bladder.
DOSAGE: 0.125–0.25 mg (1–2 tabs) 3–4 times/d, 1 capsule q12h (SR), 5–10 mL elixir 3–4 times/d or q8h.

Ibuprofen (Motrin, Rufen, Advil, Others)

COMMON USES: Control of inflammatory conditions (rheumatoid arthritis, others) arthritis and pain, fever, gout, dysmenorrhea.
DOSAGE: *Adults:* pain, fever, dysmenorrhea 200–400 mg PO q4–6h, max 1.2 g/d; inflammatory conditions 400–800 mg ID–qid, max 3.2 g/d. *Peds:* 4–10 mg/kg/dose in 3–4 divided doses; rheumatoid arthritis 30–50 mg/kg/d divided qid, max 2.4 g/d.

Ibutilide (Covert)

COMMON USES: Rapid conversion of atrial fibrillation or flutter.
DOSAGE: <60 kg: 0.01 mg/kg (max 1 mg); >60 kg: 1 mg IV over 10 min. May be repeated once if needed 10 min later.
NOTES: Do not administer class I or III antiarrhythmics concurrently or within 4 h of ibutilide infusion.

Imipenem/Cilastatin (Primaxin)

COMMON USES: Serious infections caused by a wide variety of susceptible bacteria; multiresistant infections, inactive against *S aureus,* group A and B streptococci, and others; empiric therapy of gram-negative sepsis in immunocompromised host.
DOSAGE: *Adults:* 250–500 mg (Imipenem) IV q6h. *Peds:* <3 y: 100 mg/kg/24h IV divided q6h; >3 y: 60 mg/kg/24h IV divided q6h.
NOTES: Seizures may occur if drug accumulates; adjust dose for renal insufficiency to avoid drug accumulation if creatinine clearance <70 mL/min.

Imipramine (Tofranil)

COMMON USES: Depression, enuresis.
DOSAGE: *Adults:* Hospitalized for severe depression: Start at 100 mg/24h PO or IV in divided doses, increase over several weeks to 250–300 mg/24h. Outpatient: 50–150 mg PO qhs not to exceed 200 mg/24h. *Peds:* Antidepressant: 1.5–5.0 mg/kg/24h divided tid; enuresis: 10–25 mg PO qhs; increase by 10–25 mg at 1- to 2-wk intervals, treat for 2–3 mo, then taper.
NOTES: Do not use with MAO inhibitors; less sedation than amitriptyline.

Immune Globulin, Intravenous (Gamimune N, Sandoglobulin, Gammar IV)

COMMON USES: IgG antibody deficiency diseases (congenital agammaglobulinemia, common variable hypogammaglobulinemia); idiopathic thrombocytopenic purpura.
DOSAGE: *Adults* and *Peds:* Immunodeficiency: 100–200 mg/kg IV monthly rate of 0.01–0.04 mL/kg/min to 400 mg/kg/dose max. Idiopathic thrombocytopenic purpura: 400 mg/kg/dose IV qd for 5 d. Bone marrow transplantation: 500 mg/kg/wk.
NOTES: Adverse effects associated mostly with rate of infusion.

Indapamide (Lozol)

COMMON USES: HTN and CHF.

DOSAGE: 2.5–5.0 mg PO qd.
NOTES: Doses >5 mg do not have additional effects on lowering BP.

Indomethacin (Indocin)

COMMON USES: Arthritis and closure of the ductus arteriosus.
DOSAGE: *Adults:* 25–50 mg PO bid-tid, 200 mg/d max. Infants: 0.2–0.25 mg/kg/dose IV; may be repeated in 12–24 h for up to 3 doses.
NOTES: Monitor renal function.

Infliximab (Remicade)

COMMON USES: Management of moderate to severe Crohn's disease.
DOSAGE: 5 mg/kg IV infusion, subsequent doses 2 and 6 wk after initial infusion.
NOTES: May cause hypersensitivity reaction, made up of human constant and murine variable regions.

Insulins

COMMON USES: Diabetes mellitus that cannot be controlled by diet and/or oral hypoglycemic agents.
DOSAGE: Based on serum glucose levels; usually given SC, can also be given IV or IM (only regular insulin can be given IV). See Table IX–5. General guidelines: 0.5–1U/kg/d, ⅔ dose before breakfast, ⅓ before supper; adjust based on blood sugars over several days. Regular or rapid insulin should be dosed q4–6h, NPH or intermediate q8–12h. Ketoacidosis: hydrate patient well with NS, regular insulin 10 U IV followed by infusion 0.1 U/kg/h; optimum serum glucose decrease: 50–100 mg/dL/h.

TABLE IX–5. COMPARISON OF INSULINS

Type of Insulin	Onset (h)	Peak (h)	Duration (h)
Ultra Rapid			
Humalog (Lispro)	Immediate	0.5–1.5	3–5
Novolog			
(Insulin aspart)	Immediate	0.5–1.5	3–5
Rapid			
Regular Iletin II	0.25–0.5	2.0–4.0	5–7
Humulin R	0.5	2.0–4.0	6–8
Novolin R	0.5	2.5–5.0	5–8
Velosulin	0.5	2.0–5.0	6–8
Intermediate			
NPH Iletin II	1.0–2.0	6–12	18–24
Lente Iletin II	1.0–2.0	6–12	18–24
Humulin N	1.0–2.0	6–12	14–24
Novulin L	2.5–5.0	7–15	18–24
Novulin 70/30	0.5	7–12	24
Prolonged			
Ultralente	4.0–6.0	14–24	28–36
Humulin U	4.0–6.0	8–20	24–28
Lantus (Insulin glargine)	4.0–6.0	No peak	24
Combination Insulins			
Humalog Mix (Lispro protamine/Lispro)	0.25–0.5	1–4	24

NOTES: The highly purified insulins provide an increase in free insulin; monitor these patients closely for several weeks when changing doses; most standard insulins 100 U/mL.

Interferon Alpha (Roferon-A, Intron A)

COMMON USES: Hairy cell leukemia, Kaposi's sarcoma, multiple myeloma, chronic myelogenous leukemia, renal cell carcinoma, bladder cancer, melanoma, and chronic hepatitis C.

DOSAGE: Alfa-2a (Roferon): 3 million IU daily for 16–24 wk SQ or IM. Alfa-2b (Intron): 2 million IU/m^2 IM or SQ 3 times/wk for 2–6 mo; intravesical 50–100 million IU in NS 50 mL weekly $\times$ 6.

NOTES: Systemic use may cause flu-like symptoms; fatigue is common; anorexia occurs in 20–30% of patients; neurotoxicity may occur at large doses; neutralizing antibodies can occur in up to 40% of patients receiving prolonged systemic therapy.

Interferon Alpha & Ribavirin (Roferon-A, Intron A)

COMMON USES: Chronic hepatitis C.

DOSAGE: Intron A: 3 million IU SQ 3 times with rebtrol 1000–1200 mg divided PO bid for 24 wk.

NOTES: Supplied in combination with multidose pen injector for Intron A.

Interferon Alfacon-1 (Infergen)

COMMON USES: Management of chronic hepatitis C.

DOSAGE: 9 mg SC 3 times/wk.

NOTES: $\geq$48 h should elapse between injections.

Ipecac Syrup

COMMON USES: Management of drug overdose and certain cases of poisoning.

DOSAGE: *Adults:* 15–30 mL PO followed by water 200–300 mL; if no emesis occurs in 20 min, may repeat once. *Peds:* 6–12 mo: 5–10 mL PO followed by water; 1–12 y: 15 mL PO followed by water.

NOTES: Do not use for ingestion of petroleum distillates, strong acid, base, or other corrosive or caustic agents; not for use in comatose or unconscious patients; caution in CNS depressant overdose.

Ipratropium Bromide Inhalant (Atrovent)

COMMON USES: Bronchospasm associated with COPD.

DOSAGE: *Adults* and *Children >12 y:* 2–4 puffs qid.

NOTES: Not for initial therapy of acute episodes of bronchospasm.

Irbesartan (Avapro)

COMMON USES: Management of HTN.

DOSAGE: 150 mg/d PO, may be increased to 300 mg/d.

Iron Dextran (Dexferrum)

COMMON USES: Iron deficiency when PO supplementation is not possible.

DOSAGE: Based on estimate of iron deficiency (see package insert).

NOTES: Must administer a test dose because anaphylaxis is common (adult 0.5 mL, infants 0.25 mL; may be given deep IM using "Z-track" technique, although IV route most preferred).

Isoetharine (Bronkosol, Bronkometer)

COMMON USES: Bronchial asthma and reversible bronchospasm.

DOSAGE: *Adults* and *Peds:* Nebulization: 0.25–1.0 mL diluted 1:3 with saline q4–6h. Metered dose inhaler: 1–2 inhalations q4h.

Isoniazid (INH)

COMMON USES: Control of *Mycobacterium* species infections.

DOSAGE: *Adults:* Active tuberculosis: 5 mg/kg/24h PO or IM qd (usually 300 mg/d). Prophylaxis: 300 mg PO qd for 6–12 mo. *Peds:* Active tuberculosis: 10–20 mg/kg/24H PO or IM qd to 300 mg/d max. Prophylaxis: 10 mg/kg/24H PO qd.
NOTES: Can cause severe hepatitis; given with other antituberculous drugs for active tuberculosis; IM route rarely used; to prevent peripheral neuropathy, can give pyridoxine 50–100 mg/d.

Isoproterenol (Isuprel, Medihaler-Iso)

COMMON USES: Shock, cardiac arrest, AV nodal block, antiasthmatic.
DOSAGE: *Adults:* Emergency cardiac care: 2–20 mg/min IV infusion, titrated to effect. Shock: 1–4 mg/min IV infusion, titrated to effect. AV nodal block: 20–60 mg IV push; may repeat q3–5 min; 1–5 mg/min IV infusion maintenance. Inhalation: 1–2 inhalations 4–6 times/d. *Peds:* Emergency cardiac care: 0.1–1.5 mg/kg/min IV infusion, titrated to effect. Inhalation: 1–2 inhalations 4–6 times/d.
NOTES: Contraindications: tachycardia; pulse >130 beats/min may induce ventricular arrhythmias.

Isosorbide Dinitrate (Isordil)

COMMON USES: Angina pectoris.
DOSAGE: Acute angina: 2.5–10.0 mg PO (chewable tablet) or SL prn q5–10 min; >3 doses should not be given in 15- to 30-min period. Angina prophylaxis: 5–60 mg PO tid.
NOTES: Nitrates should not be given on long-term q6h or qid basis because of development of tolerance; can cause headaches; usually need to administer a larger PO dose to achieve same results as with SL forms.

Isosorbide Monohydrate (ISMO)

COMMON USES: Prevention of angina pectoris.
DOSAGE: 20 mg PO bid, with the 2 doses given 7 h apart or extended release 30–120 mg PO qd.

Isradipine (DynaCirc)

COMMON USES: Control of HTN.
DOSAGE: 2.5–5.0 mg PO bid.

Itraconazole (Sporanox)

COMMON USES: Control of systemic fungal infections caused by *Aspergillus*, *Blastomyces*, and *Histoplasma*.
DOSAGE: 200 mg PO or IV qd–bid.
NOTES: Administer with meals or cola; should not be used concurrently with H_2-antagonist, omeprazole, antacids.

Kaolin-Pectin

COMMON USES: Control of diarrhea.
DOSAGE: *Adults:* 60–120 mL PO after each loose stool or q3–4h prn. *Peds:* 3–6 y: 15–30 mL/dose PO prn; 6–12 y: 30–60 mL/dose PO prn.

Ketoconazole (Nizoral)

COMMON USES: Systemic fungal infections: candidiasis, chronic mucocutaneous candidiasis, blastomycosis, coccidioidomycosis, histoplasmosis, and paracoccidioidomycosis; topical cream for localized fungal infections due to dermatophytes and yeast; rapid short-term therapy of prostate cancer where rapid decrease of testosterone is needed (ie, spinal cord compression).
DOSAGE: *Adults:* PO: 200 mg PO qd; increase to 400 mg PO qd for very serious infections; prostate cancer: 400 mg PO tid (short term). Topical: Apply to affected area once daily. *Peds:* 3.3–6.6 mg/kg/24H PO qd.
NOTES: Associated with severe hepatotoxicity; monitor LFTs closely throughout course of therapy; drug interaction with any agent that increases gastric pH, thus

preventing absorption of ketoconazole; may enhance oral anticoagulants; may react with alcohol to produce disulfiram-like reaction.

Ketoprofen (Orudis)

COMMON USES: Management of arthritis and pain.
DOSAGE: 25–75 mg PO tid–qid to 300 mg/d max.

Ketorolac (Toradol)

COMMON USES: Management of arthritis and pain.
DOSAGE: 15–30 mg IV/IM q6h or 10 mg PO qid.
NOTES: Do NOT use >5 d.

Labetalol (Trandate, Normodyne)

COMMON USES: HTN, hypertensive emergencies.
DOSAGE: *Adults:* HTM: Initially, 100 mg PO bid, then 200–400 mg PO bid. Hypertensive emergency: 20–80 mg IV bolus, then 2 mg/min IV infusion, titrated to effect. *Peds:* PO: 3–20 mg/kg/d in divided doses. Hypertensive emergency: 0.4–3 mg/kg/h IV continuous infusion.

Lactobacillus (Lactinex Granules)

COMMON USES: Control of diarrhea, especially after antibiotic therapy.
DOSAGE: *Adults* and *Peds >3 y:* 1 packet, 2 capsules, or 4 tablets with meals or liquids tid.

Lactulose (Chronulac, Cephulac)

COMMON USES: Hepatic encephalopathy; laxative; constipation.
DOSAGE: *Adults:* Acute hepatic encephalopathy: 30–45 mL PO q1h until soft stools are observed, then tid–qid. Long-term laxative therapy: 30–45 mL PO tid–qid; adjust the dosage every 1–2 d to produce 2–3 soft stools qd. PR: 200 g diluted with water 700 mL instilled into the rectum. *Peds:* Infants: 2.5–10 mL/24h divided tid–qid. Children: 40–90 mL/24h divided tid-qid.
NOTES: Can cause severe diarrhea.

Lamotrigine (Lamictal)

COMMON USES: Management of partial seizures.
DOSAGE: *Adults:* Initially 50 mg PO qd, then 50 mg PO bid for 2 wk, then maintenance 300–500 mg/d divided bid. *Peds:* 0.15 mg/kg in 1–2 divided doses for weeks 1 and 2, then 0.3 mg/kg for weeks 3 and 4, then maintenance dose of 1 mg/kg/d in 1–2 divided doses.
NOTES: May cause rash and photosensitivity; the value of therapeutic monitoring has not been established.

Lansoprazole (Prevacid)

COMMON USES: Management of duodenal ulcers, *H pylori* infection, erosive esophagitis, and hypersecretory conditions.
DOSAGE: 15–30 mg PO once daily.

Leflunomide (Arava)

COMMON USES: Management of active rheumatoid arthritis.
DOSAGE: 100 mg PO once daily for 3 d, followed by 10–20 mg once daily.
NOTES: Pregnancy category X: DO NOT USE; monitor alanine aminotransferase.

Lepirudin (Refludan)

COMMON USES: Management of heparin-induced thrombocytopenia.
DOSAGE: Bolus of 0.4 mg/kg IV, followed by 0.15 mg/kg continuous infusion. Dose adjustments as necessary for renal insufficiency.
NOTES: Monitor aPTT 4 h into initial infusion and at least daily; adjust dose based on aPTT ratio; maintain aPTT ratio of 1.5–2.0.

Leucovorin Calcium (Wellcovorin)

COMMON USES: Antidote for folic acid antagonist.
DOSAGE: *Adults* and *Peds:* Methotrexate rescue: 10–100 mg/m^2/dose IV or PO q3–6h. Adjunct to antimicrobials: 5–10 mg PO qd.
NOTES: Many different dosing schedules exist for Leucovorin rescue after methotrexate therapy.

Levalbuterol (Xopenex)

COMMON USES: Management and prevention of bronchospasm.
DOSAGE: 0.63 mg nebulized every 6–8 h.
NOTES: Therapeutically active R-isomer of albuterol.

Levetiracetam (Kappra)

COMMON USES: Management of partial onset seizures.
DOSAGE: 500 mg PO bid, may be increased to 3000 mg/d max.
NOTES: May cause dizziness and somnolence; may impair coordination.

Levofloxacin (Levaquin)

COMMON USES: Control of lower respiratory tract infections, sinusitises, and UTIs.
DOSAGE: 250–500 mg PO or IV once daily.
NOTES: Reliable activity against *S pneumoniae,* drug interactions with cation-containing products.

Levonorgestrel Implants (Norplant)

COMMON USES: Prevention of pregnancy.
DOSAGE: Implant 6 capsules in the mid-forearm.
NOTES: Prevents pregnancy for up to 5 y; capsules may be removed if pregnancy is desired.

Levorphanol (Levo-Dromoran) [C]

COMMON USES: Moderate to severe pain.
DOSAGE: 2 mg PO or SC prn.

Levothyroxine (Synthroid)

COMMON USES: Hypothyroidism.
DOSAGE: *Adults:* 25–50 mg/d PO or IV initially; increase by 25–50 mg/d every month; usual dose 100–200 mg/d. *Peds:* 0–1 y: 8–10 mg/kg/24h PO or IV qd; 1–5 y: 4–6 mg/kg/24h PO or IV qd; >5 y: 3–4 mg/kg/24h PO or IV qd.
NOTES: Titrate dosage based on clinical response and thyroid function tests; dosage can be increased more rapidly in young to middle-age patients.

Lidocaine (Xylocaine)

COMMON USES: Local anesthesia; management of cardiac arrhythmias.
DOSAGE: *Adults:* Arrhythmias: 1 mg/kg (50–100 mg) IV bolus, then 2–4 mg/min IV infusion, should repeat bolus after 5 min. Local anesthesia: Infiltrate a few milliliters of a 0.5–1.0% solution to 3 mg/kg/dose max. *Peds:* Arrhythmias: 1 mg/kg dose IV bolus, then 20–50 mg/kg/min IV infusion. Local anesthetic: Infiltrate a few milliliters of a 0.5–1.0% solution, with a maximum of 3 mg/kg/dose.
NOTES: Epinephrine may be added for local anesthesia to prolong effect and help decrease bleeding; for IV forms, decreased dose is required with liver disease and CHF; dizziness, paresthesias, and convulsions are associated with toxicity.

Lidocaine/Prilocaine (EMLA)

COMMON USES: Topical anesthetic; adjunct to phlebotomy or invasive dermal procedures.
DOSAGE: *Adults:* EMLA Cream and Anesthetic Disc (1 g/10 cm^2): Thick layer of cream 2–2.5 g applied to intact skin and covered with an occlusive dressing

(Tegaderm) for ≥1 h. Anesthetic Disc : 1 g/10 cm² for ≥1 h. **Peds:** Maximum dose: up to 3 mo or <5 kg: 1 g/10 cm² for 1 h; 3–12 mo and >5 kg: 2 g/20 cm² for 4 h; 1–6 y and >10 kg: 10 g/100 cm² for 4 h; 7–12 y and >20 kg: 20 g/200 cm² for 4 h.
NOTES: Longer contact time produces greater effect.

Lindane (Kwell)

COMMON USES: Control of head lice, crab lice, scabies.
DOSAGE: *Adults* and *Peds:* Cream or lotion: Apply thin layer after bathing and leave in place for 24 h; pour on laundry. Shampoo: Apply 30 mL and develop lather with warm water for 4 min; comb out nits.
NOTES: Caution with overuse, may be absorbed into blood; wash clothing and bedding to clear infestation.

Linezolid (Zyvox)

COMMON USES: Infections caused by gram-positive bacteria, including vancomycin-resistant and methicillin-resistant strains.
DOSAGE: 400–600 mg IV or PO q12h.
NOTES: A reversible, inhibitor of MAO; therefore avoid foods that contain tyramine; avoid cough and cold products that contain pseudoephedrine or phenylpropanolamine.

Liothyronine (Cytomel)

COMMON USES: Hypothyroidism.
DOSAGE: *Adults:* Initially 25 mg/24h, then titration q1–2 wk according to clinical response and thyroid function test results to maintenance of 25–75 mg PO qd. *Peds:* Initially 5 mg/24h, then titration by 5 mg/24h increments at 1- to 2-wk intervals; maintenance 25–75 mg/24h PO qd.
NOTES: Decrease dose in elderly patients; monitor thyroid function test.

Lisinopril (Prinivil, Zestril)

COMMON USES: Control of HTN, heart failure, and AMI.
DOSAGE: 5–40 mg/24h PO qd-bid. AMI: 5 mg within 24 h of MI, then 5 mg after 24 h, 10 mg after 48 h, and then 10 mg qd.
NOTES: Dizziness, headache, and cough are common side effects; DO NOT use in pregnancy.

Lithium Carbonate (Eskalith, others)

COMMON USES: Manic episodes of manic-depressive illness; maintenance therapy in recurrent disease.
DOSAGE: Acute mania: 600 mg PO tid or 900 mg slow release bid. Maintenance: 300 mg PO tid–qid.
NOTES: Dosage must be titrated; follow serum levels (see Table IX–2 page 460); common side effects are polyuria and tremor; contraindicated in patients with severe renal impairment; sodium retention or diuretic use may potentate toxicity.

Lomefloxacin (Maxaquin)

COMMON USES: Control of UTI and lower respiratory tract infections caused by gram-negative bacteria; prophylaxis in transurethral procedures.
DOSAGE: 400 mg PO qd.
NOTES: May cause severe photosensitivity.

Loperamide (Imodium)

COMMON USES: Diarrhea.
DOSAGE: *Adults:* 4 mg PO initially, then 2 mg after each loose stool, up to 16 mg/d. *Peds:* 0.4–0.8 mg/kg/24h PO divided q6–12h until diarrhea resolves or for 7 d max.
NOTES: Do not use in acute diarrhea caused by *Salmonella*, *Shigella*, or *C difficile*.

Loracarbef (Lorabid)

COMMON USES: Control of infections caused by susceptible bacteria involving the upper and lower respiratory tract, skin, bone, urinary tract, abdomen, and gynecologic system.
DOSAGE: *Adults:* 200–400 mg PO bid. *Peds:* 7.5–15 mg/kg/d PO divided bid.
NOTES: Has more gram-negative activity than first-generation cephalosporins.

Loratadine (Claritin)

COMMON USES: Management of allergic rhinitis.
DOSAGE: 10 mg PO once daily.
NOTES: Take on empty stomach.

Lorazepam (Ativan, Alzapam) [C]

COMMON USES: Anxiety and anxiety mixed with depression; preop sedation; control of status epilepticus.
DOSAGE: *Adults:* Anxiety: 0.5–1.0 mg PO bid–tid. Preop: 0.05 mg/kg up to 4 mg max IM 2 h before surgery. Insomnia: 2–4 mg PO qhs. Status epilepticus: 2.5–10 mg/dose IV repeated at 15- to 20-min intervals prn. *Peds:* Status epilepticus: 0.05 mg/kg/dose IV repeated at 15–20 min interval prn.
NOTES: Decrease dose in elderly patients; may take up to 10 min to see effect when given IV.

Losartan (Cozaar)

COMMON USES: Management of HTN.
DOSAGE: 25–50 mg PO qd–bid.
NOTES: Do not use in pregnancy; symptomatic hypotension may occur in patients on diuretics.

Lovastatin (Mevacor)

COMMON USES: Adjunct to diet to decrease total and low-density lipoprotein cholesterol levels in patients with primary hypercholesterolemia (types IIa and IIb).
DOSAGE: 20 mg PO daily with evening meal; increase at 4-wk intervals to 80 mg/d max.
NOTES: Patient should be maintained on standard cholesterol-lowering diet throughout therapy; monitor LFTs every 6 wk during first year of therapy; headache and GI intolerance common.

Magnesium Citrate

COMMON USES: Vigorous bowel prep; constipation.
DOSAGE: *Adults:* 120–240 mL PO prn. *Peds:* 0.5 mL/kg/dose, up to 200 mL max PO.
NOTES: Do not use in renal insufficiency or intestinal obstruction.

Magnesium Hydroxide (Milk of Magnesia)

COMMON USES: Constipation.
DOSAGE: *Adults:* 15–30 mL PO prn. *Peds:* 0.5 mL/kg/dose PO prn.
NOTES: Do not use in renal insufficiency or intestinal obstruction.

Magnesium Oxide (Uro-Mag, Mag-Ox 400, Maox)

COMMON USES: Replacement for low plasma magnesium levels.
DOSAGE: 400–800 mg/d divided qd–qid.
NOTES: May cause diarrhea.

Magnesium Sulfate

COMMON USES: Replacement for low plasma levels; refractory hypokalemia and hypocalcemia; pre-eclampsia and premature labor.
DOSAGE: *Adults:* Supplement: 1–2 g IM or IV; repeat dosing based on response and continued hypomagnesemia. Pre-eclampsia, premature labor: 1–4

g/h IV infusion. **Peds:** 25–50 mg/kg/dose IM or IV q4–6h for 3–4 doses; may repeat if hypomagnesemia persists.

NOTES: Decrease dose with low urine output or renal insufficiency.

Mannitol

COMMON USES: Osmotic diuresis (cerebral edema, oliguria, anuria, myoglobinuria, etc), bowel prep.

DOSAGE: **Adults:** Diuresis: 0.2 g/kg/dose IV over 3–5 min; if no diuresis within 2 h, discontinue. **Peds:** Diuresis: 0.75 g/kg/dose IV over 3–5 min; if no diuresis within 2 h, discontinue. **Adults** and **Peds:** Cerebral edema: 0.25 g/kg/dose IV push repeated at 5-min intervals prn; increase incrementally to 1 g/kg/dose prn intracranial hypertension.

NOTES: Caution with CHF or volume overload.

Meclizine (Antivert)

COMMON USES: Motion sickness, vertigo associated with diseases of the vestibular system.

DOSAGE: **Adults** and **Peds >12 y:** 25 mg PO tid–qid prn.

NOTES: Drowsiness, dry mouth, blurred vision commonly occur.

Medroxyprogesterone (Provera, Depo-Provera, Others)

COMMON USES: Secondary amenorrhea and abnormal uterine bleeding owing to hormonal imbalance, endometrial cancer, contraceptive.

DOSAGE: Secondary amenorrhea: 5–10 mg PO qd for 5–10 d. Abnormal uterine bleeding: 5–10 mg PO qd for 5–10 d beginning on the 16th or 21st day of the menstrual cycle. Endometrial cancer: 400–1000 mg IM/wk.

NOTES: Contraindicated with previous thromboembolic disorders or with hepatic disease.

Megestrol Acetate (Megace)

COMMON USES: Management of breast and endometrial cancer; appetite stimulation in cancer and HIV-related cachexia.

DOSAGE: Cancer: 40–320 mg/d PO in divided doses. Appetite: 80 mg PO qid.

Meloxicam (Mobic)

COMMON USES: Management of osteoarthritis.

DOSAGE: 7.5–15 mg PO once daily.

Meperidine (Demerol) [C]

COMMON USES: Relief of moderate to severe pain.

DOSAGE: **Adults:** 50–100 mg PO or IM q3–4h prn. **Peds:** 1–1.5 mg/kg/dose PO or IM q3–4h prn.

NOTES: 75 mg IM equivalent to morphine 10 mg IM; beware of respiratory depression. A useful preprocedure sedative, particularly in children, is a so-called cardiac cocktail consisting of (per 30–lb body weight) Demerol 30 mg, Thorazine 6.25 mg, and Phenergan 6.25 mg given IM.

Mercaptopurine (Purinethol)

COMMON USES: Management of leukemia.

DOSAGE: **Adults** and **Peds:** 2.5 mg/kg/d PO.

Meropenem (Merrem)

COMMON USES: Serious infections caused by a wide variety of bacteria including intra-abdominal and polymicrobic; bacterial meningitis.

DOSAGE: **Adults:** 1 gm IV q8h. **Peds:** 20–40 mg/kg IV q8h.

NOTES: Adjust dose for renal function; less seizure potential than with imipenem.

Mesalamine (Rowasa, Asacol, Pentasa)

COMMON USES: Management of mild to moderate distal ulcerative colitis, proctosigmoiditis, or proctitis.
DOSAGE: Retention enema at bedtime daily or insert 1 suppository bid. Oral: 800–1000 mg PO 3–4 times/d.

Mesna (Mesnex)

COMMON USES: Decrease incidence of ifosfamide-induced hemorrhagic cystitis.
DOSAGE: 20% of ifosfamide dose (w/w) IV at time of ifosfamide infusion and 4 and 8 h after, for a total dose equal to 60% of ifosfamide dose.

Metaproterenol (Alupent, Metaprel)

COMMON USES: Bronchodilator for asthma and reversible bronchospasm.
DOSAGE: *Adults:* Inhalation: 1–3 inhalations q3–4h to maximum of inhalations 12/24h; allow ≥2 min between inhalations. Oral: 20 mg q6–8h. *Peds:* Inhalation: 0.5 mg/kg/dose up to 15 mg/dose max inhaled q4–6h by nebulizer or 1–2 puffs q4–6h. PO: 0.3–0.5 mg/kg/dose q6–8h.
NOTES: Fewer beta-1 effects than with isoproterenol and longer acting.

Metformin (Glucophage)

COMMON USES: Management of non–insulin-dependent diabetes mellitus.
DOSAGE: Initial dose 500 mg PO bid; may be increased to maximum daily dose 2500 mg.
NOTES: Administer with the morning and evening meals; may cause lactic acidosis; do not use if creatinine levels >1.3 in females or >1.4 in males.

Methadone (Dolophine) [C]

COMMON USES: Severe pain; detoxification and maintenance of narcotic addiction.
DOSAGE: *Adults:* 2.5–10 mg IM q8h or 5–15 mg PO q8h (titrate as needed). *Peds:* 0.7 mg/kg/24h PO or IM divided q8h.
NOTES: Equianalgesic with parenteral morphine; long half-life; increase dose slowly to avoid respiratory depression.

Methimazole (Tapazole)

COMMON USES: Hyperthyroidism; preparation for thyroid surgery or radiation.
DOSAGE: *Adults:* Initially, 15–60 mg/d PO divided tid; maintenance of 5–15 mg PO qd. *Peds:* Initially, 0.4–0.7 mg/kg/24h PO divided tid; maintenance of 0.2 mg/kg/d divided tid.
NOTES: Follow patient clinically and with thyroid function tests.

Methotrexate (Folex)

COMMON USES: Acute lymphoblastic leukemia (ALL), acute monocytic leukemia (AML), leukemic meningitis, trophoblastic tumors (chorioepithelioma, choriocarcinoma, chorioadenoma destruens, hydatidiform mole), breast cancer, Burkitt's lymphoma, mycosis fungoides, osteosarcoma, head and neck cancer, Hodgkin's and non-Hodgkin's lymphoma, lung cancer, psoriasis, and rheumatoid arthritis.
DOSAGE: Cancer: "conventional dose": 15–30 mg PO or IV 1–2 times/wk every 1–3 wk; "intermediate dose": 50–240 mg or 0.5–1 g/m^2 IV once every 4 d to 3 wk; "high dose": 1–12 g/m^2 IV once every 1–3 wk; 12 mg/m^2 (max 15 mg) intrathecally, weekly until cerebrospinal fluid cell count returns to normal. Rheumatoid arthritis: 7.5 mg/wk PO as a single dose or 2.5 mg q12h PO for 3 doses each week.
NOTES: Toxicity includes myelosuppression, nausea and vomiting, anorexia, mucositis, diarrhea, hepatotoxicity (transient and reversible; may progress to atrophy, necrosis, fibrosis, cirrhosis), rashes, dizziness, malaise, blurred vision, renal failure, pneumonitis, and, rarely, pulmonary fibrosis. Chemical arachnoiditis and headache may occur with intrathecal delivery. "Large-dose" therapy requires leu-

covorin rescue to prevent severe hematologic and mucosal toxicity (see page 497); monitor blood counts and methotrexate levels carefully.

Methyldopa (Aldomet)

COMMON USES: Essential HTN.

DOSAGE: *Adults:* 250–500 mg PO bid–tid (max 2–3 g/d) or 250 mg to 1 g IV q4–8h. *Peds:* 10 mg/kg/24h PO in 2–3 divided doses (max 40 mg/kg/24h divided q6–12h) or 5–10 mg/kg/dose IV q6–8h to a total dose of 20–40 mg/kg/24h.

NOTES: Do not use in patients with liver disease; can discolor urine; initial transient sedation or drowsiness occurs frequently.

Methylergonovine (Methergine)

COMMON USES: Prevention and control of postpartum hemorrhage caused by uterine atony.

DOSAGE: 0.2 mg IM after delivery of placenta, may repeat at 2- to 4-h intervals or 0.2–0.4 mg PO q6–12h for 2–7 d.

NOTES: IV doses should be given over a period ≥1 min with frequent BP monitoring.

Methylprednisolone (Solu-Medrol)

See "Steroids," page 522 and see Table IX–4, page 466.

Metoclopramide (Reglan, Clopra, Octamide)

COMMON USES: Relief of diabetic gastroparesis; symptomatic gastroesophageal reflux; relief of cancer chemotherapy-induced nausea and vomiting.

DOSAGE: *Adults:* Diabetic gastroparesis: 10 mg PO 30 min ac and hs for 2–8 wk prn; or same dose given IV for 10 d, then switch to PO. Reflux: 10–15 mg PO 30 min ac and hs. Antiemetic: 1–3 mg/kg/dose IV 30 min before antineoplastic agent, then q2h for 2 doses, then q3h for 3 doses. *Peds:* Reflux: 0.1 mg/kg/dose PO qid. Antiemetic: 2 mg/kg/dose IV on same schedule as adults.

NOTES: Dystonic reactions common with large doses that can be controlled with IV Benadryl; can also be used to facilitate small bowel intubation and radiologic evaluation of the upper GI tract.

Metolazone (Diulo, Zaroxolyn)

COMMON USES: Mild to moderate essential hypertension; edema of renal disease or cardiac failure.

DOSAGE: *Adults:* HTN: 2.5–5 mg/d PO; edema: 5–20 mg/d PO. *Peds:* 0.2–0.4 mg/kg/d PO divided q12h–qd.

NOTES: Monitor fluid and electrolyte status of patient during therapy.

Metoprolol (Lopressor, Toprol XL)

Used for emergency cardiac care.

COMMON USES: Management of HTN, angina, and MI.

DOSAGE: Angina: 50–100 mg PO bid. HTN: 100–450 mg PO qd. AMI: 5 mg IV for 3 doses, then 50 mg PO q6h for 48 h, then 100 mg PO bid.

Metronidazole (Flagyl)

COMMON USES: Amebiasis, trichomoniasis, *C difficile*, and anaerobic infections.

DOSAGE: *Adults:* Anaerobic infections: 500 mg IV q6–8h. Amebic dysentery: 750 mg PO qd for 5–10 d. Trichomoniasis: 250 mg PO tid for 7 d or 2 g PO in 1 dose. *C difficile:* 500 mg PO or IV q8h for 7–10 d. *Peds:* Anaerobic infections: 30 mg/kg/24h PO or IV divided q6h. Amebic dysentery: 35–50 mg/kg/24h PO in 3 divided doses for 5–10 d.

NOTES: For *Trichomonas* infections, also treat partner; decrease dose in hepatic failure; no activity against aerobic bacteria; use in combination in serious mixed infections; may cause disulfiram-like reaction.

Metyrapone (Metopirone)

COMMON USES: Diagnostic test for hypothalamic-pituitary corticotropin function.

DOSAGE: Metapyrone test: Day 1: Control period: collect 24-h urine to measure 17-hydroxycorticosteroids (17-OHCS) or 17-ketogenic steroids (17-KSG). Day 2: Corticotropin test: Infuse corticotropin 50 U over 8 h and measure 24-h urinary steroids. Days 3–4: Rest period. Day 5: Administer metapyrone with milk or snack. *Adults:* 750 mg PO q4h for 6 doses. *Peds:* 15 mg/kg q4h for 6 doses (min 250-mg dose). Day 6: Determine 24–h urinary steroids.

NOTES: Normal 24-h urine 17-OHCS is 3–12 mg; after corticotropin therapy, it increases to 15–45 mg/24h; normal response to metapyrone is a 2- to 4-fold increase in 17-OHCS excretion; drug interactions with phenytoin, cyproheptadine, and estrogens may lead to subnormal response.

Metyrosine (Demser)

COMMON USES: Pheochromocytoma; short-term preop and long term when surgery is contraindicated.

DOSAGE: *Adults* and *Peds >12 y:* 250 mg PO qid, increase by 250–500 mg/d up to 4 g/d; maintenance dose 2–3 g/d divided qid.

NOTES: Administer ≥5–7 d preop.

Mexiletine (Mexitil)

COMMON USES: Suppression of symptomatic ventricular arrhythmias.

DOSAGE: Administer with food or antacids; 200–300 mg PO q8h, max 1200 mg/d.

NOTES: Not to be used in cardiogenic shock, second- or third-degree AV block if no pacemaker; may worsen severe arrhythmias; monitor liver function during therapy; drug interactions with hepatic enzyme inducers and suppressors requiring dosing changes.

Mezlocillin (Mezlin)

COMMON USES: Infections caused by susceptible strains of gram-negative bacteria (eg, *Klebsiella*, *Proteus*, *E coli*, *Enterobacter*, *P aeruginosa*, and *Serratia*) involving the skin, bone, respiratory tract, urinary tract, abdomen, and septicemia.

DOSAGE: *Adults:* 3 mg IV q4–6h. *Peds:* 200–300 mg/kg/d divided q4–6h.

NOTES: Often used in combination with aminoglycosides.

Miconazole (Monistat)

COMMON USES: Severe systemic fungal infections including coccidioidomycosis, candidiasis, *Cryptococcus*, and others; various tinea forms; cutaneous candidiasis; vulvovaginal candidiasis; tinea versicolor.

DOSAGE: *Adults:* Systemic: 200–3600 mg/24h IV based on diagnosis divided into 3 doses. Topical: Apply to affected area twice daily for 2–4 wk. Intravaginally: Insert 1 full applicator or suppository at bedtime for 7 d. *Peds:* 20–40 mg/kg/24h IV divided q8h.

NOTES: Antagonistic to amphotericin-B in vivo; rapid IV infusion may cause tachycardia or arrhythmias; may potentiate warfarin drug activity.

Midazolam (Versed) [C]

COMMON USES: Preoperative sedation; conscious sedation for short procedures; induction of general anesthesia.

DOSAGE: *Adults:* 1–5 mg IV or IM, titrate dose to effect. *Peds:* Conscious sedation: 0.08 mg/kg IM 3 1. General anesthesia: 0.15 mg/kg IV followed by 0.05 mg/kg/dose q2min for 1–3 doses as needed to induce anesthesia.

NOTES: Monitor patient for respiratory depression; may produce hypotension under conscious sedation.

Miglitol (Glyset)

COMMON USES: Management of type 2 diabetes mellitus.

DOSAGE: Initial 25 mg PO 3 times/d taken at the first bite of each meal; maintenance 50–100 mg 3 times/d with meals.

NOTES: May be used alone or in combination with sulfonylureas; can cause GI disturbances.

Milrinone (Primacor)

COMMON USES: Management of CHF.
DOSAGE: Loading dose of 50 mg/kg, followed by a continuous infusion of 0.375–0.75 mg/kg/min.
NOTES: Carefully monitor fluid and electrolyte status.

Mineral Oil

COMMON USES: Constipation.
DOSAGE: *Adults:* 15–45 mL PO prn. *Peds >6 y:* 10–20 mL PO bid.

Minoxidil (Loniten, Rogaine)

COMMON USES: Severe HTN; control of male- and female-pattern baldness.
DOSAGE: *Adults:* Oral: 2.5–10 mg PO bid–qid. Topical Rogaine: Apply twice daily to affected area. *Peds:* 0.2–1 mg/kg/24h divided PO q12–24h.
NOTES: Pericardial effusion and volume overload may occur; hypertrichosis after long-term use.

Mirtazapine (Remeron)

COMMON USES: Control of depression.
DOSAGE: 15 mg PO qhs, up to 45 mg qhs.
NOTES: Do not increase dose at intervals <1–2 wk.

Misoprostol (Cytotec)

COMMON USES: Prevention of nonsteroidal anti-inflammatory drug-induced gastric ulcers.
DOSAGE: 200 mg PO qid.
NOTES: Do not take if pregnant; can cause miscarriage with potentially dangerous bleeding; GI side effects are common.

Moexipril (Univasc)

COMMON USES: Control of HTN.
DOSAGE: 7.5–30 mg in 1–2 divided doses administered 1 h before meals.

Molindone (Moban)

COMMON USES: Management of psychotic disorders.
DOSAGE: 5–100 mg PO tid–qid.

Montelukast (Singulair)

COMMON USES: Prophylaxis and control of chronic asthma.
DOSAGE: *Adults >15 y:* 10 mg PO daily taken in the evening. *Peds:* 6–14 y: 5 mg PO daily taken in the evening; 2–5 y: 4 mg/d PO in the evening.
NOTES: NOT for acute asthma attacks.

Moricizine (Ethmozine)

COMMON USES: Management of ventricular arrhythmias.
DOSAGE: 200–300 mg PO tid.

Morphine Sulfate [C]

COMMON USES: Relief of severe pain.
DOSAGE: *Adults:* Oral: 10–30 mg q4h prn; SR tablets 30–60 mg q8–12h. IV/IM: 2.5–15 mg q4h prn. *Peds:* 0.1–0.2 mg/kg/dose IM/IV q2–4h prn up to 15 mg/dose max.
NOTES: Large number of narcotic side effects; may require scheduled dosing to relieve severe chronic pain.

Moxifloxacin (Avelon)

COMMON USES: Management of acute sinusitis, acute bronchitis, and community-acquired pneumonia.

DOSAGE: 400 mg once daily.

NOTES: Active against gram-negative bacteria and *S pneumoniae*; interactions with Mg^-, Ca^-, Al^-, and Fe-containing products and class IA and III antiarrhythmic agents.

Mupirocin (Bactroban)

COMMON USES: Management of impetigo; eradication of methicillin-resistant *S aureus* nasal carrier state.

DOSAGE: Topical: apply small amount to affected area. Nasal: apply twice daily in the nostrils.

NOTES: Do not use concurrently with other nasal products.

Mycophenolate Mofetil (CellCept)

COMMON USES: Prevention of organ rejection after transplantation.

DOSAGE: 1 g PO bid.

NOTES: Used in conjunction with corticosteroids and cyclosporine.

Nabumetone (Relafen)

COMMON USES: Arthritis and pain control.

DOSAGE: 1000–2000 mg/d divided qd–bid.

Nadolol (Corgard)

COMMON USES: HTN and angina, prevention of migraines.

DOSAGE: 40–80 mg qd; 160 mg/d max.

Nafcillin (Nallpen)

COMMON USES: Control of infections caused by susceptible strains of *S aureus* and *Streptococcus*.

DOSAGE: *Adults:* 250–500 mg (1 g max) PO q4–6h; 1–2 g IV q4–6h; 500 mg IM q4–6h. *Peds:* 50–200 mg/kg/d divided q4–6h (max 12 g/d); 50–100 mg/kg/d divided q6h.

NOTES: No adjustments for renal function.

Nalbuphine (Nubain)

COMMON USES: Moderate to severe pain.

DOSAGE: 10–20 mg IM, IV, SC q4–6h prn.

NOTES: Causes CNS depression and drowsiness; use with caution in patients receiving opiate drugs.

Naloxone (Narcan)

COMMON USES: Reversal of narcotic effect.

DOSAGE: *Adults:* 0.4–2.0 mg IV, IM or SC every 5 min, max 10 mg. *Peds:* 0.01 mg/kg/dose IV, IM, or SC; may repeat IV every 3 min for 3 doses prn.

NOTES: May precipitate acute withdrawal in addicts; if no response after 10 mg, suspect a non-narcotic cause.

Naproxen (Naprosyn, Anaprox)

COMMON USES: Control of arthritis and pain.

DOSAGE: *Adults* and *Peds >12 y:* 200–500 mg bid–tid to 1500 mg/d max.

Nedocromil (Tilade)

COMMON USES: Management of patients with mild to moderate asthma.

DOSAGE: 2 inhalations 4 times/d.

Nefazodone (Serzone)

COMMON USES: Management of depression.

DOSAGE: Initially, 100 mg PO bid; usual effective range is 300–600 mg/d in 2 divided doses.

NOTES: May cause postural hypotension and allergic reactions.

Neomycin

COMMON USES: Hepatic coma; preop bowel prep; minor skin infections.
DOSAGE: *Adults:* 3–12 g/24h PO in 3–4 divided doses. *Peds:* 50–100 mg/kg/24h PO in 3–4 divided doses.
NOTES: Part of Nichols-Condon bowel prep.

Neomycin, Polymyxin-B & Dexamethasone, (Maxitrol)

COMMON USES: Steroid-responsive ocular conditions with bacterial infection.
DOSAGE: 1–2 drops in eye(s) q4–6h; apply ointment in eye 3–4 times/d.
NOTES: Should be used under supervision of ophthalmologist.

Neomycin, Polymyxin-B, & Hydrocortisone (Cortisporin Ophthalmic & Otic, Others)

COMMON USES: Superficial bacterial infections of the eye or external auditory canal by organisms sensitive to neomycin or polymyxin and associated with inflammation; suspension used in management of infections in mastoidectomy and fenestration cavities.
DOSAGE: *Adults* and *Peds:* Ophthalmic: ointment, apply every 3–4 h; suspension 1 drop q3–4h. Otic: 3–4 drops into external auditory canal tid–qid.
NOTES: Use suspension in cases of ruptured ear drum. Limit use to <10 d; ocular use should be used under supervision of ophthalmologist.

Nesiritide (Natrecor)

COMMON USES: Management of acutely decompensated CHF.
DOSAGE: 2 μcg/kg IV bolus followed by infusion of 0.01 μg/kg/min. May increase infusion by 0.005 μg/kg/min no more frequently than every 3 h to 0.03 μg/kg/min max.
NOTES: Do not administer if systolic BP <90 mm Hg. Can cause hypotension and arrhythmias.

Nicardipine (Cardene)

COMMON USES: Chronic stable angina, HTN.
DOSAGE: PO: 20–40 mg PO tid. SR: 30–60 mg PO bid. IV: 0.5–15 mg/h continuous IV infusion. Titrate to desired BP.
NOTES: PO to IV conversion: 20 mg tid = 0.5 mg/h; 30 mg tid = 1.2 mg/h; 40 mg tid = 2.2 mg/h.

Nicotine, Transdermal (Habitrol, NicoDerm, Nicotrol, Prostep)

COMMON USES: Aid to smoking cessation for relief from nicotine withdrawal.
DOSAGE: Individualized to patient's needs; apply 1 patch (14–22 mg qd) and taper over 6 wk.
NOTES: Nicotrol to be worn for 16 h to mimic smoking patterns; others worn for 24 h; patients must stop smoking and perform behavior modification for maximum effect.

Nifedipine (Procardia, Procardia XL, Adalat, Adalat CC)

COMMON USES: Vasospastic or chronic stable angina; HTN.
DOSAGE: *Adults:* 10–30 mg PO q8h, max 180 mg/d, or SR tablets 30–90 mg once daily. *Peds:* 0.6–0.9 mg/kg/24h divided tid–qid.
NOTES: Headaches common on initial therapy; reflex tachycardia may occur; Adalat CC and Procardia XL are not interchangeable dosing forms. SL use not indicated secondary to profound decreases in BP.

Nimodipine (Nimotop)

COMMON USES: Prevention of vasospasms after subarachnoid hemorrhage.
DOSAGE: 60 mg PO q4h for 21 d.
NOTES: Contents of capsule may be extracted and administered through a nasogastric tube if the capsule cannot be swallowed whole.

Nisoldipine (Sular)

COMMON USES: Control of HTN.
DOSAGE: 10–60 mg PO once daily.
NOTES: Do not take with grapefruit juice or high-fat meal.

Nitrofurantoin (Macrodantin, Furadantin)

COMMON USES: Control of UTIs.
DOSAGE: *Adults:* Suppression: 50–100 mg PO qd. Management: 50–100 mg PO qid. *Peds:* 5–7 mg/kg/24h in 4 divided doses.
NOTES: GI side effects common; should be taken with food, milk, or antacid; macrocrystals (Macrodantin) cause less nausea than other forms of drug, may cause pulmonary fibrosis.

Nitroglycerin (Nitrostat, Nitrolingual, Nitro-Bid Ointment, Nitro-bid IV, Nitrodisc, Transderm-Nitro)

COMMON USES: Angina pectoris; acute and prophylactic therapy; CHF, BP control, pulmonary HTN in children.
DOSAGE: *Adults:* SL: 1 tablet (0.3, 0.4, or 0.6 mg) SL q5min prn at 3 doses. Translingual: 1–2 doses sprayed under tongue q5min prn at 3 doses. PO: 2.5-, 6.5-, or 9-mg SR capsule or tablet PO tid. IV: 5–20 mg/min titrated to effect 200 mg/min max. Topical: 1–2 inches of ointment to chest wall q6h, then wipe off at night. Transdermal: 0.2–0.4 mg/h, titrated to 0.4–0.8 mg/h; patches deliver in 24 h: 2.5, 5, 7.5, 10, or 15 mg; keep patch off 10–12 h each day. *Peds:* 1 mg/kg/min IV titrated to effect, max 5 mg/kg/min.
NOTES: Tolerance to nitrates develops with constant use after 1–2 wk; this can be avoided by providing a nitrate-free period each day; shorter-acting nitrates should be used on a tid basis, and long-acting patches and ointment should be removed before bedtime to prevent the development of tolerance.

Nitroprusside (Nipride, Nitropress)

COMMON USES: Hypertensive emergency, aortic dissection, pulmonary edema.
DOSAGE: *Adults* and *Peds:* 0.5–10 mg/kg/min IV infusion titrated to desired effect.
NOTES: Thiocyanate, the metabolite, is excreted by the kidney; thiocyanate toxicity occurs at plasma levels of 5–10 mg/dL; if used to control aortic dissection, a beta-blocker must be used concomitantly.

Nizatidine (Axid)

COMMON USES: Management of duodenal ulcers.
DOSAGE: Active ulcer: 150 mg PO bid or 300 mg PO qhs. Maintenance: 150 mg PO qhs.

Norepinephrine (Levophed)

COMMON USES: Acute hypotensive states.
DOSAGE: *Adults:* 8–12 mg/kg/min IV titrated to desired effect. *Peds:* 0.1 mg/kg/min IV titrated to desired effect.
NOTES: Correct blood volume depletion as much as possible before initiation of vasopressor therapy; drug interaction with tricyclic antidepressants leading to severe profound hypertension; infuse into large vein to avoid extravasation; phentolamine 5–10 mg/NS 10 mL injected locally is antidote to extravasation.

Norfloxacin (Noroxin, Chibroxin Ophthalmic)

COMMON USES: Complicated and uncomplicated UTIs resulting from a wide variety of gram-negative bacteria, and prostatitis; topical for ocular infections.
DOSAGE: *Adults:* 400 mg PO bid; ophthalmic 1–2 drops qid; if severe, use up to q2h. *Peds:* Not recommended for use in patients <18 y.
NOTES: Not for use in pregnancy; drug interactions with antacids, theophylline, and caffeine.

Nortriptyline (Aventyl, Pamelor)

COMMON USES: Endogenous depression.
DOSAGE: 25 mg PO tid to qid; doses >100 mg/d are not recommended.
NOTES: Many anticholinergic side effects, eg, blurred vision, urinary retention, and dry mouth.

Nystatin (Mycostatin, Nilstat)

COMMON USES: Control of mucocutaneous *Candida* infections (thrush, vaginitis).
DOSAGE: *Adults:* PO: 400,000–600,000 U PO "swish and swallow" qid or troche 200,000 U 1–2 dissolved in mouth. Vaginal: 1 tablet inserted into vagina qhs. Topical: Apply 2–3 times/d to affected area (cream, ointment, or powder). *Peds:* Infants: 200,000 U PO q6h. Children: Same as adult.
NOTES: Not absorbed orally, so not effective for systemic infections.

Octreotide Acetate (Sandostatin)

COMMON USES: Suppresses or inhibits severe diarrhea associated with carcinoid and vasoactive intestinal tumors.
DOSAGE: *Adults:* 100–600 mg/d SC in 2–4 divided doses. *Peds:* 1–10 mg/kg/24h SC in 2–4 divided doses.
NOTES: May cause nausea, vomiting, and abdominal discomfort.

Ofloxacin (Floxin, Ocuflox Ophthalmic)

COMMON USES: Infections of the lower respiratory tract, skin and skin structure, and urinary tract, prostatitis, uncomplicated gonorrhea, and chlamydia infections; topical for bacterial conjunctivitis and otitis externa.
DOSAGE: *Adults:* 200–400 mg PO bid or IV q12h. *Adults and Peds >1 y:* Ophthalmic: 1–2 drops in eye(s) q2–4h for 2 d, then qid for another 5 d. *Peds:* Systemic administration should not be used in children <18 y. *Peds 1–12 y:* Otic: 5 drops in ear bid for 10 d. *Adults and Peds >12 y:* Otic: 10 drops in ear bid for 10 d.
NOTES: May cause nausea, vomiting, diarrhea, insomnia and headache; drug interactions with antacids, sucralfate, and iron- and zinc-containing products that decrease absorption of ofloxacin; may increase theophylline levels.

Olanzapine (Zyprexa)

COMMON USES: Management of psychotic disorders.
DOSAGE: Titrate up to 20 mg/d max.
NOTES: May take many weeks to titrate to therapeutic dose; cigarette smoking will decrease levels.

Olsalazine (Dipentum)

COMMON USES: Maintenance of remission of ulcerative colitis.
DOSAGE: 500 mg PO bid.
NOTES: Take with food; may cause diarrhea.

Omeprazole (Prilosec)

COMMON USES: Management of duodenal and gastric ulcers, Zollinger-Ellison syndrome, GERD, and *H pylori* infections.
DOSAGE: 20–40 mg PO qd-bid.
NOTES: Combination therapy necessary for *H pylori*.

Ondansetron (Zofran)

COMMON USES: Prevention of nausea and vomiting associated with cancer chemotherapy and postoperative nausea and vomiting.
DOSAGE: *Adults* and *Peds:* Chemotherapy: 0.15 mg/kg/dose IV before chemotherapy, then repeated 4 and 8 h after the first dose or 4–8 mg PO tid; administer first dose 30 min before chemotherapy. *Adults:* Postop: 4 mg IV immediately before induction or postop.
NOTES: May cause diarrhea and headache.

Orpernadrine (Norflex)

COMMON USES: Control of muscle spasms.
DOSAGE: 60–100 mg bid.
NOTES: Dose dependent on route of administration.

Oseltamivir (Tamiflu)

COMMON USES: Control of influenzae A and B.
DOSAGE: 75 mg twice daily for 5 d.

Oxacillin (Bactocill, Prostaphlin)

COMMON USES: Control of infections caused by susceptible strains of *S aureus* and *Streptococcus.*
DOSAGE: *Adults:* 1–2 mg IV q4–6h. *Peds:* 150–200 mg/kg/d IV q4–6h.

Oxaprozin (Daypro)

COMMON USES: Control of arthritis and pain.
DOSAGE: 600–1200 mg qd.

Oxazepam (Serax) [C]

COMMON USES: Anxiety; acute alcohol withdrawal; anxiety with depressive symptoms.
DOSAGE: 10–15 mg PO tid–qid; severe anxiety and alcohol withdrawal may require up to 30 mg qid.
NOTES: Oxazepam is a diazepam metabolite (Valium).

Oxcarbazepine (Trileptal)

COMMON USES: Control of partial seizures.
DOSAGE: *Adults:* 300 mg, increase dose weekly to a usual dose of 1200–2400 mg/d. *Peds:* 8–10 mg/kg PO bid, 600 mg/d max; increase dose weekly to target maintenance dose.
NOTES: May cause hyponatremia.

Oxybutynin (Ditropan, Ditropan XL)

COMMON USES: Symptomatic relief of urgency, nocturia, and incontinence associated with neurogenic or reflex neurogenic bladder.
DOSAGE: *Adults* and *Peds >5 y:* 5 mg PO tid–qid. *Adults:* extended release 5 mg PO qd; can titrate up to 30 mg PO qd (5 and 10 mg/tab). *Peds 1–5 y:* 0.02 mg/kg/dose 2–4 times a day (syrup 5 mg/5 mL).
NOTES: Anticholinergic side effects (dry mouth, constipation, dry eyes, somnolence, others).

Oxycodone (OxyContin, Roxicodone, others) [C]

COMMON USES: Moderate to severe pain usually in combination with other analgesics.
DOSAGE: *Adults:* 5 mg PO q4–6h prn; 10–40 mg PO q12h SR. *Peds:* 6–12 y: 1.25 mg PO q6h prn; >12 y: 2.5 mg PO q6h prn.
NOTES: SR (OxyContin) 10, 20, 40, 80 mg; liquid 5 mg/5 mL; solution 20 mg/mL

Oxycodone & Acetaminophen (Percocet, Tylox) [C]

COMMON USES: Moderate to severe pain.
DOSAGE: *Adults:* 1–2 tablets/capsules PO q4–6h prn (specify oxycodone/acetaminophen dose). *Peds:* 0.05–0.15 mg/kg/dose q4–6h, max 5 mg/dose (based on oxycodone).
NOTES: Supplied as (Percocet: oxycodone/acetaminophen 2.5 mg/325 mg, 5 mg/325 mg, 7.5 mg/500 mg, 10 mg/500 mg; Tylox: oxycodone 5 mg, acetaminophen 500 mg) solution oxycodone 5 mg/acetaminophen 325 mg/5 mL.

Oxycodone & Aspirin (Percodan, Percodan-Demi) [C]

COMMON USES: Moderate to moderately severe pain.

DOSAGE: *Adults:* 1–2 tablets/capsules PO q4–6h prn. *Peds:* 0.05–0.15 mg/kg/dose q4–6h, max 5 mg/dose (based on oxycodone).
NOTES: Percodan: oxycodone hydrochloride 4.5 mg, oxycodone terephthalate 0.38 mg, aspirin 325 mg; Pedcodan-Demi: oxycodone hydrochloride 2.25 mg, oxycodone terephthalate 0.19 mg, aspirin 325 mg.

Oxytocin (Pitocin, Syntocinon)

COMMON USES: Induction of labor; control of postpartum hemorrhage.
DOSAGE: 0.001–0.002 U/min IV titrate to effect, max 0.02 U/min.
NOTES: Can cause uterine rupture and fetal death; monitor vital signs closely.

Pancreatin

Pancrelipase (Pancrease, Cotazym)

COMMON USES: For patients deficient in exocrine pancreatic secretions (cystic fibrosis, chronic pancreatitis, other pancreatic insufficiency) and for steatorrhea of malabsorption syndrome.
DOSAGE: *Adults* and *Peds:* 1–3 capsules (tablets) with meals and snacks may be increased up to 8 capsules (tablets).
NOTES: Avoid antacids; may cause nausea, abdominal cramps, or diarrhea; do not crush or chew enteric-coated products.

Pancuronium (Pavulon)

COMMON USES: Aids in management of patients on mechanical ventilator; intra-operative muscle relaxation.
DOSAGE: *Adults:* 2–4 mg IV q2–4h prn. *Peds:* 0.02–0.10 mg/kg/dose q2–4h prn.
NOTES: Patient must be intubated and on controlled ventilation; use adequate amount of sedation or analgesia.

Paregoric [C]

COMMON USES: Diarrhea, pain, and neonatal withdrawal syndrome.
DOSAGE: *Adults:* 5–10 mL qd–qid prn.
NOTES: Contains opium.

Paroxetine (Paxil)

COMMON USES: Depression.
DOSAGE: 20–50 mg PO as a single daily dose.

Pantoprazole (Protonix)

COMMON USES: GERD.
DOSAGE: 40 mg PO once daily.
NOTES: Delayed-release tablet, so do not crush or chew tablet.

Penbutolol (Levatol)

COMMON USES: Control of HTN.
DOSAGE: 20–40 mg qd.

Penicillin G Aqueous, Potassium or Sodium (Pfizerpen, Pentids)

COMMON USES: Most gram-positive infections (except penicillin-resistant staphylococci) including streptococci, *N meningitidis*, syphilis, clostridia, corynebacteria, and some coliforms.
DOSAGE: *Adults:* 400,000–800,000 U PO qid; IV doses greatly depend on indications; range: 1.2–24 million U/d. *Peds:* Newborns <1 wk: 25,000–50,000 U/kg/dose IV q12h. Infants 1 wk–1 mo: 25,000–50,000 U/kg/dose IV q8h. Children: 100,000–300,000 U/kg/24h IV divided q4h.
NOTES: Watch for hypersensitivity reactions; drug of choice for group A streptococcal infections and syphilis.

Penicillin G Benzathine (Bicillin)

COMMON USES: Useful as a single-dose regimen for streptococcal pharyngitis, rheumatic fever and glomerulonephritis prophylaxis, and syphilis.
DOSAGE: *Adults:* 1.2–2.4 million U deep IM injection q2–4 wk. *Peds:* 50,000 U/kg/dose to a maximum of 2.4 million U/dose deep IM injection q2–4wk.
NOTES: Sustained action with detectable levels up to 4 wk; considered drug of choice for control of noncongenital syphilis; Bicillin L-A contains the benzathine salt only; Bicillin C-R contains a combination of benzathine and procaine salts and is used for most acute strep infections (procaine 300,000 U with benzathine 300,000 U /mL or benzathine 900,000 U with procaine 300,000 U /2 mL).

Penicillin G Procaine (Wycillin, others)

COMMON USES: Moderately severe infections caused by penicillin G–sensitive organisms that respond to low persistent serum levels (syphilis, uncomplicated pneumococcal pneumonia).
DOSAGE: *Adults:* 300,000–1.2 million U/d IM divided qd–bid. *Peds:* 25,000–50,000 U/kg/d IM divided qd–bid.
NOTES: A long-acting parenteral penicillin; blood levels up to 15 h; administer probenecid ≥30 min before administration of penicillin to prolong action.

Penicillin V (Pen-Vee K, Veetids, others)

COMMON USES: Most gram-positive infections (except penicillin-resistant staphylococci) including streptococci, *N meningitidis,* syphilis, clostridia, corynebacteria, and some coliforms.
DOSAGE: *Adults:* 250–500 mg PO q6h. *Peds:* 25–50 mg/kg/24h PO in 4 divided doses.
NOTES: A well-tolerated PO penicillin; 250 mg = penicillin G 400,000 U.

Pentamidine Isethionate (Pentam 300, NebuPent)

COMMON USES: Control and prevention of *P carinii* pneumonia.
DOSAGE: *Adults* and *Peds:* 4 mg/kg/24h IV daily for 14–21 d. *Adults:* Prevention: 300 mg once every 4 wk, administered via Respirgard II nebulizer.
NOTES: Monitor patient for severe hypotension after IV administration; associated with pancreatic islet cell necrosis leading to hypoglycemia and hyperglycemia; monitor hematology laboratory results for leukopenia and thrombocytopenia.

Pentazocine (Talwin) [C]

COMMON USES: Moderate to severe pain.
DOSAGE: 30 mg IM or IV; 50–100 mg PO q3–4h prn.
NOTES: 30–60 mg IM equianalgesic to morphine 10 mg IM; associated with considerable dysphoria.

Pentobarbital (Nembutal, Others) [C]

COMMON USES: Insomnia, convulsions, induced coma after severe head injury.
DOSAGE: *Adults:* Sedative: 20–40 mg PO or PR q6–12h. Hypnotic: 100–200 mg PO or PR qhs prn. Induced coma: load 3–5 mg/kg IV, then maintenance 2–3.5 mg/kg/h IV q1h prn to keep level at 25–40 mg/mL. *Peds:* Hypnotic: 2–6 mg/kg/dose PO qhs prn. Induced coma: See adult.
NOTES: Can cause respiratory depression; may produce hypotension when used IV for cerebral edema; tolerance to sedative-hypnotic effect acquired within 1–2 wk.

Pentoxifylline (Trental)

COMMON USES: Intermittent claudication.
DOSAGE: 400 mg PO tid with meals.
NOTES: Treat for ≥8 wk to see full effect.

Pergolide (Permax)

COMMON USES: Parkinson's disease.
DOSAGE: Initially 0.05 mg PO tid, titrated every 2–3 d to desired effect.
NOTES: May cause hypotension during initiation of therapy.

Perindopril (Aceon)

COMMON USES: Control of HTN and CHF.
DOSAGE: 4–8 mg/d.
NOTES: Avoid taking with food.

Perphenazine (Trilafon)

COMMON USES: Psychotic disorders, intractable hiccups, severe nausea.
DOSAGE: Antipsychotic: 4–8 mg PO tid, max 64 mg/d. Hiccups: 5 mg IM q6h prn
or 1 mg IV at >1–2 mg/min intervals up to 5 mg.

Phenazopyridine (Pyridium)

COMMON USES: Symptomatic relief of discomfort from lower urinary tract irritation.
DOSAGE: *Adults:* 200 mg PO tid. *Peds:* 6–12 y: 12 mg/kg/24h PO in 3 divided
doses.
NOTES: GI disturbances; causes red-orange urine color, which can stain clothing.

Phenobarbital [C]

COMMON USES: Seizure disorders, insomnia, anxiety.
DOSAGE: *Adults:* Sedative-hypnotic: 30–120 mg PO or IM qd prn. Anticonvulsant: Load 10–12 mg/kg in 3 divided doses, then 1–3 mg/kg/24h PO, IM, or IV.
Peds: Sedative-hypnotic: 2–3 mg/kg/24h PO or IM qhs prn. Anticonvulsant: Load
15–20 mg/kg divided into 2 equal doses 4 h apart, then 3–5 mg/kg/24h PO divided in 2–3 doses.
NOTES: Tolerance develops to sedation; paradoxical hyperactivity seen in pediatric patients; long half-life allows single daily dosing. See levels on page 460.

Phenylephrine (Neo-Synephrine)

COMMON USES: Management of vascular failure in shock, hypersensitivity, or
drug-induced hypotension; nasal congestion; mydriatic.
DOSAGE: *Adults:* Mild to moderate hypotension: 2–5 mg IM or SC increases BP
for 2 h; 0.1–0.5 mg IV increases BP for 15 min. Severe hypotension/shock: Infusion at 100–180 mg/min; after BP stabilized, maintenance rate of 40–60 mg/min.
Nasal congestion: 1–2 sprays into each nostril prn. *Adults* and *Peds* >1 y: Mydriasis: 1 drop 2.5–10% solution in eye(s) 30 min before procedure; may repeat in
10–60 min if needed. *Peds:* Hypotension: 5–20 mg/kg/dose IV q10–15 min or
0.1–0.5 mg/kg/min IV infusion titrated to desired effect. Nasal congestion: 1 spray
into each nostril q3–4h prn. *Peds* <1 y: Mydriasis: 1 drop 2.5% solution in eye(s)
30 min before procedure.
NOTES: Promptly restore blood volume if loss has occurred; use caution in patients with hyperthyroidism, bradycardia, partial heart block, myocardial disease, or
severe arteriosclerosis; use large veins for infusion to avoid extravasation; phentolamine 10 mg in saline 10–15 mL for local injection as antidote for extravasation;
activity potentiated by oxytocin, MAO inhibitors, and tricyclic antidepressants.

Phenytoin (Dilantin)

COMMON USES: Tonic-clonic and partial seizures.
DOSAGE: *Adults* and *Peds:* Load: 15–20 mg/kg, IV at a maximum infusion rate
of 25 mg/min or PO in 400-mg doses at 4-h intervals. *Adults:* Maintenance: 200
mg PO or IV bid or 300 mg qhs initially, then follow serum level. *Peds:* Maintenance: 4–7 mg/kg/24h PO or IV divided qd–bid.
NOTES: Caution with cardiac depressant side effects, especially with IV administration; follow levels as needed (see Table IX–2, page 460); nystagmus and

ataxia are early signs of toxicity; gum hyperplasia occurs with long-term use; avoid use of PO suspension, if possible, because of erratic absorption; avoid use in pregnancy.

Physostigmine (Antilirium)

COMMON USES: Antidote for tricyclic antidepressant, atropine, and scopolamine overdose.

DOSAGE: *Adults:* 2 mg IV/IM q15min. *Peds:* 0.01–0.03 mg/kg/dose IV q15–30 min.

NOTES: Rapid IV administration associated with convulsions; cholinergic side effects; may cause asystole.

Phytonadione [Vitamin K] (AquaMEPHYTON, others)

COMMON USES: Coagulation disorders caused by faulty formation of factors II, VII, IX, and X, hyperalimentation.

DOSAGE: *Adults* and *Peds:* Anticoagulant-induced prothrombin deficiency: 2.5–10.0 mg PO or IV slowly. Hyperalimentation: 10 mg IM or IV every week. Infants: 0.5–1.0 mg/dose IM, SC, or PO.

NOTES: With parenteral therapy, usually see first change in prothrombin in 12–24 h; anaphylaxis can result from IV dosing; should be administered slowly IV.

Pindolol (Visken)

COMMON USES: Control of HTN.

DOSAGE: 5–10 mg bid.

Piperacillin (Pipracil)

COMMON USES: Infections caused by susceptible strains of gram-negative bacteria (eg, *Klebsiella*, *Proteus*, *E coli*, *Enterobacter*, *P aeruginosa*, and *Serratia*) involving the skin, bone, respiratory tract, urinary tract, abdomen, and septicemia.

DOSAGE: *Adults:* 3 g IV q4–6h. *Peds:* 200–300 mg/kg/d IV divided q4–6h.

NOTES: Often used in combination with aminoglycosides

Piperacillin/Tazobactam (Zosyn)

COMMON USES: Control of infections caused by susceptible strains of gram-negative bacteria (eg, *Klebsiella*, *Proteus*, *E coli*, *Enterobacter*, *P aeruginosa*, and *Serratia*) involving the skin, bone, respiratory tract, urinary tract, abdomen, and septicemia.

DOSAGE: *Adults:* 3.375–4.5 g IV q6h. Adjust dose for renal insufficiency.

NOTES: Often used in combination with aminoglycosides.

Pirbuterol (Maxair)

COMMON USES: Prevention and reversal of bronchospasm.

DOSAGE: *Adults* and *Peds* >12 y: 2 inhalations q4–6h, max 12 inhalations/d.

Piroxicam (Feldene)

COMMON USES: Management of arthritis and pain.

DOSAGE: 10–20 mg qd.

Pneumococcal Vaccine, Polyvalent (Pneumovax-23)

COMMON USES: Immunization against pneumococcal infections in patients predisposed to or at high risk of acquiring these infections (ie, before elective splenectomy).

DOSAGE: *Adults* and *Peds* >2 y: 0.5 mL IM.

NOTES: Do not vaccinate during immunosuppressive therapy.

Pneumococcal 7-Valent Conjugate Vaccine (Prevnar)

COMMON USES: Immunization against pneumococcal infections in infants and children.

DOSAGE: 0.5 mL IM per dose; series consists of 3 doses; first dose at 2 mo with subsequent doses every 2 mo.

Polyethylene Glycol-electrolyte Solution (Go-LYTLEY, Colyte)

COMMON USES: Bowel cleansing before examination or surgery.
DOSAGE: *Adults:* After 3–4 h fast, the patient must drink 240 mL solution every 10 min until 4 L is consumed. *Peds:* 25–40 mL/kg/h over 4–10 h.
NOTES: First bowel movement should occur in approximately 1 h; may cause some cramping or nausea.

Potassium Iodide [Lugol's solution] (SSKI, Thyro-Block)

COMMON USES: Thyroid crisis, decrease vascularity before thyroid surgery, thin bronchial secretions.
DOSAGE: Preop thyroidectomy: *Adults* and *Peds:* 50–250 mg PO tid 3 times/d (2–6 drops strong iodine solution); administer for 10 d before surgery. Thyroid crisis: *Adults* and *Peds:* >1 y: 300 mg (6 drops SSKI q8h); <1 y: 1/2 dose.
NOTES: SSKI = 1 g/mL, Lugol's solution = 100 mg/mL.

Potassium Supplements

COMMON USES: Prevention or management of hypokalemia.
DOSAGE: *Adults:* 20–100 mEq/d PO divided qd–bid; IV 10–20 mEq/h, max 40 mEq/h and 150 mEq/d (monitor frequent potassium levels when using high-dose IV infusions). *Peds:* Calculate potassium deficit; 1–3 mEq/kg/d PO divided qd–qid; IV max dose 0.5–1 mEq/kg/h.
NOTES: Dosing is based on clinical conditions. Table IX–6 lists PO agents. Can cause GI irritation; powder and liquids must be mixed with beverage (unsalted tomato juice, etc); use cautiously in renal insufficiency and with non-steroidal anti-inflammatory drugs and angiotensin-converting enzyme inhibitors; chloride salt recommended in coexisting alkalosis; for coexisting acidosis, use acetate, bicarbonate, citrate, or gluconate salt.

Pramoxine (Anusol, ProctoFoam-NS, Others)

Pramoxine With Hydrocortisone (ProctoFoam-HC, Anusol-HC, Others)

COMMON USES: Relief of pain and itching from external and internal hemorrhoids and anorectal surgery.
DOSAGE: 1 suppository every morning and bedtime and after each bowel movement; apply cream, ointment, gel, or spray freely to anal area q6–12h.
NOTES: Anusol-HC/ProctoFoam HC contains 1% hydrocortisone.

Pravastatin (Pravachol)

COMMON USES: Decrease high cholesterol levels.
DOSAGE: 10–40 mg PO qhs.

Prazepam (Centrax) [C]

COMMON USES: Anxiety disorders.
DOSAGE: 5–10 mg PO tid–qid, or 20–50 mg PO as single bedtime dose to minimize daytime drowsiness.

Prazosin (Minipres)

COMMON USES: HTF and CHF.
DOSAGE: *Adults:* 1 mg PO tid, to total daily dose of 20 mg/d prn. *Peds:* 5–25 mg/kg/dose q6h.
NOTES: Can cause orthostatic hypotension, so the patient should take the first dose at bedtime; tolerance develops to this effect; tachyphylaxis may result.

Prednisone

See "Steroids," page 522 and Table IX–4, page 466.

TABLE IX–6. SOME COMMON ORAL POTASSIUM SUPPLEMENTS

Brand Name	Salt	Form	mEq Potassium/ Dosing Unit
Glu-K	Gluconate	Tablet	2 mEq/tablet
Kaochlor 10%	KCl	Liquid	20 mEq/15 mL
Kaochlor S-F 10% (sugar-free)	KCl	Liquid	20 mEq/15 mL
Kaochlor Eff	Bicarbonate/KCl/ citrate	Effervescent tablet	20 mEq/tablet
Kaon Elixir	Gluconate	Liquid	20 mEq/15 mL
Kaon	Gluconate	Tablet	5 mEq/tablet
Kaon-Cl	KCl	Tablet, SR	6.67 mEq/tablet
Kaon-Cl 20%	KCl	Liquid	40 mEq/15 mL
KayCiel	KCl	Liquid	20 mEq/15 mL
K-Lor	KCl	Powder	15 or 20 mEq/packet
Klorvess	Bicarbonate/KCl	Liquid	20 mEq/15 mL
Klotrix	KCl	Tablet, SR	10 mEq/tablet
K-Lyte	Bicarbonate/citrate	Effervescent tablet	25 mEq/tablet
K-Tab	KCl	Tablet, SR	10 mEq/tablet
Micro-K	KCl	Capsule, SR	8 mEq/capsule
Slow-K	KCl	Tablet, SR	8 mEq/tablet
Tri-K	Acetate/bicarbonate and citrate	Liquid	45 mEq/15 mL
Twin-K	Citrate/gluconate	Liquid	20 mEq/5 mL

Prednisolone
See "Steroids," page 522 and Table IX–4, page 466.

Prednisolone, Ophthalmic (AK-Pred Ophthalmic, Pred-Forte Ophthalmic, Others)
COMMON USES: Iritis, postoperative inflammation, palpebral and bulbar conjunctivitis, chemical, radiation or thermal injury, corneal abrasion.
DOSAGE: 1–2 drops in eye(s) every hour during day and q2h at night until inflammation subsides; then 1 drop q4h.
NOTES: Can increase intraocular pressure, cause cataracts, and worsen herpes keratitis.

Probenecid (Benemid)
COMMON USES: Gout, maintenance of serum levels of penicillins or cephalosporins.
DOSAGE: *Adults:* Gout: 0.25 g bid for 1 wk, then 0.5 g PO bid. Antibiotic effect: 1–2 g PO 30 min before dose of antibiotic. *Peds:* 25 mg/kg, then 40 mg/kg/d PO divided qid.

Procainamide (Pronestyl, Procan)

COMMON USES: Management of supraventricular and ventricular arrhythmias.
DOSAGE: *Adults:* Emergency cardiac care: 100–200 mg/dose IV q5min until dysrhythmia resolves, hypotension ensues, or dose totals 1 g; then maintenance of 1–4 mg/min IV infusion. Long-term dosing: 50 mg/kg/d PO in divided doses q4–6h. *Peds:* Emergency cardiac care: 3–6 mg/kg/dose IV over 5 min, then 20–80 mg/kg/min IV infusion. Maintenance: 15–50 mg/kg/24h PO divided q3–6h.
NOTES: Can cause hypotension and a lupus-like syndrome; dose adjustment for renal impairment; see Table IX–2, page 460.

Prochlorperazine (Compazine)

COMMON USES: Nausea, vomiting, agitation, psychotic disorders.
DOSAGE: *Adults:* Antiemetic: 5–10 mg PO tid–qid or 25 mg PR bid or 5–10 mg IM q4–6h. Antipsychotic: 10–20 mg IM acutely or 5–10 mg PO tid–qid for mainte-nance. *Peds:* 0.1–0.15 mg/kg/dose IM q4–6h or 0.4 mg/kg/24h PO divided tid–qid.
NOTES: Much larger dose may be required for antipsychotic effect; extrapyrami-dal side effects common; control acute extrapyramidal reactions with diphenhy-dramine.

Procyclidine (Kemadrin)

COMMON USES: Control of Parkinson's syndrome.
DOSAGE: 2.5 mg PO tid.
NOTES: Contraindicated for glaucoma patients.

Promethazine (Phenergan)

COMMON USES: Nausea, vomiting, motion sickness.
DOSAGE: *Adults:* 12.5–50 mg PO, PR, or IM bid–qid prn. *Peds:* 0.1–0.5 mg/kg/dose PO or IM q4–6h prn.
NOTES: High incidence of drowsiness.

Propafenone (Rythmol)

COMMON USES: Control of life-threatening ventricular arrhythmias.
DOSAGE: 150–300 mg PO q8h.
NOTES: May cause dizziness, unusual taste, and first-degree heart block.

Propantheline (Pro-Banthine)

COMMON USES: Symptomatic management of small intestine hypermotility, spastic colon, ureteral spasm, bladder spasm, and pylorospasm.
DOSAGE: *Adults:* 15 mg PO ac and 30 mg PO hs. *Peds:* 1.5–3.0 mg/kg/24h PO divided tid–qid.
NOTES: Anticholinergic side effects such as dry mouth, blurred vision are com-mon.

Propofol (Diprivan)

COMMON USES: Induction or maintenance of anesthesia; continuous sedation in intubated patients.
DOSAGE: Anesthesia: 20–40 mg every 10 min until induction onset, then 50–200 mg/kg/min continuous infusion. ICU sedation: 5–50 mg/kg/min continuous infusion.
NOTES: Propofol 1 mL contains fat 0.1 g; may increase serum triglycerides when administered for extended periods.

Propoxyphene (Darvon) [C]

Propoxyphene & Acetaminophen (Darvocet) [C]

Propoxyphene & Aspirin (Darvon Compound-65, Darvon-N With Aspirin) [C]

COMMON USES: Mild to moderate pain.
DOSAGE: 1–2 PO q4h prn.

NOTES: Darvon: propoxyphene HCl capsule 65 mg. Darvon-N: propoxyphene napsylate 100-mg tablet. Darvocet-N: Propoxyphene napsylate 50 mg/acetaminophen 325 mg. Darvocet-N 100: Propoxyphene napsylate 100 mg/acetaminophen 650 mg. Darvon Compound-65: Propoxyphene HCl 65-mg/aspirin 389-mg/caffeine 32-mg capsules. Darvon-N with Aspirin: Propoxyphene napsylate 100 mg/aspirin 325 mg.

Propranolol (Inderal)

COMMON USES: Control of HTN, angina, myocardial infarction prophylaxis, arrhythmias (atrial fibrillation, atrial flutter, others) essential tremor, pheochromocytoma, thyrotoxicosis, migraine prevention.
DOSAGE: *Adults:* Angina: 80–320 mg PO qd divided bid–qid or 80–160 mg SR qd. Arrhythmia: 10–80 mg PO tid–qid or 1 mg IV slowly, repeat q5min up to 5 mg. HTN: 40 mg PO bid or 60–80 mg SR qd, increase weekly to max 640 mg/d. Hypertrophic subaortic stenosis: 20–40 mg PO tid–qid. MI: 180–240 mg PO divided tid–qid. Migraine prophylaxis: 80 mg/d divided qid–tid, increase weekly to max 160–240 mg/d divided tid–qid; wean off if no response in 6 wk. Pheochromocytoma: 30–60 mg/d divided tid–qid. Thyrotoxicosis: 1–3 mg IV single dose; 10–40 mg PO q6h. Tremor: 40 mg PO bid, increase as needed to max 320 mg/d. *Peds:* Arrhythmia 0.5–1.0 mg/kg/d divided tid–qid, increase as needed q3–7d to max 60 mg/d; 0.01–0.1 mg/kg IV over 10 min, max 1 mg. HTN: 0.5–1.0 mg/kg divided bid–qid, increase as needed q3–7d to 2 mg/kg/d max.

Propylthiouracil [PTU]

COMMON USES: Management of hyperthyroidism.
DOSAGE: *Adults:* 100 mg PO q8h increase up to 1200 mg/d); after euthyroid (6–8 wk), taper dose by ⅓ every 4–6 wk to a maintenance dose of 50–150 mg/24h; therapy is often discontinued in 2–3 y. *Peds:* Initial 5–7 mg/kg/24h PO divided q8h, then maintenance of ⅓ to ⅔ of initial dose.
NOTES: Follow patient clinically; monitor thyroid function tests.

Protamine Sulfate

COMMON USES: Reversal of heparin effect.
DOSAGE: *Adults* and *Peds:* Based on amount of heparin reversal desired; given slow IV, 1 mg will reverse heparin approximately 100 U given in the preceding 3–4 h to max 50 mg.
NOTES: Follow coagulation studies; may have anticoagulant effect if given without heparin.

Pseudoephedrine (Sudafed, Novafed, Afrinol)

COMMON USES: Decongestant.
DOSAGE: *Adults:* 30–60 mg PO q6–8h; SR capsules 120 mg PO q12h. *Peds:* 4 mg/kg/24h PO divided qid.
NOTES: Contraindicated in patients with hypertension or coronary artery disease and in those taking MAO inhibitors; an ingredient in many cough and cold preparations.

Psyllium (Metamucil, Serutan, Effer-Syllium)

COMMON USES: Constipation, diverticular disease of the colon.
DOSAGE: 1 teaspoon (7 g) in a glass of water qd–tid.
NOTES: Do not use if bowel obstruction is suspect; one of the safest laxatives; psyllium in effervescent (Effer-Syllium) form usually contains potassium and should be used with caution in patients with renal failure.

Pyrazinamide

COMMON USES: Management of active tuberculosis.
DOSAGE: *Adults:* 20–35 mg/kg/24h PO divided tid–qid, max 3 g/d. *Peds:* 15–30 mg/kg/d PO divided bid or qd.

NOTES: May cause hepatotoxicity; use in combination with other antituberculosis drugs.

Pyridoxine (Vitamin B₆)

COMMON USES: Management and prevention of vitamin B₆ deficiency.
DOSAGE: Deficiency: 2.5–10.0 mg PO qd. Drug-induced neuritis: 50 mg PO qd.

Quinapril (Accupril)

COMMON USES: Control of HTN.
DOSAGE: 10–80 mg PO qd in single dose.

Quinidine (Quinidex, Quinaglute)

COMMON USES: Prevention of tachydysrhythmia.
DOSAGE: *Adults:* Premature atrial and ventricular contractions: 200–300 mg PO tid–qid. Conversion of atrial fibrillation or flutter: Use after digitalization, 200 mg q2–3h for 8 doses, then increase daily dose to 3–4 g max or until normal rhythm. *Peds:* 30 mg/kg/24h PO in 4–5 divided doses.
NOTES: Contraindicated in digitalis toxicity, AV block; follow serum levels if available (see Table IX–2, page 460); extreme hypotension seen with IV administration. Sulfate salt contains 83% quinidine, and gluconate salt is 62% quinidine.

Quinupristin/Dalfopristin (Synercid)

COMMON USES: Infections caused by vancomycin-resistant *E faecium,* and other gram-positive organisms.
DOSAGE: *Adults* and *Peds:* 7.5 mg/kg IV q8–12h.
NOTES: Administer through central line if possible; NOT compatible with saline or heparin, so flush IV lines with dextrose.

Rabeprazole (AcipHex)

COMMON USES: Peptic ulcers, GERD, and hypersecretory conditions.
DOSAGE: 20 mg once daily; may be increased to 60 mg/d.
NOTES: Do not crush tablets.

Raloxifene (Evista)

COMMON USES: Prevention of osteoporosis.
DOSAGE: 60 mg/d.

Ramipril (Altace)

COMMON USES: Control of HTN and CHF.
DOSAGE: 2.5–20 mg/d PO divided qd-bid.
NOTES: May use in combination with diuretics; may cause a nonproductive cough.

Ranitidine (Zantac)

COMMON USES: Duodenal ulcer, active benign ulcers, hypersecretory conditions, gastroesophageal reflux.
DOSAGE: *Adults:* Ulcer: 150 mg PO bid, 300 mg PO qhs, or 50 mg IV q6–8h; or 400 mg IV/d continuous infusion. Maintenance: 150 mg PO qhs. Hypersecretion: 150 mg PO bid. *Peds:* 0.1–0.8 mg/kg/dose IV q6–8h or 1.25–2.0 mg/kg/dose PO q12h.
NOTES: Decrease dose with renal failure; note oral and parenteral doses are different.

Rimexolone (Vexol Ophthalmic)

COMMON USES: Postoperative inflammation and uveitis
DOSAGE: *Adults* and *Peds >2 y:* Uveitis: 1–2 drops q1h daytime and q2h at night, can taper to 1 drop q4h; postoperative 1–2 drops qid for up to 2 wk.
NOTES: Should taper dose to zero.

Repaglinide (Prandin)

COMMON USES: Management of type 2 diabetes mellitus.
DOSAGE: 0.5–4 mg ac.

Reteplase (Retavase)

COMMON USES: Thrombolytic after AMI.
DOSAGE: 10 U IV over 2 min, second dose 30 min later of 10 U IV over 2 min.

Ribavirin (Virazole, Rebetron)

COMMON USES: Management of infants and children with respiratory syncytial virus infection; management of hepatitis C.
DOSAGE: Respiratory syncytial virus: 6 g in sterile water 300 mL inhaled over 12–18 h. Hepatitis C: 600 mg PO bid in combination with interferon alfa-2b.
NOTES: Aerosolized by a SPAG generator; may accumulate on soft contact lenses; monitor hemoglobin and hematocrit frequently; pregnancy test every month.

Rifampin (Rifadin)

COMMON USES: Tuberculosis; management and prophylaxis of *N meningitidis*, *H influenzae*, or *S aureus* carriers.
DOSAGE: *Adults: N meningitidis* and *H influenzae* carrier: 600 mg PO qd 3–4 d. Tuberculosis: 600 mg PO or IV qd or twice weekly with combination therapy regimen. *Peds:* 10–20 mg/kg/dose PO or IV qd–bid.
NOTES: Multiple side effects; causes orange-red discoloration of bodily secretions including tears; never used as a single agent to control active tuberculosis infections.

Rifapentine (Priftin)

COMMON USES: Management of tuberculosis.
DOSAGE: Intensive phase: 600 mg PO twice weekly for 2 mo; separate doses by ≥3 d. Continuation phase: 600 mg PO once weekly.
NOTES: Has adverse effects and drug interactions similar to those of rifampin.

Rimantadine (Flumadine)

COMMON USES: Prophylaxis and management of influenza A virus infections.
DOSAGE: *Adults:* 100 mg PO bid. *Peds:* 5 mg/kg PO qd, not to exceed 150 mg/d.

Risedronate (Actonel)

COMMON USES: Prevention and control of postmenopausal osteoporosis.
DOSAGE: 5 mg PO once daily with water 6–8 oz.
NOTES: Take 30 min before first food or drink of the day; interaction with calcium supplements; may cause GI distress and arthralgia.

Risperidone (Risperdal)

COMMON USES: Management of psychotic disorders.
DOSAGE: 1–8 mg PO bid.

Rofecoxib (Vioxx)

COMMON USES: Osteoarthritis, acute pain, and primary dysmenorrhea.
DOSAGE: 12.5–50 mg/d.
NOTES: Alert patients to be aware of GI ulceration or bleeding.

Ropinirole (Requip)

COMMON USES: Management of Parkinson's disease.
DOSAGE: 0.75–24 mg/d divided in 3 doses.

Rosiglitazone (Avandia)

COMMON USES: Management of type 2 diabetes mellitus.

DOSAGE: 4–8 mg PO once daily or in 2 divided doses.
NOTES: May be taken with or without meals.

Rosuvastatin (Crestor)

COMMON USES: Control high cholesterol levels.
DOSAGE: 5–40 mg once daily.

Salmeterol (Serevent)

COMMON USES: Management of asthma and exercise-induced bronchospasm.
DOSAGE: 2 inhalations twice daily.

Sargramostim [GM-CSF] (Prokine, Leukine)

COMMON USES: Management of myeloid recovery after bone marrow transplantation.
DOSAGE: *Adults* and *Peds:* 250 mg/m^2/d IV for 21 d.
NOTES: May cause bone pain.

Scopolamine

Scopolamine, Transdermal (Transderm-Scop)

COMMON USES: Prevention of nausea and vomiting associated with motion sickness; preop control of secretions.
DOSAGE: Transderm-Scop: Apply 1 patch behind the ear every 3 d; 0.3–0.65 IM/IV/SC repeat prn q4–6h.
NOTES: May cause dry mouth, drowsiness, and blurred vision.

Secobarbital (Seconal) [C]

COMMON USES: Insomnia.
DOSAGE: *Adults:* 100 mg PO, or IM qhs prn. *Peds:* 3–5 mg/kg/dose PO or IM qhs prn.
NOTES: Beware of respiratory depression; tolerance acquired within 1–2 wk.

Selegiline (Eldepryl)

COMMON USES: Parkinson's disease.
DOSAGE: 5 mg PO bid.
NOTES: May cause nausea and dizziness.

Sertraline (Zoloft)

COMMON USES: Management of depression.
DOSAGE: 50–200 mg PO qd.
NOTES: Can activate manic/hypomanic state; has caused weight loss in clinical trials.

Sildenafil (Viagra)

COMMON USES: Erectile dysfunction.
DOSAGE: 25–100 mg 1 h before sexual activity, maximum dosing is once daily.
NOTES: Do not take with nitrates in any form; adjust dose in persons >65 y.

Silver Nitrate

COMMON USES: Prevention of ophthalmia neonatorium due to GC; removal of granulation tissue cauterization of wounds.
DOSAGE: *Adults* and *Peds:* Apply to moist surface 2–3 times/wk for several weeks or until desired effect. *Peds:* Newborns receive 2 drops into conjunctival sac immediately after birth.

Silver Sulfadiazine (Silvadene)

COMMON USES: Prevention of sepsis in second-degree and third-degree burns.
DOSAGE: *Adults* and *Peds:* Aseptically cover affected area with thin coating bid.
NOTES: Can have systemic absorption with extensive application; must be aggressively debrided daily.

Simethicone (Mylicon)

COMMON USES: Symptomatic management of flatulence.
DOSAGE: *Adults* and *Peds:* 40–125 mg PO pc and hs prn.

Simvastatin (Zocor)

COMMON USES: Decrease high cholesterol levels.
DOSAGE: 5–40 mg PO qhs.

Sirolimus (Rapamune)

COMMON USES: Prophylaxis of organ rejection.
DOSAGE: 2 mg/d PO.
NOTES: Dilute in water or orange juice; do NOT drink grapefruit juice while on sirolimus; take 4 h after cyclosporin.

Sodium Bicarbonate

COMMON USES: Alkalinization of urine, renal tubular acidosis (RTA), control of metabolic acidosis.
DOSAGE: *Adults:* Emergency cardiac care: initiate adequate ventilation, 1 mEq/kg/dose IV; can repeat 0.5 mEq/kg in 10 min once or based on acid/base status. Metabolic acidosis: 2–5 mEq/kg IV over 8 h and prn based on acid/base status. Alkalinize urine: 4 g (48 mEq) PO, then 1–2 g q4h; adjust based on urine pH. Chronic renal failure: 1–3 mEq/kg/d. Distal RTA: 1 mEq/kg/d PO. *Peds:* >1 y: Emergency cardiac care: see Adult. <1 y: Emergency cardiac care: initiate adequate ventilation, 1:1 dilution 1 mEq/mL dosed 1 mEq/kg IV; can repeat with 0.5 mEq/kg in 10 min once or based on acid/base status. Chronic renal failure: see Adult. Distal RTA: 2–3 mEq/kg/d PO. Proximal RTA: 5–10 mEq/kg/d titrate based on serum bicarbonate levels. Urine alkalinization: 84–840 mg/kg/d (1–10 mEq/kg/d) divided doses; adjust based on urine pH.
NOTES: 1 g neutralizes acid 12 mEq; in infants, do not exceed 10 mEq/min infusion; supplied as IV infusion, powder, and tablets: 300 mg = 3.6 mEq, 325 mg = 3.8 mEq, 520 mg = 6.3 mEq, 600 mg = 7.3 mEq, 650 mg = 7.6 mEq.

Sodium Citrate (Bicitra)

COMMON USES: Alkalinization of urine; dissolve uric acid and cysteine stones.
DOSAGE: *Adults:* 2–6 teaspoonfuls (10–30 mL) diluted in water 1–3 oz pc and hs. *Peds:* 1–3 teaspoonfuls (5–15 mL) diluted in water 1–3 oz pc and hs. Supplied: 15- or 30-mL unit dose: 16 (473 mL) or 4 (118 mL) fluid ounces.
NOTES: Should not be given to patients on aluminum-based antacids. Contraindicated in patients with severe renal impairment and on sodium-restricted diets.

Sodium Polystyrene Sulfonate (Kayexalate)

COMMON USES: Management of hyperkalemia.
DOSAGE: *Adults:* 15–60 g PO or 30–60 g PR q6h based on serum K. *Peds:* 1 g/kg/dose PO or PR q6h based on serum K.
NOTES: Can cause hypernatremia; given with agent such as sorbitol (mixed in 70% solution 20–100 mL) to promote movement through bowel.

Sorbitol

COMMON USES: Constipation.
DOSAGE: *Adults* and *Peds >12 y:* 20–70% solution 30–150 mL prn.

Sotalol (Betapace)

COMMON USES: Management of ventricular arrhythmias.
DOSAGE: 80 mg PO bid; may be increased to 240–320 mg/d.
NOTES: Dose should be adjusted for renal insufficiency.

Spironolactone (Aldactone)

COMMON USES: Management of hyperaldosteronism, essential hypertension, edematous states (CHF, cirrhosis), polycystic ovary.

DOSAGE: *Adults:* 25–100 mg PO qid. *Peds:* 1–3.3 mg/kg/24h PO divided bid–qid.
NOTES: Can cause hyperkalemia and gynecomastia; avoid prolonged use; diuretic of choice for cirrhotic edema and ascites.

Steroids, Systemic

(See also Table IX–4, page 466)
The following relates only to the commonly used systemic glucocorticoids.
COMMON USES: Endocrine disorders (adrenal insufficiency), rheumatoid disorders, collagen-vascular diseases, dermatologic diseases, allergic states, edematous states (cerebral, nephrotic syndrome), immunosuppression for transplantation, hypercalcemia, malignancies (breast, lymphomas), preoperatively (in any patient who has been on steroids in the previous year, known hypoadrenalism, preop for adrenalectomy); injection into joints/tissue.
DOSAGE: Varies with use and institutional protocols. Some commonly used doses are: Adrenal insufficiency, acute (Addisonian crisis): *Adults:* hydrocortisone 100 mg IV q8h, then 300 mg/d divided q8h; convert to 50 mg PO q8h for 6 doses, taper to 30–50 mg/d divided bid. *Peds:* hydrocortisone: 1–2 mg/kg IV, then 150–250 mg/d divided tid. Adrenal insufficiency, chronic (physiologic replacement): may also need mineralocorticoid supplementation such as DOCA. *Adults:* Hydrocortisone 20 mg PO qAM, 10 mg PO qPM; cortisone 0.5–0.75 mg/kg/d divided bid; cortisone 0.25–0.35 mg/kg IM qd; dexamethasone: 0.03–0.15 mg/kg/d or 0.6–0.75 mg/m^2/d divided q6–12h PO, IM, IV. *Peds:* Hydrocortisone: 0.5–0.75 mg/kg/d PO tid; hydrocortisone succinate: 0.25–0.35 mg/kg/d IM. Asthma, acute: *Peds:* prednisolone 1–2 mg/kg/d or prednisone 1–2 mg/kg/d divided qd–bid for up to 5 d; prednisone 2–4 mg/kg/d IV divided tid. Congenital adrenal hyperplasia: *Peds:* Initially hydrocortisone 30–36 mg/m^2/d PO divided ⅔ dose qAM, ⅓ dose qPM; maintenance: 20–25 mg/m^2/d divided q6–8h; 1–5 mg/kg/d IM/IV divided bid/qd. Nephrotic syndrome: *Children:* prednisolone or prednisone 2 mg/kg/d PO divided tid–qid until urine is protein free for 5 d, use up to 28 d; for persistent proteinuria, 4 mg/kg/dose PO qod max 120 mg/d for an additional 28 d; maintenance: 2 mg/kg/dose qod for 28 d; taper over 4–6 wk (max 80 mg/d). Septic shock: *Adults:* Hydrocortisone 500 mg–1 g IM/IV q2–6h. *Peds:* Hydrocortisone 50 mg/kg IM/IV, repeat q4–24h prn. Status asthmaticus: *Adults* and *Peds:* Hydrocortisone 1–2 mg/kg/dose IV q6h, then 0.5–1 mg/kg q6h. Rheumatic disease: *Adults:* Intra-articular: hydrocortisone acetate 25–37.5 mg in large joint, 10–25 mg in small joint; methylprednisolone acetate 20–80 mg in large joint, 4–10 mg in small joint. Intrabursal: Hydrocortisone acetate 25–37.5 mg. Intraganglia: Hydrocortisone acetate 25–37.5 mg. Tendon sheath: Hydrocortisone acetate 5–12.5 mg. Perioperative steroid coverage: Hydrocortisone 100 mg IV night before surgery, 1 h preop, intraoperatively, and 4, 8, and 12 h postoperatively; POD No. 1: 100 mg IV q6h; POD No. 2: 100 mg IV q8h; POD No. 3: 100 mg IV q12h; POD No. 4: 50 mg IV q12h; POD No. 5: 25 mg IV q12h; then resume previous PO dosing if long-term use or discontinue if only perioperative coverage is required. Cerebral edema: Dexamethasone 10 mg IV, then 4 mg IV q4–6h.
NOTES: See Table IX–4, page 466. All can cause hyperglycemia, "steroid psychosis," adrenal suppression; never acutely stop steroids, especially if long-term therapy; taper dose. Hydrocortisone succinate administered systemically, acetate form intra-articular.

Steroids, Topical

COMMON USES: Topical therapy for different inflammatory and pruritic dermatologic conditions that respond to corticosteroid therapy.
DOSAGE: Application based on individual agent (Table IX–7, page 524).

Streptokinase (Streptase, Kabikinase)

COMMON USES: Coronary artery thrombosis; acute massive pulmonary embolism; DVT; some occluded vascular grafts.
DOSAGE: Pulmonary embolus: Loading dose 250,000 IU IV through a peripheral vein over 30 min, then 100,000 IU/h IV for 24–72 h. DVT or arterial embolism: Load as with pulmonary embolus, then 100,000 IU/h for 72 h.
NOTES: If maintenance infusion is not adequate to maintain thrombin clotting time 2–5 times control, refer to package insert, PDR, or Hospital Formulary Service for adjustments.

Succinylcholine (Anectine, Quelicin, Sucostrin)

COMMON USES: Adjunct to general anesthesia to facilitate endotracheal intubation and to induce skeletal muscle relaxation during surgery or mechanically supported ventilation.
DOSAGE: *Adults:* 0.6 mg/kg IV over 10–30 s followed by 0.04–0.07 mg/kg as needed to maintain muscle relaxation. *Peds:* 1–2 mg/kg/dose IV followed by 0.03–0.06 mg/kg/dose at 10- to 20-min intervals.
NOTES: May precipitate malignant hyperthermia; respiratory depression or prolonged apnea may occur; many drug interactions potentiating activity of succinylcholine; observe for cardiovascular effects; use only freshly prepared solutions.

Sucralfate (Carafate)

COMMON USES: Management of duodenal ulcers, gastric ulcers.
DOSAGE: *Adults:* 1 g PO qid, 1 h before meals and hs. *Peds:* 40–80 mg/kg/d divided q6h.
NOTES: Therapy should be continued for 4–8 wk unless healing is demonstrated by radiograph or endoscopy; constipation is the most frequent side effect.

Sufentanil (Sufenta) [C]

COMMON USES: Analgesic adjunct to maintain balanced general anesthesia.
DOSAGE: Adjunctive: 1–8 mg/kg with nitrous oxide/oxygen; maintenance of 10–50 mg prn. General anesthesia: 8–30 mg/kg with oxygen and a skeletal muscle relaxant; maintenance of 25–50 mg prn.
NOTES: Respiratory depressant effects persist longer than the analgesic effects; 80 times more potent than morphine.

Sulfasalazine (Azulfidine)

COMMON USES: Ulcerative colitis.
DOSAGE: *Adults:* 1–2 g PO initially, increase to max 8 g/d in 3–4 divided doses; maintenance 500 mg PO qid. *Peds:* 40–60 mg/kg/24h PO divided q4–6h initially; maintenance 20–30 mg/kg/24h PO divided q6h.
NOTES: Can cause severe GI upset; discolors urine.

Sulfinpyrazone (Anturane)

COMMON USES: Acute and chronic gout.
DOSAGE: 100–200 mg PO bid for 1 wk, then increase as needed to maintenance of 200–400 mg bid.

Sulindac (Clinoril)

COMMON USES: Control of arthritis and pain.
DOSAGE: 150–200 mg bid.

Tacrolimus [FK 506] (Prograf)

COMMON USES: Prophylaxis of organ rejection.

TABLE IX–7. TOPICAL STEROID PREPARATIONS

Agent	Common Trade Names	Potency	Apply
Alclometasone dipropionate	Aclovate, cream, ointment 0.05%	Low	bid/tid
Betamethasone valerate	Valisone cream, lotion 0.01%	Low	qd/bid
	Valisone cream 0.01, 0.1%, ointment, lotion 0.1%	Intermediate	qd/bid
Betamethasone dipropionate	Diprosone cream, lotion, ointment 0.05%	High	qd/bid
	Diprosone aerosol (0.1%)		
Betamethasone dipropionate, augmented	Diprolene ointment, gel 0.05%	Ultrahigh	qd/bid
Clobetasol propionate	Temovate cream, gel, ointment, solution 0.05%	Ultrahigh	Scalp, bid (2 weeks max)
Clocortolone pivalate	Cloderm cream 0.1%	Intermediate	qd/qid
Desonide	DesOwen, cream, ointment, lotion 0.05%	Low	bid/qid
Desoximetasone	Topicort LP cream, gel 0.05%	Intermediate	bid/tid
	Topicort cream, ointment 0.25%	High	
Dexamethasone base	Aeroseb-Dex aerosol 0.01%	Low	bid/qid
	Decadron cream 0.1%		
Diflorasone diacetate	Psorcon cream, ointment 0.05%	Ultrahigh	bid/qid
Fluocinolone	Fluocinolone acetonide 0.01%		
	Synalar cream, solution 0.01%	Low	bid/tid
	Synalar ointment, cream 0.025%	Intermediate	bid/tid
	Synalar-HP cream 0.2%	High	bid/tid
Fluocinonide 0.05%	Lidex, anhydrous cream, gel, ointment, solution 0.05%	High	bid/tid
	Lidex-E aqeous cream 0.05%		
Flurandrenolide	Cordran cream, ointment 0.025%	Intermediate	bid/tid
	cream, lotion, ointment 0.05%	Intermediate	bid/tid
	tape, 4 μg/cm^2	Intermediate	qd
Fluticasone propionate	Cutivate cream 0.05%, ointment 0.005%	Intermediate	bid

TABLE IX–7. TOPICAL STEROID PREPARATIONS. (*continued*)

Agent	Common Trade Names	Potency	Apply
Halobetasol	Ultravate cream, ointment 0.05%	Very HIgh	bid
Halcinonide	Halog cream 0.025%, emollient base 0.1% Cream, ointment, solution 0.1%	High	qd/tid
Hydrocortisone	Hydrocortisone Cortizone, Caldecort, Hycort, Hytone, others Aerosol: 1%; Cream: 0.5, 1, 2.5%; Gel 0.5%; Ointment 0.5, 1, 2.5% Lotion 0.5, 1.25%; Paste 0.5%; Solution 1%	Low	tid/qid
			(*continued*)
Hydrocortisone acetate	Corticaine cream, ointment 0.5, 1%	Low	tid/qid
Hydrocortisone butyrate	Locoid ointment, solution 0.1%	Intermediate	bid/tid
Hydrocortisone valerate	Westcort cream, ointment 0.2%	Intermediate	bid/tid
Mometasone furoate	Elocon 0.1% cream, ointment, lotion	Intermediate	qd
Prednicarbate	Dermatop 0.1% cream	Intermediate	bid
Triamcinolone acetonide	Aristocort, Kenalog cream, ointment, lotion 0.025%	Low	tid/qid
	Aristocort, Kenalog cream, ointment, lotion 0.1% Aerosol 0.2 mg/2s spray	Intermediate	tid/qid
Triamcinolone acetonide	Aristocort, Kenalog cream, ointment 0.5%	High	tid/qid

DOSAGE: IV: 0.05–0.1 mg/kg/d as continuous infusion; PO: 0.15–0.3 mg/kg/d divided into 2 doses.
NOTES: May cause neurotoxicity and nephrotoxicity.

Tamsulosin (Flomax)
COMMON USES: Management of BPH.
DOSAGE: 0.4–0.8 mg qd

Telmisartan (Micardis)
COMMON USES: Management of HTN.
DOSAGE: 40–80 mg once daily.
NOTES: Avoid use during pregnancy.

Temazepam (Restoril) [C]

COMMON USES: Insomnia.
DOSAGE: 15–30 mg PO qhs prn.
NOTES: Decrease dose in elderly patients.

Tenecteplase (TNKase)

COMMON USES: Decrease of mortality associated with AMI.
DOSAGE: 30–50 mg IV; see product information for weight-based dosing.

Terazosin (Hytrin)

COMMON USES: Management of HTN and BPH.
DOSAGE: Initially 1 mg PO hs; titrate up to max 20 mg PO qhs.
NOTES: Hypotension and syncope after first dose; dizziness, weakness, nasal congestion, peripheral edema common; often used with thiazide diuretic.

Terbutaline (Brethine, Bricanyl)

COMMON USES: Reversible bronchospasm (asthma, COPD); inhibition of labor.
DOSAGE: *Adults:* Bronchodilator: 2.5–5 mg PO qid or 0.25 mg SC, may repeat in 15 min (max 0.5 mg in 4 h). Metered dose inhaler: 2 inhalations q4–6h. Premature labor: 10–80 mg/min IV infusion for 4h, then 2.5 mg PO q4–6h until term. *Peds:* Oral: 0.05–0.15 mg/kg/dose PO tid; max 5 mg/24h.
NOTES: Caution with diabetes, HTN, hyperthyroidism; high doses may precipitate beta-1-adrenergic effects.

Tetanus Immune Globulin

COMMON USES: Passive immunization against tetanus for any person with a suspect contaminated wound and unknown immunization status (see Appendix).
DOSAGE: *Adults* and *Peds:* 250–500 U IM (larger doses if delay in initiation of therapy).
NOTES: May begin active immunization series at different injection site if required.

Tetanus Toxoid

COMMON USES: Protection against tetanus.
DOSAGE: See Appendix for tetanus prophylaxis.

Tetracycline (Achromycin V, Sumycin)

COMMON USES: Broad-spectrum antibiotic therapy against *Staphylococcus*, *Streptococcus*, *Chlamydia*, *Rickettsia*, and *Mycoplasma*.
DOSAGE: *Adults:* 250–500 mg PO bid–qid. *Peds >8 y:* 25–50 mg/kg/24h PO q6–12h. Do not use in children <8 y.
NOTES: Can stain enamel and depress bone formation in children; caution with use in pregnancy; do not use in presence of impaired renal function (see Doxycycline, page 481).

Theophylline (Theolair, Theo-Dur, Somophyllin, Others)

COMMON USES: Asthma, bronchospasm.
DOSAGE: *Adults:* 24 mg/kg/24h PO divided q6h; SR products may be divided q8–12h. *Peds:* 16 mg/kg/24h PO divided q6h; SR products may be divided q8–12h.
NOTES: See drug levels in Table IX–2 on page 460; many drug interactions; side effects include nausea, vomiting, tachycardia, and seizures.

Thiamine (Vitamin B₁)

COMMON USES: Thiamine deficiency (beriberi); alcoholic neuritis; Wernicke's encephalopathy.

DOSAGE: *Adults:* Deficiency: 100 mg IM qd for 2 wk, then 5–10 mg PO qd for 1 mo. Wernicke's encephalopathy: 100 mg IV 3 1 dose, then 100 mg IM qd for 2 wk. *Peds:*10–25 mg IM qd for 2 wk, then 5–10 mg/24h PO qd for 1 mo.
NOTES: IV thiamine administration associated with anaphylactic reaction; must be given slowly IV.

Thiethylperazine (Torecan)

COMMON USES: Nausea and vomiting.
DOSAGE: 10 mg PO, PR or IM qd–tid.
NOTES: Extrapyramidal reactions may occur.

Thioridazine (Mellaril)

COMMON USES: Psychotic disorders; short-term therapy of depression, agitation, or organic brain syndrome.
DOSAGE: *Adults:* Initially 50–100 mg PO tid; maintenance 200–800 mg/24h PO in 2–4 divided doses. *Peds* >2 y: 1–2.5 mg/kg/24h PO divided bid–tid.
NOTES: Low incidence of extrapyramidal effects.

Thiothixene (Navane)

COMMON USES: Psychotic disorders.
DOSAGE: *Adults* and *Peds:* >12 y: Mild to moderate psychosis: 2 mg PO tid. Severe psychosis: 5 mg PO bid; increase to max 60 mg/24h prn. IM use: 16–20 mg/24h divided bid–qid; max 30 mg/d. <12 y: 0.25 mg/kg/24h PO divided q6–12h.
NOTES: Drowsiness and extrapyramidal side effects most common.

Thyroid (Desiccated Extract)

COMMON USES: Replacement in hypothyroidism.
DOSAGE: 30 mg/d PO, titrate 30 mg/d over several weeks; maintenance 60–120 mg/d.

Tiagabine (Gabitril)

COMMON USES: Adjunctive therapy of partial seizures.
DOSAGE: Initially 4 mg once daily, increase by 4 mg during second week; increase by 4–8 mg/d until clinical response is achieved; max 32 mg/d.
NOTES: Withdraw gradually; used in combination with other anticonvulsants.

Ticarcillin (Ticar)

COMMON USES: Infections caused by susceptible strains of gram-negative bacteria (eg *Klebsiella*, *Proteus*, *E coli*, *Enterobacter*, *P aeruginosa*, and *Serratia*) involving the skin, bone, respiratory tract, urinary tract, abdomen, and septicemia.
DOSAGE: *Adults:* 3 g IV q4–6h. *Peds:* 200–300 mg/kg/d IV divided q4–6h.
NOTES: Often used in combination with aminoglycosides.

Ticarcillin/Potassium Clavulanate (Timentin)

COMMON USES: Infections caused by susceptible strains of gram-negative bacteria (*Klebsiella*, *Proteus*, *E coli*, *Enterobacter*, *P aeruginosa*, and *Serratia*) involving the skin, bone, respiratory tract, urinary tract, abdomen, and septicemia.
DOSAGE: *Adults:* 3.1 g IV q4–6h. *Peds:* 200–300 mg/kg/d IV divided q4–6h.
NOTES: Often used in combination with aminoglycosides.

Ticlopidine (Ticlid)

COMMON USES: Decrease risk of thrombotic stroke.
DOSAGE: 250 mg PO bid.
NOTES: Should be administered with food.

Timolol (Blocadren, Timoptic)

COMMON USES: Management of HTN and MI; glaucoma.

DOSAGE: HTN: 10–20 mg bid. MI: 10 mg bid. Ophthalmic: 0.25% 1 drop bid; decrease to qd when controlled; use 0.5% if needed; 1 drop gel qd.
NOTES: Timoptic XE (0.25, 0.5%) is a gel-forming solution.

Tioconazole (Vagistat)

COMMON USES: Vaginal fungal infections.
DOSAGE: 1 applicator intravaginally at bedtime (single dose).

Tirofiban (Aggrastat)

COMMON USES: Management of acute coronary syndrome.
DOSAGE: Initial 0.4 mg/kg/min for 30 min, followed by 0.1 mg/kg/min.
NOTES: Adjust dose in renal insufficiency; use in combination with heparin.

Tobramycin (Nebcin)

COMMON USES: Serious gram-negative infections, especially *Pseudomonas*.
DOSAGE: Based on renal function 2 mg/kg IV load followed by 1.5 mg/kg IV q8h; refer to Aminoglycoside Dosing on page 459.
NOTES: Nephrotoxic and ototoxic; decrease dose with renal insufficiency; monitor creatinine clearance and serum concentrations for dosing adjustments; see Table IX–2, page 460.

Tocainide (Tonocard)

COMMON USES: Suppression of ventricular arrhythmias including premature ventricular contractions and ventricular tachycardia.
DOSAGE: 400–600 mg PO q8h.
NOTES: Properties similar to lidocaine; decrease dose in renal failure; CNS and GI side effects are common.

Tolazamide (Tolinase)

COMMON USES: Management of non–insulin-dependent diabetes mellitus.
DOSAGE: 100–500 mg qd.

Tolazoline (Priscoline)

COMMON USES: Persistent pulmonary vasoconstriction and HTN in the newborn, peripheral vasospastic disorders.
DOSAGE: *Adults:* 10–50 mg IM/IV/SC qid. *Neonates:* 1–2 mg/kg IV over 10–15 min, followed by 1–2 mg/kg/h.

Tolbutamide (Orinase)

COMMON USES: Management of non–insulin-dependent diabetes mellitus.
DOSAGE: 500–1000 mg bid.

Tolmetin (Tolectin)

COMMON USES: Management of arthritis and pain.
DOSAGE: 200–600 mg tid to 2000 mg/d max.

Topiramate (Topamax)

COMMON USES: Management of partial onset seizures.
DOSAGE: Total dose 400 mg/d. See product information of 8-wk titration schedule.
NOTES: May precipitate kidney stones.

Torsemide (Demadex)

COMMON USES: Edema, HTN, CHF, and hepatic cirrhosis.
DOSAGE: 5–20 mg PO or IV once daily.

Tramadol (Ultram)

COMMON USES: Management of moderate to severe pain.
DOSAGE: 50–100 mg PO q4–6h prn, not to exceed 400 mg/d.

Trandolapril (Mavik)

COMMON USES: Management of HTN, CHF, left ventricular systolic dysfunction, after AMI.
DOSAGE: HTN: 2–4 mg/d; CHF/left ventricular dysfunction: 4 mg/d.

Trazodone (Desyrel)

COMMON USES: Major depression.
DOSAGE: 50–150 mg PO qd–qid; max 600 mg/d.
NOTES: May take 1–2 wk for symptomatic improvement; anticholinergic side effects.

Triamterene (Dyrenium)

COMMON USES: Edema associated with CHF, cirrhosis.
DOSAGE: 100–300 mg/24h PO divided qd–bid.
NOTES: Can cause hyperkalemia; blood dyscrasias, liver damage, and other reactions.

Triazolam (Halcion) [C]

COMMON USES: Insomnia.
DOSAGE: 0.125–0.5 mg PO qhs prn.
NOTES: Additive CNS depression with alcohol and other CNS depressants.

Trifluoperazine (Stelazine)

COMMON USES: Psychotic disorders.
DOSAGE: *Adults:* 2–10 mg PO bid. *Peds 6–12 y:* 1 mg PO qd–bid, gradually increase up to 15 mg/d.
NOTES: Decrease dose in elderly and debilitated patients; PO concentrate must be diluted to ≥60 mL before administration.

Trihexyphenidyl (Artane)

COMMON USES: Parkinson's disease.
DOSAGE: 2–5 mg PO qd–qid.
NOTES: Contraindicated in narrow-angle glaucoma.

Trimethobenzamide (Tigan)

COMMON USES: Nausea and vomiting.
DOSAGE: *Adults:* 250 mg PO or 200 mg PR or IM tid–qid prn. *Peds:* 20 mg/kg/24h PO or 15 mg/kg/24h PR or IM in 3–4 divided doses (not recommended for infants).
NOTES: In the presence of viral infections, may contribute to Reye's syndrome; may cause parkinsonian-like syndrome.

Trimethoprim (Trimpex, Proloprim)

COMMON USES: Urinary tract infections caused by susceptible gram-positive and gram-negative organisms.
DOSAGE: 100 mg PO bid or 200 mg PO qd.
NOTES: Decrease dose in renal failure.

Trimethoprim-Sulfamethoxazole [Co-trimoxazole] (Bactrim, Septra)

COMMON USES: Urinary tract infections, otitis media, sinusitis, bronchitis, *Shigella*, *P carinii*, Nocardia.
DOSAGE: *Adults:* 1 double strength (DS) tablet PO bid or 5–10 mg/kg/24h (based on trimethoprim component) IV in 3–4 divided doses. *P carinii:* 15–20 mg/kg/d IV or PO (trimethoprim component) in 4 divided doses. *Peds:* 8–10 mg/kg/24h (trimethoprim) PO divided into 2 doses or 3–4 doses IV; do not use in newborn.
NOTES: Synergistic combination; decrease dosage in renal failure.

Trimipramine (Surmontil)

COMMON USES: Management of depression.
DOSAGE: 75–300 mg PO qhs.

Urokinase (Abbokinase)

COMMON USES: Pulmonary embolism, DVT, restore patency to IV catheters, coronary artery thrombosis.
DOSAGE: *Adults* and *Peds:* Systemic effect: 4400 IU/kg IV over 10 min, followed by 4400 IU/kg/h for 12 h. Restore catheter patency: Inject 5000 IU into catheter and gently aspirate.
NOTES: Do not use systemically within 10 d of surgery, delivery, or organ biopsy.

Valacyclovir (Valtrex)

COMMON USES: Management of herpes zoster.
DOSAGE: 1 g PO tid.

Valproic Acid & Divalproex (Depakene & Depakote)

COMMON USES: Epilepsy, mania, and prophylaxis of migraines.
DOSAGE: *Adults* and *Peds:* Seizures: 30–60 mg/kg/24h PO divided tid. Mania: 750 mg in 3 divided doses, increased to 60 mg/kg/d max. Migraines: 250 mg bid, increased to 1000 mg/d.
NOTES: Monitor LFTs and follow serum levels; concurrent use of phenobarbital and phenytoin may alter serum levels of these agents.

Valsartan (Diovan)

COMMON USES: Control of HTN.
DOSAGE: 80 mg once daily.
NOTES: Use with caution with potassium-sparing diuretics or potassium supplements.

Vancomycin (Vancocin, Vancoled)

COMMON USES: Serious infections resulting from methicillin-resistant staphylococci and in enterococcal endocarditis in combination with aminoglycosides in penicillin-allergic patients; PO therapy of *C difficile* pseudomembranous colitis.
DOSAGE: *Adults:* 1 g IV q12h; for colitis 250–500 mg PO q6h. *Peds (not neonates):* 40 mg/kg/24h IV in divided doses q12–6h.
NOTES: Ototoxic and nephrotoxic; not absorbed PO, provides local effect in gut only; IV dose must be given slowly over 1 h to prevent "red-man syndrome"; adjust dose in renal failure; see Table IX–2, page 460.

Vasopressin (Antidiuretic Hormone) (Pitressin)

COMMON USES: Management of diabetes insipidus; gaseous GI tract distention; severe GI bleeding; septic shock.
DOSAGE: *Adults* and *Peds:* Diabetes insipidus: 2.5–10 U SC or IM tid–qid or 1.5–5.0 U IM q1–3d of the tannate. GI hemorrhage: 20 U in 50–100-mL D5W or NS given IV over 15–30 min. Septic shock: 0.04 U/min to titrate off other vasopressors.
NOTES: Should be used with caution with any vascular disease.

Vecuronium (Norcuron)

COMMON USES: Skeletal muscle relaxation during surgery or mechanical ventilation.
DOSAGE: *Adults* and *Peds:* 0.08–0.1 mg/kg IV bolus; maintenance of 0.010–0.015 mg/kg after 25–40 min followed with additional doses every 12–15 min.
NOTES: Drug interactions leading to increased effect of vecuronium include aminoglycosides, tetracycline, and succinylcholine; fewer cardiac effects then pancuronium.

Venlafaxine (Effexor)

COMMON USES: Management of depression.
DOSAGE: 75–225 mg/d divided into 2–3 equal doses.

Verapamil (Calan, Isoptin)

COMMON USES: Supraventricular tachyarrhythmias (PAT, Wolff-Parkinson-White syndrome, atrial flutter or fibrillation); vasospastic (Prinzmetal's) and unstable (crescendo, preinfarction) angina; chronic stable angina (classic effort-associated); HTN.
DOSAGE: *Adults:* Tachyarrhythmias: 5–10 mg IV over 2 min (may repeat in 30 min). Angina: 240–480 mg/24h divided in 3–4 doses. HTN: 80–180 mg PO tid or SR tablet 240 mg PO qd. *Peds:* <1 y: 0.1–0.2 mg/kg IV over 2 min (may repeat in 30 min); 1–15 y: 0.1–0.3 mg/kg IV over 2 min (may repeat in 30 min); do not exceed 5 mg.
NOTES: Use caution with elderly patients; decrease dose in renal failure; constipation is a common side effect.

Vitamin B$_{12}$

See "Cyanocobalamin," page 476.

Vitamin K

See "Phytonadione," page 513.

Voriconazole (Vefend)

COMMON USES: Management of invasive aspergillosis infections, esophageal candidiasis, *Fusarium* and *Scedosporium* infections.
DOSAGE: Initial dosing IV: 6 mg/kg q12hrs for 2 doses followed by 4 mg/kg q12h. May convert to PO as tolerated. PO dosing: 200–300 mg q12h for patients >40 kg, 150-200 mg q12hrs for those <40 kg.
NOTES: May cause transient visual disturbances.

Warfarin Sodium (Coumadin)

COMMON USES: Prophylaxis and management of pulmonary embolism and venous thrombosis, atrial fibrillation with embolization, other postop uses.
DOSAGE: *Adults:* Need to individualize dose to keep INR level at 2–3; some mechanical heart valves require INR to be 2.5–3.5; initially, 10–15 mg PO, IM, or IV qd for 1–3 d; then maintenance, 2–10 mg PO, IV, or IM qd; follow INR levels during initial phase to guide dosing. *Peds:* 0.05–0.34 mg/kg/24h PO, IM, or IV qd. Follow PT closely to adjust dose.
NOTES: Follow INR while on maintenance dose; beware of bleeding caused by over anticoagulation (PT >3 times control); caution patient on effects of taking Coumadin with other medications, especially aspirin; to rapidly correct over coumadinization, use vitamin K or fresh frozen plasma or both; highly teratogenic, do not use in pregnancy.

Witch Hazel (Tucks Pads)

COMMON USES: After bowel movement cleansing to decrease local irritation or relieve hemorrhoids; after anorectal surgery and episiotomy.
DOSAGE: Apply as needed.

Zafirlukast (Accolate)

COMMON USES: Prophylaxis and long-term therapy of asthma.
DOSAGE: 20 mg bid.
NOTES: Not for acute exacerbations of asthma, contraindicated in nursing women.

Zanamivir (Relenza)

COMMON USES: Control of influenza.

DOSAGE: 2 inhalations (10 mg) twice daily.
NOTES: Uses a Diskhaler for administration.

Zidovudine (Retrovir)

COMMON USES: Management of patients with HIV infections.
DOSAGE: *Adults:* 200 mg PO tid or 300 mg PO bid or 1–2 mg/kg/dose IV q4h. Pregnancy: 100 mg PO 5 times/d until labor; during labor 2 mg/kg over 1 h followed by 1 mg/kg/h until clamping of the umbilical cord. *Peds:* 720 mg/m^2/24h PO divided 5 times/d.
NOTES: Not a cure for HIV infections.

Zileuton (Zyflo)

COMMON USES: Prophylaxis and long-term therapy of asthma.
DOSAGE: 600 mg qid.
NOTES: MUST take on a regular basis; does not control acute exacerbation.

Zoledronic Acid (Zometa)

COMMON USES: Management of hypercalcemia of malignancy.
DOSAGE: 4 mg IV over 15 min in 1 dose.
NOTES: Hydrate well. Not recommended in patients with bone metastases with severe renal impairment.

Zolpidem (Ambien) [C]

COMMON USES: Short-term therapy of insomnia.
DOSAGE: 5–10 mg PO qhs prn.

Zonisamide (Zonegran)

COMMON USES: Partial seizures.
DOSAGE: Initial 100 mg once daily; may be increased to 400 mg/d.
NOTES: Contraindicated in persons with hypersensitivity to sulfonamides.

Appendix

BODY SURFACE AREA: ADULT (SEE FIGURE A–1)

BODY SURFACE AREA: ADULT

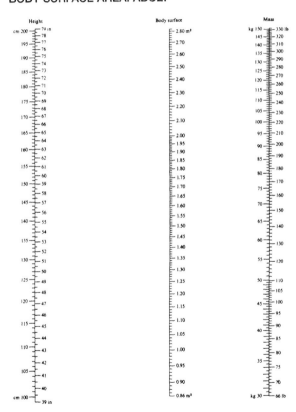

Figure A–1. To determine the body surface area in an adult, use a straight edge to connect the height and mass. The point of intersection on the body surface line gives the area in square meters. *(From Lentner C, ed. Geigy Scientific Tables, 8th ed. CIBA-GEIGY 1981;1:226.)*

BODY SURFACE AREA:
CHILDREN (SEE FIGURE A–2)

BODY SURFACE AREA: CHILDREN

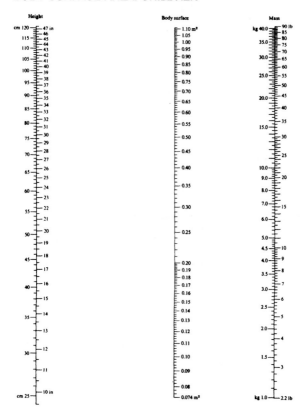

Figure A–2. To determine the body surface area in a child, use a straight edge to connect the height and mass. The point of intersection on the body surface line gives the area in square meters. *(From Lentner C, ed. Geigy Scientific Tables, 8th ed. CIBA-GEIGY 1981;1:227.)*

BOWEL PREPS

The purpose of a bowel preparation is the removal of all solid material from the bowel and the reduction of the bacterial population to decrease the incidence of complications of surgical procedures and to provide a clean bowel for endoscopic procedures.

A. Noncolonic surgery.
    1. The patient should remain NPO after midnight before surgery.
    2. Bowel preparation may be indicated for upper gastrointestinal surgical procedures.
        a. Surgery may involve the colon (eg, extensive surgery for gynecologic malignancy or large gastric tumors).
        b. Achlorhydria, gastric carcinoma, prolonged H_2-receptor blocker use, and obstructive peptic ulcer disease will allow bacterial growth in the stomach. Consider using an oral antibiotic prep (eg, neomycin) for gastric surgery in these patients (see below).

B. Colonic surgery mechanical or whole gut lavage prep with or without oral antibiotic prep. Many variations exist.
    1. Mechanical prep.
        a. Day 1: Diet should consist of clear liquids; administer a laxative of choice (castor oil 60 mL, milk of magnesia 30 mL, magnesium citrate 250 mL), and a tap water or a soap-suds enema until bowel is clear.
        b. Day 2: Diet should consist of clear liquids, administer IV fluids, a laxative of choice, and an enema (AM and PM).
        c. Day 3: Operation.
        An alternative mechanical bowel prep:
        a. Day 1: Diet should consist of clear liquids; administer IV fluids, Fleets Phospho-soda 1–2 oz with water (repeat × 1), a Dulcolax suppository in the evening, and an enema × 1.
        b. Day 2: Operation.
    2. Whole gut lavage (GoLYTELY, a polyethylene glycol electrolyte-balanced solution).
        a. Day 1: GoLYTELY 4 L PO or per NG tube over 4 h.
        b. Administer metoclopramide 10 mg PO to decrease bloating and nausea.
        c. Day 2: Operation.
    3. Oral antibiotic prep, mechanical prep, or whole gut lavage should be completed before administration of oral antibiotic prep.
        a. Nichols-Condon prep: On day before surgery, administer neomycin 1 g and erythromycin base 1 g of

each PO at 1 PM, 2 PM, and 11 PM for a patient scheduled at 8 AM.

   b. Metronidazole (500 mg) PO: This may be substituted for erythromycin base in the Nichols-Condon prep (causes less nausea than with erythromycin base).

4. Perioperative IV antibiotics may be used in conjunction with, or instead of, the oral antibiotic prep, depending on the preference of the attending surgeon. For patients undergoing operations in which preoperative antibiotics are indicated (eg, clean-contaminated or contaminated procedures) the literature is clear that antibiotics should be given within 1 h of the start of the surgical procedure.

   a. These antibiotics should be administered immediately preoperatively (see above) and intraoperatively for prolonged operations. Any further postoperative doses reportedly are not effective in preventing wound infection; nevertheless, most surgeons administer ≥1 dose of antibiotic postoperatively.

   b. Choice of antibiotic (Table A–1): The key here is to obtain broad coverage of enteric organisms (gram-negatives, anaerobes, eg, gentamicin and clindamycin, cefazolin and metronidazole, or cefotetan).

(Printed, with permission, from Preoperative preparation. In: Koutlas TC, ed. *The Mont Reid Surgical Handbook.* St. Louis: Mosby; 1994.)

CHARTWORK

Preoperative Note

The specific items in the preoperative note depend on institutional guidelines, the nature of the procedure, and the age and health of the patient. For example, an elecardiogram and blood setup may not be necessary for a 2-year-old child about to undergo a herniorrhaphy, but it is essential for a 70-year-old patient scheduled for vascular surgery.

   Preop diagnosis: State the preop diagnosis, eg, "acute appendicitis."

   Procedure: Indicate what the planned procedure is, eg, "exploratory laparotomy."

   Laboratory results: Note results of the complete blood cell count, electrolytes, urinalysis, etc.

   Chest radiograph: Note the results.

   Electrocardiogram: Note the results.

TABLE A–1. PREVENTION OF WOUND INFECTION AND SEPSIS IN SURGICAL PATIENTS

Nature of Operation	Likely Pathogens	Recommended Drugs	Adult Dosage Before Surgery[a]
Cardiac			
Prosthetic valve, coronary artery bypass, other open-heart surgery, pacemaker or defibrillator implant	*Staphylococcus epidermidis, S aureus, Corynebacterium*, enteric gram-negative bacilli	cefazolin or cefuroxime or vancomycin[c]	1–2 g IV[b] 1–2 g IV[b] 1 g IV
Gastrointestinal			
Esophageal, gastroduodenal	Enteric gram-negative bacilli, gram-positive cocci	*High risk*[d] *only:* cefazolin[e]	1–2 g IV
Biliary tract	Enteric gram-negative bacilli, enterococci, clostridia	*High risk*[f] *only:* cefazolin[e]	1–2 g IV
Colorectal	Enteric gram-negative bacilli, anaerobes, enterococci	*Oral:* neomycin + erythromycin base[g]	
		Parenteral: cefoxitin or cefatetan or cefazolin + metronidazole	1–2 g IV 1–2 g IV 1–2 g IV 0.5 g IV
Appendectomy, non-perforated	Enteric gram-negative bacilli, anaerobes, enterococci	cefoxitin or cefotetan	1–2 g IV 1–2 g IV
Genitourinary	Enteric gram-negative bacilli, enterococci	*High risk*[h] *only:* ciprofloxacin	500 mg PO or 400 mg IV
Gynecologic and Obstetric			
Vaginal or abdominal hysterectomy	Enteric gram-negatives, anaerobes, group B strep, enterococci	cefazolin or cefotetan or cefoxitin	1–2 g IV 1–2 g IV 1 g IV
Cesarean section	Same as for hysterectomy	*High risk*[i] *only:* cefazolin	1 g IV after cord clamping

TABLE A-1. PREVENTION OF WOUND INFECTION AND SEPSIS IN SURGICAL PATIENTS (continued)

Nature of Operation	Likely Pathogens	Recommended Drugs	Adult Dosage Before Surgery[1]
Abortion	Same as for hysterectomy	*First trimester, high risk*[l]: aqueous penicillin G or doxycycline	2 mill U IV 300 mg PO[k]
		Second trimester: cefazolin	1 g IV
Head and Neck Surgery			
Incisions through oral or pharyngeal mucosa	Anaerobes, enteric gram-negative bacilli, *S. aureus*	Clindamycin + gentamicin	600–900 mg IV 1.5 mg/kg IV
Neurosurgery			
Craniotomy	*S aureus, S epidermidis*	Cefazolin *or* vancomycin[c]	1–2 g IV 1 g IV
Ophthalmic	*S epidermidis, S aureus*, streptococci, enteric gram-negative bacilli, Pseudomonas	Gentamicin, tobramycin, ciprofloxacin, ofloxacin or neomycin-gramicidin-polymyxin B	Multiple drops topically over 2–24 h
		Cefazolin	100 mg subconjunctivally
Orthopedic			
Total joint replacement, internal fixation of fractures	*S aureus, S epidermidis*	Cefazolin *or* vancomycin[c]	1–2 g IV 1 g IV
Thoracic (Non-Cardiac)	*S aureus, S epidermidis*, streptococci, enteric gram-negative bacilli	Cefazolin or cefuroxime *or* vancomycin[c]	1–2 g IV 1–2 g IV 1 g IV
Vascular			
Arterial surgery involving a prosthesis, the abdominal aorta, or a groin incision	*S aureus, S epidermidis*, enteric gram-negative bacilli	Cefazolin *or* vancomycin[c]	1–2 g IV 1 g IV
Lower extremity amputation for ischemia	*S aureus, S epidermidis*, enteric gram-negative bacilli, clostridia	Cefazolin[e] *or* vancomycin[c]	1–2 g IV 1 g IV

CONTAMINATED SURGERY[l]

Condition	Likely pathogens	Prophylaxis	Dose
Ruptured viscus	Enteric gram-negative bacilli, anaer-obes, enterococci	Cefoxitin or cefotetan ± gentamicin *or* clindamycin + gentamicin	1–2 g IV q6h 1–2 IV q12h 1.5 mg/kg IV q8h 600 mg IV q6h 1.5 mg/kg IV q8h
Traumatic wound	*S aureus*, group A strep, clostridia	cefazolin[m]	1–2 g IV q8h

[a] Parenteral prophylactic antimicrobials can be given as a single intravenous dose just before the operation. For prolonged operations, additional intraoperative doses should be given q4–8h for the duration of the procedure.

[b] Some consultants recommend an additional dose when patients are removed from bypass during open-heart surgery.

[c] For hospitals in which methicillin-resistant *S. aureus* and *S. epidermidis* are a frequent cause of postoperative wound infection, or for patients allergic to penicillins or cephalosporins. Rapid IV administration may cause hypotension, which could be especially dangerous during induction of anesthesia. Even if the drug is given over 60 minutes, hypotension may occur; treatment with diphenhydramine (*Benadryl* and others) and further slowing of the infusion rate may be helpful (DG Maki et al. *J Thorac Cardiovasc Surg*, 104:1423, 1992). For procedures in which enteric gram-negative bacilli are likely pathogens, such as vascular surgery involving a groin inci-sion, cefazolin should be included in the prophylaxis regimen for patients not allergic to cephalosporins.

[d] Morbid obesity, esophageal obstruction, decreased gastric acidity, or gastrointestinal motility.

[e] Some Medical Letter consultants favor cefoxitin for better anaerobic coverage in this setting.

[f] Age > 70 years, acute cholecystitis, non-functioning gall bladder, obstructive jaundice or common duct stones.

[g] After appropriate diet and catharsis, 1 g of each at 1 PM, 2 PM and 11 PM the day before an 8 AM operation.

[h] Urine culture positive or unavailable, preoperative catheter, transrectal prostatic biopsy.

[i] Active labor or premature rupture of membranes.

[j] Patients with previous pelvic inflammatory disease, previous gonorrhea or multiple sex partners.

[k] Divided into 100 mg 1h before the abortion and 200 mg 30 min after.

[l] For contaminated or "dirty" surgery, therapy should usually be continued for about five days. Ruptured viscus in postoperative setting (dehiscence) requires antibate-rials to include coverage of nosocomial pathogens.

[m] For bite wounds, in which likely pathogens may also include oral anaerobes, *Eikenella corrodens* (human), or *Pasteurella multocida* (dog and cat), some Medical Let-ter consultants recommend use of amoxicillin/clavulanic acid (*Augmentin*) or ampicillin/sulbactam (*Unasyn*).

(Reproduced with permission from The Medical Letter 1999;41:76.)

Blood: Type and cross packed red cells 2 U, blood not needed, etc.

History & physical examination: Note specifically pertinent items in the preoperative note.

Orders: Note special preop orders written, eg, preoperative colon preps, and prophylactic antibiotics.

Permit: If this has been completed, write "signed and on chart."

Operative Note

The operative note is written immediately after surgery to summarize the operation for those who were not present and is meant to complement the formal operative summary that is dictated by the surgeon.

Preop diagnosis: Indicate why the patient was taken to surgery, eg, "acute appendicitis."

Postop diagnosis: This should be based on the operative findings, eg, "mesenteric lymphadenitis."

Procedure: Indicate what procedure was actually performed, eg, "appendectomy."

Surgeons: List the attending physicians, residents, and students who scrubbed on the case and their titles (eg, MD, CCIV, MSII). It is often helpful to identify the dictating surgeon.

Findings: Briefly note operative findings, eg, "normal appendix with marked lymphadenopathy."

Anesthesia: State type of anesthesia used (local, spinal, general, endotracheal, etc). Also write the name of the anesthesiologist.

Fluids: Indicate amount and type used during case (eg, normal saline, blood, or albumin). This is usually obtained from the anesthesia records.

Estimated blood loss: This is usually obtained from the anesthesia or nursing records.

Drains: State location and type of drain, eg, "Jackson-Pratt drain in left upper quadrant" or "T-tube in midline."

Specimens: State whether any specimens were sent to the pathology laboratory and indicate the test results of any intraoperative frozen sections.

Complications: Usually "none" but anything significant should be written here after talking to the surgeon in charge.

Condition: Note where the patient is taken immediately after surgery and indicate the patient's condition (eg, "transferred to the recovery room in stable condition").

Night of Surgery Note (Postoperative Note)

This is a specific type of progress note that is written several hours after surgery or on the same night.

Procedure: Indicate the operation performed.

Level of consciousness: Note whether the patient is alert, drowsy, etc.

Vital signs: Indicate blood pressure, pulse, and respiration.

Intake & output: Calculate IV fluids, urine output, and other drainage and attempt to assess fluid balance.

Labs: Review results, if any were obtained since surgery.

Physical examination: Examine and note the findings for the chest, heart, abdomen, extremities, and any other part as needed; examine the dressing for bleeding.

Assessment: Evaluate the postop course thus far (stable, etc).

Plan: Note any changes in orders.

Glasgow Coma Scale (Table A–2)

The Glasgow Coma Scale (EMV Scale) is a fairly reliable, objective method of monitoring changes in levels of consciousness. It is based on eye opening, motor responses, and verbal responses (EMV). A person's EMV score is based on the total of the 3 different responses. The score ranges from 3 (lowest) to 15 (highest).

SBE Prophylaxis

The following recommendations (Tables A–3, A–4, and A–5) are based on guidelines published by the American Heart Association (*JAMA* 277:1794, 1997). These updated guidelines currently specify those patients who are at high, moderate, and low risk of bacteremia, and they provide general guidelines for procedures that are more likely to be associated with bacterial endocarditis.

TABLE A–2. GLASGOW COMA SCALE.

Parameter	Response		Score
Eyes	Open: spontaneously		4
	To verbal command		3
	To pain		2
	No response		1
Best motor response	To verbal command	Obeys	6
	To painful stimulus	Localizes pain	5
		Flexion-withdrawal	4
		Decorticate (flex)	3
		Decerebrate (extend)	2
		No response	1
Best verbal response	Oriented, converses		5
	Disoriented, converses		4
	Inappropriate responses		3
	Incomprehensible sounds		2
	No response		1

TABLE A–3. SBE PROPHYLAXIS BASED ON PROCEDURE

Dental: Dental extractions, periodontal procedures, dental implants; reimplantation of avulsed teeth; endodontic instrumentation only beyond the apex; subgingival placement of antibiotic fibers or strips; placement of orthodontic bands (not brackets); intraligamentary anesthetic injections; cleaning of teeth or implants where bleeding likely

Respiratory: Tonsillectomy and/or adenoidectomy; surgery on the respiratory mucosa; rigid bronchoscopy

Gastrointestinal tract: Sclerotherapy for esophageal varices; esophageal stricture dilation; ERCP with biliary obstruction; biliary tract surgery; operations involving intestinal mucosa

Genitourinary: Prostate surgery, cystoscopy, urethral dilation

ERCP = endoscopic retrograde cholangiopancreatography.

SBE prophylaxis is recommended for patients with high- or moderate-risk conditions.

High risk: Prosthetic cardiac valves, history of bacterial endocarditis; complex cyanotic congenital heart disease, surgically constructed systemic pulmonary shunts.

Moderate risk: Most other congenital cardiac malformations (other than above and below), acquired valvar disease (eg, rheumatic heart disease), hypertrophic cardiomyopathy, mitral valve prolapse with regurgitation and/or thickened leaflets.

TABLE A–4. SBE PROPHYLAXIS FOR ORAL, RESPIRATORY OR ESOPHAGEAL PROCEDURES

	Agent	Regimen[a]
Standard prophylaxis	Amoxicillin	Adults: 2.0 g; children: 50 mg/kg PO 1 h before procedure
Unable to take oral medications	Ampicillin	Adults: 2.0 g IM or IV; children: 50 mg/kg IM or IV 30 min before procedure
Allergic to penicillin	Clindamycin **or**	Adults: 600 mg; children 20 mg/kg PO 1 h before procedure
	Cephalexin **or** Cefadroxil	Adults: 2.0 g; children: 50 mg/kg PO 1 h before procedure
	Azithromycin **or** Clarithromycin	Adults: 500 mg; children: 15 mg/kg PO 1 h before procedure
Penicillin allergic and unable to take oral medications	Clindamycin **or** Cefazolin	Adults: 600 mg; children: 20 mg/kg IV 30 min before procedure Adults: 1.0 g; children: 25 mg/kg IM or IV 30 min before procedure

[a]Total children's dose should not exceed adult dose.

**TABLE A–5. SBE PROPHYLAXIS FOR GU/GI
(EXCLUDING ESOPHAGEAL) PROCEDURES**

	Agents	Regimen[a]
High-risk patients	Ampicillin + gentamicin	Adults: ampicillin 2.0 g IM/IV + gentamicin 1.5 mg/kg (max 120 mg) within 30 min of procedure; 6 h later, ampicillin 1 g IM/IV or amoxicillin 1 g PO
		Children: ampicillin 50 mg/kg IM or IV (2.0 g max) + gentamicin 1.5 mg/kg within 30 min of procedure; 6 h later, ampicillin 25 mg/kg IM/IV or amoxicillin 25 mg/kg PO
High-risk patients allergic to ampicillin/ amoxicillin	Vancomycin + gentamicin	Adults: vancomycin 1.0 g IV over 1–2 h + gentamicin 1.5 mg/kg IV/IM (120 mg max); dose within 30 min of starting procedure
		Children: vancomycin 20 mg/kg IV over 1–2 h + gentamicin 1.5 mg/kg IV/IM; complete dose within 30 min of starting procedure
Moderate-risk patients	Amoxicillin or ampicillin	Adults: amoxicillin 2.0 g PO 1 h before procedure, or ampicillin 2.0 g IM/IV within 30 min of starting procedure
		Children: amoxicillin 50 mg/kg PO 1 h before procedure, or ampicillin 50 mg/kg IM/IV within 30 min of starting procedure
Moderate-risk patients allergic to ampicillin/ amoxicillin	Vancomycin	Adults: vancomycin 1.0 g IV over 1–2 h complete infusion within 30 min of starting procedure
		Children: vancomycin 20 mg/kg IV over 1–2 h; complete infusion within 30 min of starting procedure

[a]Total children's dose should not exceed adult dose.

Low risk: Isolated atrial septal defect secundum; repair of atrial/ventricular septal defect or patent ductus arteriosus; previous coronary artery bypass grafting; mitral valve prolapse without regurgitation; innocent heart murmurs; previous Kawasaki's disease or rheumatic fever without valve dysfunction; pacemakers or implanted defibrillator.

Index

Page numbers followed by *f* and *t* refer to figures and tables, respectively.